NEUROPROTECTIVE AGENTS

SEVENTH INTERNATIONAL CONFERENCE

ANNALS OF THE NEW YORK ACADEMY OF SCIENCES
Volume 1053

NEUROPROTECTIVE AGENTS

SEVENTH INTERNATIONAL CONFERENCE

Edited by William Slikker, Jr., Russell J. Andrews, and Bruce Trembly

The New York Academy of Sciences
New York, New York
2005

Library of Congress Cataloging-in-Publication Data

International Conference on Neuroprotective Agents: Clinical and
Experimental Aspects (7th: 2004: Pacific Grove, Calif.)
Neuroprotective agents: seventh international conference / edited
by William Slikker, Jr., Russell J. Andrews, and Bruce Trembly.
p.; cm. — (Annals of the New York Academy of Sciences, ISSN
0077-8923; v. 1053)
Includes bibliographical references and index.
ISBN 1-57331-578-8 (cloth: alk. paper) — ISBN 1-57331-579-6 (pbk.: alk. paper)
1. Nervous system—Degeneration—Chemoprevention—Congresses.
2. Neuropharmacology—Congresses. 3. Neurotoxicology—Congresses.
I. Slikker, William. II. Andrews, Russell J. III. Trembly, Bruce.
IV. Title. V. Series.
[DNLM: 1. Nerve Degeneration—prevention & control—Congresses.
2. Neuroprotective Agents—therapeutic use—Congresses. 3. Neuro-
toxicity Syndromes—therapy—Congresses. W1 AN626YL v.1053
2005 / WL 102.5 I59na 2005]
Q11.N5 vol. 1053
[RC365]
500 s—dc22
[616.8]

2005017244

GYAT / PCP

Printed in the United States of America
ISBN 1-57331-578-8 (cloth)
ISBN 1-57331-579-6 (paper)
ISSN 0077-8923

ANNALS OF THE NEW YORK ACADEMY OF SCIENCES

Volume 1053
August 2005

NEUROPROTECTIVE AGENTS

SEVENTH INTERNATIONAL CONFERENCE

Editors

WILLIAM SLIKKER, JR., RUSSELL J. ANDREWS, AND BRUCE TREMBLY

This volume is the result of the **Seventh International Conference on Neuroprotective Agents**, held November 14–19, 2004, in Pacific Grove, California.

CONTENTS

Session II. Mechanisms of Neuroprotection (1)

Session III. Neuroprotection in Inflammation-Related Neurodegenerative Diseases

Session IV. Role of Carnitines and Other Agents in Neuroprotection

Session V. Neuroprotective Approaches and Models

Session VI. Neuroprotective Agents and Mechanisms

Session VII. The NMDA Receptor as a Target for Neurotoxicity and Neuroprotection

Session VIII. Mechanisms of Neuroprotection (2)

Session IX. Sensitive Targets for Neurotoxicity and Neuroprotection

Session X. Novel Approaches to Neuroprotection

Session XI. Workshop PBPK/PD Models for Developing Humans: Risk Assessment Strategies and Research Recommendations

Financial assistance was received from:

- CENTRAL ARKANSAS CHAPTER OF SIGMA XI
- THE NATIONAL CENTER FOR TOXICOLOGICAL RESEARCH/FDA
- UNITED STATES ENVIRONMENTAL PROTECTION AGENCY

Preface

This volume contains papers, abstracts, and questions/answers from the Seventh International Conference on Neuroprotective Agents held in Pacific Grove, California, November 14–19, 2004. Previous conferences were held in Rockland, Maine, in 1991; Lake George, New York, in 1994 (*Annals* Vol. 765); Lake Como, Italy, in 1996 (*Annals* Vol. 825); Annapolis, Maryland, in 1998 (*Annals* Vol. 890); Lake Tahoe, California, in 2000 (*Annals* Vol. 939); and Hilton Head, South Carolina, in 2002 (*Annals* Vol. 993).

It has been the aim of these conferences to bring together clinicians, regulators, and basic science researchers from many disciplines and many parts of the world in a congenial and informal setting. The clinical focus of this seventh conference centered on the proposed mechanistic pathways to produce neuroprotection, the need to understand the developmental stage of susceptibility and prevention of neurotoxicity, and the need for combinational and time-course application of multiple therapies. New technologies were introduced for describing both the insult and the treatment necessary for neuroprotection, including physiological monitoring, gene express assays (genomics), and the use of endogenous agents as therapeutics.

Several papers were devoted to the examination of the predictive value of models for outcome measures in clinical ischemic stroke neuroprotective trials. The need to move from *in vitro* models to more predictive *in vivo* approaches was addressed. Others papers emphasized the role of existing agents (e.g., lithium, antioxidants) and endogenous agents such as vitamin D, melatonin, L-carnitine, estrogens, and growth factors in acute and chronic spinal cord and brain injury and therapy. The wide range of presentations, from a detailed paper on the very precise use of neurophysiological monitoring to aid in recovery from cardiac surgery to a comprehensive presentation of the importance of measurements of function as a guiding force in the next generation of preventive measures, served to illustrate the overall scientific scope of these conferences.

We are grateful to the New York Academy of Sciences for the opportunity to share these proceedings with other clinicians and scientists.

The Eighth International Conference on Neuroprotective Agents will be held on the eastern coast of the United States during the fall of 2006.

—William Slikker, Jr.
—Russell J. Andrews
—Bruce Trembly

Ann. N.Y. Acad. Sci. 1053: xi (2005). © 2005 New York Academy of Sciences.
doi: 10.1196/annals.1344.070

Neuroprotection Trek—The Next Generation

The Measurement Is the Message

RUSSELL J. ANDREWS

Smart Systems and Nanotechnology, NASA Ames Research Center, Moffett Field, California, USA

ABSTRACT: Animal trials of many pharmacological neuroprotective agents have been quite successful, whereas trials in humans have been uniformly disappointing. A major difference between laboratory research in animals and clinical research in humans is the amount and/or quality of data obtained. The goal of this presentation is to argue that when clinical studies consist of more valid, objective data—that is, as our measurement capabilities in clinical research become as robust as they are in laboratory research—we are likely to gain new insights into both (1) injury to the nervous system and (2) neuroprotective treatment strategies. Technological advances (in data acquisition and analysis)—often novel even in the laboratory—will be the "scale" that will enable progress in measurement. As examples of such technological advances, two projects initiated at NASA Ames Research Center are cited. The NASA Smart Probe Project, with the goal of combining multiple microsensors and neural networks for real-time tissue identification (e.g., for tumor detection), has recently moved into the clinical realm, with a prototype being used to diagnose breast cancer in women "on the spot". The NASA Nanoelectrode Array Project has fabricated nanoscale devices that can simultaneously monitor electrical activity and neurotransmitter concentrations, while providing electrical stimulation focally and precisely (and potentially in a closed-loop fashion based on the input from the nanosensors). The large amounts of data that such techniques can acquire and analyze—separated spatially and temporally throughout the nervous system, if necessary—will provide insights not only into neuroprotective strategies, but also into the workings of the nervous system itself.

KEYWORDS: cancer diagnosis; deep brain stimulation; electrical stimulation; nanotechnology; neuromodulation; neuroprotection; optical spectroscopy

INTRODUCTION

Why have so many pharmacological neuroprotective agents that appeared quite effective in stroke or brain injury in animal models proven to be so ineffective in human trials? This topic was addressed in part by my contribution to the Fourth International Conference on Neuroprotective Agents (1998), where the argument was made that failure to achieve neuroprotection in humans was in large part due to

Address for correspondence: Russell J. Andrews, 555 Knowles Drive (#112), Los Gatos, CA 95032. Voice: 408-829-1700; fax: 408-866-8842.
rja@russelljandrews.org

**Ann. N.Y. Acad. Sci. 1053: 1–11 (2005). © 2005 New York Academy of Sciences.
doi: 10.1196/annals.1344.001**

(1) our failure to understand the complexity of the "ischemic cascade"—the almost certain need for a multidrug "cocktail" approach to neuroprotection—and (2) the politics of the pharmaceutical industry in betting on short-term success with a single agent "magic bullet" drug that might turn a substantial profit before patent expiration. At that time (1998), it appeared that technological advances were making a greater contribution to clinical neuroprotection than pharmacological advances—two examples given were cardiovascular stenting and deep brain stimulation for movement disorders.[1]

The present contribution carries on that theme of technology driving neuroprotection. The argument is that, in the laboratory, the data are "cleaner" (if not more accurate) and the endpoints are more quantitative (e.g., "percent of the rat hemisphere infarcted", in contrast to "Uncle Harry's ability to function independently after his stroke"). However, we are now gaining some tools that may enable us to realize more substantial progress in clinical neuroprotection. The theme is that dramatic improvements in our ability to *measure* the events of neural injury and neurodegeneration, as well as *measure* the neurorepair and neuroregeneration following intervention, should result in substantial improvement in clinical neuroprotection for a variety of disorders from stroke to movement disorders to Alzheimer's disease.

MARSHALING THE EVIDENCE FOR MEASUREMENT

"Evidence-based" has become a mantra of modern medicine, an incantation chanted by the medical literati and the health maintenance organizations (HMOs) alike. Research "evidence" has been categorized into four classes:[2]

- Class I: prospective, randomized, controlled trials;
- Class II: case control, cohort, prevalence studies;
- Class III: retrospective series, registries, databases;
- Class IV: case reports, "expert" opinions.

In class I, measurement accuracy is certain; in contrast, in class IV, measurement accuracy is uncertain. Laboratory studies entail well-controlled, well-measured research conditions, well-measured treatments (e.g., amount of drug, blood/brain levels, duration of treatment), and well-measured outcomes (e.g., volume of brain infarcted). Clinical studies tend to be messy (even if not tainted by political or economic pressures)—or, if well measured, very expensive.

Consider the following quote, and the adaptation—by substituting *measurement* for *electric light*:

> "The *electric light* is pure information. It is a medium without a message.... Whether the *light* is being used for brain surgery or night baseball is a matter of indifference. It could be argued that these activities are in some way the 'content' of the *electric light*, since they could not exist without the *electric light*. This fact merely underlines the point that 'the medium is the message' because it is the medium that shapes and controls the scale and form of human association and action."[3]
>
> MARSHALL MCLUHAN, *Understanding Media: The Extensions of Man*, 1964

"*Measurement* is pure information. It is a medium without a message.... Whether *measurement* is being used for brain surgery or night baseball is a matter of indifference. It could be argued that these activities are in some way the 'content' of *measurement*, since they could not exist without *measurement*. This fact merely underlines the point that '*measurement* is the message' because it is *measurement* that shapes and controls the scale and form of human association and action."

With Apologies to Marshall McLuhan

The effect of the "information explosion" (e.g., the Internet) needs little elaboration. With a click, we can "google" any notion that can be expressed as keystrokes. The ability to marshal large amounts of objectively acquired data has fueled the move toward evidence-based medicine. To adapt another quote:

"In the fields of observation, chance favors only the prepared mind."

LOUIS PASTEUR, *Inaugural Lecture, University of Lille,* 1854

"In research, publication and funding favor only the well-measured data (and lots of it!)."

With Apologies to Louis Pasteur

In the following sections, two projects at NASA Ames Research Center are considered. The common theme is the use of "cutting-edge" technology to gather large amounts of data—objectively, accurately, minimally invasively, and dispersed spatially and temporally—which enables us to measure with much more validity the various processes that are occurring in tissues that are undergoing (or have undergone) undesirable changes (e.g., ischemic, neoplastic, neurodegenerative). The first is the NASA Smart Probe Project, originating with the Smart Systems Group at NASA Ames and carried into clinical trials by the start-up company, BioLuminate (Dublin, CA). The second is the NASA Nanoelectrode Array Project, involving the Nanotechnology Group at NASA Ames and the nearby Parkinson's Institute (Sunnyvale, CA).

THE SMART PROBE PROJECT FOR REAL-TIME TISSUE RECOGNITION

The NASA Smart Probe Project and the refinements developed by the NASA technology licensee, BioLuminate (Dublin, CA), demonstrate that a unique "signature" for any tissue—indeed, a unique "signature + address" (e.g., the substantia nigra pars compacta of the brain)—can be acquired in real time.[4]

The Smart Probe combines continuous data streams from multiple microsensors, with the data being processed in real time by neural network/fuzzy logic algorithms (FIG. 1). Various "off-the-shelf" microsensors, each < 1 mm in diameter, have been tested at NASA Ames in rodents: a microstrain gauge, a laser-Doppler blood flow probe (Vasamedics, St. Paul, MN), a fiber-optic neuroendoscope (Codman/Johnson & Johnson, Raynham, MA), a combination CO_2/O_2/pH monitor probe (NeuroTrend, Codman/Johnson & Johnson, Raynham, MA), a standard microelectrode, and a light-scattering spectroscopy probe (PC2000, Ocean Optics, Dunedin, FL). Various types of optical spectroscopy have been shown to be extremely powerful in differentiating tissues *in vivo*; typical spectra for several tissues using light-scattering spectroscopy are illustrated in FIGURE 2.

The BioLuminate probe for breast cancer diagnosis is illustrated in FIGURE 3. Breast "biopsies" in 24 women with suspected breast cancer have been performed at

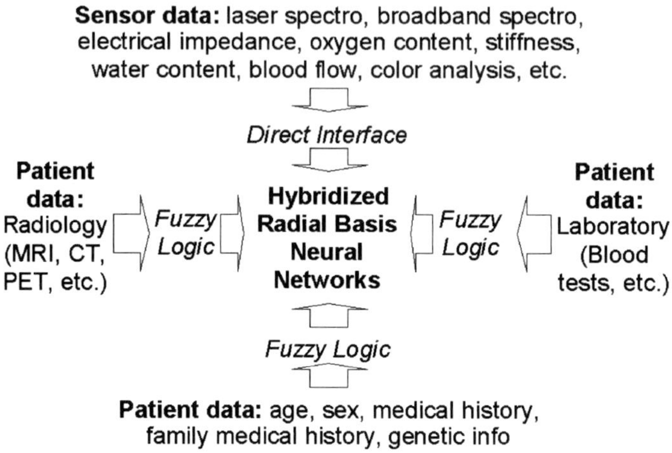

FIGURE 1. NASA Smart Probe schematic.

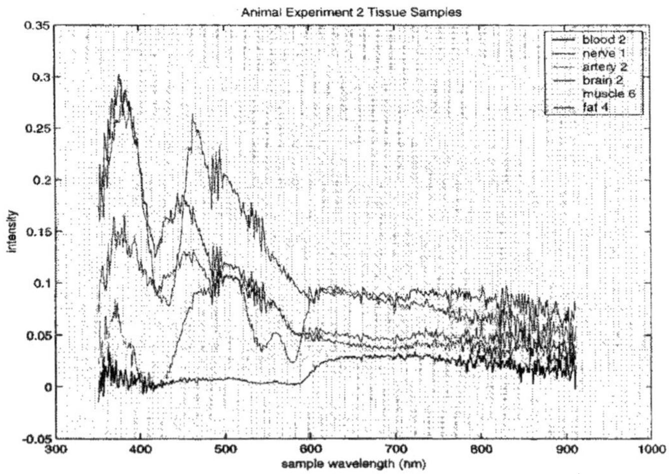

FIGURE 2. Rodent *in vivo* tissue spectra, 350–900 nm. From top to bottom at 475 nm: brain, nerve, fat, artery, muscle, blood.

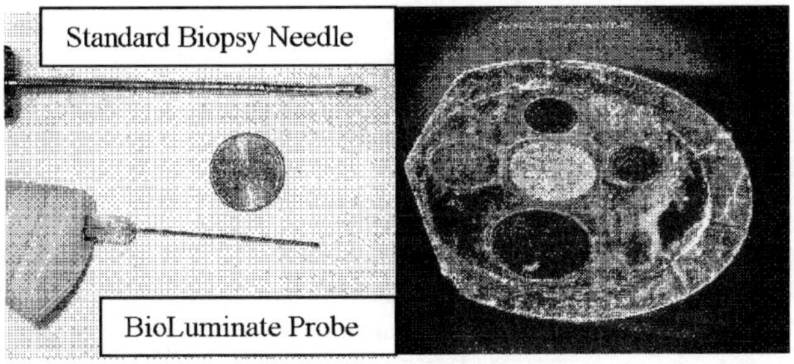

FIGURE 3. BioLuminate probe for breast biopsy: (*left*) comparison with standard breast biopsy needle; (*right*) end view of beveled tip of needle (<1 mm diameter).

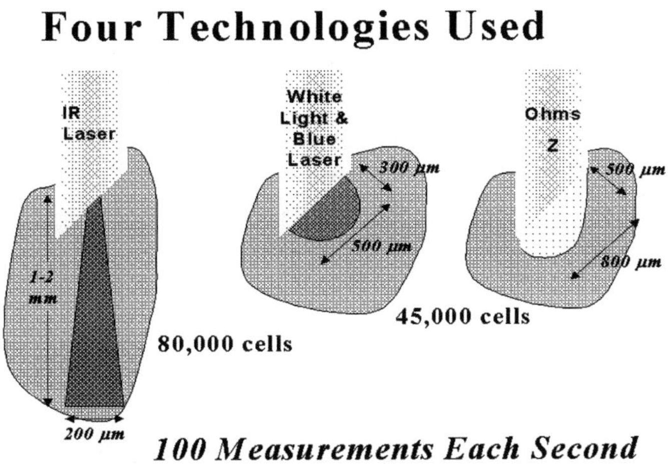

FIGURE 4. BioLuminate probe sensors. Left to right: infrared laser spectroscopy sensor, white light (broadband) and blue laser spectroscopy sensors, and electrical impedance sensor.

the University of California, Davis and San Francisco, Medical Centers; the results were compared with histopathological samples acquired by standard breast biopsy techniques. The probe simultaneously assesses (1) oxy- and deoxyhemoglobin concentrations (using infrared and blue laser spectroscopy), (2) broadband (white light) spectroscopy, and (3) electrical impedance (FIG. 4). With a repetition rate of 100 times per second, more than 500 MB of data are collected for each patient (from three or more probe tracks per patient through the lesion and adjacent tissues).

FIGURES 5–7 present data collected by BioLuminate. FIGURE 5 presents white (broadband) spectroscopy data for 2 women with breast carcinoma, contrasting tumor oxyhemoglobin at the edge versus the center. FIGURE 6 presents data contrasting the edge and the center for both blue laser (fluorescence) and white (broadband, oxyhemoglobin fraction) spectroscopy. FIGURE 7 presents impedance data in normal

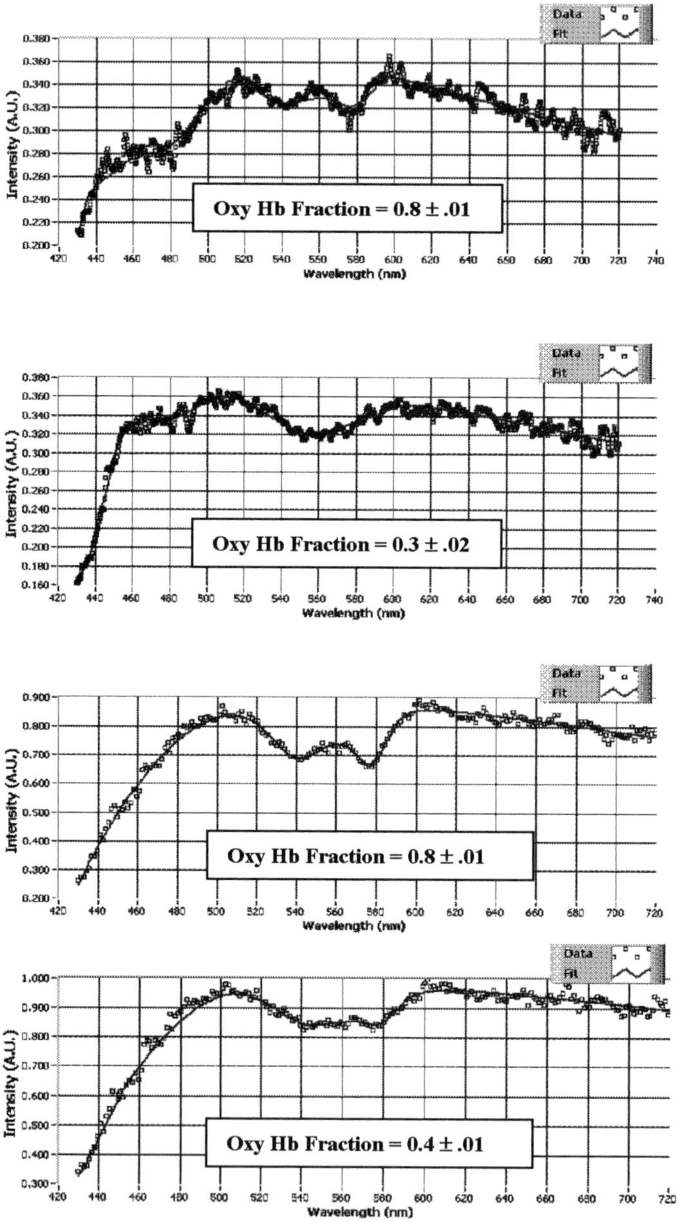

FIGURE 5. Broadband spectroscopy data from 2 patients (D-007 and D-012) with histologically verified breast carcinoma.

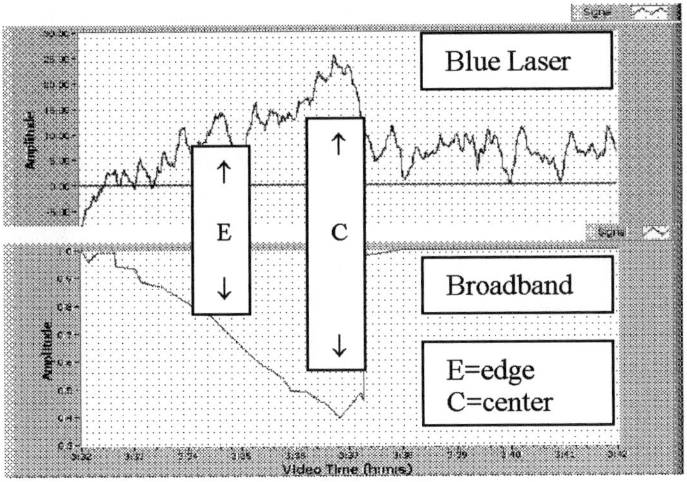

FIGURE 6. Patient with histologically verified infiltrating ductal breast carcinoma, grade III, 2.2 cm diameter: (*top*) blue laser (fluorescence); (*bottom*) white/broadband (oxy-Hb fraction).

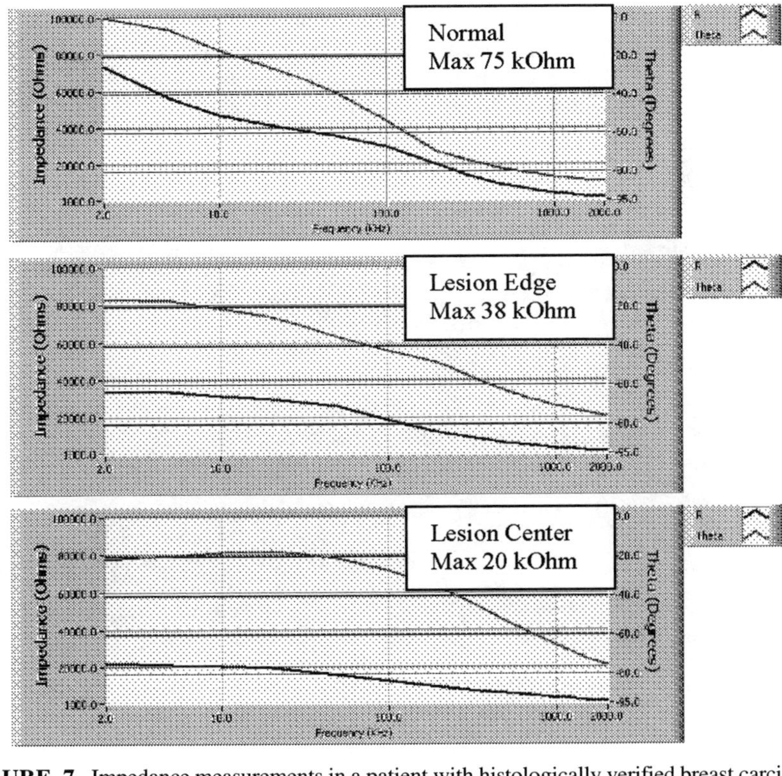

FIGURE 7. Impedance measurements in a patient with histologically verified breast carcinoma.

breast, edge of breast carcinoma, and center of breast carcinoma over the frequency range of 2 to 2000 kHz, with the maximum tissue differentiation being at the lowest frequency (2 kHz).

NANOELECTRODE ARRAYS FOR SIMULTANEOUS NEUROTRANSMITTER AND ELECTRICAL ACTIVITY MONITORING, PLUS ELECTRICAL STIMULATION

Neuromodulation—the use of controlled electrical stimulation of the central or peripheral nervous system—is a treatment modality being explored for various nervous system disorders, for example, movement disorders, epilepsy, chronic pain, depression, and eating disorders. Three of the most common forms of neuromodulation—deep brain stimulation, vagus nerve stimulation, and transcranial magnetic stimulation—were reviewed in the last conference.[5] At present, each of these techniques is an "open-loop" system, that is, the stimulation is performed without the benefit of input from the brain to guide the timing or characteristics of the stimulation. There is evidence from neuromodulation for intractable epilepsy that a "closed-loop" system (with monitoring of the brain's electrical activity—to detect an impending seizure) can greatly increase the effectiveness of neuromodulation.[6]

Combining continuous monitoring of neurotransmitter levels and electrical activity with precise focal electrical stimulation [electrochemical closed-loop neuromodulation (ECN)] would be a significant advance over currently available techniques. Additionally, reducing the scale to the nanolevel (1) improves signal-to-noise ratios, (2) permits greater precision (down to the subnuclei level), and (3) opens the possibility of multiple recording/monitoring and stimulation sites throughout the central nervous system.

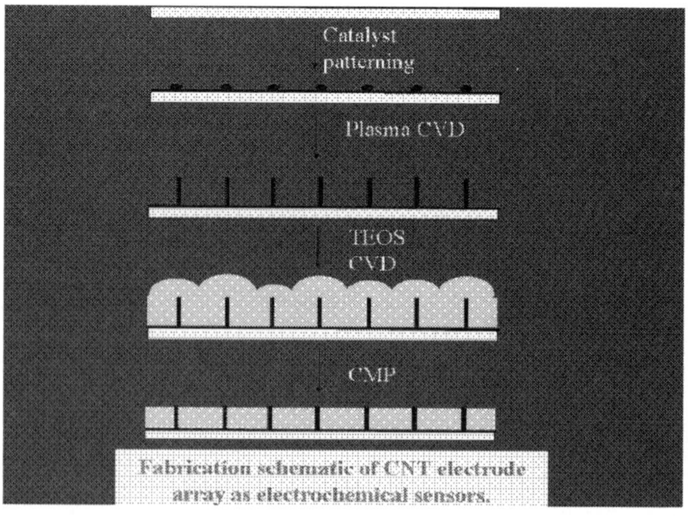

FIGURE 8. Nanoelectrode array fabrication. See text for abbreviations and details.

The NASA Ames Nanotechnology Center is developing microchip nanoelectrode arrays for neuromodulation that exhibit the above properties.[7] The microchip consists of two types of vertically aligned multiwalled carbon nanotube (MWCNT) arrays on multiple individually addressed microelectrode pads. The first type is a forestlike MWCNT array that presents a large surface area and is used as a stimulation electrode. The second type is encapsulated with an insulator, leaving only the very end of the MWCNTs exposed at the surface to form an inlaid nanodisk electrode array.

A schematic for the fabrication of the nanoelectrode arrays is given in FIGURE 8. To a silicon wafer, a nickel catalyst film is deposited. The vertically aligned MWCNT arrays are grown on the nickel catalyst by a plasma carbon vapor deposition (CVD) process. For the uninsulated stimulation electrode, the fabrication stops at this point. For the insulated recording electrode (electrical and electrochemical), two more steps are required. First, a silicon oxide layer is created by tetraethylorthosilicate (TEOS) CVD. Next, chemical mechanical polishing (CMP) removes the insulation so that only the tips of the MWCNT arrays are exposed. FIGURE 9 illustrates both the insulated and uninsulated electrodes, plus one potential configuration with a single recording electrode surrounded by eight stimulating electrodes.

The insulated nanodisk electrode array has shown extraordinary electrochemical properties, with a detection limit of redox species down to a few nanomolars and an extremely high temporal resolution down to milliseconds, which are ideal for measuring simultaneously (1) extracellular neurotransmitters (e.g., dopamine) and (2) focal electrical activity. The uninsulated array is ideal for focal electrical stimulation, potentially as a focal (or regional) closed-loop stimulation system depending upon variations in the monitored electrical activity and/or neurotransmitter concentration (ECN). FIGURE 10 summarizes these advantages of nanoelectrode arrays.

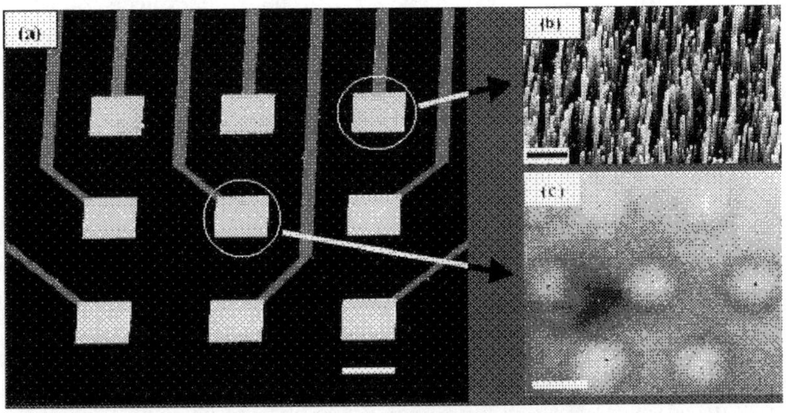

FIGURE 9. Uninsulated and insulated carbon nanotube (CNT) arrays. Scanning electron micrograph (SEM) image of **(a)** a 3×3 microelectrode array, **(b)** a high-magnification image of exposed CNT array electrodes used for electrical stimulation, and **(c)** an embedded low-density CNT array used for recording changes in local neurotransmitter concentrations. Scale bars: (a) 200 μm; (b) 1 μm; (c) 2 μm.

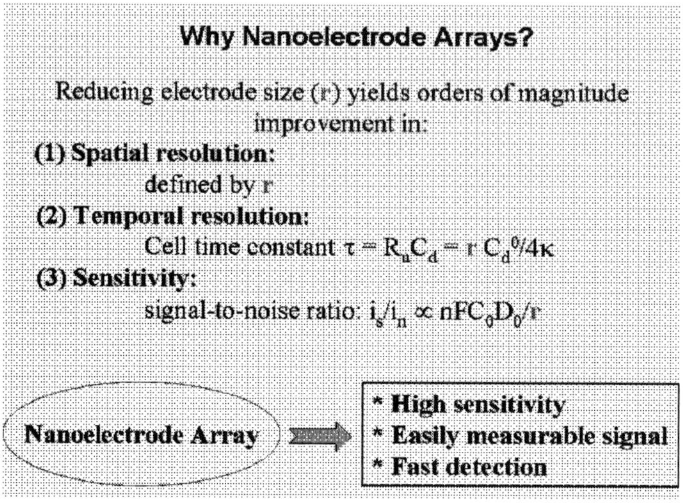

FIGURE 10. The spatial, temporal, and sensitivity advantages of nanoelectrodes in comparison with microelectrodes.

CONCLUSIONS

The NASA Ames Smart Probe and Nanoelectrode Array Projects represent steps toward the goal of using "cutting-edge" technology to gather large amounts of data—objectively, accurately, minimally invasively, and dispersed spatially and temporally. The Smart Probe is primarily a software concept of employing neural networks and fuzzy logic techniques to integrate multiple data streams in real time to provide immediate feedback—in the form of either a tissue diagnosis or information to guide an intervention (e.g., a closed-loop neuromodulation system). The Nanoelectrode Array allows the simultaneous and continuous gathering of data—both electrical and electrochemical (e.g., neurotransmitters)—from multiple sites in the brain. When combined with neural network software, the Nanoelectrode Array also can form both the recording and stimulation ends of a closed-loop neuromodulation system (ECN).

A major difference between laboratory and clinical neuroprotection trials is the quantity and precision of the data collected in the former in comparison with the latter. With advances such as the Smart Probe and the Nanoelectrode Array, the measurement of neuroprotection processes and outcomes in clinical trials may eventually rival those of laboratory studies. As we trek beyond the neuroprotection "base camp", advances in measurement may prove to be one of the trustiest "guides". Importantly, just as a seasoned guide may lead to unexpected vistas, advances in measurement will likely lead to novel neuroprotection insights and strategies.

ACKNOWLEDGMENTS

The projects reported here involved the following individuals: R. Mah, S. Jeffrey, M. Guerrero, R. Papasin, and C. Reed from NASA Ames Smart Systems; J. Li, H. Chen, B. Nguyen-Vu, M. Meyyappan, A. Cassell, J. Koehne, H. Purewal, and O. Ye from NASA Ames Nanotechnology; L. DaSilva and U. Kasthuri from Bio-Luminate (Dublin, CA); and N. Huang and L. Chen from the Parkinson's Institute (Sunnyvale, CA).

REFERENCES

1. ANDREWS, R.J. 1999. Neuroprotective "agents" in surgery: secret "agent" man, or common "agent" machine? Ann. N.Y. Acad. Sci. **890:** 59–72.
2. KNOPMAN, D.S., S.T. DEKOSKY, J.L. CUMMINGS *et al.* 2001. Practice parameter: diagnosis of dementia (an evidence-based review)—Report of the Quality Standards Subcommittee of the American Academy of Neurology. Neurology **56:** 1143–1153.
3. MCLUHAN, M. 1964. Understanding Media: The Extensions of Man. McGraw–Hill. New York.
4. ANDREWS, R., R. MAH & L. DASILVA. 2004. The NASA Smart Probe for real time multiple microsensor tissue recognition. Proc. SPIE (Prog. Biomed. Opt. Imag. Opt. Biop. V) **5326:** 92–97.
5. ANDREWS, R.J. 2003. Neuroprotection trek—the next generation: Neuromodulation I. Techniques—deep brain stimulation, vagus nerve stimulation, and transcranial magnetic stimulation. Ann. N.Y. Acad. Sci. **993:** 1–13.
6. ANDREWS, R.J. 2003. Neuroprotection trek—the next generation: Neuromodulation II. Applications—epilepsy, nerve regeneration, neurotrophins. Ann. N.Y. Acad. Sci. **993:** 14–24.
7. NGUYEN-VU, B., H. CHEN, A. CASSELL *et al.* 2004. Carbon nanotube nanoelectrode array for electrophysiology. Presented at the NIH Workshop on Neural Interfaces, Washington, D.C.

Protective Effect of Neuromonitoring during Cardiac Surgery

HARVEY L. EDMONDS, JR.

Neuromonitoring Associates, Incorporated, Louisville, Kentucky, USA

ABSTRACT: This study was a retrospective examination of the influence of multimodality neuromonitoring on the incidence of serious brain injury associated with a common type of adult cardiac surgery, coronary artery bypass grafting (CABG). Multichannel EEG, cerebral oximetry, and transcranial Doppler ultrasound were used to detect and correct imbalances in cerebral perfusion and oxygenation. Imbalances were detected in 59% of the cases and successfully corrected in all but 2%. In the absence of neuromonitoring, the expected incidence of serious brain injury is 6.1%. With neuromonitoring, the actual observed incidence was 3.0% (P = 0.03). The apparent improvement can be attributed primarily to a reduction in the number of nonembolic diffuse injuries.

KEYWORDS: cardiac surgery; brain injury; neuroprotection; EEG; cerebral oximetry; transcranial Doppler ultrasound; outcome

The landmark prospective multicenter study of Roach *et al.*[1] established the incidence of overt brain injury resulting from a common cardiac surgical procedure. In the study population of 2108 patients undergoing coronary artery bypass graft (CABG) surgery, the incidence of type I injury (focal injury, stupor, or coma at discharge) was 3.1%, while type II injury (deterioration in intellectual function, memory deficit, or seizures) occurred in 3.0%. The authors' conservative estimate of direct cost of injury was approximately $8000 per patient (in 1996 dollars), while total indirect cost to the U.S. health care delivery system was thought to be ten times greater.[2] Thus, the current national economic impact of this potentially preventable cardiac surgery–related brain injury exceeds $2 billion annually.

Brain injury associated with cardiac surgery appears to have three major causes: hypo- or hyperperfusion, embolization, and/or a systemic inflammatory response.[3] In principle, the first two of these causes should be detectable by neurophysiologic monitoring. Recent technologic developments have turned this theoretical principle into a practical reality. Continuous monitoring of cerebral blood flow, oxygenation, and neuronal function has facilitated the rapid detection and correction of neurophysiologic imbalance or emboli generation. Therefore, the goal of this study was to compare the expected incidence of overt neurologic injury in patients without neuromonitoring (i.e., the study of Roach *et al.*)[1] with the observed incidence in a demographically similar group of patients receiving multimodality neuromonitoring.

Address for correspondence: Harvey L. Edmonds, Jr., Ph.D., Neuromonitoring Associates, Inc., 3712 Plymouth Road, Louisville, KY 40207. Voice: 502-262-3976; fax: 502-290-1751.
lharvo@louisville.edu

Ann. N.Y. Acad. Sci. 1053: 12–19 (2005). © 2005 New York Academy of Sciences.
doi: 10.1196/annals.1344.002

Although such comparison cannot be used as proof of cause and effect, it is an essential first step in the development of an adequately powered, randomized, prospective study.

METHODS

Subjects: With local IRB approval, the records of 332 patients undergoing CABG surgery at a single hospital from 2001 through 2004 were reviewed. Transcranial Doppler ultrasound data from an additional 286 revascularization procedures obtained between 1994 and 1996 were also reviewed for additional historical comparison.

Surgery: All surgeries were performed by a single group of cardiothoracic surgeons and cardiac anesthesiologists who had a consistent approach to patient management. Of the 332 surgeries, 30 were performed without cardiopulmonary bypass. None of the patients had concomitant intracardiac or vascular procedures.

Neuromonitoring: Four-channel EEG was recorded from gold disk electrodes located bilaterally in the fronto-temporal and centro-parietal scalp regions to assess changes in cerebral cortical synaptic activity. The recording montage was designed to detect ischemic EEG slowing in the anterior and posterior cortical vascular watershed regions, both of which are particularly susceptible to injury during cardiac sur-

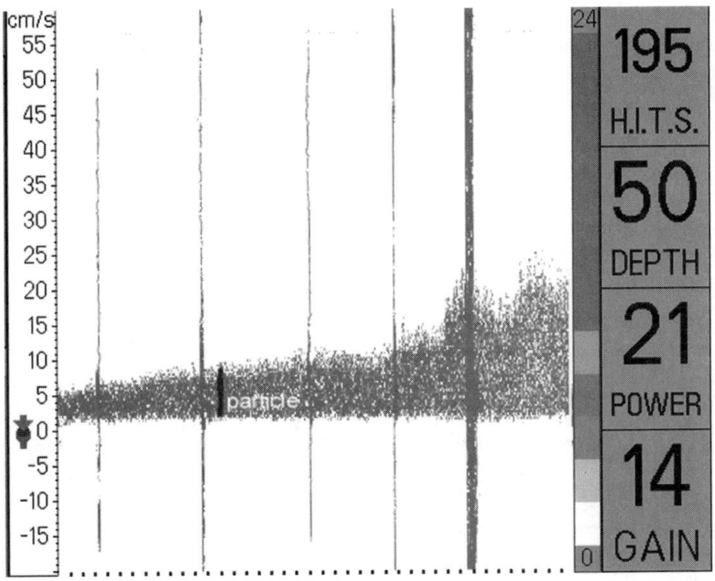

FIGURE 1. The display shows large changes in the right middle cerebral artery flow-velocity spectrum over a 20-s interval during cardiopulmonary bypass. Flow-velocity increase to the preincision baseline was accomplished by increasing bypass pump flow. Also shown are the high-intensity transient signals representing emboli. The single particulate embolus is shown as a dark vertical bar completely within the flow-velocity spectrum adjacent to the particle label. In contrast, five gaseous emboli are seen as full-scale vertical lines, representing their higher acoustic impedance.

gery.[4] Computer-processed digital EEG (A-1000 monitor, Aspect Medical Systems, Newton, MA) yielded compressed spectral trended displays as well as numeric EEG descriptors (total power, median frequency, 95% spectral edge frequency, and suppression ratio). Transcranial Doppler ultrasound (TCD) was used to continuously measure change in middle cerebral artery blood flow velocity. The TCD spectral displays (Companion, Nicolet Vascular, Madison, WI) were obtained from 2 MHz ultrasound probes held in place in the temporal region with an elastic headband fixation system. TCD also detected the presence of high-intensity transient signals (HITS) indicative of particulate or gaseous emboli. Cerebral oximetry based on transcranial near-infrared spectroscopy (INVOS 4100, Somanetics Corp., Troy, MI) was used to quantify change in microvascular oxygen balance bilaterally within the anterior vascular watershed of the frontal cortex.

Intervention criteria: Standardized criteria were used to objectively detect physiologic imbalance. Cerebral hypoperfusion was characterized by a decline in middle cerebral artery blood flow velocity to <20% of preincision baseline (FIG. 1), while hyperperfusion was indicated by a >200% increase. Ultrasonic HITS were defined as transients of >10 ms, but <200 ms duration, with an intensity of >12 db above spectral background (FIG. 1). A decline in regional cerebral oxygen saturation (rSO_2) of >20% below awake baseline signified cerebral hypoxia (FIG. 2).[5] Cerebral cortical synaptic suppression suggestive of ischemia was identified using the established criteria of a >50% reduction below preincision baseline in either amplitude (i.e., total power) or frequency (i.e., median or 95% spectral edge) (FIG. 3).[6]

Based on this information, patient management was systematically altered to correct the imbalance. The immediate success of each intervention was determined by prompt resolution of the detected imbalance. If the initial intervention was ineffec-

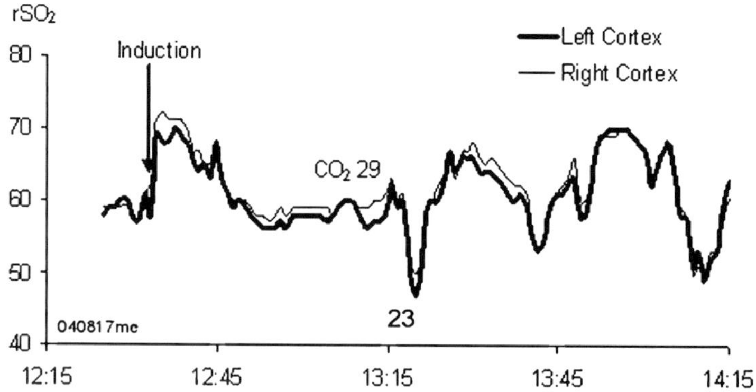

FIGURE 2. The graph illustrates regional cerebral oxygen saturation (rSO_2) changes from the initiation of monitoring in the awake patient until the onset of cardiopulmonary bypass at 14:00 h. The transient decline to the intervention threshold at 13:18 was precipitated by progressive hypocapnia. The desaturation was promptly corrected by increasing arterial CO_2 partial pressure towards normocapnia. The transient desaturation at the onset of cardiopulmonary bypass reflected the passage of pump priming solution through the cerebral vasculature. Because of its transient nature, no intervention was necessary.

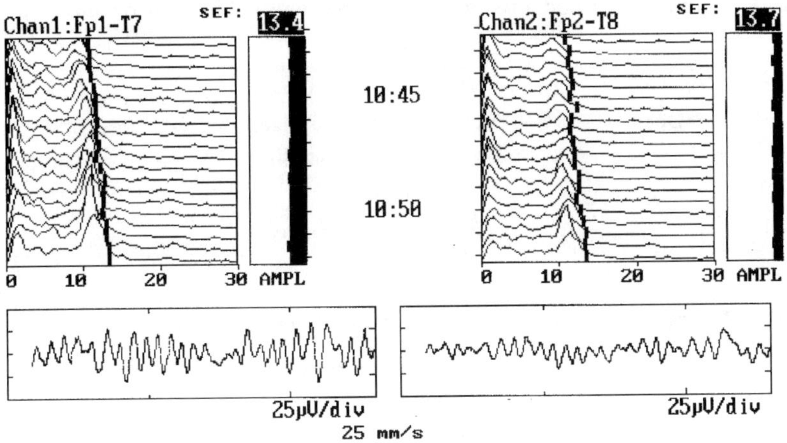

FIGURE 3. The lower boxed waveforms depict 2.5-s EEG segments obtained from the left (channel 1: Fp1-T7) and right (channel 2: Fp2-T8) fronto-temporal regions at 10:55 h. The upper compressed spectral array displays illustrate the time course of EEG frequency changes. The upper boundary of the frequency spectrum (i.e., 95% spectral edge frequency) is shown as a series of vertical bars and as a numeric value next to the box labeled SEF. The narrow vertical boxes labeled AMPL provide a trend of the total power contained in the EEG signal. EEG evidence of right hemisphere suppression is manifested most prominently by left vs. right amplitude asymmetry most evident in both the waveform and total power displays.

tive, additional physiologic variables were successively altered until resolution was achieved. The standardized intervention technique was similar to that utilized by Murkin *et al.*[7] Specific interventions included increases in (1) arterial CO_2 tension if < 35 mmHg, (2) mean arterial pressure, or (3) pump flow (or cardiac output). If these measures were ineffectual, cerebral oxygen demand was reduced by continuous infusion of propofol. During rewarming, normothermia was restored if nasopharyngeal temperature rose above 37.5°C. As a last resort, blood products were administered if the hematocrit was <20%.

RESULTS

Compared with the study of Roach *et al.*,[1] the demographics of the patient population receiving neuromonitoring were very similar [age > 70 years (32% vs. 33%); hypertension (57% vs. 52%); diabetes mellitus (25% vs. 22%); history of stroke or transient ischemic attack (8% vs. 5%)]. In contrast, the combined type I and II brain injury incidence was significantly lower ($P = 0.03$) in the neuromonitored population (6.1% expected vs. 3.0% observed). Most of the apparent benefit was obtained by a reduction of type II injury (3.0% expected vs. 0.3% observed, $P < .001$).

TABLE 1 summarizes the physiologic imbalances detected by neuromonitoring. The most common physiologic imbalance was regional cerebral hypoxia—inadequate oxygen delivery to meet metabolic demand—which occurred in 43% of cases.

TABLE 1. Physiologic and anesthetic imbalance detected by neuromonitoring

Modality	Imbalance	Incidence
Cerebral oximetry	Desaturation > 20%	42%
Transcranial Doppler	Velocity < 20% baseline	13%
	Velocity > twice baseline	2%
	Air leak	1%
EEG	New focal abnormality	1%

TABLE 2. Neuromonitoring-directed interventions to correct physiologic or anesthetic imbalance

Blood pressure increase	23%
CO_2 increase	13%
Pump flow increase	17%
Miscellaneous	
Blood product administration	1%
CO_2 decrease	<1%
Air leak repair & de-air	1%
Reposition heart	1%
Resume cardiopulmonary bypass	1%
Inspired O_2 increase	1%

NOTE: Results are shown as % of cases monitored.

Low saturation was associated with neurologic injury. The minimum saturation experienced by injured patients (rSO_2 44 ± 11, n = 10) was significantly lower (P = 0.02) than that observed in uninjured patients (rSO_2 54 ± 11, n = 322). Adjustment for cerebral hypoxia duration did not improve intergroup discrimination. The other common (i.e., 13% incidence) physiologic imbalance was hypoperfusion, a marked reduction in middle cerebral artery flow velocity. Thus, potentially injurious and readily correctable deficiencies in delivery of oxygen or nutrients to the brain occurred in more than half of the surgeries.

TABLE 2 summarizes the relative frequency of interventions employed to correct physiologic imbalances. In only 2% of the attempted interventions did the imbalance remain uncorrected. In many cases, cerebral hypoxia or hypoperfusion was readily corrected with small increases in systemic perfusion pressure or cardiac output (pump flow) or normalization of hypocapnia to increase cerebral blood flow.

The progressive influence of TCD monitoring on cerebral embolization may be appreciated by comparison with historical data. Over the past decade, the gradual introduction of a series of simple TCD-guided strategies aimed at emboli reduction has resulted in a 13-fold decrease in the embolic load delivered through the middle cerebral arteries during myocardial revascularization. These strategies include the (1) epiaortic ultrasonic scanning of the ascending aorta and arch to select plaque-free

TABLE 3. Reduction in ultrasonic HITS indicative of cerebral microemboli

	1994–1995	2001–2004
Sample size (no. of cases)	286	332
Zero HITS/case	0% of cases	15% of cases[a]
Median HITS (interquartile range)	274 (110–627)	21 (6–65)[a]
>200 HITS/case	59% of cases	8% of cases[a]

[a] $P < .001$.

cannulation and occlusion sites,[8] (2) avoidance of the reinfusion of unwashed cardiotomy suction material,[9] and (3) use of disposable cardiopulmonary bypass circuit components with a low propensity for emboli production.[10] (See TABLE 3.)

DISCUSSION

The findings of this study challenge the widely held notion that cardiac surgery–related brain injury is exclusively embolic and therefore unpreventable. Type I injury often does appear to be of macroembolic origin with a course that is difficult to influence. However, the more diffuse type II injury involves both microemboli and hypoperfusion—injurious processes that are detectable and correctable. The predominantly type II reduction observed in the present study is consistent with this view.

TCD and cerebral oximetry demonstrate that large and potentially injurious reductions in cerebral perfusion and oxygenation occur frequently during coronary artery bypass grafting with or without cardiopulmonary bypass. Thus, the present results are consistent with numerous studies that have found association between low cerebral oxygen saturation and signs of brain injury.[11–14] The results of the current study also agree with the observation that correction of cerebral oxygen imbalance is associated with reduction in overt brain injury and its consequences.[7,15,16]

Nevertheless, TCD and cerebral oximetry have noteworthy limitations. A TCD intervention threshold based on a 70% flow-velocity reduction has been established for conscious[5] and anesthetized[17] patients with normothermic pulsatile perfusion. However, the hemodilution, hypothermia, and alpha-stat acid-base management accompanying cardiopulmonary bypass require threshold adjustment because of the altered relationship between cerebral blood flow and velocity. Our experience during cardiopulmonary bypass in thousands of near-normothermic patients has demonstrated that flow-velocity decreases of >80% below baseline consistently result in cerebral oxygen desaturation and EEG suppression suggestive of cerebral ischemia.

Although many studies have documented an association between ultrasonic HITS and neurologic or cognitive injury,[18] the precise nature of the relationship is controversial.[19] Current TCD technology is unable to determine emboli size or composition. In addition, despite the recommendations of a consensus panel,[20] the manufacturer- and laboratory-specific ultrasonic criteria for emboli detection remain nonstandard. Consequently, ultrasonic quantification of cerebral microemboli during cardiac surgery may be viewed as a semiquantitative process.

The major limitation of cerebral oximetry is that sensor placement is restricted to glabrous skin (i.e., forehead). Thus, cerebral ischemia occurring in the susceptible posterior watershed territory is not often detectable.

Quantitative EEG monitoring enables objective detection of ischemia involving the cerebral convexity. The measurement has high sensitivity,[6] but relatively low specificity, because synaptic suppression may have a benign cause (i.e., excessive anesthesia or cooling).

In the present study, the strength of evidence in favor of apparent neuromonitoring benefit rests with the appropriateness of the comparison with the historical cohort described by Roach *et al.*[1] The relevance of this cohort to our local practice has been established previously. We reported a nearly identical 6.2% incidence of major neurologic complications in a demographically similar group of CABG surgery patients from 1999–2000 who did not receive any form of neuromonitoring.[21]

Clinically and economically significant neuroprotection can be achieved with multimodality neurophysiologic monitoring coupled with a standardized intervention protocol. The success of this approach has now been demonstrated in pediatric cardiac surgery,[22] aortic arch aneurysm repair,[23] and myocardial revascularization.[21,24] Since the risks of monitoring are nil, the cost modest, and the benefit substantial, there is compelling justification for its routine integration into the perioperative management of the cardiac surgical patient.

REFERENCES

1. Roach, G.W. *et al.* 1996. Adverse cerebral outcomes after coronary bypass surgery. N. Engl. J. Med. **335**(25): 1857–1863.
2. Mangano, D.T. 1995. Cardiovascular morbidity and CABG surgery—a perspective: epidemiology, costs, and potential therapeutic solutions. J. Card. Surg. **10**(suppl.): 366–368.
3. Taylor, K.M. 1998. Brain damage during cardiopulmonary bypass. Ann. Thorac. Surg. **65:** S20–S26.
4. Barbut, D. *et al.* 1998. Posterior distribution of infarcts in strokes related to cardiac operations. Ann. Thorac. Surg. **65:** 1656–1659.
5. Singer, I. & H.L. Edmonds, Jr. 1998. Head-up tilt testing predicts syncope during ventricular tachycardia in implantable cardioverter-defibrillator patients. J. Interven. Cardiol. **11**(3): 205–211.
6. Minicucci, F. *et al.* 2000. Computer-assisted EEG monitoring during carotid endarterectomy. J. Clin. Neurophysiol. **17**(1): 101–107.
7. Murkin, J.M. *et al.* 2004. Monitoring cerebral oxygen saturation significantly decreases major organ morbidity in CABG patients: a randomized blinded study [abstract]. Heart Surg. Forum **7:** 515.
8. Waering, T.H. *et al.* 1992. Management of the severely atherosclerotic ascending aorta during cardiac operations: a strategy for detection and treatment. J. Thorac. Cardiovasc. Surg. **103:** 453–462.
9. Brooker, R.F. *et al.* 1998. Cardiotomy suction: a major source of brain lipid emboli during cardiopulmonary bypass. Ann. Thorac. Surg. **65:** 1651–1655.
10. Jones, T.J.J. *et al.* 2000. The propagation of entrained air during cardiopulmonary bypass is affected by circuit design, but not by vacuum assisted venous drainage [abstract]. Anesth. Analg. **90:** SCA39.
11. Basker-Rao, B. *et al.* 1998. Evidence for improved cerebral function after minimally invasive bypass surgery. J. Cardiac Surg. **13:** 27–31.
12. Edmonds, H.L., Jr. *et al.* 1998. Cerebral oxygen desaturation during myocardial revascularization is associated with frontal lobe injury [abstract]. Anesth. Analg. **86:** SCA13.

13. EDMONDS, H.L., JR. *et al.* 2000. Neuromonitoring for cardiac and vascular surgery. *In* The Brain and Cardiac Surgery, pp. 143–164. Harwood. London.
14. CAO, L., Q-J. YU & H.L. EDMONDS, JR. 2000. Application of eye movement test in the assessment of central nervous system dysfunction after cardiac surgery in elderly patients. Chin. J. Geriatr. Cardiovasc. Cerebrovasc. Dis. **2**(5)**:** 322–324.
15. MONK, T.G., K.A. RENO & B.S. OLSEN. 2000. Post-operative cognitive dysfunction is associated with cerebral oxygen desaturations [abstract]. Anesthesiology **93:** A167.
16. ALEXANDER, J.C., JR., M.A. KRONEFELD & G.R. DANCE. 2002. Reduced post-operative length of stay may result from using cerebral oximetry monitoring to guide treatment [abstract]. Ann. Thorac. Surg. **73:** 373C.
17. SPENCER, M.P. 1997. Transcranial Doppler monitoring and causes of stroke from carotid endarterectomy. Stroke **28**(4)**:** 685–691.
18. STUMP, D. *et al.* 1996. Cerebral emboli and cognitive outcome after cardiac surgery. J. Cardiothorac. Vasc. Anesth. **10:** 113–119.
19. NEVILLE, M.J. *et al.* 2001. Similar neurobehavioral outcome after valve or coronary artery operations despite differing carotid embolic counts. J. Thorac. Cardiovasc. Surg. **121:** 125–136.
20. RINGELSTEIN, E.B. *et al.* 1998. Consensus on microembolus detection by TCD. Stroke **29**(3)**:** 725–729.
21. EDMONDS, H.L., JR. 2002. Multi-modality neurophysiologic monitoring. Heart Surg. Forum **5**(3)**:** 225–228.
22. AUSTIN, E.H., III *et al.* 1997. Benefit of neurophysiologic monitoring for pediatric cardiac surgery. J. Thorac. Cardiovasc. Surg. **114:** 707–717.
23. GANZEL, B.L. *et al.* 1997. Neurophysiological monitoring to assure delivery of retrograde cerebral perfusion. J. Thorac. Cardiovasc. Surg. **113:** 748–757.
24. LASCHINGER, J. *et al.* 2003. Cardiac surgery: value of neuromonitoring [abstract]. Heart Surg. Forum **6:** 204.

Neuropsychiatric Alterations in MDMA Users

Preliminary Findings

RONALD I. HERNING, WARREN BETTER, KIMBERLY TATE, AND JEAN L. CADET

Molecular Neuropsychiatry Branch, National Institute on Drug Abuse, Intramural Research Program, Baltimore, Maryland 21224, USA

ABSTRACT: The use of marijuana is rampant among 3,4-methylenedioxymethamphetamine (MDMA) users. The co-occurrence of abuse of these two drugs has made it difficult to assess the specific residual effects of MDMA alone. As a first step toward identifying the effects of long-term MDMA use, we studied 8 MDMA abusers, 8 marijuana/MDMA abusers, 15 marijuana abusers (matched in marijuana use without MDMA use), and 17 control subjects. EEG, cerebral blood velocity by pulsed transcranial Doppler (TCD), and psychological measures were collected. Three-minute resting eyes-closed EEG recordings were obtained from 16 electrodes. The EEG was converted to 6 frequency bands (delta, theta, alpha-1, alpha-2, beta-1, and beta-2) using a fast Fourier transformation. Blood flow velocity was determined using a temporal window for the right and left middle cerebral arteries using TCD. Absolute log delta power in the EEG of MDMA abusers at central electrode sites was significantly higher than that of the MDMA/marijuana, marijuana abusers, and control subjects. There were also increases in alpha-2 EEG power observed only in marijuana abusers. The blood flow measure, diastolic velocity, was increased in MDMA abusers whether they used marijuana or not. Because increases in delta power and perfusion deficits are associated with some chronic disorders, our findings in these ecstasy abusers suggest that MDMA use may be associated with a drug-induced neuropathological state. More research is necessary to test these ideas.

KEYWORDS: MDMA; ecstasy; marijuana; polysubstance abuse; EEG deficits; cerebral perfusion deficits; transcranial Doppler; medical complications

INTRODUCTION

MDMA (3,4-methylenedioxymethamphetamine) abuse among young individuals has increased.[1] MDMA is a serotonin (5-HT) releaser and uptake inhibitor[2] whose long-term use in animals causes severe 5-HT depletion,[3] downregulation of 5-HT_2 receptors,[4] and loss of 5-HT nerve terminals.[3] In humans, MDMA abuse was reported to be associated with depression,[5] panic and anxiety attacks,[6] seizures,[7,8] cerebrovascular accidents,[9] and memory deficits.[10]

Address for correspondence: Ronald I. Herning, Ph.D., Molecular Neuropsychiatry Branch, NIDA/IRP, 5500 Nathan Shock Drive, Baltimore, MD 21224. Voice: 410-550-1551.
rherning@intra.nida.nih.gov

Ann. N.Y. Acad. Sci. 1053: 20–27 (2005). © 2005 New York Academy of Sciences.
doi: 10.1196/annals.1344.003

The cause of these neuropsychiatric side effects is being actively studied. For example, cognitive impairments were observed in abstinent MDMA abusers by some researchers,[10–12] whereas no deficits in cognitive performance were reported by other investigators.[13,14] Similarly, cerebral blood flow and glucose metabolism were reported as altered in abstinent MDMA abusers by some,[9,15] but not by all researchers.[13,14] Using fMRI, the blood oxygenation level–dependent (BOLD) response was found to be greater in MDMA abusers compared to control subjects during working memory tasks by one group,[16] but decreased in MDMA abusers by another group.[17] Abstinent MDMA abusers were reported to show increases in theta, alpha-1, and beta EEG power by two research groups.[18,19]

These conflicting results might be due to a number of issues including different study populations reported in the various studies. For example, the use of cocaine, amphetamine, LSD, and heroin was prevalent among the MDMA users.[10,11,13–16,20] Marijuana use was reported in MDMA users in most studies.[15,21–26] The presence of comorbid states might explain why marijuana abusers and MDMA/marijuana abusers are reported to show similar cognitive deficits.[15,23] Other studies have indeed attributed cognitive deficits and neuroendocrine abnormalities observed in MDMA/marijuana abusers to their use of marijuana.[17,27,28] In an attempt to clarify some of these issues further, we have used EEG and TCD (transcranial Doppler sonography) physiological indices in MDMA abusers by controlling for marijuana abuse and excluding subjects with other illicit substance abuse.

METHODS

Subjects

Four groups of subjects were tested as outpatients: MDMA group (8 subjects), marijuana group (15 subjects), MDMA/marijuana group (8 subjects), and control group (17 subjects). Before undergoing blood flow velocity assessment by TCD and EEG, all volunteers had undergone medical, neurological, psychological, and laboratory evaluations. Exclusion criteria that applied to all subjects include (1) major medical and psychiatric illnesses including history of hypertension, (2) head injuries with loss of consciousness for greater than 5 minutes, (3) evidence of any neurological abnormalities by history or examination, (4) HIV seropositivity, and (5) illicit drug use (cocaine, heroin, etc.) or excessive alcohol use by DSM-IV criteria for alcohol abuse or dependence.[29] The research protocol was approved by the National Institute on Drug Abuse and Johns Hopkins Bayview Medical Center Institutional Review Boards for Human Research. Informed consent was obtained from all subjects.

Demographic information (see TABLE 1) and drug-use history information (see TABLE 2) were obtained from the addiction severity index (ASI).[30] Illicit drug use other than MDMA, alcohol, tobacco, and marijuana use was not self-reported nor observed in urine toxicologies obtained during the screening process. Subjects with a lifetime diagnosis of alcohol abuse or dependence by DSM-IV criteria[29] were also screened out of the study. Drug abusers were tested during 1–7 days of abstinence. Any possible acute effects of nicotine on TCD and EEG measures were eliminated by testing subjects for 20 minutes or longer after cigarette smoking. Caffeinated beverages were not allowed for 2 hours or more before the recording session.

TABLE 1. Demographic measures and drug history

Measure	Control ($n = 17$) (mean ± SD)	MDMA ($n = 8$) (mean ± SD)	Marijuana ($n = 15$) (mean ± SD)	MDMA + marijuana ($n = 8$) (mean ± SD)
Age (years)	23.7 ± 5.5	22.4 ± 1.3	21.1 ± 1.0	23.7 ± 1.3
Shipley IQ	104.5 ± 2.4	103.7 ± 3.6	95.8 ± 2.9	99.8 ± 3.6
Education (years)	12.5 ± 1.4	12.7 ± 0.5	11.3 ± 0.5	12.8 ± 0.6
Women (%)	47.0%	60.0%	20.0%	50.0%
African-Americans (%)	58.8%	75.0%	100.0%	25.0%

TABLE 2. Drug history measures

Measure	Control (mean ± SD)	MDMA (mean ± SD)	Marijuana (mean ± SD)	MDMA + marijuana (mean ± SD)
MDMA: days/30 days[a]		2.6 ± 0.8		3.2 ± 0.8
MDMA: pills/90 days		18.6 ± 3.8		17.5 ± 3.8
MDMA: years[b]		2.4 ± 1.3		1.6 ± 1.3
Alcohol: days/30 days	1.2 ± 1.3	3.5 ± 1.9	5.5 ± 1.7	7.4 ± 1.9
Alcohol: years	1.2 ± 0.7	1.7 ± 1.1	3.0 ± 1.0	3.4 ± 1.1
Marijuana: days/30 days		1.4 ± 1.1	28.6 ± 1.1	20.6 ± 1.7
Marijuana: years		3.5 ± 1.1	6.4 ± 0.8	5.9 ± 2.2
Cigarettes/day	2.1 ± 1.8	7.7 ± 2.8	7.2 ± 2.4	9.0 ± 2.7
Cigarettes: years	1.6 ± 1.4	3.6 ± 2.1	8.8 ± 1.8	6.5 ± 2.0

[a]Number of days of substance use in the last 30 days from the ASI.[30]
[b]Years of substance use calculated from the ASI.[30]

Psychological and Neurological Tests

Psychological tests included Symptom Checklist-90R (SCL-90R).[31] A structured neurological history and exam was also obtained.

TCD Procedures

Blood flow velocity was determined using a temporal window for right and left middle cerebral arteries (MCA) using pulsed TCD (Nicolet, Model TC2000). TCD uses a handheld ultrasound transducer applied over the cerebral artery of interest using the correct placement on the skull, angle, and depth setting. A shift in frequency in the reflected sound indicates the blood flow velocity in that artery. Mean velocity (Vm: cm/s), systolic velocity (Vs: cm/s), diastolic velocity (Vd: cm/s), and pulsatility index [PI = (Vs − Vd)/Vm] were obtained for each artery. Resting heart rate and blood pressure were measured at the time of TCD recording.

EEG Recording Procedures

Participants sat in a reclining chair in a sound-attenuated, electronically shielded chamber. A 3-minute eyes-closed recording was obtained. The EEG was recorded from the following 16 international 10/20 scalp sites: Fp1, F3, C3, P3, O1, F7, T3, T5, Fp2, F4, C4, P4, O2, F8, T4, and T6. The EEG recording used the ear tips as reference. Eye movement was recorded from above and to the side of the left eye. Silver/silver chloride electrodes were used at all locations. The EEG was amplified with Grass (Model 7P511) amplifiers and processed with a 1- to 50-Hz half-amplitude band-pass and notch filter at 60 Hz. The EEG was sampled at the rate of 104 samples per second per channel. Artifacts in the EEG were removed by computer-assisted visual inspection by an operator blind to the subject group. EEG power was then determined for delta (0.4–3.9 Hz), theta (4.0–7.9 Hz), alpha-1 (8.0–9.9 Hz), alpha-2 (10.0–13.9 Hz), beta-1 (14.0–24.9 Hz), and beta-2 (25.0–40.0 Hz) EEG bands using the fast Fourier transformation using 256 points per epoch and averaging the spectra over epochs. The logarithm (log) of EEG power was calculated for each EEG band.

Statistical Analyses

A group-by-side analysis of variance (ANOVA) was performed on the TCD parameters for the MCA. A group-by-electrode ANOVA was performed on the log power for each EEG band. When assumptions of the model were violated as revealed by Mauchly's test, the Greenhouse-Geisser corrected P value ($P_{G\text{-}G}$) or the Huynh-Feldt corrected P value ($P_{H\text{-}F}$) is given.[32] When assumptions of the model were not violated, the unadjusted P value (P) is presented. After each ANOVA, post-hoc tests were made using a Newman-Keuls procedure for multiple tests on the appropriate means.

RESULTS

Psychological and Neurological Testing

The drug groups (MDMA, marijuana, and MDMA/marijuana) had 8 of the 9 SCL-90R scales significantly elevated compared to the control group, but the drug groups did not differ among themselves on any scale. The subjects in the MDMA/marijuana group rated themselves significantly less well than any of the other groups ($P < 0.05$). The MDMA group reported more headaches than the other groups.

EEG

Regional differences between the groups were observed in the EEG band as indicated by significant group-by-electrode interactions for log delta power [$F(45,600) = 1.70$, $P_{H\text{-}F} < 0.004$, $P_{G\text{-}G} < 0.016$] and log alpha-2 power [$F(45,600) = 1.51$, $P_{H\text{-}F} < 0.027$, $P_{G\text{-}G} < 0.056$], while approaching significance for alpha-1 power [$F(45,600) = 1.48$, $P_{H\text{-}F} < 0.035$, $P_{G\text{-}G} < 0.067$]. These regional changes among groups are shown in brain maps in FIGURES 1 and 2. Increases in log delta EEG power are observed in MDMA abusers at central electrode sites (FIG. 1). Increases in log alpha-2 EEG power in the frontal area are observed in marijuana abusers (FIG. 2).

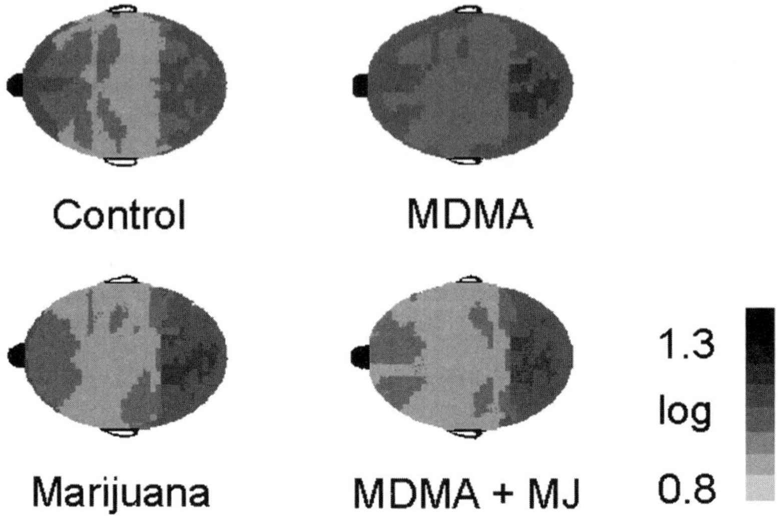

FIGURE 1. Topographical maps of log delta power. The MDMA group has significantly ($P < 0.05$) more delta power at central electrode sites than the other groups.

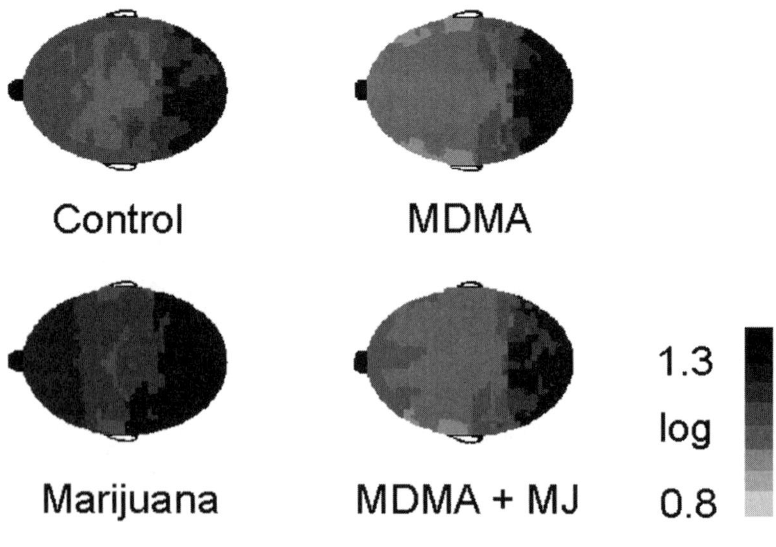

FIGURE 2. Topographical maps of log alpha-2 power. The marijuana group has significantly ($P < 0.05$) more alpha-2 power at frontal electrode sites than the other groups.

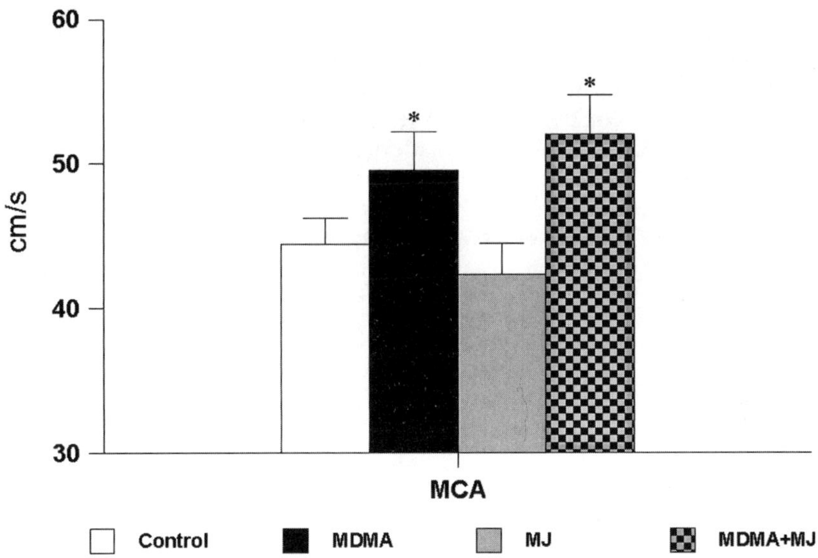

FIGURE 3. Diastolic velocity for the middle arteries (mean of the right and left sides). The MDMA and MDMA/marijuana groups have significantly ($*P < 0.05$) faster velocities than the control and marijuana groups.

Cerebral Flow Velocity

Vd was significantly different among the groups [$F(3,43) = 6.38$, $P < 0.001$]. The means for Vd are plotted in FIGURE 3. Both groups of subjects who used MDMA have elevated diastolic velocities compared to the marijuana and control groups. No differences among groups were observed for systolic velocity and pulsatility. Likewise, no significant differences among groups were observed for heart rate or blood pressure.

DISCUSSION

With the exclusion of MDMA subjects with illicit drug use other than marijuana and using a control group that used only marijuana, it was possible to determine the residual effects of MDMA abuse. MDMA abusers had increases in log delta EEG power at central electrode sites and increased diastolic velocity in the middle cerebral arteries.

Gamma and associates[19] reported that abstinent MDMA abusers had increases in theta, alpha, and beta power, whereas we found no increases in these EEG power bands in the MDMA abusers compared to the control subjects. However, the MDMA abusers in the study by Gamma and associates[19] used illicit substances other than marijuana. Their findings might be due to the use of marijuana, cocaine, and heroin. Increases in alpha-2 power at frontal sites were observed only in the marijuana group and have been observed by other researchers in chronic marijuana abusers.[33]

Increased diastolic velocity in the MDMA abusers might be due to vasoconstriction of the middle cerebral artery produced by MDMA since blood pressure was similar among the four groups. This idea is consistent with the report of decreases in cerebral blood in abstinent MDMA abusers by some researchers,[9,15] but other researchers report no such deficits.[13,14] Here again, the MDMA abusers tested by these latter researchers also abused illicit drugs such as cocaine and heroin, which was not the case in our study.

Because increases in EEG delta[34] and impaired cortical blood flow[35] are associated with chronic neurological disorders such as dementia, our findings in these ecstasy abusers suggest that MDMA use may be associated with a drug-induced neuropathological state. More research is necessary to test these ideas.

REFERENCES

1. BANKEN, J.A. 2004. Drug abuse trends among youth in the United States. Ann. N.Y. Acad. Sci. **1025:** 465–471.
2. HUETHER, G., D. ZHOU & E. RUTHER. 1997. Long-term modulation of presynaptic 5-HT-output: experimentally induced changes in cortical 5-HT-transporter density, tryptophan hydroxylase content, and 5-HT innervation density. J. Neural. Transm. **104:** 993–1004.
3. RICAURTE, G.A., L.E. DELANNEY, S.G. WIENER *et al.* 1988. 5-Hydroxyindoleacetic acid in cerebrospinal fluid reflects serotonergic damage induced by 3,4-methylenedioxymethamphetamine in CNS of non-human primates. Brain Res. **474:** 359–363.
4. SCHEFFEL, U., J.R. LEVER, M. STATHIS & G.A. RICAURTE. 1992. Repeated administration of MDMA causes transient down-regulation of serotonin 5-HT2 receptors. Neuropharmacology **31:** 881–893.
5. BENAZZI, F. & M. MAZZOLI. 1991. Psychiatric illness associated with "ecstasy". Lancet **338:** 1520.
6. PALLANTI, S. & D. MAZZI. 1992. MDMA (ecstasy) precipitation of panic disorder. Biol. Psychiatry **32:** 91–95.
7. THEUNE, M., W. ESSER, K.E DRUSCHKY *et al.* 1999. Grand mal series after ecstasy abuse. Nervenarzt **70:** 1094–1097.
8. FINSTERER, J., C. STOLLBERGER, C. STEGER & A. KROISS. 2003. Long lasting impaired cerebral blood flow after ecstasy intoxication. Psychiatry Clin. Neurosci. **57:** 221–225.
9. RENEMAN, L., J.B. HABRAKEN, C.B. MAJOIE *et al.* 2000. MDMA ("ecstasy") and its association with cerebrovascular accidents: preliminary findings. Am. J. Neuroradiol. **21:** 1001–1007.
10. BOLLA, K.I., U.D. MCCANN & G.A. RICAURTE. 1998. Memory impairment in abstinent MDMA ("ecstasy") users. Neurology **51:** 1532–1537.
11. WAREING, M., J.E. FISK, P. MURPHY & C. MONTGOMERY. 2004. Verbal working memory deficits in current and previous users of MDMA. Hum. Psychopharmacol. **19:** 225–234.
12. MCCANN, U.D., M. MERTL, V. ELIGULASHVILI & G.A. RICAURTE. 1999. Cognitive performance in (±)3,4-methylenedioxymethamphetamine (MDMA, "ecstasy") users: a controlled study. Psychopharmacology (Berl.) **143:** 417–425.
13. GAMMA, A., A. BUCK, T. BERTHOLD & F.X. VOLLENWEIDER. 2001. No difference in brain activation during cognitive performance between ecstasy (3,4-methylenedioxymethamphetamine) users and control subjects: a [H2(15)O]-positron emission tomography study. J. Clin. Psychopharmacol. **21:** 66–71.
14. CHANG, L, C.S. GROB, T. ERNST *et al.* 2000. Effect of ecstasy [3,4-methylenedioxymethamphetamine (MDMA)] on cerebral blood flow: a co-registered SPECT and MRI study. Psychiatry Res. **98:** 15–28.
15. BUCHERT, R., J. OBROCKI, R. THOMASIUS *et al.* 2001. Long-term effects of "ecstasy" abuse on the human brain studied by FDG PET. Nucl. Med. Commun. **22:** 889–897.
16. MOELLER, F.G., J.L. STEINBERG, G.M. DOUGHERTY *et al.* 2004. Functional MRI study of working memory in MDMA users. Psychopharmacology (Berl.) **177:** 185–194.

17. DAUMANN, J., JR., T. FISCHERMANN, K. HEEKEREN *et al.* 2004. Neural mechanisms of working memory in ecstasy (MDMA) users who continue or discontinue ecstasy and amphetamine use: evidence from an 18-month longitudinal functional magnetic resonance imaging study. Biol. Psychiatry **56:** 349–355.
18. DAFTERS, R.I., F. DUFFY, P.J. O'DONNELL & C. BOUQUET. 1999. Level of use of 3,4-methylenedioxymethamphetamine (MDMA or ecstasy) in humans correlates with EEG power and coherence. Psychopharmacology (Berl.) **145:** 82–90.
19. GAMMA, A., E. FREI, D. LEHMANN *et al.* 2000. Mood state and brain electric activity in ecstasy users. Neuroreport **11:** 157–162.
20. PARROTT, A.C., E. SISK & J.J. TURNER. 2000. Psychobiological problems in heavy "ecstasy" (MDMA) polydrug users. Drug Alcohol Depend. **60:** 105–110.
21. RODGERS, J. 2000. Cognitive performance amongst recreational users of "ecstasy". Psychopharmacology (Berl.) **151:** 19–24.
22. CROFT, R.J., A. KLUGMAN, T. BALDEWEG & J.H. GRUZELIER. 2001. Electrophysiological evidence of serotonergic impairment in long-term MDMA ("ecstasy") users. Am. J. Psychiatry **158:** 1687–1692.
23. SIMON, N.G. & R.P. MATTICK. 2002. The impact of regular ecstasy use on memory function. Addiction **97:** 1523–1529.
24. DAFTERS, R.I., R. HOSHI & A.C. TALBOT. 2004. Contribution of cannabis and MDMA ("ecstasy") to cognitive changes in long-term polydrug users. Psychopharmacology (Berl.) **173:** 405–410.
25. BOYD, C.J., S.E. MCCABE & H. D'ARCY. 2003. Ecstasy use among college undergraduates: gender, race, and sexual identity. J. Subst. Abuse Treat. **24:** 209–215.
26. SINGER, L.T., T.L. LINARES, S. NTIRI *et al.* 2004. Psychosocial profiles of older adolescent MDMA users. Drug Alcohol Depend. **74:** 245–252.
27. DAUMANN, J., S. PELZ, S. BECKER *et al.* 2001. Psychological profile of abstinent recreational ecstasy (MDMA) users and significance of concomitant cannabis use. Hum. Psychopharmacol. **16:** 627–633.
28. FISK, J.E., C. MONTGOMERY, P. MURPHY & M. WAREING. 2004. Evidence for executive deficits among users of MDMA (ecstasy). Br. J. Psychol. **95:** 457–466.
29. ROBINS, L.N., L. COTTLER, K. BUCHOLZ & W. COMPTON. 1995. Diagnostic Interview Schedule for DSM-IV. Washington University Press. St. Louis.
30. MCLELLAN, A.T., L. LUBORSKY, J. CACCIOLA *et al.* 1986. Guide to the Addiction Severity Index: Background, Administration, and Field Testing Results. National Institute on Drug Abuse, Treatment Research Reports. Rockville, MD.
31. DEROGATIS, L.R. 1983. Administration, Scoring, and Procedures for SCL-90R: Manual II. Clinical Psychometric Research. Towson, MD.
32. GREENHOUSE, S.W. & S. GEISSER. 1959. On methods in the analysis of profile data. Psychometrika **24:** 95–112.
33. STRUVE, F.A., J.J. STRAUMANIS, G. PATRICK *et al.* 1999. Topographic quantitative EEG sequelae of chronic marihuana use: a replication using medically and psychiatrically screened normal subjects. Drug Alcohol Depend. **56:** 167–179.
34. BRUNOVSKY, M., M. MATOUSEK, A. EDMA *et al.* 2003. Objective assessment of the degree of dementia by means of EEG. Neuropsychobiology **48:** 19–26.
35. SATTEL, H., S. BIEDERT & H. FORSTL. 1996. Senile dementia of Alzheimer type and multi-infarct dementia investigated by transcranial Doppler. Dementia **7:** 41–46.

Intraoperative Monitoring during Aneurysm Surgery as a Neuroprotective Activity with Reference to Evoked Potential and Microvascular Doppler Techniques

KARL E. SANZENBACHER

EEG/Clinical Neurophysiology and Neuromonitoring Laboratory, Eastern Maine Medical Center, Bangor, Maine, USA

KEYWORDS: monitoring; intraoperative; microvascular Doppler; modalities; evoked potentials

As neuroprotective modalities, successful intraoperative monitoring techniques confer multiple benefits including improvements in patient outcomes and quality of life. The aim is to detect impairments of central nervous system circulation as well as effects of instrumentation and systemic problems, which may occur during the operative procedure. Early detection of complications gives warning to the surgeon, allowing corrective actions to be taken.

Monitoring modalities include different types of somatosensory evoked potentials (SSEPs), electrical motor evoked potentials (eMEPs), and microvascular Doppler studies. Each contributes information regarding patient status with varying sensitivity during different phases of the procedure. This paper describes the benefits and limitations of these modalities in different types and locations of cerebral aneurysms, as well as comparing them with each other. Overall, eMEPs are superior to SSEPs in most situations. However, eMEPs may require an intermittent temporary halt in the procedure due to induced patient movement. A longer experience with SSEP changes in cases of immediately detected vascular impairment demonstrates a strong corresponding correlation with the postoperative patient status. SSEP changes not related to the event of vascular occlusion result in an increased incidence of clinical impairment as compared to eSEPs, which were unchanged.

Microvascular Doppler utilizes a 16- or 20-MHz Doppler probe of approximately 1-mm size to detect flow in vessels down to 1-mm size. The availability of microvascular Doppler allows the neurosurgeon to detect the status and inadvertent occlusion of vessels and subsequently modify clip position.

Address for correspondence: Karl E. Sanzenbacher, M.D., M.S., Medical Director of EEG/Clinical Neurophysiology and Neuromonitoring Laboratory, Eastern Maine Medical Center, Bangor, ME 04401.

ksanzenbacher@eemh.org

Ann. N.Y. Acad. Sci. 1053: 28–29 (2005). © 2005 New York Academy of Sciences.
doi: 10.1196/annals.1344.050

With the detection of abnormalities, interventions have been undertaken in 8–10% of cases. These include modification of retraction and other instrumentation as well as removing temporary clips with subsequent repositioning. In some cases, blood pressure was elevated. Although morbidity and mortality may be reduced, interventions have not done away with all deficits.

Panel of Biomarkers Predicts Stroke

D. T. LASKOWITZ, R. BLESSING, J. FLOYD, W. D. WHITE, AND J. R. LYNCH

Department of Medicine (Neurology), Duke University Medical Center, Durham, North Carolina, USA

KEYWORDS: **biomarker; stroke; ischemic stroke; symptoms; patients**

The absence of a widely available and sensitive diagnostic test limits the management of patients with acute cerebral ischemia. Here, we validate that a panel of biomarkers can be used to diagnose stroke with high sensitivity and specificity in patients presenting with the acute onset of neurological symptoms.

Blood samples were drawn from 130 patients with suspected stroke presenting at Duke University Medical Center within 6 h from onset of symptoms. Patients with intracranial hemorrhage (ICH) were excluded. Plasma levels of different biomarkers involved in the ischemic cascade were determined by immunoassay. The primary outcome was the clinical diagnosis of ischemic stroke, defined as focal neurological symptoms of vascular origin persisting for greater than 24 h with compatible imaging studies. Logistic regression was performed on each biomarker, and a 5-variable multiple logistic regression model was generated. In a separate analysis, blood samples were drawn from 68 patients with ischemic stroke and 23 patients with primary ICH presenting within 24 h from onset of symptoms. A 3-variable multiple logistic regression model was generated to differentiate ICH from ischemic stroke.

In the 0- to 6-h time window, 41 patients (32%) were diagnosed with ischemic stroke. Demographic characteristics were similar between stroke and control patients ($P > 0.05$ for age, gender, and ethnicity). The final predictive model for the diagnosis of ischemic stroke included BNP, CRP, D-Dimer, MMP-9, and S100B. This model had a concordance index of 0.81, with a corresponding sensitivity of 81% and a specificity of 70%. The final predictive model to distinguish ICH from ischemic stroke included caspase-3 ($P = 0.005$), monocyte chemoattractant protein-1, and neural cell adhesion molecule. This model had a concordance index of 0.78, with a corresponding sensitivity of 93% and a specificity of 65%.

A panel of biomarkers was able to predict the diagnosis of ischemic stroke with high sensitivity and specificity in patients presenting acutely with neurological symptoms, as well as distinguish ICH from ischemic stroke. These data suggest that such a panel may serve as a useful point-of-care screening test and may also serve as surrogate markers in future neuroprotection trials.

D. T. Laskowitz is a consultant for Biosite, Inc., which also provided funding for this study.

Address for correspondence: D. T. Laskowitz, M.D., Department of Medicine (Neurology), Duke University Medical Center, Durham, NC 27710. Voice: 919-684-0056; fax: 919-684-6514. danl@neuro.duke.edu

Ann. N.Y. Acad. Sci. 1053: 30 (2005). © 2005 New York Academy of Sciences.
doi: 10.1196/annals.1344.051

Evaluating Neuroprotective Agents in Coronary Artery Bypass Surgery

STANTON NEWMAN

Department of Medicine, University College London, London, United Kingdom

Keywords: coronary artery bypass grafting (CABG); neuroprotective agents; surgery; stroke; macroemboli

Coronary artery bypass grafting (CABG) is associated with a small, but important, risk of perioperative stroke of between 1.5% and 5.2% (McKhann *et al.*, 1997). Neurologic complications of cardiac surgery are generally considered to be the result of hemodynamic changes with inadequate brain perfusion or macroembolism. The pathological evidence indicates that strokes are ischemic rather than hypoxic, suggesting that macroemboli are the most important causal agent (Harrison and Newman, 1999).

Neuropsychological (NP)–assessed change from before to after surgery has indicated that a significant proportion of patients have enduring changes in cognitive function (Newman *et al.*, 2000). The cause of these changes appears to be multifactorial, but is related to the occurrence of microemboli during surgery, altered brain blood flow or perfusion pressure, and the systemic inflammatory response. A number of different successful techniques have been introduced to reduce the incidence of NP problems following CABG surgery, such as the use of arterial line filtration (Pugsely *et al.*, 1994) and leukocyte depleting filtration (Whitaker *et al.*, 2004). In addition, pharmacological agents have been used in an attempt to reduce the impact of CABG on the brain (Arrowsmith *et al.*, 1998; Kong *et al.*, 2000).

The use of CABG to examine neuroprotective agents has a number of potential advantages to other approaches in humans. These include before and after NP measurement, relatively small sample sizes and consequent reduced costs, information on the microembolic load of each patient, and a relatively short time course for the study. The design of these studies, however, does require careful planning. This presentation will examine the issues in designing such studies and present the recent research findings on a number of neuroprotective agents in CABG surgery.

Address for correspondence: Professor Stanton Newman, Department of Medicine, University College London, Wolfson Building, 48 Riding House Street, London W1W 7EY, United Kingdom. Voice: +44-20-7679-9468.

s.newman@ucl.ac.uk

Ann. N.Y. Acad. Sci. 1053: 31 (2005). © 2005 New York Academy of Sciences.
doi: 10.1196/annals.1344.052

Questions and Answers

Session I: The Human Experience of Neuroprotection

QUESTIONS FOR STANTON NEWMAN

From William Slikker, Jr.

How do you select the domains for the optimal neuropsychological test?

ANSWER: The selection of domains is first governed by the theoretical considerations of the possible nature of the insult. Essentially, in an area of diffuse cortical damage, the key areas to be assessed should include memory and attention and concentration. There are other issues that govern test selection and these include the sensitivity of the test to detect change, the possibility of repeat assessments (as in this context change scores can be calculated), and the practicalities of performing a test within the clinical constraints of patients attending for cardiac surgery.

From Chia Yi Kuan

Your neuropsychological assessment appears to be very sensitive, which is excellent. Have you compared your neuropsychological assessment with functional MRI in the sensitivity of detecting deficit?

ANSWER: The neuropsychological assessment has been done in parallel with MRI studies where we have found a significant relationship between the likelihood of obtaining a change on the MRI and the evidence of deterioration in cognitive function. To date, we have not compared it with functional MRI.

From Merle Paule

You mentioned two of the tasks that you used to assess cognitive function in your patients (digit symbol substitution and visual pattern recognition/memory). What other tests do you include in your assessment battery and how long does it take to administer?

ANSWER: The range of other areas that we examine include verbal memory, reaction time, perceptuo-motor skills, and other tests of attention and concentration. Overall, we tend to use a battery of 9 or 10 tests that we have found to be sensitive to interventions to reduce the impact of cardiac surgery on the brain.

From Kenneth Maynard

Are neurocognitive tests robust and sensitive to acute neurologic injury (e.g., stroke and brain trauma) as well as chronic neurodegenerative diseases (e.g., AD, PD, ALS, HD) so as to determine neuroprotective effects with drugs? How does one account for natural history of disease course of the cognitive deficit in terms of testing neuroprotective drugs?

Ann. N.Y. Acad. Sci. 1053: 32–38 (2005). © 2005 New York Academy of Sciences.
doi: 10.1196/annals.1344.060

ANSWER: The test selected will differ according to the clinical domain and the nature of the brain damage that one is assessing. Neuropsychological or neurocognitive tests, if selected appropriately, are sensitive to acute and chronic conditions. They have been used to assess the cognitive deterioration of individuals who have neurodegenerative conditions.

A design to examine the impact of a neuroprotective agent in a neurodegenerative condition would be to have a standard placebo randomized control trial. The outcome would be the change in cognitive performance measured over time. The control group should reflect the natural history, and the group receiving the intervention should reflect the impact of the natural history and the potential neuroprotective effects of the agent.

QUESTIONS FOR HARVEY EDMONDS, JR.

From William Slikker, Jr.

What was your best measurement for prediction? Is the method to noninvasively measure brain oxygenation widely available?

ANSWER: In our adult cardiac surgery experience, multimodality neuromonitoring detected cerebral physiologic imbalance in need of correction during 88% of the cases. All but 3% of these imbalances were corrected by simple physiologic adjustments. From a statistical perspective, cerebral oximetry had the highest utility since it identified imbalance in half of the surgeries. EEG signs of inappropriate cortical synaptic depression were observed in one-quarter of the cases, while transcranial Doppler ultrasound detection of flow imbalance or embolization occurred in 13%.

Noninvasive cerebral oximetry was cleared by the FDA in 1996 for use in adults and in 2000 for pediatric applications. The manufacturer states that their product is now used in approximately 20% of adult cardiac surgery centers and 50% of pediatric centers in the United States.

From Russell J. Andrews

Is there a company planning to integrate the neuromonitoring devices you described?

ANSWER: Several manufacturers now provide monitors that incorporate into a single display the output from devices using each of these technologies. The next step is to functionally integrate all three modalities into a single monitor. There are at least two companies developing this capability and they expect to provide multimodality monitors for evaluation within a year.

QUESTIONS FOR KARL SANZENBACHER

From William Slikker, Jr.

With SSEPs, are the measurements quantitative? Are velocity and magnitude useful measurements?

ANSWER: The measurement of somatosensory evoked potentials is quantitative in terms of amplitude and latencies of waveforms. A 10% increase in latency is cause for warning to the surgeon if this cannot be accounted for by other factors. Similarly, a 50% decrease in amplitude of the waveform is also considered a cause for warning, provided these changes cannot be accounted for by technical or physiological factors not related to the surgical intervention.

Amplitudes and even the presence or absence of cortical SSEP potentials are sensitive to anesthetic agents. Subcortical potentials are more resistant to these effects. Latencies also vary with body temperature so that tracking of this is important. With tibial nerve SSEPs, we monitor popliteal nerve potentials at the knees; with median nerve SSEPs, we monitor Erb's point potentials to track some of these factors as well as the adequacy of stimulation.

Motor evoked potentials are even more sensitive to agents used to induce anesthesia. Halogenated gases are taboo in most cases. Some will allow other gases such as nitrous oxide. We prefer a constant intravenous infusion of propofol and a narcotic agent such as remifentanyl to be substituted after induction and intubation. Etomidate has been used by some centers for spine cases, but is not used in aneurysm cases.

Neuromuscular blocking agents are completely avoided if the endpoint for giving a warning is an EMG threshold difference of greater than 100 volts for a particular muscle being monitored. This is the methodology advocated by Calancie *et al.* Deletis and others use an endpoint for warning based on EMG latency and amplitude; changes in amplitude may vary more widely than latency changes. They allow some neuromuscular blockade by monitoring the degree of blockade with a "train-of-four" stimulation getting down to one twitch. They do this in attempting to decrease or prevent patient movement caused by the stimulus train.

Therefore, in addition to tracking the quantitative data of the evoked potentials, it is also important to track blood pressure, heart rate, body temperature, and end-tidal concentrations of gaseous anesthetic agents to make certain that a quantitative change being reported is truly due to the surgical intervention itself.

From Russell J. Andrews

Electrocardiogram machines automatically interpret the EKG: normal vs. abnormal. Has the same been done for SSEPs or MEPs? If anesthetic concentration, etc., were incorporated, automated interpretation might be more rapid and more accurate than subjective interpretation.

ANSWER: Currently, automatic interpretation has not proved to be adequate. One can program into axon and other neurophysiology intraoperative monitoring equipment the accumulated waveforms in a rastered or overlapping display over time. The peak latency and amplitude values can be detected by the program automatically, but they often require manual correction.

Interpretation of EEG can be given by direct observation of the raw EEG data, but also can be done automatically using FFT/spectral analysis, wavelet analysis, and other techniques. These all require someone to look back at the raw data to confirm the absence of artifact and the adequacy of the interpretation. These digital analysis techniques can alert personnel that something may be happening, but are not adequate by themselves.

Some companies have made claims that their equipment can give automated data interpretations with a minimal number of channels. One of the most popular systems is the BIS system, which samples only a minimal number of locations and makes claims to detect anesthetic levels as well as CNS status. I have personally reviewed much of their literature. Most of the data are antidotal and the claims are usually unsubstantiated by control studies. The point of my paper is to point out the different sensitivities of monitoring techniques during intracranial aneurysm surgery, including SSEPs, MEPs, and microvascular Doppler (MVD) studies. Each is of value during phases of this surgery. Each also has drawbacks. Each can give data to warn the surgeon of problems. Altogether, they are more protective than each alone. To overcome the problem that MVD sampling is usually only intermittent and not continuous, we are currently looking into adding multiple microvascular probes. At least one could be fixed on a distal vessel by being threaded down a microsuction unit that is clamped in place and another for free hand use. The first could be used for constant monitoring with an automatic alarm to detect determined threshold changes in flow velocity. This would still require ascertaining that vessel contact and angle were adequate.

In summary, the state of the art has not yet been reached that I would want to be a patient being monitored by an automated system without a trained neurophysiologist being there to constantly observe the data and confirm or negate what the automated system was saying. This may come in the future, but unfortunately is not here yet.

QUESTIONS FOR DANIEL LASKOWITZ

From Merle Paule

Do you have any idea what percentage of penumbral cell death is apoptotic versus necrotic?

ANSWER: The mechanism of cell death following clinical ischemia remains an active source of controversy. It is generally assumed that cells undergo necrotic death in the ischemic core, whereas apoptotic death may play a more important role in the tenuously perfused—but still viable—penumbral area. Certainly, both apoptosis and necrosis contribute to postischemic neuronal death, and often a combination of these two processes may be evident in the same cell. Although there are many reports of apoptotic death of neurons in experimental models of ischemic stroke, few of them display the characteristic morphological features of apoptosis nor DNA laddering [YAMASHIMA, T. 2004. Cell Calcium **36**(3/4): 285–293].

From Kenneth Maynard

Does the panel of markers differentiate between hemorrhagic versus ischemic stroke? Might the panel be used by paramedics to determine immediate course of treatment based upon the type of stroke detected?

ANSWER: The current panel effectively differentiates mimics of stroke from ischemic and hemorrhagic stroke. The sensitivity of this test is slightly higher in detecting hemorrhagic stroke from this high-risk mimic population (patients presenting to the Emergency Department with the acute onset of neurological deficit). However, our current panel not been optimized to differentiate hemorrhagic from ischemic stroke. This may be theoretically possible in the future, though, as systemic elevation of markers such as MMP-9 has been associated with hemorrhagic transformation (ROSENBERG, G.A. *et al.* 1998. Stroke **29:** 2189–2195). A combination approach may also be effective at discriminating ischemic from hemorrhagic stroke, and we have presented data at the 2004 International Stroke Conference demonstrating that a panel of three biomarkers, including caspase-3, MCP-1, and VEGF, could discriminate hemorrhagic from ischemic stroke with a sensitivity of 93%.

As a practical matter, however, an unenhanced CT scan is readily available in a timely fashion at most institutions and is more sensitive than a biomarker approach at detecting intracranial hemorrhage. Given the risk of potentially fatal bleeding if a patient with intracranial hemorrhage is treated inappropriately with a thrombolytic such as tissue plasminogen activator (tPA), CT will probably remain the standard of care prior to treatment with tPA. It is reasonable to speculate that a noninvasive test may ultimately play an important role in screening patients with suspected stroke in the prehospital setting. Such a test may also ultimately play an important role in deciding whether to initiate a therapeutic intervention not associated with bleeding risk, such as neuroprotective strategies currently under development.

From William Slikker, Jr.

What is the evidence for blood-brain barrier (BBB) opening with acute stroke? Does it occur 100% of the time? Does caspase-3, when activated, always indicate neuronal cell death?

ANSWER: There is strong experimental and clinical evidence suggesting that the BBB is breached following focal stroke, although the time course has not been well defined [KUROIWA, T. *et al.* 1985. Acta Neuropathol. **68:** 122–129; LATOUR, L.L. *et al.* 2004. Ann. Neurol. **56**(4)**:** 468–477]. Although we were able to detect biochemical markers associated with brain injury in the peripheral circulation within 3 h of ischemia, it is not certain that these markers originated within the CNS. It is certainly possible, for example, that elevation of acute inflammatory markers such as D-dimer or interleukin-6 originated in the periphery in response to CNS insult.

From Naren Banik

Does the intracellular calcium level increase in the penumbra? Have you looked at calpain activity and expression, or would you expect to see any increase since calpain is know to cause cell death in ischemia and spinal cord injury?

ANSWER: Calpain, a calcium-dependent cysteine protease is an interesting target in neurological disease, and has been associated with brain ischemia and reperfusion in experimental models [YAMASHIMA, T. *et al.* 2003. Hippocampus **13**(7)**:** 791–800]. There is also recent evidence that calpain is present in the cerebrospinal fluid following rodent MCA occlusion [PIKE, B.R. *et al.* 2004. J. Cereb. Blood Flow Metab. **24**(1)**:** 98–106], and calpain inhibition is being investigated as a therapeutic target. However, we have not yet evaluated calpain in the peripheral blood following ischemic stroke.

From Chia Yi Kuan

Your rationale seems to be that brain neuronal injury markers can be detected in the blood if there is damage to the BBB. How fast does the BBB breakdown occur after ischemic stroke? If the BBB damage occurs late, how do you explain that you can detect early changes in the peripheral blood?

ANSWER: The BBB is variably affected after the onset of focal ischemia, although the exact time course has not been defined. In animal models of focal ischemia/reperfusion, breach of the BBB is a consistent finding (KUROIWA, T. *et al.* 1985. Acta Neuropathol. **68:** 122–129). Recent clinical data suggest that significant disruption of the BBB occurs in approximately one-third of patients assessed acutely after stroke, with a median latency estimated to be less than 4 h after symptom onset. Time to reperfusion was an important predictor of BBB disruption [LATOUR, L.L. *et al.* 2004. Ann. Neurol. **56**(4)**:** 468–477]. Several of the markers that we are evaluating, such as MMP-9, have previously been associated with opening of the BBB and subsequent hemorrhagic transformation (ROSENBERG, G.A. *et al.* 1998. Stroke **29:** 2189–2195).

In addition to the extent of BBB compromise. there are many factors that influence whether a biochemical marker of brain injury can be detected in the peripheral circulation acutely after the onset of cerebral ischemia. For example, the size and lipophilicity of the marker may affect passage from the CNS into the systemic circulation. In our study, we were able to identify biochemical markers of brain injury in the peripheral circulation within the first 3 h of ischemia. Although our results suggest that biochemical markers of injury are released from the CNS compartment, perhaps facilitated by breach of the BBB, we cannot rule out the possibility that these markers originated outside the CNS, where they were secondarily upregulated in response to CNS injury.

QUESTION FOR RUSSELL J. ANDREWS

From Xiaoyang Qi

I am very interested in your presentation about the bioluminal sensor: (1) Does the sensor measure O_2 level in the intracellular or intercellular region? (2) Does the sensor measure pH value?

ANSWER: The BioLuminate probe as presently configured uses optical spectroscopy and electrical impedance microsensors. It does not measure O_2 directly nor pH, but there are sensors for measuring either O_2 or pH. Such sensors could certainly be added to the spectroscopy and impedance sensors if desired for a specific application.

QUESTIONS FOR RON HERNING

From Karl Sanzenbacher

My recall is that some of the patients with sudden death had little or no pathology at autopsy. My guess would be that the patients had seizures with autonomic features resulting in cardiac standstill or arrest.

ANSWER: In terms of the case histories of MDMA-associated death, the causes have included hyperthermia, hyponatremia, seizures, hepatitis, cerebrovascular accidents, and arrhythmias. There does not seem to be a single cause of death, but certainly you are right in the case of seizures.

From Ashraf Virmani

There are sudden deaths associated with MDMA use. What is the underlying mechanism for this?

ANSWER: Rhabdomyolysis involving the myocardium is thought to be responsible for sudden death in cases of acute MDMA toxicity (GESI, M. *et al.* 2002. Pharmacol. Toxicol. **91:** 29–33).

Delineating and Understanding Cerebellar Neuroprotective Pathways

Potential Implication for Protecting the Cortex

XUAN WU,[a] XUEYING JIANG,[a] ANN M. MARINI,[a] AND ROBERT H. LIPSKY[b]

[a]*Department of Neurology, Uniformed Services University of the Health Sciences, Bethesda, Maryland 20814, USA*

[b]*Section on Molecular Genetics, Laboratory of Neurogenetics, National Institute on Alcohol Abuse and Alcoholism, National Institutes of Health, Rockville, Maryland 20892, USA*

ABSTRACT: The cerebellum is a brain region that is resistant to many of the neurodegenerative disorders such as stroke and Alzheimer's disease. In contrast, the neocortex (cerebrum, cerebral cortex) is vulnerable to these disorders. While there may be many reasons for the differences in vulnerability to acute and chronic neurodegenerative disorders, the cerebellum appears to be equipped with the tools necessary to protect itself against these types of insults. Over the last century, evidence has accumulated to suggest that the cerebellum is also involved in memory and higher cognitive function. We have discovered that intrinsic survival pathways exist in cerebellar granule cells that are regulated by low level stimulation of *N*-methyl-D-aspartate (NMDA) receptors. Activation of NMDA receptors protects vulnerable neurons against glutamate-mediated excitotoxicity acting on NMDA receptors. This report focuses on how modulation of neuronal survival by NMDA receptors through a brain-derived neurotrophic factor (BDNF)–mediated pathway may be incorporated into a network of cerebellar function, particularly in light of recent findings suggesting that the cerebellum plays a vital role in learning, memory, fear conditioning, and cognitive processing.

KEYWORDS: NMDA receptors; cultured neurons; cognition; NF-κB; neuroprotection; ERK 1/2

INTRODUCTION

The cerebellum has traditionally been regarded as a structure that coordinates voluntary movement. Literature dating back to the nineteenth century suggests that the cerebellum plays a much more fundamental role. Clinical reports of mental retardation, low intelligence, impaired intellect, and mild cognitive impairment

Address for correspondence: Robert H. Lipsky, Ph.D., Chief, Unit on Molecular Genetics, Laboratory of Neurogenetics, National Institute on Alcohol Abuse and Alcoholism, National Institutes of Health, 5625 Fishers Lane, Room 3S32, MSC 9412, Bethesda, MD 20892. Voice: 301-402-5591; fax: 301-480-2839.
rlipsky@mail.nih.gov

Ann. N.Y. Acad. Sci. 1053: 39–47 (2005). © 2005 New York Academy of Sciences.
doi: 10.1196/annals.1344.004

describe various cerebellar lesions.[1] Neuropsychiatric symptoms including dementia, schizophrenia, and manic depression have been associated with cerebellar agenesis.[1]

The cerebellum exhibits a unique form of synaptic plasticity termed long-term depression (LTD). It is known that Purkinje cells receive two distinct excitatory inputs: climbing fibers that come from the inferior olive in the brain stem and granule cell axons that relay information from the mossy fibers, which are also located in the brain stem. Purkinje cells constitute the sole inhibitory output from the cerebellar cortex.[2,3] The arrangement of several granule cell axons and a single climbing fiber to a single Purkinje cell is a characteristic and distinct feature of cerebellar neuronal circuitry.[4] It was Albus,[5] an electrical engineer, who viewed the cerebellum as a "learning pattern recognition system", along with complementary work of David Marr.[6] These investigators put together a cogent theory of cerebellar function based upon a conjunction of presynaptic and postsynaptic excitatory input, but it was Albus[5] who suggested that the conjunction results in a depression and not a potentiation. Thus, LTD is induced at the granule cell axon–Purkinje cell synapse.

PARALLEL FIBERS OF CEREBELLAR GRANULE CELLS REVISITED

The anatomical features of the cerebellar cortex consist of Purkinje cells (PCs), which are in turn activated by granule cells through the parallel fibers; granule cells exert excitatory influences on many PCs.[7] As the parallel fibers extend along the cerebellar cortex perpendicular to the long axis, they synapse on the PC dendritic tree to elicit a response from the PC. This concept has been challenged. Recent data suggest that stimulating granule cell axons below the cortex results in localized activation of cortex in the immediate surrounding area.[8] Thus, mossy fiber activity produces localized responses in the cerebellar cortex; the parallel fiber organization increases responsiveness at a distant area as opposed to spreading the information throughout their path.[8]

ANATOMICAL RELATIONSHIPS BETWEEN THE CEREBELLUM AND THE CORTEX

The cerebellum is robustly interconnected with the contralateral cerebral hemispheres in a bidirectional manner. The cerebrocerebellar circuit consists of the feedforward or afferent limb and the feedback or efferent limb.[9] Information from various cortical association areas is carried from the cerebral cortex to neurons in the pons, which is located in the brain stem. Pontine axons transmit the information from the cortex to the opposite cerebellar cortex. The feedback circuit comprises the cerebellar cortex, which makes connections with the deep cerebellar nuclei. Axons from the deep cerebellar nuclei travel to the red nucleus in the midbrain and then to the opposite thalamus. The thalamus feeds back to the same side of the cortex to complete the circuit.[9] The association areas of the cerebral cortex are known to be areas where integrative processing takes place. Knowledge and other cognitive functions can be stored in various locations across multiple cortical and subcortical locations, and specific sites of information may act as neural hubs that allow access to the network of locations that store the information.[10] Evidence has accumulated to suggest that the cerebellum is connected to these higher cognition areas through the cerebrocerebellar circuit.[1,9]

Connections between the cerebellum and the limbic system also exist. Electrical stimulation of the cerebellum resulted in responses in the hippocampus and amygdala,[11] a brain structure known to consolidate emotional memory.[12] A recent report indicates that the cerebellum itself is crucial for consolidating memories for tone and contextual fear conditioning and does so several days longer than the basolateral amygdala.[13] Thus, anatomical and physiological studies of the cerebellum and its strong connections to the opposite cerebral cortex and limbic structures have set the stage for the cogent hypothesis that the cerebellum plays a role in cognitive and behavioral processes.

The cerebellum contains more than half of all the neurons in the brain.[14] Cortical association areas and the prefrontal cortex are connected to the cerebellum through the pons, and the cerebellum connects to various higher cortical function areas from the deep cerebellar nuclei via the red nucleus and thalamus. Because there are many more afferents that project to the cerebellum compared to efferents, it is possible that the cerebellum serves as an integrative structure.[15]

CEREBELLAR LESIONS AND COGNITIVE DYSFUNCTION

Mental deficiency was found in a family with cerebellar degeneration, and neuropathological analysis demonstrated loss of granule cells with some involvement of the PCs and inferior olives, whereas the remainder of the brain appeared normal.[16] About one-third of patients with olivopontocerebellar degeneration were found to have deficiencies in verbal and nonverbal intelligence, memory, and frontal lobe function; these deficits were directly correlated with their cerebellar ataxia symptoms.[17] A significant number of patients with ataxia-telangiectasia were shown to exhibit below-normal mental capacity without cerebral abnormalities.[18,19] In a recent study, patients with cerebellar lesions on either the right or left side exhibited impairment in executive function, working memory, and attention.[15] Interestingly, right-sided cerebellar lesions caused more verbal impairment than left-sided lesions. Since the feedback loop from the cerebellum projects to the opposite cerebral cortex, then right-sided cerebellar lesions would affect the left side of the cortex, the dominant hemisphere for language and thus verbal fluency in most people. Evidence supporting a role of the cerebellum in language and cognition in children[20] and impaired water maze learning[21] has also been documented. Recently, 20 patients with only cerebellar lesions were found to have difficulties with executive function, including problems with working memory, impaired visual-spatial memory, personality changes, and language difficulties, and this syndrome is now referred to as the cerebellar cognitive affective syndrome (CCAS).[22]

CEREBELLAR GRANULE CELLS AND NEUROPROTECTION

Glutamate is the endogenous excitatory amino acid in brain that is responsible for normal physiological excitatory neurotransmission. Glutamate is also involved in the pathophysiology of hypoxic-ischemic neuronal injury.[23–25] The *N*-methyl-D-aspartate (NMDA) receptor is thought to play a major role in this neuropathological progess. In addition, NMDA receptors mediate adaptive responses important for synaptic plasticity.[26,27] The mechanisms that differentiate these opposing effects remain largely unclear. Cerebellar granule cells are relatively homogeneous in culture and express all of the glutamate receptor subtypes, including the NMDA receptor. Excitotoxic concentrations of glutamate kill cerebellar granule cells through an NMDA receptor–mediated mechanism.[28] In addition to exerting neuronal cell death, low-level stimulation of NMDA receptors protects against hypoglycemic culture conditions[29] and NMDA receptor–mediated excitotoxicity.[30] NMDA receptors have a voltage-gated calcium channel that is physiologically blocked by magnesium.[31] In cerebellar granule cells, pretreatment with a neuroprotective concentration of NMDA followed by an excitotoxic concentration of glutamate was not associated with a change in the intracellular calcium level compared with an excitotoxic concentration of glutamate alone.[32]

Increases in intracellular calcium result in complex responses in neurons. Activation of signaling pathways such as cAMP response element binding protein (CREB), extracellular signal–regulated kinase (ERK), and direct calcium/calmodulin actions are known to occur in neurons. NMDA receptor activation activates calcium/calmodulin-dependent kinase II [CaM KII],[33] calcium/calmodulin IV,[34] and calcineurin.[35] CaM KII interacts with NR2B, a subunit of the NMDA receptor,[36] and is involved in memory, a form of synaptic plasticity.[37] Because NMDA receptors mediate plastic responses and activate CaM KII, we tested whether a neuroprotective concentration of NMDA (100 μM) increases activated (phosphorylated) CaM KII in cultured rat cerebellar neurons. Preliminary results suggest that NMDA increases activated CaM KII within 20 min (FIG. 1). Binding of the calcium/calmodulin complex to the subunits of CaM KII activates the enzyme by displacing an autoinhibitory domain from the active site of the enzyme phosphorylation of Thr[286] and is required for long-term potentiation.[38] CaM KII has also been implicated in LTD.[39] Calmodulin activates the Ras pathway and by so doing affects the activity of the mitogen-activated protein kinase (MAPK) pathway.[40] The MAPK cascade is also involved in synaptic

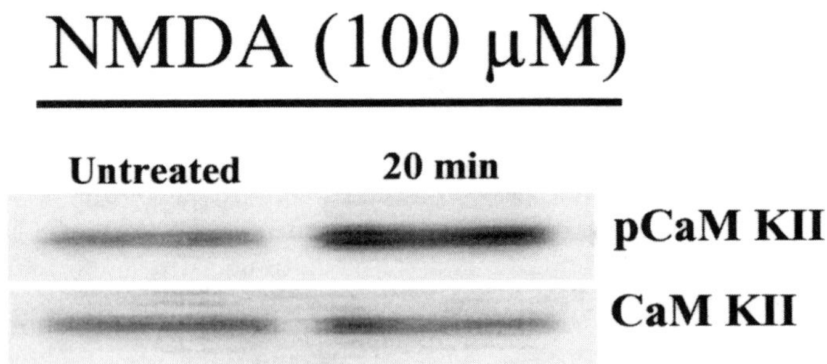

FIGURE 1. A maximum neuroprotective concentration of NMDA increases phosphorylated CaM KII in cultured cerebellar granule cells. Cultured cerebellar granule cells were treated with a maximum neuroprotective concentration of NMDA (100 μM) for 20 min. Cell lysates were prepared and the proteins were resolved by gel electrophoresis.[53] After transfer of the proteins to nitrocellulose, the blot was probed with a CaM KII phospho-specific antibody that recognizes phospho-Tyr[286] (Cell Signaling, Beverly, MA).

plasticity.[41] We have also shown that the ERK 1/2 pathway, a subclass of the MAPK cascade, is required for NMDA to mediate its neuroprotective effect.[42] Taken together, these results suggest that activation of calcium-mediated signaling pathways by a neuroprotective concentration of NMDA may provide the substrate to not only promote survival, but to mediate plastic responses in the cerebellum. Thus, the mossy fiber–granule cell axon–PC synapse may be the network where these pathways may play an important role in mediating synaptic plasticity in the cerebellum. NMDA receptor activation of these same pathways either directly or indirectly, that is, through brain-derived neurotrophic factor (BDNF) release, may also be involved in the contribution of the cerebellum to the neural networks that are involved in cognition and/or plasticity. Thus, "movement is intricately bound with sensation, and with intellectual and emotional growth".[43]

There are other molecules that are involved in similar neuronal responses. Survival and plastic responses of neurons are greatly affected by the availability of growth factors, particularly the neurotrophins. BDNF is a member of the neurotrophin family that functions in long-term potentiation (LTP) presynaptically[44] and postsynaptically[45] and in the maintenance of high-frequency stimulation-induced LTP in the adult rat brain.[46] We have shown previously that a neuroprotective concentration of NMDA increases BDNF mRNA levels.[47] We now show that activation of NMDA receptors increases exon 4–specific BDNF mRNA in a time-dependent

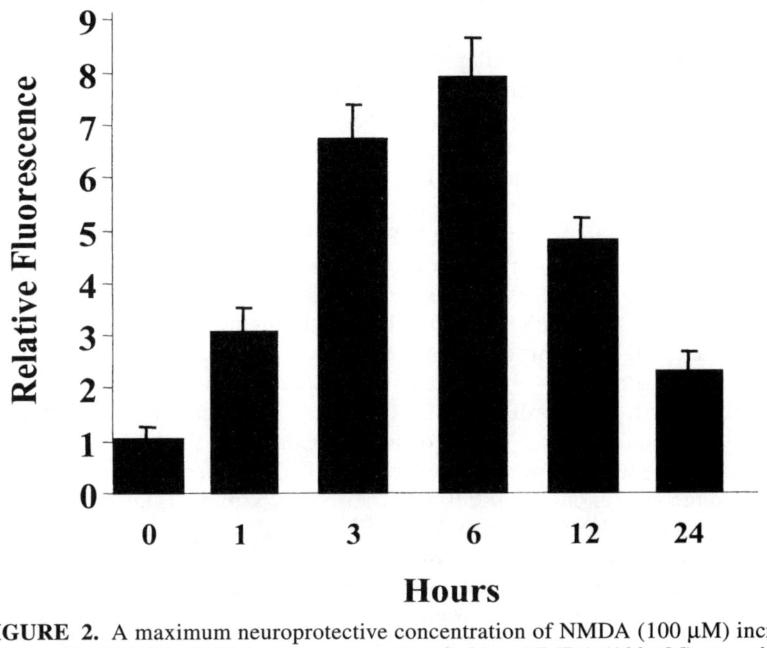

FIGURE 2. A maximum neuroprotective concentration of NMDA (100 μM) increases exon 4–specific BDNF mRNA in a time-dependent fashion. NMDA (100 μM) was added to cultured rat cerebellar granule cells *in vitro* at various times at 8 days after seeding. At the indicated time, the cells were disrupted and total RNA isolated and purified. Exon 4–specific BDNF mRNA was determined by the 5′ nuclease assay.[53]

manner in cultured rat cerebellar granule cells (FIG. 2). We discovered a nuclear factor kappa-B (NF-κB) binding site in the 5′ flanking region of exon 4 of the *bdnf* gene and showed that NF-κB plays an important role in NMDA receptor–mediated neuroprotection.[48] How do these results compare with neurons derived from the cortex, a brain region highly vulnerable to neurodegeneration in acute and chronic neurodegenerative disorders?

We determined the role of physiological preconditioning with NMDA in hippocampal neurons cultured from embryonic day 20 fetuses. We find that low-level stimulation of NMDA receptors can protect up to 40% of the neurons that would otherwise die from an excitotoxic concentration of glutamate acting on NMDA receptors. Moreover, the immediate release and later synthesis of BDNF plays a major role in NMDA neuroprotection.[49] Thus, neurons from an early stage of development from a cortical brain region have the identical mechanism of neuroprotection as the cerebellum.[49] Interestingly, a neuroprotective concentration of NMDA increases activated NF-κB and cAMP response element binding protein (CREB) (data not shown) in cultured hippocampal neurons. Whether NMDA neuroprotection requires both of these transcription factors is currently under investigation.

Currently, we do not understand why the cerebellum is more resistant than the cortex to acute and chronic neurodegenerative disorders. However, results from our laboratory as well as others suggest that physiological preconditioning with glutamate or NMDA protects neurons against excitotoxicity by a BDNF-dependent mechanism. Acute and chronic neurodegenerative disorders involve glutamate excitotoxicity. We propose that developing innovative strategies to stimulate inotropic glutamate receptors to maintain and sustain intracellular survival pathways may pave the way toward protecting the brain against the devastating neurological disability associated with acute and chronic neurodegenerative disorders.

In summary, low-level NMDA receptor activation results in the influx of calcium leading to the activation of CREB, NF-κB, and ERK 1/2. Activation of calcium-mediated signal transduction pathways results in the activation of NF-κB through the phosphorylation of I-κB; phosphorylation of I-κB destines the molecule for ubiquination and degradation via the 26S proteosome. In addition to the intracellular signal cascade and activation of the transcription factors, NMDA receptor activation evokes the release of BDNF, which in turn binds to and activates TrkB receptors. A later increase in BDNF mRNA occurs in part through binding of activated CREB (pCREB) and NF-κB to promoter binding sites. These coordinated actions protect neurons against glutamate-mediated excitotoxicity in cerebellar granule cells through ERK 1/2, NF-κB, and possibly CaM KII (FIG. 3). It is unknown whether CaM KII activation is required for NMDA to protect neurons against glutamate-mediated excitotoxicity or whether increases in activated ERK 1/2 are required for NF-κB activation to increase exon-specific BDNF transcripts. While it is known that activated CREB increases BDNF transcription,[50–52] its role is NMDA neuroprotection is unclear. Also unknown is the role of other neuroprotective molecules that NMDA may activate, evoke the release of, or alter their synthesis. Further delineation of the pathways involved in NMDA neuroprotection may lead to the development of novel strategies to prevent neurodegenerative disorders. Moreover, because NMDA neuroprotection is a phenomenon that was discovered under physiological conditions, understanding these mechanisms may also provide insight into why millimolar concentrations of glutamate in the synaptic cleft do not kill neurons *in vivo*.

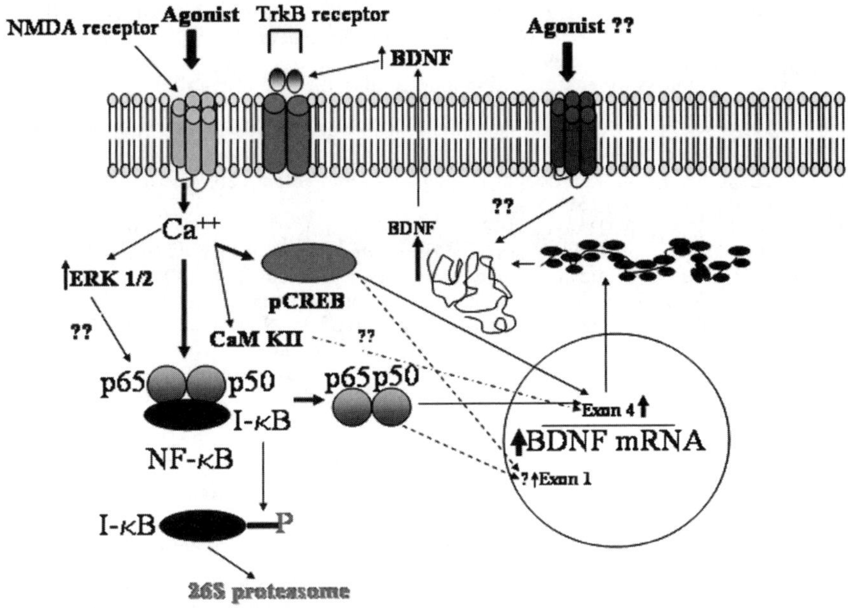

FIGURE 3. Current overview of intracellular events that may be involved in NMDA neuroprotection. Activation of NMDA receptors results in the influx of calcium, which leads to the activation of ERK 1/2, CREB, CaM KII, and NF-κB. Activated NF-κB and CREB bind to sequences in DNA to regulate BDNF transcription. The possible role of other neuroprotective molecules is indicated ("Agonist??"). Possible interactions or effects are indicated with question marks and/or dashed arrows.

ACKNOWLEDGMENTS

This work was funded by Intramural Research Grant No. Z01-AA00325 from the National Institute on Alcohol Abuse and Alcoholism, NIH (to R. H. Lipsky); and by Grant Nos. F292BU, Defense Brain and Spinal Cord Injury Program (DBSCIP), Department of Defense, and HO92BI, USUHS (to A. M. Marini).

REFERENCES

1. SCHMAHMANN, J.D. & D.A. PANDYA. 1997. The cerebrocerebellar system. *In* The Cerebellum and Cognition. Vol. 41, pp. 31–60. Academic Press. San Diego.
2. ITO, M. & M. YOSHIDA. 1964. The cerebellar-evoked monosynaptic inhibition of Deiters' neurons. Experientia **20:** 515–516.
3. ITO, M. & M. YOSHIDA. 1966. The origin of cerebellar-induced inhibition of Deiters' neurons: monosynaptic initiation of the inhibitory postsynaptic potentials. Exp. Brain Res. **2:** 330–349.
4. PALAY, S.L. & V. CHAN-PALAY. 1974. The Cerebellar Cortex. Springer-Verlag. New York/Berlin.
5. ALBUS, J.S. 1971. A theory of cerebellar function. Math. Biosci. **10:** 25–61.
6. MARR, D. 1969. A theory of cerebellar cortex. J. Physiol. (Lond.) **202:** 437–470.

7. ECCLES, J.C., M. ITO & J. SZENTAGOTHAI. 1967. The Cerebellum as a Neuronal Machine. Springer-Verlag. New York/Berlin/Heidelberg.
8. COHEN, D. & Y. YAROM. 1998. Patches of synchronized activity in the cerebellar cortex evoked by mossy-fiber stimulation: questioning the role of parallel fibers. Proc. Natl. Acad. Sci. USA **95:** 15032–15036.
9. SCHMAHMANN, J.D. 1991. An emerging concept: the cerebellar contribution to higher function. Arch. Neurol. **48:** 1178–1187.
10. MESULAM, M. 1994. Neurocognitive networks and selectively distributed processing. Rev. Neurol. (Paris) **150:** 564–569.
11. HEATH, R.G. & J.W. HARPER. 1974. Ascending projections of the cerebellar fastigial nucleus to the hippocampus amygdala and other temporal lobe sites: evoked potential and histological studies in monkeys and cats. Exp. Neurol. **45:** 2482–2487.
12. FANSELOW, M.S. & J.E. LEDOUX. 1999. Why we think plasticity underlying Pavlovian fear conditioning occurs in the basolateral amygdala. Neuron **23:** 229–232.
13. SACCHETTI, B., E. BALDI, C.A. LORENZINI & C. BUCHERELLI. 2002. Cerebellar role in fear-conditioning consolidation. Proc. Natl. Acad. Sci. USA **99:** 8406–8411.
14. RAPOPORT, M., R. VAN REEKUM & H. MAYBERG. 2000. The role of the cerebellum in cognition and behavior: a selective review. J. Neuropsychiatry Clin. Neurosci. **12:** 193–198.
15. GOTTWALD, B., B. WILDE, Z. MIHAJLOVIC & H.M. MEHDORN. 2004. Evidence for distinct cognitive deficits after focal cerebellar lesions. J. Neurol. Neurosurg. Psychiatry **75:** 1524–1531.
16. JERVIS, G.A. 1950. Early familial cerebellar degeneration. J. Nerv. Ment. Dis. **111:** 398–407.
17. LANDIS, D.M., R.N. ROSENBERG, S.C. LANDIS *et al.* 1974. Olivopontocerebellar degeneration: clinical and ultrastructural abnormalities. Arch. Neurol. **31:** 295–307.
18. MCFARLIN, D.E., W. STROBER & T.A. WALDMAN. 1972. Ataxia-telangiectasia. Medicine **51:** 281–314.
19. AGUILAR, M.J., S. KAMOSHITA, B.H. LANDING *et al.* 1968. Pathological observations in ataxia-telangiectasia: a report of five cases. J. Neuropathol. Exp. Neurol. **27:** 659–676.
20. VANDEINSE, D. & J.E. HORNYAK. 1997. Linguistic and cognitive deficits associated with cerebellar mutism. Pediatr. Rehabil. **1:** 41–44.
21. LALONDE, R. & C. STRAZIELLE. 2003. The effects of cerebellar damage on maze learning in animals. Cerebellum **2:** 300–309.
22. SCHMAHMANN, J.D. 2004. Disorders of the cerebellum: ataxia, dysmetria of thought, and the cerebellar cognitive affective syndrome. Neuropsychiatric Practice Opin. **16:** 367–378.
23. OLNEY, J.W., O.L. HO & V. RHEE. 1971. Cytotoxic effects of acidic and sulphur containing amino acids on the infant mouse central nervous system. Exp. Brain Res. **14:** 61–76.
24. CHOI, D.W. 1988. Glutamate neurotoxicity and diseases of the nervous system. Neuron **1:** 623–634.
25. MATTSON, M.P. 2003. Excitotoxic and excitoprotective mechanisms: abundant targets for the prevention and treatment of neurodegenerative disorders. Neuromol. Med. **3:** 65–94.
26. GHOSH, A. & M.E. GREENBERG. 1995. Calcium signaling in neurons: molecular mechanisms and cellular consequences. Science **268:** 239–247.
27. KATZ, L.C. & C.J. SHATZ. 1996. Synaptic activity and the construction of cortical circuits. Science **274:** 1133–1138.
28. NOVELLI, A., J.A. REILLY, P.G. LYSKO & R.C. HENNEBERRY. 1988. Glutamate becomes neurotoxic via the *N*-methyl-D-aspartate receptor when intracellular energy levels are reduced. Brain Res. **451:** 205–212.
29. MARINI, A.M. & A. NOVELLI. 1991. The glutamate uptake blocker DL-threo-3-hydroxy-aspartate reduces NMDA receptor activation by glutamate in cultured neurons. Eur. J. Pharmacol. **194:** 131–132.
30. MARINI, A.M. & S.M. PAUL. 1992. *N*-Methyl-D-aspartate receptor–mediated neuroprotection in cerebellar granule cells requires new RNA and protein synthesis. Proc. Natl. Acad. Sci. USA **89:** 6555–6559.

31. MacDermott, A.B., M.L. Mayer, G.L. Westbrook *et al.* 1986. NMDA-receptor activation increases cytoplasmic calcium concentration in cultured spinal cord neurones. Nature **321:** 519–522.
32. Marini, A.M., Y. Ueda & C.H. June. 1999. Intracellular survival pathways against glutamate receptor agonist excitotoxicity in cultured neurons: intracellular calcium responses. Ann. N.Y. Acad. Sci. **890:** 421–437.
33. Shen, K. & T. Meyer. 1999. Dynamic control of CaMKII translocation and localization in hippocampal neurons by NMDA receptor stimulation. Science **284:** 162–166.
34. Deisseroth, K., E.K. Heist & R.W. Tsien. 1998. Translocation of calmodulin to the nucleus supports CREB phosphorylation in hippocampal neurons. Nature **392:** 198–202.
35. Mulkey, R.M., S. Endo, S. Shenolikar & R.C. Malenka. 1994. Involvement of a calcineurin/inhibitor-1 phosphatase cascade in hippocampal long-term depression. Nature **369:** 486–488.
36. Bayer, K-U., P. De Konlock, A.S. Leonard *et al.* 2001. Interaction with the NMDA receptor locks CaMKII in an active conformation. Nature **411:** 801–805.
37. Limback-Stokin, K., E. Korzus, R. Nagaoka-Yasuda & M. Mayford. 2004. Nuclear calcium/calmodulin regulates memory consolidation. J. Neurosci. **24:** 10858–10867.
38. Giese, K.P., N.B. Fedorov, R.K. Filipkowski & A.J. Silva. 1998. Autophosphorylation at Thr286 of the alpha calcium-calmodulin kinase II in LTP and learning. Science **279:** 870–873.
39. Stevens, C.F., S. Tonegawa & Y. Wang. 1994. The role of calcium-calmodulin kinase II in three forms of synaptic plasticity. Curr. Biol. **4:** 687–693.
40. Gawler, D.J. 1998. Points of convergence between Ca2+ and Ras signaling pathways. Biochim. Biophys. Acta **1448:** 171–182.
41. Sweatt, J.D. 2004. Mitogen-activated protein kinases in synaptic plasticity and memory. Curr. Opin. Neurobiol. **14:** 311–317.
42. Zhu, D., X. Wu, K.I. Strauss *et al.* 2005. *N*-Methyl-D-aspartate and TrkB receptors protect neurons against glutamate excitotoxicity through an extracellular signal–regulated kinase pathway. J. Neurosci. Res. **80:** 104–113.
43. Schmahmann, J.D. 2004. The cerebellum and cognition. Education Program Syllabus. American Academy of Neurology Fifty-sixth Annual Meeting (April 24 – May 1, 2004).
44. Xu, B., W. Gottschalk, A. Chow *et al.* 2000. The role of brain-derived neurotrophic factor receptors in the mature hippocampus: modulation of long-term potentiation through a presynaptic mechanism involving TrkB. J. Neurosci. **20:** 6888–6897.
45. Kovalchuk, Y., E. Hanse, K.W. Kafitz & A. Konnerth. 2002. Postsynaptic induction of BDNF-mediated long-term potentiation. Science **295:** 1729–1734.
46. Messaoudi, E., S.W. Ying, T. Kanhema *et al.* 2002. Brain-derived neurotrophic factor triggers transcription-dependent, late phase long-term potentiation *in vivo*. J. Neurosci. **22:** 7453–7461.
47. Marini, A.M., S.J. Rabin, R.H. Lipsky & I. Mocchetti. 1998. Activity-dependent release of brain-derived neurotrophic factor underlies the neuroprotective effect of *N*-methyl-D-aspartate. J. Biol. Chem. **273:** 29394–29399.
48. Lipsky, R.H., K. Xu, D. Zhu *et al.* 2001. NF-κB is a critical determinant for NMDA receptor–mediated neuroprotection. J. Neurochem. **78:** 254–264.
49. Jiang, X., F. Tian, K.M. Mearow *et al.* 2005. The excitoprotective effect of *N*-methyl-D-aspartate receptors is mediated by a BDNF autocrine loop. J. Neurochem. In press.
50. Finkbeiner, S., S.F. Tavazoie, A. Maloratsky *et al.* 1997. CREB: a major mediator of neuronal neurotrophin responses. Neuron **19:** 1031–1047.
51. Tao, X., S. Finkbeiner, D.B. Arnold *et al.* 1998. Ca2+ influx regulates BDNF transcription by a CREB family transcription factor–dependent mechanism. Neuron **20:** 709–726.
52. West, A.E., W.G. Chen, M.B. Dalva *et al.* 2001. Calcium regulation of neuronal gene expression. Proc. Natl. Acad. Sci. USA **98:** 11024–11031.
53. Wu, X., D. Zhu, X. Jiang *et al.* 2004. AMPA protects cultured neurons against glutamate excitotoxicity through a phosphatidylinositol 3-kinase–dependent activation in extracellular signal–regulated kinase to upregulate BDNF gene expression. J. Neurochem. **90:** 807–818.

A Role for Calpain in Optic Neuritis

M. KELLY GUYTON,[a] ERIC A. SRIBNICK,[b] SWAPAN K. RAY,[b]
AND NAREN L. BANIK[b]

Departments of [a]Microbiology/Immunology and [b]Neuroscience/Neurology, Medical University of South Carolina, Charleston, South Carolina 29425, USA

ABSTRACT: Optic neuritis (ON) is one of the most commonly presenting symptoms of multiple sclerosis (MS), which is a neurodegenerative disease of the central nervous system (CNS) thought to be caused by an attack on myelin by autoreactive T cells and other immune cells. Experimental autoimmune encephalomyelitis (EAE) is a widely used model for MS and ON, which are characterized by demyelination, axonal damage, and neuronal death. The mechanisms of neurodegeneration are unclear; however, the calcium (Ca^{2+})–dependent neutral protease calpain is thought to be involved. The focus of this article is to summarize the evidence suggesting that calpain plays a role in the development of EAE-ON in Lewis rats.

KEYWORDS: calpain; optic neuritis (ON); multiple sclerosis (MS); experimental autoimmune encephalomyelitis (EAE)

INTRODUCTION

Multiple sclerosis (MS) is an autoimmune, demyelinating disease of the central nervous system (CNS) resulting in myelin breakdown, axonal damage, and death of neurons and glial cells. MS is thought to occur due to an attack by myelin-specific T cells and other immune cells on the myelin sheath affecting the brain, spinal cord, and optic nerve, with clinical symptoms of fatigue, paralysis, and vision loss.[1] In fact, optic neuritis (ON), an inflammation of the optic nerve, is one of the most commonly presented symptoms of MS, resulting in vision impairment.[2] MS patients demonstrate a decrease in both visual-evoked potentials (VEPs) and electroretinogram (ERG) recordings, indicating that both the optic nerve and the retina are affected.[3] The mechanisms leading to axonal damage and cell death in autoimmune ON are unclear; however, investigations in our laboratory and others have suggested that the calcium (Ca^{2+})–dependent protease calpain may play an important role.

EXPERIMENTAL ON IN EAE

Experimental autoimmune encephalomyelitis (EAE) is an animal model commonly used for studying the pathophysiology of MS and ON (EAE-ON). EAE can

Address for correspondence: Naren L. Banik, Ph.D., Department of Neurology, Medical University of South Carolina, 96 Jonathan Lucus Street, Charleston, SC 29425. Voice: 843-792-7605; fax: 843-792-8626.
baniknl@musc.edu

Ann. N.Y. Acad. Sci. 1053: 48–54 (2005). © 2005 New York Academy of Sciences.
doi: 10.1196/annals.1344.005

be induced in rodents by administering spinal cord homogenate and myelin proteins, including myelin basic protein (MBP), myelin oligodendrocyte protein (MOG), and proteolipid protein (PLP), or by adoptive transfer of MBP-specific T cells to generate a relapsing/remitting model of MS.[4–7] Our laboratory studied an acute EAE-ON model in which male Lewis rats (200–230 g) were injected with an emulsion of complete Freund's adjuvant (CFA) containing *Mycobacterium tuberculosis* (10 mg/mL) plus guinea pig spinal cord homogenate (10 mg/rat) and MBP (10 μg/rat).[8] Animals lose weight and develop clinical symptoms of paralysis at days 9–12 post-EAE induction, and then recover with no further episode of the disease. As observed in MS patients, EAE-ON animals also demonstrate decreased VEP and ERG recordings, implicating visual dysfunction due to pathophysiological changes in the optic nerve and retina.[9–11] Perivascular cuffing of immune cells, splitting of the myelin lamellae, and cleavage of myelin and cytoskeletal proteins, such as α-spectrin and neurofilament protein (NFP), have been shown in optic nerve from EAE-ON animals.[12,13] Unfortunately, the molecular events leading to axonal damage and apoptotic cell death in MS and EAE-ON are not fully understood, but studies have demonstrated that Ca^{2+}-associated events, including calpain activation, may be at least partially responsible.

ROLE OF Ca^{2+}-ASSOCIATED EVENTS IN EAE-ON

Increased levels of intracellular free Ca^{2+} have been implicated in many vision disorders, including cataract formation,[14] photoreceptor degeneration,[15,16] retinal ischemia,[17] and EAE-ON.[8,18] Selenite cataract formation in rats was shown to be dependent on increased intracellular Ca^{2+} levels.[14] Increased levels of intracellular free Ca^{2+} led to neuronal apoptosis through mitochondrial depolarization and caspase-3 activation in the rd mouse, which is a mouse strain containing a recessive mutation in the rd gene that encodes for a cGMP phosphodiesterase, causing rapid degeneration of photoreceptors,[16] and in chemical-induced photoreceptor degeneration.[15] Treatment with Ca^{2+} channel blockers actually blocked much of the damage associated with Ca^{2+} toxicity in patients with retinal ischemia and improved visual function.[17]

The mechanisms of Ca^{2+} influx in MS and EAE-ON are unclear; however, membrane damage, glutamate neurotoxicity, and alterations in Ca^{2+} channels may be involved. For instance, treatment with a voltage-gated Ca^{2+} channel blocker inhibited apoptosis of retinal ganglion cells (RGCs) in EAE-ON.[18] Once Ca^{2+} influx occurs, signaling pathways are activated that lead to axonal damage and cell death in the optic nerve and retina. One Ca^{2+}-induced event, which is upregulated in EAE-ON, is increased expression and activation of the Ca^{2+}-dependent protease calpain, which has been shown to cause cell death.[16]

ROLE OF CALPAIN IN EAE-ON

A total of 15 ubiquitous and tissue-specific calpains have been identified to date.[19] Of the ubiquitous forms, the two major isoforms are micro-calpain (μ-calpain) and milli-calpain (m-calpain), which require μM and mM concentrations for activation, respectively. Each calpain is formed by an 80-kDa catalytic subunit and

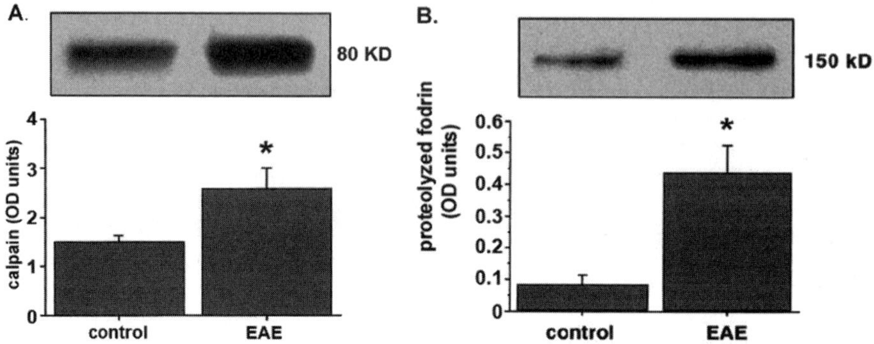

FIGURE 1. Increased calpain expression and activity in EAE-ON. Western blot analysis of **(A)** calpain expression in control and EAE-ON optic nerve from Lewis rats using calpain-specific antibody against the 80-kDa calpain subunit or **(B)** calpain activity using an antibody against α-spectrin (fodrin) that detects the 150-kDa calpain-cleaved fodrin breakdown product. One representative Western blot and a graph of the average scanning densitometry from at least three independent experiments are shown. $^{*}P < 0.05$ compared to control. Figure reproduced with permission from reference 8.

a 30-kDa regulatory subunit, and regulation is controlled by calpastatin (endogenous inhibitor), lipids, and an activator protein.[19,20] Calpain cleaves many proteins in optic nerve and RGCs, including myelin proteins [MBP, myelin-associated glycoprotein (MAG)], cytoskeletal proteins (α-spectrin, actin), NFPs, and cell signaling proteins (caspase-3).[19]

Biochemical studies in our laboratory have demonstrated that, while calpain transcriptional expression was not altered in EAE-ON optic nerve from Lewis rats (data not shown), translational expression was significantly increased (FIG. 1A). The increase in calpain expression correlated with an increase in the calpain-specific α-spectrin (fodrin) breakdown product in EAE-ON (FIG. 1B). A decrease in MAG was also found in EAE-ON.[8] However, no significant changes in transcriptional or translational expression of calpastatin, the endogenous inhibitor of calpain, were found, suggesting that increases in calpain expression and activity in EAE-ON were not due to decreased calpastatin expression.[8] Calpain-dependent degradation of NFP, a marker for axonal damage, in optic nerve *in vitro* was also demonstrated.[21] Immunohistolabeling of calpain expression in EAE-ON indicated that both inflammatory (T cell, macrophages) and glial (astrocytes) cells expressed increased levels of calpain, as compared to controls.[13] Since calpain has been shown to be involved in apoptosis in many CNS diseases,[16,22] the data suggest that calpain upregulation may also play a role in apoptosis of many cell types in EAE-ON.

In many MS patients, ON is the first presenting clinical symptom. While not all patients diagnosed with ON develop MS, at least 50% of all MS patients will experience vision loss. In support of this notion, visual dysfunction due to axonal damage and loss of RGCs had been documented before the onset of clinical symptoms.[11] Thus, we hypothesized that since calpain is associated with axonal damage and cell death, calpain expression may be upregulated in optic nerve before the onset

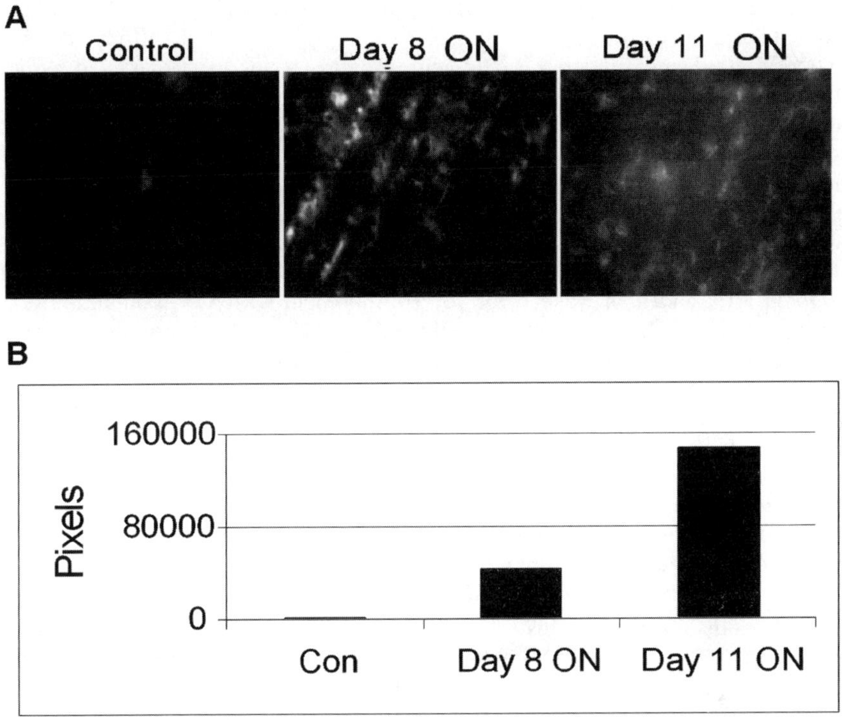

FIGURE 2. Increased calpain expression in EAE-ON before the onset of clinical symptoms. **(A)** Representative picture of calpain expression in optic nerve from control and EAE-ON Lewis rats as demonstrated by immunofluorescent labeling using calpain-specific IgG antibody (green). Magnification: ×400. **(B)** Quantification of calpain expression by counting green pixels ($n = 2$).

of clinical symptoms. To test the hypothesis, optic nerve from control and EAE-ON Lewis rats were stained with antibody against m-calpain both before (day 8) and after (day 11) onset of clinical symptoms of EAE (tail limpness, paralysis). We found that, compared to control optic nerve, calpain expression was increased at days 8 and 11 post-EAE induction (FIG. 2). Axonal damage, as assessed by increases in dephosphorylated NFP, was also increased at days 8 and 11 (data not shown). These studies suggest that increased calpain expression in optic nerve in EAE-ON animals occurred before the onset of clinical symptoms of EAE.

MATERIALS AND METHODS

Protein Extraction and Western Blot Analysis

Sodium dodecyl sulfate polyacrylamide gel electrophoresis (SDS-PAGE) and Western blot methods were used for determination and separation of protein. Briefly, optic nerve tissue was homogenized in 4°C protein homogenization buffer (50 mM Tris-HCl buffer, pH 7.4, 320 mM sucrose, 0.1 mM phenyl-methyl-sulfonyl-flouride, and 1 mM ethylenediaminetetraacetic acid). Total proteins were extracted by centrifugation. Coomassie Blue® Plus Protein Assay Reagent (Pierce, Rockford, IL) was used for protein concentration by measuring color density at 595 nm via spectrophotometer (Spectronic Instruments, Rochester, NY). Protein samples were equally loaded onto SDS-PAGE (4–20% gradient) gels (BioRad Laboratories, Hercules, CA). Gels were transferred to Immobilon™-P membranes (Millipore Corp., Bedford, MA), and the blots were blocked overnight at 4°C in blocking buffer containing Tris-buffered saline (TBS; Tris-HCl, pH 7.6, 137 mM NaCl) and 5% (w/v) nonfat powdered milk and then washed 3×, for 10 min each, with TBS containing 0.1% Tween-20 (TBST). Blots were then incubated for 24 h with antibodies against m-calpain (1:100) or fodrin (1:5000) diluted in TBST plus 5% (w/v) nonfat powdered milk. The blot was washed 2× (10 min) with 0.1% TBST and then incubated for 45 min with horseradish peroxidase (HRP)–conjugated anti-rabbit IgG antibody (1:2000) (ICN Pharmaceuticals, Aurora, OH) in 0.1% TBST. Blots were then washed 3× (10 min) and protein bands were detected by alkaline HRP-catalyzed oxidation of luminol in the presence of H_2O_2 using enhanced chemiluminescence (ECL, Amersham Life Science, Buckinghamshire, U.K.). Blots were exposed immediately to X-OMAT XAR-2 film (Eastman Kodak Co., Rochester, NY) for autoradiography. The ECL autoradiograms were scanned using a PowerLook Scanner (UMAX, Fremont, CA), and then imaged and digitized using Adobe Photoshop software (Adobe Systems, Seattle, WA). Bands were quantitated using *NIH Image* software.

Double-Immunofluorescent Labeling

For detection of calpain expression, optic nerve tissue sections (10 μm) were blocked for 1 h with blocking buffer containing 2% horse serum and 2% goat serum in phosphate-buffered serum (PBS). Then, the sections were incubated for 1 h in blocking buffer containing rabbit anti-rat m-calpain IgG antibody (1:100, generated in our laboratory).[23] The sections were washed 2× with PBS for 5 min and then incubated for 30 min in the dark with goat anti-rabbit IgG antibody conjugated to FITC (1:100; Vector Laboratories, Burlingame, CA) to detect calpain. The slides were washed 2× with PBS and 1× with double-distilled H_2O, and then mounted with one drop of Vectashield Mounting Media (Vector Laboratories) and covered with a coverslip. The slides were immediately viewed under a fluorescent microscope at 40× magnification.

SUMMARY

Calpain expression and activity in optic nerve of Lewis rats with EAE-ON was associated with loss of myelin proteins and axonal damage.[8,21] Calpain overexpression in immune and glial cells in the optic nerve suggests that calpain may also play a role in cell death, resulting in vision loss.[13] While calpain expression in RGCs has not been demonstrated in EAE-ON, increased calpain-mediated apoptosis of RGCs in other retinal disorders indicates that calpain may play a role in RGC loss in EAE-ON as well. Treatment with calpain inhibitors blocked damage in retinal ischemia,[24] cataract formation,[25] and photoreceptor degeneration,[16] suggesting that blocking calpain activity with calpain inhibitors may attenuate the pathophysiological events and prevent visual dysfunction in EAE-ON animals and eventually MS patients.

REFERENCES

1. WILLIAMS, K.C., E. ULVESTAD & W.F. HICKEY. 1994. Immunology of multiple sclerosis. Clin. Neurosci. **2:** 229.
2. COMPSTON, A. & A.D. SADOVNICK. 1992. Epidemiology and genetics of multiple sclerosis. Curr. Opin. Neurol. Neurosurg. **5:** 175.
3. COUPLAND, S.G. & T.H. KIRKHAM. 1982. Flash electroretinogram abnormalities in patients with clinically definite multiple sclerosis. Can. J. Neurol. Sci. **9:** 325.
4. BULLINGTON, S.J. & B.H. WAKSMAN. 1958. Uveitis in rabbits with experimental allergic encephalomyelitis; results produced by injection of nervous tissue and adjuvants. AMA Arch. Ophthalmol. **59:** 435.
5. RAO, N.A. 1981. Chronic experimental allergic optic neuritis. Invest. Ophthalmol. Vis. Sci. **20:** 159.
6. SHIELDS, D.C., W.R. TYOR, G.E. DEIBLER *et al.* 1998. Increased calpain expression in activated glial and inflammatory cells in experimental allergic encephalomyelitis. Proc. Natl. Acad. Sci. USA **95:** 5768.
7. DASGUPTA, S., Y. ZHOU, M. JANA *et al.* 2003. Sodium phenylacetate inhibits adoptive transfer of experimental allergic encephalomyelitis in SJL/J mice at multiple steps. J. Immunol. **170:** 3874.
8. SHIELDS, D.C. & N.L. BANIK. 1998. Putative role of calpain in the pathophysiology of experimental optic neuritis. Exp. Eye Res. **67:** 403.
9. BILBOOL, N., M. KAITZ, M. FEINSOD *et al.* 1983. Visual evoked potentials in experimental allergic encephalomyelitis. J. Neurol. Sci. **60:** 105.
10. MEYER, R., R. WEISSERT, R. DIEM *et al.* 2001. Acute neuronal apoptosis in a rat model of multiple sclerosis. J. Neurosci. **21:** 6214.
11. HOBOM, M., M.K. STORCH, R. WEISSERT *et al.* 2004. Mechanisms and time course of neuronal degeneration in experimental autoimmune encephalomyelitis. Brain Pathol. **14:** 148.
12. VON SALLMANN, L., R.E. MYERS, E.M. LERNER II & S.H. STONE. 1967. Vasculo-occlusive retinopathy in experimental allergic encephalomyelitis. Arch. Ophthalmol. **78:** 112.
13. BANIK, N.L. & D. C. SHIELDS. 1999. A putative role for calpain in demyelination associated with optic neuritis. Histol. Histopathol. **14:** 649.
14. SHEARER, T.R. & L.L. DAVID. 1982. Role of calcium in selenium cataract. Curr. Eye Res. **2:** 777.
15. FOX, D.A., A.T. POBLENZ & L. HE. 1999. Calcium overload triggers rod photoreceptor apoptotic cell death in chemical-induced and inherited retinal degenerations. Ann. N.Y. Acad. Sci. **893:** 282.
16. SHARMA, A.K. & B. ROHRER. 2004. Calcium-induced calpain mediates apoptosis via caspase-3 in a mouse photoreceptor cell line. J. Biol. Chem. **279:** 35564.
17. NIHARD, P. 1982. Effect of calcium-entry-blockers on arterioles, capillaries, and venules of the retina. Angiology **33:** 37.
18. DIEM, R., M. HOBOM, K. MAIER *et al.* 2003. Methylprednisolone increases neuronal apoptosis during autoimmune CNS inflammation by inhibition of an endogenous neuroprotective pathway. J. Neurosci. **23:** 6993.
19. RAY, S.K. & N.L. BANIK. 2003. Calpain and its involvement in the pathophysiology of CNS injuries and diseases: therapeutic potential of calpain inhibitors for prevention of neurodegeneration. Curr. Drug Targets CNS Neurol. Disord. **2:** 173.
20. MURACHI, T. 1984. Calcium-dependent proteinases and specific inhibitors: calpain and calpastatin. Biochem. Soc. Symp. **49:** 149.
21. SHIELDS, D.C., C. LEBLANC & N.L. BANIK. 1997. Calcium-mediated neurofilament protein degradation in rat optic nerve *in vitro*: activity and autolysis of calpain proenzyme. Exp. Eye Res. **65:** 15.

22. RAY, S.K., G.G. WILFORD, D.C. MATZELLE *et al.* 1999. Calpeptin and methylprednisolone inhibit apoptosis in rat spinal cord injury. Ann. N.Y. Acad. Sci. **890:** 261.
23. CHAKRABARTI, A.K., N.L. BANIK, J.M. POWERS & E.L. HOGAN. 1989. The regional and subcellular distribution of calcium activated neutral proteinase (CANP) in the bovine central nervous system. Neurochem. Res. **14:** 259.
24. SAKAMOTO, Y.R., T.R. NAKAJIMA, C.R. FUKIAGE *et al.* 2000. Involvement of calpain isoforms in ischemia-reperfusion injury in rat retina. Curr. Eye Res. **21:** 571.
25. FUKIAGE, C., M. AZUMA, Y. NAKAMURA *et al.* 1997. SJA6017, a newly synthesized peptide aldehyde inhibitor of calpain: amelioration of cataract in cultured rat lenses. Biochim. Biophys. Acta **1361:** 304.

Activation of Neuroprotective Pathways by Metabotropic Group I Glutamate Receptors: A Potential Target for Drug Discovery?

ANDRIUS BASKYS,[a,b,c] LIWEI FANG,[a] AND ILDAR BAYAZITOV[a,c]

[a]*Southern California Institute for Research and Education, Long Beach, California 90822, USA*

[b]*Mental Illness Research and Education Clinical Center (MIRECC), VA Health Care System, Long Beach, California 90822, USA*

[c]*Department of Psychiatry and Human Behavior, University of California, Irvine, California 92668, USA*

ABSTRACT: **Stroke neuroprotection trials suggest that pharmacological manipulations of a single neuroprotective mechanism are generally ineffective and that new approaches, possibly involving simultaneous manipulations of multiple mechanisms, need to be sought. To identify optimal components for such a multipronged approach, we studied NMDA receptor activation-induced cell death in organotypic hippocampal culture preparations as a model of excitotoxicity. Metabotropic group I glutamate receptor (mGluR) activation by their selective agonist, (*S*)-3,5-dihydroxyphenylglycine (DHPG), resulted in concentration-dependent reduction of nerve cell susceptibility to NMDA-mediated injury (neuroprotective effect). The neuroprotection was mediated primarily by mGluR1, required phospholipase C activation, was inhibited by cholesterol-containing methyl-β-cyclodextrin treatment, and occluded by antipsychotic quetiapine. It was associated with suppression of NMDA currents and prolongation of $GABA_A$ receptor–mediated currents in DHPG-treated cultures. cDNA microarray analysis of 1128 brain-relevant genes revealed that mGluR-mediated neuroprotection was associated with simultaneous activation of endocytosis, and inactivation of inflammation, cell adhesion, cell death, and transcription-related genes. Antisense inhibition of Rab5b, a gene coding for a small GTPase associated with endocytosis, significantly reduced the mGluR-mediated neuroprotection. These findings expand our understanding of the role that mGluRs play in regulation of nerve cell susceptibility to injury and should facilitate the design of novel therapeutic strategies for stroke and other neurodegenerative diseases.**

KEYWORDS: **neuroprotection; organotypic; DHPG; Rab5b; GABARAP; cholesterol; quetiapine**

Address for correspondence: Andrius Baskys, M.D., Ph.D., 5901 East 7th Street, 06/116A, Long Beach, CA 90822. Voice: 562-826-8000, ext. 4313; fax: 562-826-5969.
abaskys@uci.edu; andrius.baskys@med.va.gov

Ann. N.Y. Acad. Sci. 1053: 55–73 (2005).
doi: 10.1196/annals.1344.006

WHY STUDY NEUROPROTECTION?

In adult brain, nerve cell death can be caused by a variety of insults, most common of which is the sudden interruption of blood flow to the brain or ischemia. Brain tissue ischemia is commonly associated with such events as stroke. It has been estimated that there are 400,000 strokes in the United States each year and approximately 150,000 deaths are attributable to cerebrovascular disease.[1] Those who survive suffer from long-term physical, emotional, and cognitive disabilities, a treatment of which carries a great financial burden.

There have been numerous attempts to develop drugs that prevent ischemic brain tissue death, most of them unsuccessful. For example, out of 178 controlled clinical trials of acute stroke therapies reported in English language literature in the 20th century, only 4 produced positive results. Among them, clot-dissolving treatments were more likely to be successful. In contrast, out of 49 neuroprotective drugs tested in 114 stroke studies, none was successful.[2] The numerous reasons for this failure range from clinical trial design issues to failure to fully appreciate the complexity of mechanisms controlling nerve cell death and survival.[2]

Ischemic nerve cell death is thought to occur via excitotoxicity. This excitotoxicity appears to be mediated primarily by excessive release of glutamate, which overactivates the *N*-methyl-D-aspartate receptor/channel complex (NMDAR), allowing the influx of toxic levels of Ca^{2+} into nerve cells.[3,4] This knowledge has, however, not yet resulted in effective ischemic stroke treatment or prevention strategies. Although blockade of NMDARs is very effective in reducing ischemic cell death in experimental models, the clinical use of this approach has been negligible mainly due to psychotogenic side effects[5] of NMDAR antagonists.

A BRIEF OVERVIEW OF EXCITOTOXICITY

Olney initially described excitotoxicity in 1969 when he found that treatment of mice with monosodium glutamate caused brain lesions.[6] (*S*)-Glutamic acid (IUPAC nomenclature, also referred to as L-glutamate or merely glutamate) is the most abundant excitatory neurotransmitter in the central nervous system (CNS).[7] Glutamate exerts its effect on two main groups of receptors. One group comprises ligand-gated ion channels termed ionotropic glutamate receptors (iGluRs); the other comprises the G-protein-coupled metabotropic glutamate receptors (mGluRs). The iGluRs are further subdivided into *N*-methyl-D-aspartate (NMDA), 2-alpha-amino-3-hydroxy-5-methyl-4-isoxazolepropionic acid (AMPA), and kainic acid (kainate; KA) receptors based on their high affinity for these ligands.[8] It is generally believed that excessive stimulation of iGluRs triggers an influx of Na^+ and Ca^{2+} through the receptor-controlled channels and subsequently leads to cell death. It has been proposed that Ca^{2+} entering through NMDARs may be especially lethal due to colocalization of these channels with particularly sensitive intracellular targets (e.g., calpain-induced cytoskeletal breakdown, phospholipase-A_2-induced formation of arachidonic acid and metabolites, membrane translocation of protein kinase C (PKC), Ca^{2+}-activated endonuclease destruction of cellular DNA, and other Ca^{2+}-dependent processes). There have been numerous reports on glutamate toxicity in a variety of preparations, and several excellent reviews have been published on this topic[9–11] recognizing the critical role of NMDARs in pathophysiology of ischemic nerve cell death. The nature of cell death (necrosis vs. apoptosis) remains a subject of debate (as perhaps is the definition of the term "apoptosis"[12]). Morphological and other features of both apoptotic and necrotic cell death have been reported following ischemic damage.[13,14]

Based on this scenario, it is not surprising that the focus in treating ischemic brain damage has been on designing drugs that are iGluR antagonists, in particular NMDAR antagonists (such as phencyclidine, ketamine, or MK-801), thereby inhibiting the increase in intracellular Ca^{2+}. In animal models, these drugs have proved to be very effective against ischemic damage; however, in human clinical trials, the results have been very disappointing, mainly due to severe side effects such as psychosis, nausea, vomiting, impaired memory, and in some cases even neurotoxicity.[5] Because of their modulatory effects on glutamate neurotransmission and their extrasynaptic placement, discovery of mGluRs opens a promising new opportunity for pharmacological interventions.

METABOTROPIC GLUTAMATE RECEPTORS IN THE BRAIN

The first evidence on the existence of mGluRs came in 1985, when it was reported that quisqualate could induce formation of inositol phosphates in striatal neurons,[15] a phenomenon later found in the hippocampus[16] and cerebellar granule cells.[17] In 1991, the first mGluR was eventually cloned by two different groups and designated mGluR1; in the following years, 7 additional mGluRs (mGluR2–8) were cloned.[18] The 8 cloned mGluRs belong to superfamily C of the G-protein-coupled receptors, together with the calcium-sensing receptors, two γ-amino-butyric acid type B ($GABA_B$) receptors, and some putative pheromone and taste receptors.[19] Within superfamily C, the mGluRs are further subdivided into three groups based on their sequence homology, signal transduction, and agonist pharmacology. Group I contains mGluR1 and 5 (splice variants mGluR1a, b, d, e; and mGluR5a, b). Group II receptors are mGluR2 and 3, and group III are mGluR4, 6, 7, and 8 (splice variants mGluR4a, b; mGluR7a, b; and mGluR8a, b).

NEUROPROTECTION BY GLUTAMATE INVOLVES GROUP I mGluRs

Glutamate can be both an excitotoxin and a neuroprotectant. It has been well established that moderate levels of glutamate agonists can protect neurons from damage caused by their subsequent exposure to glutamate at excitotoxic concentrations.[20–22] Recent evidence suggests that stimulation of mGluRs is crucial for neuroprotection,[23–25] particularly against ischemic nerve cell death.[26–28] The $G_{\alpha q/11}$ family of G-proteins couples group I mGluRs to multiple isoforms of PLC.[29] PLC activation typically results in production of second messengers, inositol 1,4,5-trisphosphate (IP3) and 1,2-diacylglycerol (DAG), which in turn release intracellular Ca^{2+} and activate PKC. Group II (mGluR2 and 3) and group III (mGluR4–8) receptors are negatively coupled to forskolin-sensitive cAMP production and to voltage-dependent Ca^{2+} channels.[30] Glutamate is also an agonist at several poorly characterized mGluRs that appear to be coupled to phospholipase D (PLD) and/or the IP3/DAG system.[31]

There is evidence supporting both neurotoxic and neuroprotective actions of group I mGluRs. Most of the evidence favoring neurotoxic actions of mGluRs comes from studies showing that group I agonists potentiate NMDA effects[32–35] and that antagonists for this group are neuroprotective[36,37] or that mGluRs support or promote epileptiform activity.[38] In addition, simultaneous application of the nonselective mGluR agonist ACPD [(1*S*,3*R*)-1-aminocyclopentane-1,3-dicarboxylic acid] or the group I–specific agonist DHPG and NMDA was toxic to cortical neurons and hippocampal slice cultures.[39]

There is an equally abundant and credible body of evidence, though, that group I mGluR stimulation could be neuroprotective. Support for this viewpoint comes from studies of nitric oxide (NO)– or ischemia-induced cell death,[40,41] the associated reduction of apoptosis markers,[42–44] and NMDA toxicity.[45,46] Bruno *et al.* reported that the group I agonist DHPG was protective when coapplied with NMDA, despite an increase in NMDAR-mediated currents.[47] Neuroprotection by mGluRs requires PKC activation,[27] suggesting that group I mGluRs coupled to the PLC-dependent signaling pathway may be involved.

Among the mGluRs, group II and III receptors act presynaptically to decrease Ca^{2+}-dependent release of glutamate and have also been implicated in neuroprotection.[48] However, accumulation of extracellular glutamate in ischemic nerve tissue is in part caused by reverse operation of glutamate transporters,[49] which suggests that the presynaptic mechanism of action of these mGluRs may limit their effectiveness as neuroprotectants.[48] Although some pharmacological studies did not support the role of group II and group III receptors in neuroprotection against direct NMDA toxicity,[50,51] the ability of these mGluRs to regulate adenylate cyclase activity could be conducive to neuroprotection against NMDA toxicity.[52]

REDUCTION OF THE NMDA-STIMULATED MEMBRANE CURRENT AS A MECHANISM OF GROUP I mGluR-MEDIATED PROTECTION

Using propidium iodide (PI) uptake measurements as an indicator of cell death, we have shown that treatment of organotypic hippocampal slice cultures with a selective group I mGluR agonist, (*S*)-3,5-dihydroxyphenylglycine (DHPG), protects neurons from NMDA-induced excitotoxicity in hippocampal CA1 and CA3 subfields in a concentration-dependent manner (FIG. 1).[53] Neuroprotection required a prolonged exposure to the agonist: DHPG (10 μM) did not induce significant neuroprotection after short-term (10 min) exposure (91.1±28.1% vs. NMDA alone, $P > 0.05$, $n = 12$ cultures per group); application of 100 μM for 10 min produced a marked reduction in NMDA toxicity, which was not statistically significant however. Treatment of cultures with 10 μM DHPG for 2 h induced a significant protection, suggesting that a prolonged mGluR stimulation is required for the neuroprotection to occur. Neuroprotection was long-lasting, that is, cultures treated for up to 21 days still showed reduced sensitivity to NMDA as compared to control cultures of the same age. Neuroprotection occurred only if the mGluR stimulation was prior to the NMDA exposure, but not if DHPG was applied for 2 h immediately afterwards.[53] Thus, conflicting reports on the role of glutamate in neuroprotection and neurodegeneration, discussed earlier, may be due to the varying duration and timing of agonist application in different studies. Interestingly, immunohistochemistry experi-

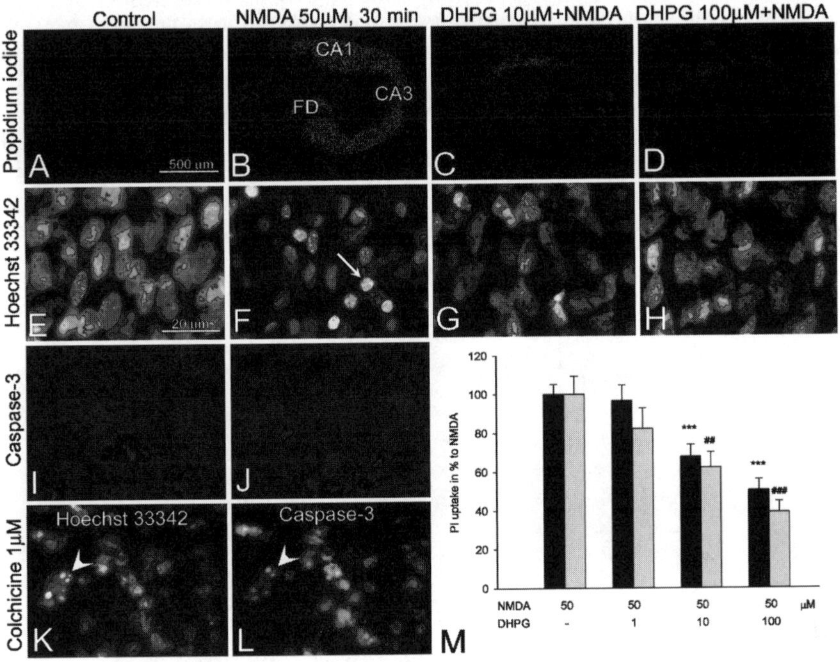

FIGURE 1. DHPG-induced neuroprotection against NMDA excitotoxicity. **A–D** show PI uptake after 24 h in organotypic hippocampal slice cultures exposed to NMDA (50 μM for 30 min) compared to slices pretreated with DHPG before the NMDA exposure. **E–H** show high magnification (×100) of CA1 pyramidal cells after similar treatment. **I** and **J** correspond to **E** and **F**, but in caspase-3 staining. As a positive control for the caspase-3 staining, sections from cultures treated with colchicine (1 μM for 48 h) were included (**K** and **L**). Untreated age-matched control cultures displayed a small baseline level of PI uptake (**A**), normal nuclear morphology (**E**), and no caspase-3 activity (**I**). Cultures treated with NMDA had increased PI uptake in hippocampal subfields (**B**) with nuclei appearing pyknotic and densely stained (**F**; *arrow*), but without caspase-3 activity (**J**). In contrast, nuclei in cultures treated with colchicine showed fragmentation (**K**; *arrowhead*) and increased caspase-3 activation (**L**; *arrowhead*). Pretreatment with DHPG for 2 h before the NMDA exposure reduced the NMDA-induced PI uptake (**C, D**) as well as the number of pyknotic nuclei (**G, H**). Graph **M** shows quantification of PI uptake in CA1 (*black columns*) and CA3 subfields (*gray columns*) after 24 h, with NMDA set to 100%. Pretreatment for 2 h with DHPG at 1 μM had no effect on NMDA-induced PI uptake, whereas pretreatment with DHPG at 10 and 100 μM significantly reduced PI uptake in both CA1 and CA3 in a concentration-dependent manner. Data are shown as mean ± SEM; $^{***}P < 0.001$ (compared to NMDA in CA1 alone), $^{\#\#}P < 0.01$, $^{\#\#\#}P < 0.001$ (compared to NMDA in CA3 alone), with n = 21–42 cultures per group. (Reprinted with permission from ref. 53.) [Figure reduced to 85%.]

ments showed that there was no evidence of caspase-3 staining in cultures treated with NMDA within the time window between 24 to 48 h after the treatment. To make sure that our caspase-3 staining method was sensitive enough, we treated cultures with colchicine, which is known to cause apoptotic cell death and caspase-3 activation. In these cultures, we detected a clear signal, suggesting that our method was sensitive enough to detect caspase-3 activation. On the basis of these observations, we concluded that cell death caused by NMDA in our preparation is not associated with caspase-3 activation and thus is most likely to be not apoptotic, but necrotic. These data also suggest that group I activation can reduce what appears to be a necrotic type of neuronal death.

Examination of the mGluR subtype involved in the protective effect of DHPG with a selective antagonist of mGluR1 receptor LY367385 and an antagonist for mGluR5 receptor MPEP [2-methyl-6-(phenylethynyl)pyridine] showed that only LY367385 [(*S*)-(+)α-amino-4-carboxy-2-methylbenzeneacetic acid] abolished neuro-

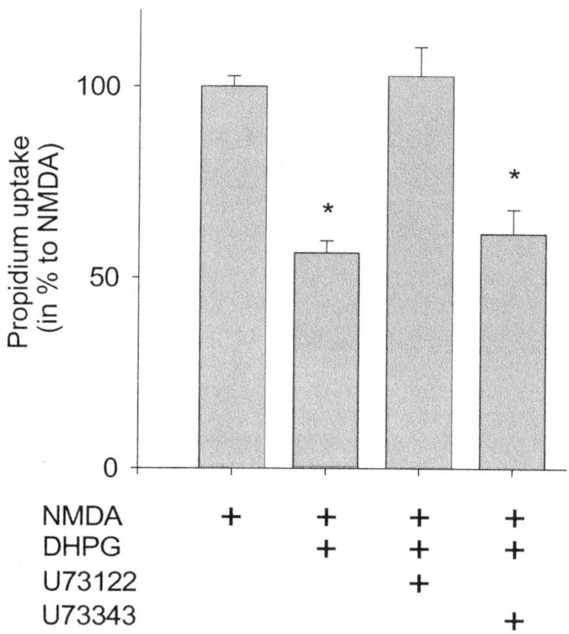

FIGURE 2. Selective inhibitor of PLC, U73122, blocks the protective effect of the group I mGluR agonist, DHPG, on organotypic hippocampal slice cultures exposed to excitotoxic concentrations of NMDA. Each column shows the relative level of cell death measured using propidium iodide uptake as a cell death marker. "+" indicates the presence of a particular compound listed on the left. An *asterisk* indicates a statistical difference ($P < 0.05$) between the adjacent columns (one-way analysis of variance with Bonferroni correction for multiple comparisons). Each experiment was performed at least in triplicate on 5–12 cultures. Note that cultures treated with DHPG (10 μM) for 2 h prior to exposure to 50 μM NMDA for 30 min displayed a marked reduction in propidium iodide uptake compared to cultures exposed to NMDA only. The protective effect of DHPG was abolished by the U73122 (10 μM). The inactive, but structurally similar compound, U73343, had no effect on DHPG protection.[54b]

protection in a concentration-dependent manner (tested at 1, 5, and 10 μM), whereas the MPEP (up to 1 μM) had no significant effect. These data suggest that, to induce neuroprotection, DHPG acts primarily on the mGluR1 receptor subtype.[53]

The neuroprotective effect seen in our studies could, in theory, be PLC-dependent or PLC-independent.[54a] To distinguish between these possibilities, we applied a selective PLC inhibitor, U73122 (1-[6[[17beta-3-methoxyestra-1,3,5(10)-triene-17-yl]amino]hexyl]-1H-pyrrole-dione), together with DHPG. Preliminary data suggest that U73122 significantly ($P < 0.05$, t test) reduced the DHPG protection (FIG. 2), while its inactive analogue, U73343 (analogue 1-[6[[17beta-3-methoxyestra-1,3,5(10)-triene-17-yl]amino]hexyl]-2,5-pyrrolidine dione, 10 μM), was ineffective.

Our next step was to examine whether the NMDA receptor/channel function was attenuated following neuroprotective DHPG treatment. To answer this question, we compared NMDA-induced membrane currents in control and DHPG-treated (10 μM, 2 h) cultures. NMDA produced a robust inward current in controls, but not in the DHPG-treated cultures (FIG. 3). The mean values of the NMDA-stimulated inward current were significantly ($P < 0.05$, two-sided t test) different between the two groups at 5, 6, and 7 min after the start of NMDA application.[53] These experiments strongly suggest that NMDA receptor function in DHPG-treated neurons was diminished, which can explain the mechanism of the DHPG neuroprotection. In order to understand whether DHPG treatment also altered synaptic AMPAR-mediated currents, we measured spontaneous excitatory synaptic current potentials (EPSCs) in

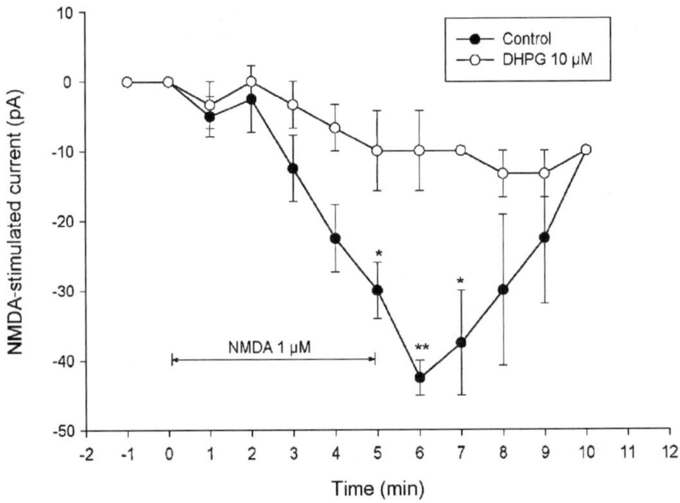

FIGURE 3. NMDA stimulated inward current in CA1 pyramidal cells from hippocampal slice cultures. In control cultures (*filled circles*), NMDA induced a clear inward current measured as holding current (I_{hold}). This current was strongly suppressed in cultures treated with DHPG (10 μM, 2 h, *open circles*). The difference between the DHPG-treated and control cultures reached significance after 5, 6, and 7 min. Data are shown as mean ± SEM; *$P < 0.05$, **$P < 0.01$ using a Student's t test, with n = 3–4 neurons from individual cultures per group. (Reprinted with permission from ref. 53.)

cultures exposed to a prolonged 2-h treatment with DHPG. DHPG treatment induced a small (20–30%), but highly significant ($P < 0.001$, Kolmogorov-Smirnoff test) decrease in both amplitude and half-width of AMPA-mediated spontaneous EPSCs, suggesting that AMPARs may be regulated by DHPG stimulation. Similar observations have been made in cerebellar granule cells, in which treatment with a mixed group I–II mGluR agonist ACPD or (*RS*)-DHPG significantly reduced Ca^{2+} influx induced by application of NMDA or glutamate,[55] and in mouse cortical cultures, where DHPG reduced NMDAR-mediated whole cell currents.[56]

cDNA MICROARRAY ANALYSIS OF NEUROPROTECTIVE ACTIVATION

In an attempt to understand molecular mechanisms of the mGluR-mediated neuroprotection, two main scenarios of the I_{NMDA} reduction were considered. One scenario included group I mGluR-mediated iGluR internalization[57] and the other was based on an idea that downregulation of NMDA receptors or their subunits could be responsible for the I_{NMDA} reduction. To distinguish between these possibilities, we used cDNA microarray analysis to compare gene expression patterns in DHPG-treated (10 μM, 2-h protocol known to induce neuroprotection) organotypic hippocampal slice cultures with untreated control cultures. A specially designed microarray ("neuroarray") consisted of ~1100 known sequence-verified genes whose expression has been associated with the CNS (see ref. 58 for methodological details).

Results of these experiments revealed that the neuroprotective treatment was associated with a simultaneous change in expression of several seemingly unrelated genes: genes associated with regulation of intracellular transport (e.g., Rab5b, GABARAP), reduction of inflammation (e.g., IL2RG, IL2RB), reduction of signaling through cell death pathways (e.g., SEMA3C, DTNA), reduction of cell adhesion (e.g., ITGAX, ITGA3), proliferation (e.g., BMP1, BMP7), and changes in transcriptional activation.[58] There was no change in the expression of NMDAR subunits (NR1, NR2A, and NR2C) on the array.[58] These findings did not support reduced NMDAR or its subunits synthesis hypothesis as an explanation of reduced I_{NMDA}. Thus, we focused on endocytosis gene Rab5b, hypothesizing that it may be responsible for increased NMDAR endocytosis, reduced I_{NMDA}, and neuroprotection. In addition, we hypothesized that GABARAP downregulation may increase $GABA_A$ receptor–mediated synaptic inhibition and further contribute to reduction of tissue excitability, which could increase hippocampal neuron resistance to excitotoxic injury.

THE RAB5B HYPOTHESIS OF DHPG-INDUCED NEUROPROTECTION

Rab5b codes for Ras-associated protein, which is a ubiquitous, small GTPase that facilitates endocytosis.[59] It belongs to the family of proteins that coordinates membrane trafficking by oscillating between guanosine-5′-triphosphate (GTP) (active) and guanosine-5′-diphosphate (GDP) (inactive) bound states.[60] Rab5 is essential for the transport of clathrin-coated vesicles from the plasma membrane to the early endosome, attachment of the vesicles to microtubules, as well as their motility along microtubules. Since both NMDA and AMPA receptors are internalized by a clathrin-dependent mechanism,[61,62] an increase in Rab5b could lead to internalization of NMDA and AMPA receptors. In light of this, Rab5b, which is highly expressed in the brain, appeared as an extremely attractive candidate gene whose increased expression could contribute to neuroprotection and I_{NMDA} reduction through a regulation of NMDAR trafficking and internalization.[57]

ANTISENSE DOWNREGULATION OF RAB5B

To confirm the gene array data, we measured Rab5b expression using real-time quantitative PCR (RT-PCR).[58] The DHPG-treated group of cultures showed higher concentration of Rab5b mRNA (0.22 ± 0.04 mg/mL, mean ± SEM) compared to the control (untreated) group (0.05 ± 0.03 mg/mL, mean ± SEM, $P = 0.012$). There was no significant difference for the housekeeping gene GAPDH concentrations between the DHPG pretreatment (27.0 ± 5.8 mg/mL, mean ± SEM) and the control group (36.5 ± 2.0 mg/mL, mean ± SEM) after correction for the RT sample ($P = 0.17$). To investigate whether Rab5b was also upregulated at the protein level, we performed Western blotting experiments. Cultures were treated with 10 and 100 µM DHPG for 2 h, the treatment paradigm known to result in concentration-dependent neuroprotection.[53] Western blot analysis performed immediately after the treatment revealed a concentration-dependent upregulation of Rab5b protein levels in response to mGluR stimulation with its agonist.

To further define the Rab5b role in the mGluR-mediated neuroprotection, we treated cultures with antisense oligonucleotides against Rab5b for 24 h prior to subjecting them to the neuroprotective treatment with DHPG.[63] The Rab5b antisense sequence was based on known human and mouse Rab5b sequences, and was designed to bind the translation initiation codon on hRab5b mRNA. Two control sequences of oligonucleotides were used: a "scrambled" sequence in which the proportion of each type of nucleotide was identical to that of the original Rab5b antisense sequence, and a sequence targeting the coding Rab5b gene region (it has been reported that antisense targeting coding sequences may be less or not effective at all).[64] Antisense treatment blocked DHPG-induced Rab5b upregulation and blocked neuroprotection (FIG. 4). Both control sequences were ineffective. These results strongly support the idea that Rab5b upregulation by DHPG is a critical element responsible for the neuroprotection.

Rab5b facilitates endocytosis by the regulation of clathrin-mediated transport from the plasma membrane to the early endosome.[65–67] DHPG treatment has been shown to result in clathrin-dependent internalization of NMDA and AMPA receptors,[57] a process that can be inhibited by hypotonic shock followed by K^+ depletion.[68] To test for clathrin-mediated endocytosis in the DHPG-mediated neuroprotection, we measured DHPG-induced neuroprotection in cultures subjected to hypotonic shock and K^+ depletion. A brief (5 min) hypotonic shock combined with K^+ depletion completely blocked DHPG-induced neuroprotection without affecting NMDA toxicity.[63] These data further support the idea of NMDAR endocytosis responsible for the neuroprotection and reduction of I_{NMDA}. A model of mGluR-mediated neuroprotection encompassing the above elements (mGluR1, PLC, Rab5b, endocytosis of NMDA, and possibly AMPA receptors) is shown in FIGURE 5.

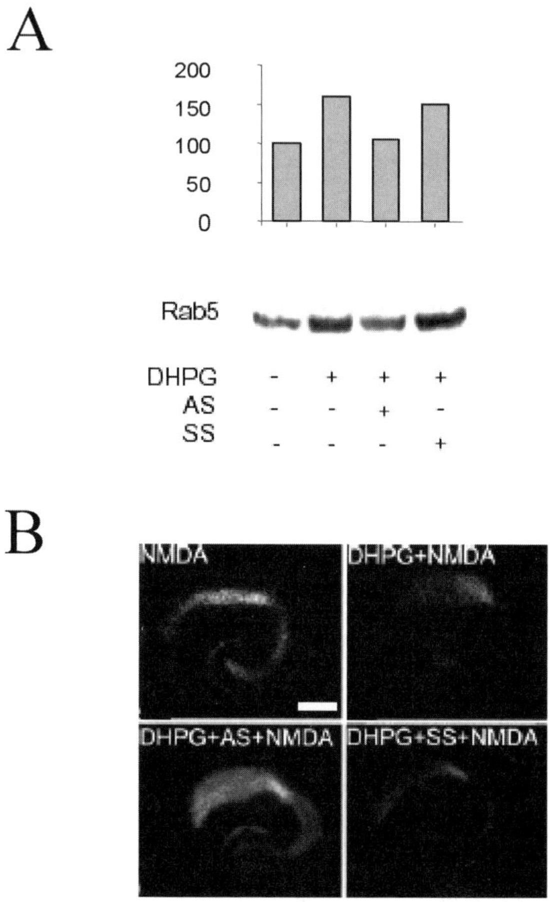

FIGURE 4. Suppression of DHPG-induced protection of NMDA toxicity by antisense to Rab5b. **(A)** Western blot analysis of Rab5b protein expression following application of DHPG (10 μM, 2 h) in either the presence (+) or absence (–) of AS (antisense) or SS (scrambled sequence) oligonucleotides. Results of densitometer scanning of the blots were as follows (in arbitrary units): control, 100; DHPG, 160; AS + DHPG, 105; SS + DHPG, 151. Experiments were performed two times with similar results. **(B)** Confocal microscope images of propidium iodide (PI) uptake in individual cultures. Bright areas correspond to higher level of PI uptake and more dead or injured cells. *Horizontal bar*: 500 μm. Note a marked reduction of PI uptake in DHPG + NMDA–treated culture in comparison to the culture treated with NMDA alone. No such reduction is seen in the culture treated with antisense to Rab5b, indicating a lack of the DHPG protection. Scrambled sequence oligonucleotide was without effect. (From ref. 63, modified with permission.)

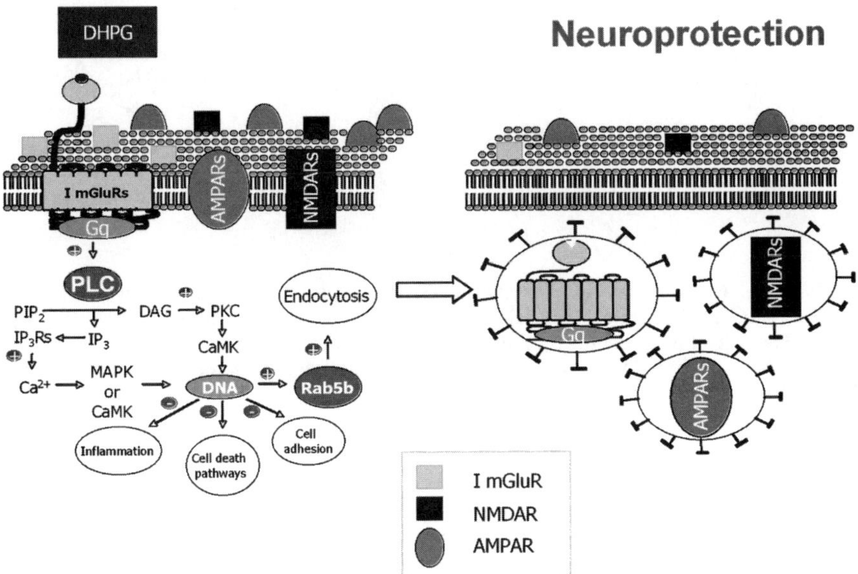

FIGURE 5. Hypothesis of DHPG-induced neuroprotection by Rab5b-stimulated endocytosis of NMDA and possibly AMPA and mGluR1,5 receptors. (*Left*) A nerve cell before DHPG exposure. In the event of significant glutamate release such as occurs in ischemia or hypoxic conditions, AMPA, NMDA, and mGluR receptors will become overactivated, causing Ca^{2+} overflow and cell death. Stimulation of group I mGluRs will (possibly through a PLC-dependent pathway) lead to changes in gene expression, including increased expression of the endocytosis-related gene, Rab5b. Increases in Rab5b protein will facilitate endocytosis and internalization of NMDA, AMPA, and mGluR membrane receptors (*right*), which will render the neuron less sensitive to high concentrations of extracellular glutamate. Downregulation of GABARAP will further reduce the spread of excitation by unclustering $GABA_A$ receptors and increasing $GABA_A$ receptor affinity to GABA (not shown).

GABARAP AND NEUROPROTECTION

A second gene that came to our attention as a result of the microarray analysis was GABARAP. GABARAP codes for $GABA_A$ receptor–associated protein (hence the name GABARAP), which is a member of the membrane trafficking and/or fusion protein family.[69] It binds to the γ2 subunit of the $GABA_A$ receptor and is ubiquitously expressed in the brain.[70] Clustering of $GABA_A$ receptors can dramatically modulate kinetic properties of these receptors and can significantly reduce their affinity for GABA.[71,72] We hypothesized, on the basis of these reports, that DHPG-induced downregulation of GABARAP could contribute to neuroprotection by unclustering $GABA_A$ receptors with a resulting increase in receptor affinity for GABA and possibly decreased excitability of neurons.

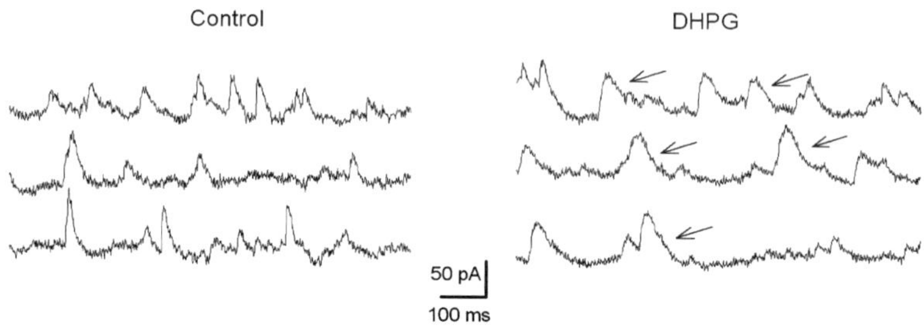

FIGURE 6. Prolongation of synaptic $GABA_A$ responses following neuroprotective DHPG treatment. Examples of IPSCs recorded before (*left*) and after (*right*) DHPG application. The role of this phenomenon in the mGluR-mediated neuroprotection is still unclear, but it could be associated with GABARAP downregulation and increased $GABA_AR$ affinity for GABA (I. Bayazitov, unpublished).

To begin addressing this question, we first conducted experiments to clarify whether $GABA_A$ receptors are involved in the DHPG-mediated neuroprotection in the organotypic hippocampal culture preparation. Addition of $GABA_A$ receptor Cl^- channel blocker picrotoxin (100 μM) to the medium at the time of DHPG treatment resulted in a significant ($P < 0.001$, t test, $n = 23$ cultures) loss of DHPG-mediated neuroprotection (DHPG and NMDA, 53±4% from NMDA alone, mean ± SEM; vs. picrotoxin + DHPG + NMDA, 114±8% from NMDA alone, mean ± SEM). This finding is in agreement with published reports showing that enhancing GABA-ergic inhibition could be neuroprotective.[73] Together, these data suggest that $GABA_A$ receptor–dependent mechanisms may be involved in DHPG protection.

To test a possibility that downregulation of GABARAP could alter $GABA_A$ receptor–mediated inhibitory postsynaptic currents (IPSCs), we electrophysiologically recorded $GABA_A$ receptor–mediated IPSCs in cultures subjected to neuroprotective DHPG treatment. Recordings were done in whole-cell configuration and voltage-clamp mode at $V_{hold} = 0$ mV in the presence of AMPA antagonist CNQX (10 μM). The nature of responses was confirmed by testing for the IPSC sensitivity to $GABA_A$ receptor channel blocker picrotoxin and insensitivity to 10 μM NMDA receptor channel blocker MK-801. Treatment with DHPG (100 μM, 10 min) induced a significant increase in half-width of IPSCs (FIG. 6). These data suggest that DHPG treatment alters synaptic $GABA_A$ receptor function. To implicate GABARAP in this interaction, we added γ2 subunit fragment peptide[74] in the recording pipette to block the interaction between GABARAP and γ2-$GABA_A$ receptor subunit. Results from 5 neurons indicate an increase in the IPSC amplitude (and half-width; not shown) over time in neurons recorded with the active inhibitory peptide, but not the scrambled sequence peptide–filled electrodes (FIG. 7). Although the difference between the two groups did not reach statistical significance, these findings lend support to the idea of GABARAP involvement in the mGluR-mediated neuroprotection and should be examined further.

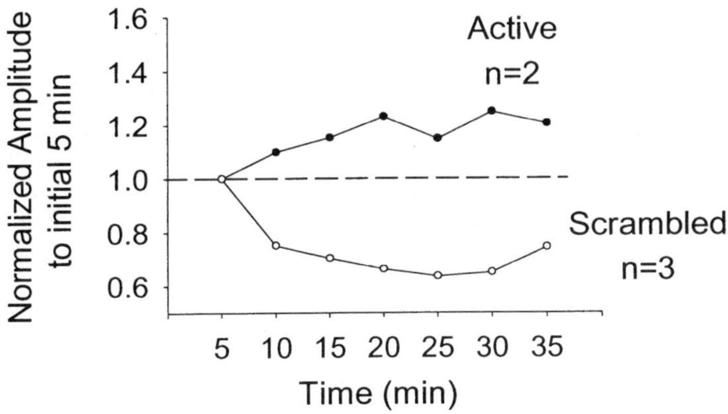

FIGURE 7. Presence of γ2 peptide fragment ("active") in the patch electrode increased $GABA_A$ receptor–mediated IPSCs, while a scrambled sequence peptide ("scrambled") had no effect.

PHYSIOLOGICAL REGULATION OF THE mGluR-MEDIATED NEUROPROTECTIVE MECHANISM: THE ROLE OF CHOLESTEROL

Influence of cholesterol as a modulator of membrane receptor function has already been established.[75,76] We therefore tested a possibility that mGluR-mediated neuroprotection could be regulated by membrane cholesterol by using, as a cholesterol donor, a cholesterol-saturated methyl-β-cyclodextrin (Chol-MβCD). Treatment of cultures with Chol-MβCD (0.1 mM) blocked the DHPG-mediated neuroprotection without affecting NMDA toxicity per se (FIG. 8). These findings suggest that physiological mechanisms such as membrane cholesterol saturation could affect the group I mGluR-mediated neuroprotection. The mechanism of cholesterol action remains unknown; however, it could represent interference with the receptor endocytosis process and/or intracellular membrane traffic in general. It is not impossible then that reduction of the neuroprotection by cholesterol could contribute to the development of ischemic strokes or to their outcome.

PSYCHOTROPIC DRUG INTERACTIONS WITH NEUROPROTECTIVE mGluR SIGNALING

Psychosis is a nonspecific syndrome associated with schizophrenia, bipolar disorder, dementias, and a variety of other psychiatric or neurological conditions. Its etiopathogenesis is not yet clearly understood, but indirect evidence suggests that regulation of nerve cell loss and survival could be among the important determinants. For example, nerve cell loss has been implicated in early-onset schizophrenia[77] and epidemiological studies lend support to an idea that schizophrenia onset and severity may be associated with nerve cell susceptibility to injury.[78] This idea is further supported by findings of ventricular enlargement and hippocampal volume reduction on

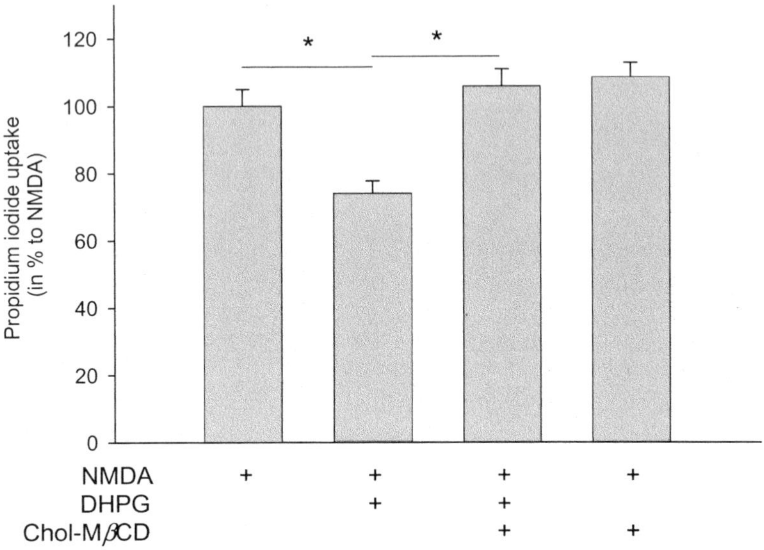

FIGURE 8. Enrichment of nerve cell membrane with cholesterol using methyl-β-cyclodextrin (Chol-MβCD) as cholesterol donor reduces DHPG-mediated neuroprotection against NMDA toxicity. Columns show the relative level of cellular death measured as cellular uptake of propidium iodide (PI). Cultures pretreated with DHPG (10 μM) for 2 h prior to exposure to 50 μM NMDA for 30 min displayed reduced PI uptake (74±3.7%, $P < 0.001$, $n = 3$ experiments, 36 cultures), compared to cultures exposed to NMDA only (100±5.0%, $n = 3$ experiments, 36 cultures). Treatment of cultures with the cholesterol-enriched medium (0.1 mM cholesterol) at 1 h prior to DHPG application and throughout the DHPG and NMDA applications abolished the protective effect of DHPG (106±5.1%, $P > 0.05$, $n = 3$ experiments, 34 cultures). The cholesterol-enriched medium did not affect the NMDA toxicity level (108±4.3%, $P > 0.05$, $n = 3$ experiments, 36 cultures). "+" indicates the presence of compounds listed on the left.

magnetic resonance images of the brain in first-onset schizophrenia patients.[79,80] It has been proposed that this loss may be caused, among other reasons, by abnormally abundant glutamatergic innervation and degeneration of fronto-temporal projections.[81]

There are several reports on antipsychotic drug interaction with the glutamatergic neurotransmitter system[82–85] and some studies indicate that novel antipsychotics could be neuroprotective in some models.[86,87] Because quetiapine is effective in suppressing symptoms of psychosis associated with a variety of conditions (schizophrenia, bipolar psychosis, dementia-associated psychosis), we used our model of NMDA-induced excitotoxic cell death in the hippocampus to examine its effects on nerve cell death.

Treatment of cultures with quetiapine (1–100 nM) for 24–96 h significantly reduced NMDA toxicity, suggesting that quetiapine may have a neuroprotective effect (FIG. 9). This effect was lost, however, after 2-h treatment of cultures with DHPG. Blockade of either mGluR1 with its selective antagonist LY367385 or mGluR5 with its antagonist MPEP did not abolish quetiapine-induced neuroprotection. Coapplica-

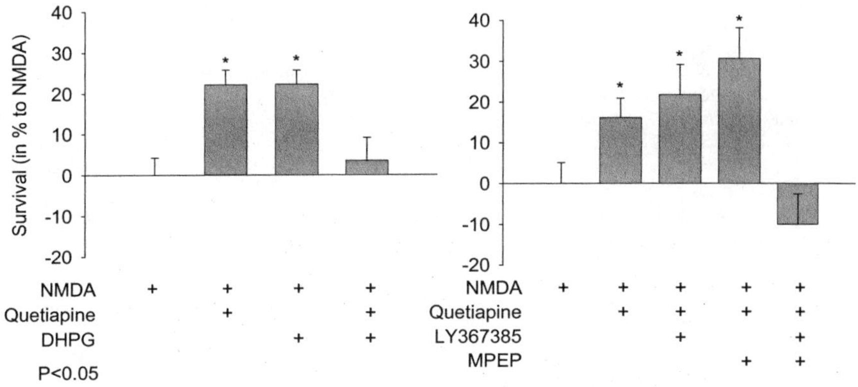

FIGURE 9. (*Left*) Application of antipsychotic quetiapine (10 nM) for 24–96 h induced a neuroprotective effect comparable to that of group I mGluR agonist DHPG (10 μM, 2 h). However, there was no neuroprotection in cultures treated with quetiapine and then subjected to DHPG treatment. (*Right*) Blockade of group I mGluR receptor 1 and 5 subtypes also abolished quetiapine neuroprotection, suggesting that the neuroprotective effect of quetiapine requires functional group I mGluR receptor to occur. "+" indicates the presence of compounds listed on the left. Each column and the vertical bars are the mean ± SEM values of PI intensity normalized to NMDA (50 nM, 30 min). Data from 2 experiments (10–12 cultures each). $*P < 0.05$, one-way analysis of variance with Bonferroni correction for multiple comparisons.

tion of both mGluR1 and 5 antagonist blockade of both mGluR1 and 5 subtypes did block the quetiapine-induced neuroprotection (FIG. 9). These findings suggest that the neuroprotective action of quetiapine may require functional group I mGluRs to occur. It remains to be established whether it contributes to the therapeutic effects of quetiapine.

CONCLUSIONS

The mechanisms of metabotropic glutamate receptor or mGluR-mediated neuroprotection are complex. They involve a multitude of seemingly unrelated pathways, of which only a minuscule portion has yet been examined. Stroke neuroprotection trials suggest that pharmacological manipulations of a single neuroprotective mechanism are generally ineffective. This study provides a rationale for clinical trials to test hypotheses of whether simultaneous manipulations of multiple mechanisms will reduce the probability of excitotoxic injury in individuals at risk.

REFERENCES

1. WOLF, P.A. 1997. Epidemiology and risk factor management. *In* Primer on Cerebrovascular Diseases. Academic Press. San Diego.

2. Gladstone, D.J., S.E. Black & A.M. Hakim. 2002. Toward wisdom from failure: lessons from neuroprotective stroke trials and new therapeutic directions. Stroke **33:** 2123–2136.
3. Choi, D.W. & S.M. Rothman. 1990. The role of glutamate neurotoxicity in hypoxic ischemic neuronal death. Annu. Rev. Neurosci. **13:** 171–182.
4. Coyle, J.T. & P. Puttfarken. 1993. Oxidative stress, glutamate, and neurodegenerative disorders. Science **262:** 689–695.
5. Muir, K.W & K.R. Lees. 1995. Clinical experience with excitatory amino acid antagonist drugs. Stroke **26:** 503–513.
6. Olney, J.W. 1969. Brain lesions, obesity, and other disturbances in mice treated with monosodium glutamate. Science **164:** 719–721.
7. Watkins, J.C. & R.H. Evans. 1981. Excitatory amino acid transmitters. Annu. Rev. Pharmacol. Toxicol. **21:** 165–204.
8. Dingledine, R. *et al.* 1999. The glutamate receptor ion channels. Pharmacol. Rev. **51:** 7–61.
9. Budd, S.L. 1998. Mechanisms of neuronal damage in brain hypoxia/ischemia: focus on the role of mitochondrial calcium accumulation. Pharmacol. Ther. **80:** 203–229.
10. Martin, L.J. *et al.* 1998. Neurodegeneration in excitotoxicity, global cerebral ischemia, and target deprivation: a perspective on the contributions of apoptosis and necrosis. Brain Res. Bull. **46:** 281–309.
11. Portera-Cailliau, C., D.L. Price & L.J. Martin. 1997. Excitotoxic neuronal death in the immature brain is an apoptosis-necrosis morphological continuum. J. Comp. Neurol. **378:** 70–87.
12. Sloviter, R.S. 2002. Apoptosis: a guide for the perplexed. Trends Pharmacol. Sci. **23:** 19–24.
13. Nitatori, T. *et al.* 1995. Delayed neuronal death in the CA1 pyramidal cell layer of the gerbil hippocampus following transient ischemia is apoptosis. J. Neurosci. **15:** 1001–1011.
14. Endres, M. *et al.* 1998. Attenuation of delayed neuronal death after mild focal ischemia in mice by inhibition of caspase family. J. Cereb. Blood Flow Metab. **18:** 238–247.
15. Sladeczek, F. *et al.* 1985. Glutamate stimulates inositol phosphate formation in striatal neurones. Nature **317:** 717–719.
16. Nicoletti, F. *et al.* 1986. Coupling of inositol phospholipid metabolism with excitatory amino acid recognition sites in rat hippocampus. J. Neurochem. **46:** 40–46.
17. Nicoletti, F. *et al.* 1986. The activation of inositol phospholipid metabolism as a signal-transducing system for excitatory amino acids in primary cultures of cerebellar granule cells. J. Neurosci. **6:** 1905–1911.
18. Baskys, A. 1994. Metabotropic Glutamate Receptors. R. G. Landes Press. Austin, TX.
19. Brauner-Osborne, H. *et al.* 2000. Ligands for glutamate receptors: design and therapeutic prospects. Med. Chem. **43:** 2609–2645.
20. Balazs, R. *et al.* 1989. *N*-Methyl-D-aspartate promotes the survival of cerebellar granule cells: pharmacological characterization. Neurosci. Lett. **101:** 241–246.
21. Marini, A.M. & S.M. Paul. 1992. *N*-Methyl-D-aspartate receptor–mediated neuroprotection in cerebellar granule cells requires new RNA and protein synthesis. Proc. Natl. Acad. Sci. USA **89:** 6555–6559.
22. Pantazis, N.J. *et al.* 1995. NMDA prevents alcohol-induced neuronal cell death of cerebellar granule cells in culture. Alcohol Clin. Exp. Res. **19:** 846–853.
23. Koh, J.Y., E. Palmer & C.W. Cotman. 1991. Activation of metabotropic glutamate receptors attenuates *N*-methyl-D-aspartate neurotoxicity in cortical cultures. Proc. Natl. Acad. Sci. USA **88:** 9431–9435.
24. Chiamulera, C. *et al.* 1992. Activation of metabotropic receptors has a neuroprotective effect in a rodent model of focal ischemia. Eur. J. Pharmacol. **216:** 335–336.
25. Opitz, T. & G. Reyman. 1993. (1*S*,3*R*)-ACPD protects synaptic transmission from hypoxia in hippocampal slices. Neuropharmacology **32:** 103–113.
26. Sagara, Y. & D. Schubert. 1998. The activation of metabotropic glutamate receptors protects nerve cells from oxidative stress. J. Neurosci. **18:** 6662–6671.

27. Schroder, U.H. *et al.* 1999. Protective effect of group I metabotropic glutamate receptor activation against hypoxic/hypoglycemic injury in rat hippocampal slices: timing and involvement of protein kinase C. Neuropharmacology **38:** 209–216.
28. Kalda, A. *et al.* 2000. Neuroprotective action of group I metabotropic glutamate receptor agonists against oxygen-glucose deprivation–induced neuronal death. Brain Res. **853:** 370–373.
29. Rebecchi, M.J. & S.N. Pentyala. 2000. Structure, function, and control of phosphoinositide-specific phospholipase C. Physiol. Rev. **80:** 1291–1335.
30. MacDonald, J.F., J.M. Wojtowicz & A. Baskys. 1996. Glutamate receptors. *In* Brain Mechanisms and Psychotropic Drugs. CRC Press. Boca Raton, FL.
31. Pellegrini-Giampietro, D.E., S.A. Torregrossa & F. Moroni. 1996. Pharmacological characterization of metabotropic glutamate receptors coupled to phospholipase D in the rat hippocampus. Br. J. Pharmacol. **118:** 1035–1043.
32. Pisani, A. *et al.* 2001. Metabotropic glutamate receptor 5 mediates the potentiation of *N*-methyl-D-aspartate responses in medium spiny striatal neurons. Neuroscience **106:** 579–587.
33. Skeberdis, V.A. *et al.* 2001. mGluR1-mediated potentiation of NMDA receptors involves a rise in intracellular calcium and activation of protein kinase C. Neuropharmacology **40:** 856–865.
34. Bandrowski, A.E. *et al.* 2001. Metabotropic glutamate receptors modify ionotropic glutamate responses in neocortical pyramidal cells and interneurons. Exp. Brain. Res. **136:** 25–40.
35. Awad, H. *et al.* 2000. Activation of metabotropic glutamate receptor 5 has direct excitatory effects and potentiates NMDA receptor currents in neurons of the subthalamic nucleus. J. Neurosci. **20:** 7871–7879.
36. O'Leary, D.M. *et al.* 2000. Selective mGluR5 antagonists MPEP and SIB-1893 decrease NMDA or glutamate-mediated neuronal toxicity through actions that reflect NMDA receptor antagonism. Br. J. Pharmacol. **131:** 1429–1437.
37. Rao, A.M., J.F. Hatcher & R.J. Dempsey. 2000. Neuroprotection by group I metabotropic glutamate receptor antagonists in forebrain ischemia of gerbil. Neurosci. Lett. **293:** 1–4.
38. Chuang, S.C. *et al.* 2001. Group I metabotropic glutamate receptors elicit epileptiform discharges in the hippocampus through PLCβ1 signaling. J. Neurosci. **21:** 6387–6394.
39. Bruno, V. *et al.* 1995. Activation of metabotropic glutamate receptors coupled to inositol phospholipid hydrolysis amplifies NMDA-induced neuronal degeneration in cultured cortical cells. Neuropharmacology **34:** 1089–1098.
40. Maiese, K. *et al.* 1995. Activation of the metabotropic glutamate receptor is neuroprotective during nitric oxide toxicity in primary hippocampal neurons of rats. Neurosci. Lett. **194:** 173–176.
41. Vincent, A.M. *et al.* 1997. Metabotropic glutamate receptors prevent nitric oxide–induced programmed cell death. J. Neurosci. Res. **50:** 549–564.
42. Vincent, A.M., M. TenBroeke & K. Maiese. 1999. Metabotropic glutamate receptors prevent programmed cell death through the modulation of neuronal endonuclease activity and intracellular pH. Exp. Neurol. **155:** 79–94.
43. Vincent, A.M. & K. Maiese. 2000. The metabotropic glutamate system promotes neuronal survival through distinct pathways of programmed cell death. Exp. Neurol. **166:** 65–82.
44. Allen, J.W., S.M. Knoblach & A.I. Faden. 2000. Activation of group I metabotropic glutamate receptors reduces neuronal apoptosis, but increases necrotic cell death *in vitro*. Cell Death Differ. **7:** 470–476.
45. Colwell, C.S., K.L. Altemus & M.S. Levine. 1996. Metabotropic glutamate receptor activation selectively limits excitotoxic damage in the intact neostriatum. Brain Res. **726:** 223–226.
46. Adamchik, Y. & A. Baskys. 2000. Glutamate-mediated neuroprotection against *N*-methyl-D-aspartate toxicity: a role for metabotropic glutamate receptors. Neuroscience **99:** 731–736.

47. BRUNO, V. *et al.* 2001. An activity-dependent switch from facilitation to inhibition in the control of excitotoxicity by group I metabotropic glutamate receptors. Eur. J. Neurosci. **13:** 1469–1478.
48. CALABRESI, P. *et al.* 2000. Is pharmacological neuroprotection dependent on reduced glutamate release? Stroke **31:** 766–772.
49. ROSSI, D.J., T. OSHIMA & D. ATTWELL. 2000. Glutamate release in severe brain ischaemia is mainly by reversed uptake. Nature **403:** 316–321.
50. BEHRENS, M.M. *et al.* 1999. Selective activation of group II mGluRs with LY354740 does not prevent neuronal excitotoxicity. Neuropharmacology **38:** 1621–1630.
51. LAFON-CAZAL, M. *et al.* 1999. mGluR7-like receptor and GABA(B) receptor activation enhance neurotoxic effects of *N*-methyl-D-aspartate in cultured mouse striatal GABAergic neurones. Neuropharmacology **38:** 1631–1640.
52. LAFON-CAZAL, M. *et al.* 1999. mGluR7-like metabotropic glutamate receptors inhibit NMDA-mediated excitotoxicity in cultured mouse cerebellar granule neurons. Eur. J. Neurosci. **11:** 663–672.
53. BLAABJERG, M., L. FANG, J. ZIMMER & A. BASKYS. 2003. Neuroprotection against NMDA excitotoxicity by group I metabotropic glutamate receptors is associated with reduction of NMDA stimulated currents. Exp. Neurol. **183:** 573–580.
54. (a) IRELAND, D.R. & W.C. ABRAHAM. 2002. Group I mGluRs increase excitability of hippocampal CA1 pyramidal neurons by a PLC-independent mechanism. J. Neurophysiol. **88:** 107–116; (b) BAYAZITOV, I.T., L. FANG & A. BASKYS. 2004. Neuroprotection by group I metabotropic glutamate receptor agonist DHPG requires activation of phospholipase C. Program no. 952.7 [online]. Abstract Viewer/Itinerary Planner. Society for Neuroscience. Washington, D.C.
55. PIZZI, M. 1996. Activation of multiple metabotropic glutamate receptor subtypes prevents NMDA-induced excitotoxicity in rat hippocampal slices. Eur. J. Neurosci. **8:** 1516–1521.
56. YU, S.P. *et al.* 1997. Membrane-delimited modulation of NMDA currents by metabotropic glutamate receptor subtypes 1/5 in cultured mouse cortical neurons. J. Physiol. **499:** 721–732.
57. SNYDER, E.M. *et al.* 2001. Internalization of ionotropic glutamate receptors in response to mGluR activation. Nat. Neurosci. **4:** 1079–1085.
58. BLAABJERG, M. *et al.* 2003. Changes in hippocampal gene expression after neuroprotective activation of group I metabotropic glutamate receptors. Mol. Brain Res. **117:** 196–205.
59. ZERIAL, M. & H. MCBRIDE. 2001. Rab proteins as membrane organizers. Nat. Rev. Mol. Cell. Biol. **2:** 107–117.
60. BASKYS, M. & M. BLAABJERG. 2005. Understanding regulation of nerve cell death by mGluRs as a method for development of successful neuroprotective strategies. J. Neurol. Sci. In press.
61. ROCHE, K.W. *et al.* 2001. Molecular determinants of NMDA receptor internalization. Nat. Neurosci. **4:** 794–802.
62. MAN, H.Y. *et al.* 2000. Regulation of AMPA receptor–mediated synaptic transmission by clathrin-dependent receptor internalization, Neuron **25:** 649–662.
63. ARNETT, A.L.H. *et al.* 2004. Antisense oligonucleotide against GTPase Rab5b inhibits metabotropic agonist DHPG-induced neuroprotection. Brain Res. **1028:** 59–65.
64. DIAS, N. & C.A. STEIN. 2002. Potential roles of antisense oligonucleotides in cancer therapy: the example of Bcl-2 antisense oligonucleotides. Eur. J. Pharm. Biopharm. **54:** 263–269.
65. BUCCI, C. *et al.* 1995. Cooperative regulation of endocytosis by three Rab5 isoforms, FEBS Lett. **366:** 65–71.
66. CHAVRIER, P., K. SIMONS & M. ZERIAL. 1992. The complexity of the Rab and Rho GTP-binding protein subfamilies revealed by a PCR cloning approach. Gene **112:** 261–264.
67. WILSON, D.B. & M.P. WILSON. 1992. Identification and subcellular localization of human Rab5b, a new member of the Ras-related superfamily of GTPases. J. Clin. Invest. **89:** 996–1005.
68. KJEKEN, R. *et al.* 2001. Fluid phase endocytosis of [^{125}I]iodixanol in rat liver parenchymal, endothelial, and Kupffer cells. Cell Tissue Res. **304:** 221–230.

69. Bavro, V.N. *et al.* 2002. Crystal structure of the GABA(A)-receptor-associated protein, GABARAP. EMBO Rep. **3:** 183–189.
70. Coyle, J.E. *et al.* 2002. Structure of GABARAP in two conformations: implications for GABA(A) receptor localization and tubulin binding. Neuron **33:** 63–74.
71. Chen, L. *et al.* 2000. The γ-aminobutyric acid type A ($GABA_A$) receptor–associated protein (GABARAP) promotes $GABA_A$ receptor clustering and modulates the channel kinetics. Proc. Natl. Acad. Sci. USA **97:** 11557–11562.
72. Kennedy, M.B. 2000. Sticking together. Proc. Natl. Acad. Sci. USA **97:** 11135–11136.
73. Kristensen, B.W., J. Noraberg & J. Zimmer. 2003. The $GABA_A$ receptor agonist THIP is neuroprotective in organotypic hippocampal slice cultures. Brain Res. **973:** 303–306.
74. Nyman-Andersen, J. *et al.* 2002. Subunit specificity and interaction domain between $GABA_A$ receptor–associated protein (GABARAP) and $GABA_A$ receptors. J. Neurochemistry **80:** 815–823.
75. Gimpl, G., K. Burger & F. Fahrenholz. 1997. Cholesterol as modulator of receptor function. Biochemistry **36:** 10959–10974.
76. Sooksawate, T. & M.A. Simmonds. 2001. Influence of membrane cholesterol on modulation of the GABA(A) receptor by neuroactive steroids and other potentiators. Br. J. Pharmacol. **134:** 1303–1311.
77. Thompson, P.M. *et al.* 2001. Mapping adolescent brain change reveals dynamic wave of accelerated gray matter loss in very early-onset schizophrenia. Proc. Natl. Acad. Sci. USA **98:** 11650–11655.
78. Seeman, M.V. 1997. Psychopathology in women and men: focus on female hormones. Am. J. Psychiatry **154:** 1641–1647.
79. Copolov, D. *et al.* 2000. Neurobiological findings in early phase schizophrenia. Brain Res. Brain Res. Rev. **31:** 157–165.
80. Lieberman, J.A. *et al.* 2002. The early stages of schizophrenia: speculations on pathogenesis, pathophysiology, and therapeutic approaches. Biol. Psychiatry **50:** 884–897. (Erratum: Biol. Psychiatry **51:** 346.)
81. Deakin, J.F. & M.D. Simpson. 1997. A two-process theory of schizophrenia: evidence from studies in post-mortem brain. J. Psychiatry Res. **31:** 277–295.
82. Geyer, M.A. 1998. Behavioral studies of hallucinogenic drugs in animals: implications for schizophrenia research. Pharmacopsychiatry **31**(suppl. 2)**:** 73–79.
83. Ninan, I., K.E. Jardemark & R.Y. Wang. 2003. Olanzapine and clozapine but not haloperidol reverse subchronic phencyclidine-induced functional hyperactivity of *N*-methyl-D-aspartate receptors in pyramidal cells of the rat medial prefrontal cortex. Neuropharmacology **44:** 462–472.
84. Tarazi, F.I. *et al.* 2003. Long-term effects of olanzapine, risperidone, and quetiapine on ionotropic glutamate receptor types: implications for antipsychotic drug treatment. J. Pharmacol. Exp. Ther. **306:** 1145–1151.
85. Kinney, G G. *et al.* 2004. A novel selective positive allosteric modulator of metabotropic glutamate receptor subtype 5 (mGluR5) has *in vivo* activity and antipsychotic-like effects in rat behavioral models. J. Pharmacol. Exp. Ther. [Epub ahead of print].
86. Li, X.M. *et al.* 1999. Differential effects of olanzapine on the gene expression of superoxide dismutase and the low affinity nerve growth factor receptor. J. Neurosci. Res. **56:** 72–75.
87. Xu, H. *et al.* 2002. Quetiapine attenuates the immobilization stress-induced decrease of brain-derived neurotrophic factor expression in rat hippocampus. Neurosci. Lett. **321:** 65–68.

Antiapoptotic and Anti-inflammatory Mechanisms of Heat-Shock Protein Protection

MIDORI A. YENARI,[a] JIALING LIU,[b] ZHEN ZHENG,[a] ZINAIDA S. VEXLER,[a,c] JONG EUN LEE,[d] AND RONA G. GIFFARD[e]

Departments of [a]Neurology, [b]Neurosurgery, and [c]Pediatrics, University of California, San Francisco, and San Francisco Veterans Affairs Medical Center, San Francisco, California, USA

[d]Department of Anatomy and BK21 Project, Yonsei University, Seoul, Korea

[e]Department of Anesthesia, Stanford University School of Medicine, Stanford, California, USA

ABSTRACT: We and others have previously shown that heat-shock proteins (HSPs) are involved in protecting the brain from a variety of insults including stroke, epilepsy, and other related insults. While the mechanism of this protection has largely been thought to be due to their chaperone functions (i.e., preventing abnormal protein folding or aggregation), recent work has shown that HSPs may also directly interfere with other cell death pathways such as apoptosis and inflammation. Using models of cerebral ischemic and ischemia-like injury, we overexpressed the 70-kDa heat-shock protein (HSP70) using gene transfer or by studying a transgenic mouse model. HSP70 protected neurons and astrocytes from experimental stroke and stroke-like insults. HSP70 transgenic mice also had better neurological scores following experimental stroke compared to their wild-type littermates. Overexpressing HSP70 was associated with less apoptotic cell death and increased expression of the antiapoptotic protein, Bcl-2. Furthermore, HSP70 suppressed microglial/monocyte activation following experimental stroke. HSP70 overexpression also led to the reduction of matrix metalloproteinases. We suggest that HSPs are capable of protecting brain cells from lethal insults through a variety of mechanisms and should be explored as a potential therapy against stroke and other neurodegenerative diseases.

KEYWORDS: heat-shock proteins; neuroprotection; apoptosis; cerebral ischemia; inflammation

INTRODUCTION

The stress response results in gene expression following such environmental challenges such as high temperatures, ischemia, excitotoxin exposure, and other stresses that result in protein denaturation (see refs. 1 and 2). Inducible heat-shock

Address for correspondence: Midori A. Yenari, M.D., University of California, San Francisco, and San Francisco VAMC, Neurology (127), 4150 Clement Street, San Francisco, CA 94121. Voice: 415-750-2011; fax: 415-750-2273.
yenari@alum.mit.edu

Ann. N.Y. Acad. Sci. 1053: 74–83 (2005). © 2005 New York Academy of Sciences.
doi: 10.1196/annals.1344.007

proteins (HSPs) are induced by stressful stimuli and are thought to assist in the maintenance of cellular integrity and viability, and HSPs are thought to prevent protein denaturation and incorrect polypeptide aggregation during exposure to physiochemical insults. However, they are also involved in antigen presentation, steroid receptor function, intracellular trafficking, nuclear receptor binding, and apoptosis,[3,4] making it clear that they may also be involved in various cell signaling pathways.

In the nervous system, the HSPs are induced in a variety of pathologic states, including cerebral ischemia, neurodegenerative diseases, epilepsy, and trauma. Expression has been detected in a variety of cell populations within the nervous system, including neurons, glia, and endothelial cells.[5] Although the 70-kDa heat-shock protein (HSP70) has been long thought to protect cells by preserving tertiary protein structure and preventing protein aggregation, direct evidence has been lacking. Gene transfer techniques and transgenic animal strains have now made it possible to selectively overexpress HSPs to better understand the precise role they play in cellular injury. This review will focus on recent findings that help to elucidate new roles of HSP70 in neuroprotection.

NEUROPROTECTION WITH HSP70 OVEREXPRESSION

Several studies have been published showing that HSP70 can protect against numerous stresses, including heat shock,[6] oxidative stress,[7] apoptotic stimuli,[8,9] and ischemia.[10,11] In the nervous system, HSP70 overexpression in cultured hippocampal[12,13] and peripheral[14–17] neurons and glia[14,15] can also protect against insults such as heat shock and metabolic stresses. Conversely, when HSP70 expression is suppressed using antisense oligonucleotides, protection from induced tolerance could be reversed with HSP70 blockade.[18]

HSP70 is also effective against cerebral ischemic and ischemia-like insults such as oxygen-glucose deprivation (OGD),[19,20] excitotoxin exposure,[13] or exposure to chemical ischemia.[17] At the *in vivo* level, HSP70 overexpression using a herpes simplex viral vector led to improved striatal neuron survival following transient middle cerebral artery occlusion,[21] and this protection could be observed even if gene transfer occurred hours after injury onset.[22] Robust protection against permanent middle cerebral artery occlusion has also been observed in a transgenic mouse model of HSP70 overexpression.[23] HSP70 appears to protect against global cerebral ischemia as well using gene transfer to hippocampal or striatal neurons in rodents.[24,25] Conversely, mice deficient in HSP70 also have increased infarct size and worsened outcome after experimental stroke.[26]

POTENTIAL MECHANISMS OF PROTECTION

The mechanism of protection with HSP70 has largely been believed to be related to its chaperone functions, leading to prevention of protein malfolding and aggregation. Following both focal[27] and global[28] cerebral ischemia, protein aggregates have been described within vulnerable cell populations. HSPs appear to interfere with the formation of such aggregates following global cerebral ischemia.[2] However, HSPs may protect by mechanisms unrelated to their chaperone function as well. Here, we review mechanisms of HSP70 protection as they pertain to the broad areas of apoptosis and inflammation.

HSP70 and Apoptosis

Recent studies in nonneuronal cell lines have shown that HSP70's protective effect may also be due to antiapoptotic mechanisms. Apoptosis, or programmed cell death, is known to occur in pathological states either by activation of specific death receptors or internally via mitochondrial release of cytochrome c. Central to mitochondria-based apoptosis is the assembly of the so-called apoptosome. This occurs when procaspase-9 binds to apoptosis protease activating factor-1 (Apaf-1) in the cytosol and becomes activated when cytochrome c is released from the mitochondria to the cytosol. This release of cytochrome c is blocked by the antiapoptotic protein, Bcl-2. Activated caspase-9 then leads to activation of various effector caspases including caspase-3. Caspase-independent pathways have also been identified via apoptosis inducing factor (AIF).[29] Under appropriate conditions, AIF is released from the mitochondria and translocates to the nucleus, where apoptosis occurs in the absence of caspase activation. Like cytochrome c, AIF release can also be antagonized by Bcl-2.[30] Other mediators of apoptosis include second mitochondria-derived activator of caspases (Smac)/direct inhibitor-of-apoptosis protein (IAP)–binding protein with low pI, which is also released from the mitochondria and reverses apoptosomal inhibition by IAPs (FIG. 1).

Several papers have now established that HSPs can interfere with apoptosis at various points in the death cascade (FIG. 1). Overexpression of HSP70 in lymphoid tumor cell lines appears to inhibit apoptosis by blocking caspase activation and activity.[6,31,32] It has recently been shown that HSP70 can inhibit caspase activation by interfering with Apaf-1 and prevent the recruitment of procaspase-9 to the apoptosome.[33,34] How this occurs is not yet clear, but has been hypothesized to be due to a direct competition between HSP70 and procaspase-9 for Apaf-1 binding.[33–35] However, Mosser *et al.*[6] demonstrated that HSP70 did not appear to interfere with caspase-3 processing, and other data suggest that HSP70 interferes with apoptosis downstream of caspase activation.[8] Yet other studies in tumor cell lines have shown that HSP70 may block stress kinase (SAPK/JNK) activation when HSP70 overexpression is induced.[6] HSP70 also appears to prevent chromatin condensation independent of Apaf-1, and specifically interacts with AIF.[36] However, HSPs do not appear to block Fas-mediated, receptor-activated apoptosis.[35,37] Together, these studies suggest that HSP70 probably acts at multiple sites to confer protection in models of apoptosis.

Recent studies now indicate that HSP70 can also prevent apoptosis from occurring in the brain. Cells with DNA fragmentation (detected by DNA nick end labeling) following focal cerebral ischemia rarely express HSP70 protein,[38] and transgenic mice overexpressing HSP70 have fewer apoptotic cells and less DNA laddering.[39] This was also associated with less cytochrome c release. Consistent with observations in cell-free systems,[36] recent data in an *in vivo* model of neonatal hypoxia/ischemia indicate that HSP70 is not only protective, but also binds and sequesters AIF.[40] Interestingly, even though HSP70 overexpression prevented both cytochrome c and AIF translocation, it did not appear to have any effect on Smac/DIABLO, which remained in the mitochondria up to 24 h after the hypoxic/ischemic insult, even

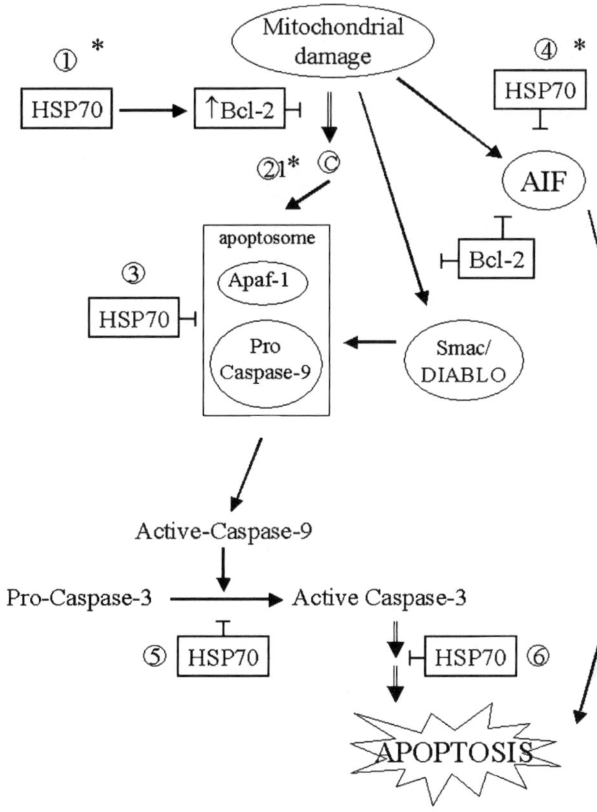

FIGURE 1. Protection from apoptosis by HSP70. HSP70 appears to have effects at several different steps in the apoptosis death cascade. Apoptosis can be activated via mitochondrial damage, leading to cytosolic release of cytochrome c (C). Cytochrome c then activates complexes of procaspase-9 and Apaf-1 (which constitute the so-called apoptosome), leading to activation of caspase-9. Caspase-9 then activates caspase-3, an effector caspase that triggers downstream enzymes to execute DNA damage. Mitochondria also release other apoptogenic factors such as Smac/DIABLO and AIF. Smac/DIABLO is thought to promote apoptosis by reversing inhibitors of apoptosis proteins (IAPs), which prevent activation of the apoptosome. AIF can also cause apoptosis in the absence of caspase activation. Once released from the mitochondria, AIF translocates to the nucleus and leads to chromatin condensation. The antiapoptotic protein, Bcl-2, has been shown to antagonize mitochondrial release of all of these factors. HSP70 appears to interfere with these pathways at multiple sites. HSP70 can increase Bcl-2 expression[25] (1) and can inhibit cytochrome c release[60] (2). HSP70 has also been shown to interfere with Apaf-1 to prevent recruitment of procaspase-9 into the apoptosome[33,34] (3), and also binds to and sequesters AIF (4).[36,40] Finally, HSP70 has been shown to interfere with caspase-3 both immediately upstream (5)[6] and at an unknown point downstream of caspase activation (6).[8] Interestingly, HSP70 does not appear to influence mitochondrial release of Smac/DIABLO.[40] *Asterisks* indicate points in the cascade where HSP70 has been shown to inhibit events following cerebral ischemia.

when cytochrome c and AIF were already released. HSP70 also appears to have upstream antiapoptotic effects as well. Following viral vector–mediated HSP70 overexpression, HSP70 was also associated with increased levels of Bcl-2 protein.[25] In this scenario, it is conceivable that HSPs, by an as yet unknown mechanism, could increase Bcl-2 expression, which in turn could block cytochrome c and AIF release and effector caspase activation.

HSP70 and Inflammation

HSP70 may also alter other proteins or genes known to be involved in inflammatory responses. It is now known that the immune response is, in part, regulated by the transcription factor, nuclear factor kappa B (NFκB)[41] (FIG. 2). Normally found in the cytosol and bound to its inhibitory protein, IκB, NFκB is activated by a variety of factors including ischemia, oxidative stress, and endotoxin exposure. This leads to activation of the IκB kinase (IKK), of which there are three isoforms (α, β, γ), which phosphorylates IκB, allowing degradation by the proteasome, and liberates NFκB to translocate to the nucleus where it can bind to its consensus sequences. Many genes involved in the inflammatory response are rapidly activated in this manner. These genes include iNOS, the inflammatory cytokines TNF and IL-1, inducible cyclooxygenase (COX-2), chemokines, and adhesion molecules. NFκB also induces IκB, leading to its own downregulation.

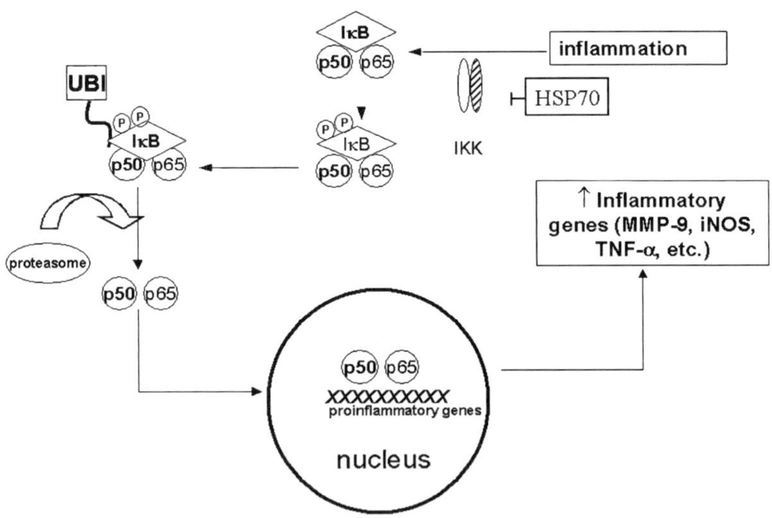

FIGURE 2. Interaction of HSP70 and NFκB: NFκB normally exists in the cytosol as heterodimer consisting of p50 and p65 subunits. It is tethered to this compartment by its inhibitor protein, IκB. When challenged by an appropriate inflammatory stimulus, IKK phosphorylates IκB, allowing IκB ubiquitination (UBI) and degradation in the proteasome. This liberates NFκB to enter the nucleus and bind to its DNA consensus sequence, leading to upregulation of various inflammatory genes. HSP70 overexpression in various model systems has been shown to inhibit inflammatory responses by preventing NFκB activation, by interfering with IKK activity.[45]

Others have shown that prior thermal stress leads to inhibition of the inflammatory response, and this inhibition was associated with increased levels of HSP70 induction and decreased nuclear NFκB translocation.[42,43] It has been speculated that HSP70 could interact with NFκB's inhibitor protein, IκB, and prevent IκB phosphorylation and NFκB dissociation.[44] A recent study by Ran *et al.*[45] showed that HSP70 can, in fact, interact with IKK, thereby preventing IκB's phosphorylation and activation.

Various studies indicate that HSP70 also has anti-inflammatory effects in pathologically relevant settings. Prior induction of HSP70 decreases the release of inflammatory mediators in a porcine model of recurrent endotoxemia,[46] protects against TNF–induced lethal inflammatory shock,[47] and attenuates the cardiopulmonary bypass–induced inflammatory response.[48] Overexpression of HSP70 inhibits bacterial endotoxin (LPS, lipopolysaccharide)–induced production of cytokines[49] and ameliorates experimental acute respiratory distress syndrome.[50] Induction of HSP70 by heat stress in peripheral leukocytes has also been shown to reduce NADPH oxidase (a major enzyme involved in inflammatory cell generation of superoxide) and increase superoxide dismutase, an endogenous antioxidant.[51] Conversely, inhibition of HSP70 expression by antisense HSP70 partially reverses such anti-inflammatory functions.[49,52,53] These anti-inflammatory properties of HSP70 are thought to be due, in part, to inhibition of NFκB.[43,48,54,55] Feinstein and colleagues[55] showed that glial cells exposed to heat shock or transfected with HSP70 followed by stimulation with LPS experienced less nuclear NFκB translocation and consequently less inducible nitric oxide synthase (iNOS) expression, an NFκB -regulated gene. Meng and Harken[54] reported that HSP70 induction in monocytes or during myocardial ischemia led to reduced upregulation of yet another NFκB-regulated gene, the inflammatory cytokine TNF-α. Similarly, in a model of brain inflammation, heat stress led to less microglial/macrophage activation and NFκB activity.[43]

Whether HSP70 plays an anti-inflammatory role in brain ischemia has not been extensively studied. Soriano and colleagues have documented HSP70 expression in microglia following experimental stroke.[56] Our labs recently showed that matrix metalloproteinase-9 (MMP-9), one of several genes regulated by NFκB, was reduced in cultured HSP70-overexpressing astrocytes exposed to OGD.[57] Consistent with the notion that HSP70 may regulate inflammatory protein expression at the transcriptional level, MMP-9 mRNA was also lower in HSP70-transfected cells.

Preliminary data in our lab now links an anti-inflammatory role for HSP70 in brain ischemia. After replicating earlier findings that HSP70 transgenic mice subjected to 2-h middle cerebral artery occlusion (MCAO) have smaller infarcts compared to wild-type mice,[23] we examined brain sections for microglia/monocytes and MHC class II antigen and found that HSP70 transgenic mice had fewer activated microglia compared to wild-type mice.[58] This was also associated with fewer ischemic brain cells in which NFκB had translocated to the nucleus. Furthermore, HSP70 overexpression in inflammatory cells is also protective. Using cocultures of astrocytes and microglia, it is possible to mix and match transgenic and wild-type cells. When we cultured transgenic or wild-type microglia with wild-type astrocytes, and exposed them to hydrogen peroxide, we found that cultures containing HSP70 transgenic microglia suffered less injury following hydrogen peroxide exposure than wild-type microglia cultured with wild-type astrocytes.[59] These data suggest that HSP70 in inflammatory cells reduces their cytotoxicity. However, the mechanism of this observed protection is unknown. It is likely that HSP70 prevents inflammatory cell generation of one or more cytotoxic mediators. Work by others suggests that, following inflammatory cell stimulation by bacterial endotoxin, substances such as nitric oxide[55] and inflammatory cytokines[49] are reduced in the presence of HSP70. Whether this is also the case for ischemic and ischemia-like insults is still unknown.

CONCLUSIONS

Recent studies from different laboratories have now established that the stress response provides the organism with a cellular process for self-preservation and that stress proteins themselves can directly protect cells from death. The specific mechanisms underlying this protection indicate that they are likely multifactorial, encompassing a wide range of cellular chaperone functions from the prevention of protein aggregation to interfering with various death cascades, including apoptosis and inflammation. Capitalizing on the cell's natural response to stress is an attractive therapeutic target for a variety of nervous system diseases.

ACKNOWLEDGMENTS

This work was funded in part by National Institutes of Health Grants NS40516 (M. A. Yenari), GM49831 (R. G. Giffard), NS40469 (J. Liu), NS44025 (Z. S. Vexler), NS35902 (Z. S. Vexler), and P01 NS37520 (R. G. Giffard and M. A. Yenari); American Heart Association (AHA) Established Investigator Award 0540066N (M. A. Yenari) and AHA SDG003007 (J. Liu); AHA Western States Affiliate Postdoctoral Fellowship 0325089Y (Z. Zheng); Korea Research Foundation Grant KRF-2001-FP0009 (J. E. Lee); and the Department of Veterans Affairs Merit Review Program (J. Liu). The authors would like to thank Donna Ferriero and Phillip Weinstein for guidance and support, and Beth Hoyte for assistance with the figures. The authors declare that they have no competing financial interests.

REFERENCES

1. Sharp, F.R., S.M. Massa & R.A. Swanson. 1999. Heat-shock protein protection. Trends Neurosci. **22:** 97–99.
2. Giffard, R.G. *et al.* 2004. Chaperones, protein aggregation, and brain protection from hypoxic/ischemic injury. J. Exp. Biol. **207:** 3213–3220.
3. Kiang, J.G. & G.C. Tsokos. 1998. Heat shock protein 70 kDa: molecular biology, biochemistry, and physiology. Pharmacol. Ther. **80:** 183–201.
4. Giffard, R.G. & M.A. Yenari. 2004. Many mechanisms for hsp70 protection from cerebral ischemia. J. Neurosurg. Anesthesiol. **16:** 53–61.
5. Foster, J.A. & I.R. Brown. 1997. Differential induction of heat shock mRNA in oligodendrocytes, microglia, and astrocytes following hyperthermia. Brain Res. Mol. Brain Res. **45:** 207–218.
6. Mosser, D.D. *et al.* 1997. Role of the human heat shock protein hsp70 in protection against stress-induced apoptosis. Mol. Cell. Biol. **17:** 5317–5327.
7. Bellmann, K. *et al.* 1996. Heat shock protein hsp70 overexpression confers resistance against nitric oxide. FEBS Lett. **391:** 185–188.

8. JAATTELA, M. *et al.* 1998. Hsp70 exerts its anti-apoptotic function downstream of caspase-3-like proteases. EMBO J. **17:** 6124–6134.
9. BUZZARD, K.A. *et al.* 1998. Heat shock protein 72 modulates pathways of stress-induced apoptosis. J. Biol. Chem. **273:** 17147–17153.
10. MESTRIL, R. *et al.* 1994. Expression of inducible stress protein 70 in rat heart myogenic cells confers protection against simulated ischemia-induced injury. J. Clin. Invest. **93:** 759–767.
11. WILLIAMS, R.S. *et al.* 1993. Human heat shock protein 70 (hsp70) protects murine cells from injury during metabolic stress. J. Clin. Invest. **92:** 503–508.
12. BEAUCAMP, N. *et al.* 1998. Overexpression of hsp70i facilitates reactivation of intracellular proteins in neurones and protects them from denaturing stress. FEBS Lett. **441:** 215–219.
13. FINK, S.L. *et al.* 1997. Defective herpes simplex virus vectors expressing the rat brain stress-inducible heat shock protein 72 protect cultured neurons from severe heat shock. J. Neurochem. **68:** 961–969.
14. UNEY, J.B. *et al.* 1993. Transfection-mediated expression of human Hsp70i protects rat dorsal root ganglion neurones and glia from severe heat stress. FEBS Lett. **334:** 313–316.
15. UNEY, J.B. *et al.* 1994. Transfection with hsp70i protects rat dorsal root ganglia neurones and glia from heat stress. Gene Ther. **1**(suppl. 1)**:** S65.
16. MAILHOS, C., M.K. HOWARD & D.S. LATCHMAN. 1994. Heat shock proteins hsp90 and hsp70 protect neuronal cells from thermal stress, but not from programmed cell death. J. Neurochem. **63:** 1787–1795.
17. WAGSTAFF, M.J. *et al.* 1998. Delivery of a constitutively active form of the heat shock factor using a virus vector protects neuronal cells from thermal or ischaemic stress, but not from apoptosis. Eur. J. Neurosci. **10:** 3343–3350.
18. SATO, K., H. SAITO & N. MATSUKI. 1996. HSP70 is essential to the neuroprotective effect of heat-shock. Brain Res. **740:** 117–123.
19. PAPADOPOULOS, M.C. *et al.* 1996. Over-expression of HSP-70 protects against combined oxygen-glucose deprivation. Neuroreport **7:** 429–432.
20. LEE, J. *et al.* 2001. Differential neuroprotection from human heat shock protein 70 overexpression in *in vitro* and *in vivo* models of ischemia and ischemia-like conditions. Exp. Neurol. **170:** 129–139.
21. YENARI, M.A. *et al.* 1998. Gene therapy with HSP72 is neuroprotective in rat models of stroke and epilepsy. Ann. Neurol. **44:** 584–591.
22. HOEHN, B. *et al.* 2001. Overexpression of HSP72 after induction of experimental stroke protects neurons from ischemic damage. J. Cereb. Blood Flow Metab. **21:** 1303–1309.
23. RAJDEV, S. *et al.* 2000. Mice overexpressing rat heat shock protein 70 are protected against cerebral infarction. Ann. Neurol. **47:** 782–791.
24. KELLY, S., J.B. UNEY & J. MCCULLOCH. 2001. Adenovirus HSP70 gene transfer ameliorates damage following global ischaemia. J. Cereb. Blood Flow Metab. **21:** S23.
25. KELLY, S. *et al.* 2002. Gene transfer of HSP72 protects cornu ammonis 1 region of the hippocampus neurons from global ischemia: influence of Bcl-2. Ann. Neurol. **52:** 160–167.
26. LEE, S.H. *et al.* 2001. Targeted hsp70.1 disruption increases infarction volume after focal cerebral ischemia in mice. Stroke **32:** 2905–2912.
27. HU, B.R. *et al.* 2001. Protein aggregation after focal brain ischemia and reperfusion. J. Cereb. Blood Flow Metab. **21:** 865–875.
28. HU, B.R. *et al.* 2000. Protein aggregation after transient cerebral ischemia. J. Neurosci. **20:** 3191–3199.
29. SUSIN, S.A. *et al.* 1999. Molecular characterization of mitochondrial apoptosis-inducing factor. Nature **397:** 441–446.
30. ZHAO, H. *et al.* 2004. Bcl-2 transfection via herpes simplex virus blocks apoptosis-inducing factor translocation after focal ischemia in the rat. J. Cereb. Blood Flow Metab. **24:** 681–692.
31. GABAI, V.L. *et al.* 1997. Hsp70 prevents activation of stress kinases: a novel pathway of cellular thermotolerance. J. Biol. Chem. **272:** 18033–18037.

32. GABAI, V.L. *et al.* 1998. Role of Hsp70 in regulation of stress-kinase JNK: implications in apoptosis and aging. FEBS Lett. **438:** 1–4.
33. SALEH, A. *et al.* 2000. Negative regulation of the Apaf-1 apoptosome by Hsp70. Nat. Cell Biol. **2:** 476–483.
34. BEERE, H.M. *et al.* 2000. Heat-shock protein 70 inhibits apoptosis by preventing recruitment of procaspase-9 to the Apaf-1 apoptosome. Nat. Cell Biol. **2:** 469–475.
35. BEERE, H.M. & D.R. GREEN. 2001. Stress management—heat shock protein-70 and the regulation of apoptosis. Trends Cell Biol. **11:** 6–10.
36. RAVAGNAN, L. *et al.* 2001. Heat-shock protein 70 antagonizes apoptosis-inducing factor. Nat. Cell Biol. **3:** 839–843.
37. CREAGH, E.M. & T.G. COTTER. 1999. Selective protection by hsp 70 against cytotoxic drug-, but not Fas-induced T-cell apoptosis. Immunology **97:** 36–44.
38. STATES, B.A. *et al.* 1996. DNA fragmentation and HSP70 protein induction in hippocampus and cortex occurs in separate neurons following permanent middle cerebral artery occlusions. J. Cereb. Blood Flow Metab. **16:** 1165–1175.
39. TSUCHIYA, D. *et al.* 2003. Overexpression of rat heat shock protein 70 is associated with reduction of early mitochondrial cytochrome c release and subsequent DNA fragmentation after permanent focal ischemia. J. Cereb. Blood Flow Metab. **23:** 718–727.
40. MATSUMORI, Y. *et al.* 2005. Hsp70 overexpression sequesters AIF and reduces neonatal hypoxic/ischemic brain injury. J. Cereb. Blood Flow Metab. **25**(7)**:** 899–910.
41. BARNES, P.J. & M. KARIN. 1997. Nuclear factor-kappaB: a pivotal transcription factor in chronic inflammatory diseases. N. Engl. J. Med. **336:** 1066–1071.
42. GUZHOVA, I.V. *et al.* 1997. Major stress protein Hsp70 interacts with NF-kB regulatory complex in human T-lymphoma cells. Cell Stress Chaperones **2:** 132–139.
43. HENEKA, M.T. *et al.* 2000. The heat shock response inhibits NF-kappaB activation, nitric oxide synthase type 2 expression, and macrophage/microglial activation in brain. J. Cereb. Blood Flow Metab. **20:** 800–811.
44. FEINSTEIN, D.L., E. GALEA & D.J. REIS. 1997. Suppression of glial nitric oxide synthase induction by heat shock: effects on proteolytic degradation of IkappaB-alpha. Nitric Oxide **1:** 167–176.
45. RAN, R. *et al.* 2004. Hsp70 promotes TNF-mediated apoptosis by binding IKK gamma and impairing NF-kappa B survival signaling. Genes Dev. **18:** 1466–1481.
46. KLOSTERHALFEN, B. *et al.* 1996. Influence of heat shock protein 70 and metallothionein induction by zinc-bis-(DL-hydrogenaspartate) on the release of inflammatory mediators in a porcine model of recurrent endotoxemia. Biochem. Pharmacol. **52:** 1201–1210.
47. VAN MOLLE, W. *et al.* 2002. HSP70 protects against TNF-induced lethal inflammatory shock. Immunity **16:** 685–695.
48. HAYASHI, Y. *et al.* 2002. Preoperative glutamine administration induces heat-shock protein 70 expression and attenuates cardiopulmonary bypass–induced inflammatory response by regulating nitric oxide synthase activity. Circulation **106:** 2601–2607.
49. DING, X.Z. *et al.* 2001. Over-expression of hsp-70 inhibits bacterial lipopolysaccharide-induced production of cytokines in human monocyte-derived macrophages. Cytokine **16:** 210–219.
50. WEISS, Y.G. *et al.* 2002. Adenoviral transfer of HSP-70 into pulmonary epithelium ameliorates experimental acute respiratory distress syndrome. J. Clin. Invest. **110:** 801–806.
51. POLLA, B.S. *et al.* 1995. Differential induction of stress proteins and functional effects of heat shock in human phagocytes. Inflammation **19:** 363–378.
52. SCHROEDER, S. *et al.* 1999. Endotoxin inhibits heat shock protein 70 (HSP70) expression in peripheral blood mononuclear cells of patients with severe sepsis. Intensive Care Med. **25:** 52–57.
53. BHAGAT, L. *et al.* 2000. Heat shock protein 70 prevents secretagogue-induced cell injury in the pancreas by preventing intracellular trypsinogen activation. J. Clin. Invest. **106:** 81–89.
54. MENG, X. & A.H. HARKEN. 2002. The interaction between Hsp70 and TNF-alpha expression: a novel mechanism for protection of the myocardium against post-injury depression. Shock **17:** 345–353.

55. FEINSTEIN, D.L. *et al.* 1996. Heat shock protein 70 suppresses astroglial-inducible nitric-oxide synthase expression by decreasing NFkappaB activation. J. Biol. Chem. **271:** 17724–17732.
56. SORIANO, M.A. *et al.* 1994. Early 72-kDa heat shock protein induction in microglial cells following focal ischemia in the rat brain. Neurosci. Lett. **182:** 205–207.
57. LEE, J.E. *et al.* 2004. The 70 kDa heat shock protein suppresses matrix metalloproteinases in astrocytes. Neuroreport **15:** 499–502.
58. ZHENG, Z. *et al.* 2004. Overexpression of the 70-kD heat shock protein in transgenic mice attenuates glial cell activation and nuclear translocation of the transcription factor, NK(kappa)B [abstract]. Stroke **35:** 275.
59. ZAMBRANO, G. *et al.* 2004. Influence of the 70 kD heat shock protein in astrocytes and microglia under injury conditions [abstract]. J. Neurochem. **90:** 60.
60. CREAGH, E.M., R.J. CARMODY & T.G. COTTER. 2000. Heat shock protein 70 inhibits caspase-dependent and -independent apoptosis in Jurkat T cells. Exp. Cell Res. **257:** 58–66.

Neuroprotection by NGF in the PC12 *In Vitro* OGD Model

Involvement of Mitogen-Activated Protein Kinases and Gene Expression

RINAT TABAKMAN,[a] HAO JIANG,[b] IRIS SHAHAR,[c] HADAR ARIEN-ZAKAY,[a] ROBERT A. LEVINE,[b] AND PHILIP LAZAROVICI[a]

[a]*Department of Pharmacology and Experimental Therapeutics, School of Pharmacy, Faculty of Medicine, The Hebrew University of Jerusalem, Jerusalem 91120, Israel*

[b]*William T. Gossett Neurology Laboratories, Henry Ford Health System, Detroit, Michigan 48202, USA*

[c]*Functional Genomics Unit, Sheba Medical Center, Tel Hashomer 52621, Israel*

ABSTRACT: Neurodegenerative disorders and chronic disability due to stroke in the brain or spinal cord afflict a large sector of the population. To investigate the mechanism involved in ischemic stroke and to develop neuroprotective drugs/therapies, *in vivo* and *in vitro*, pharmacological models are needed. To investigate the cellular and molecular neuroprotective mechanisms of nerve growth factor (NGF), a member of the nervous system neurotrophin family of growth factors, under ischemia, we used an oxygen-glucose-deprivation (OGD) device and pheochromocytoma PC12 cells exposed to a paradigm of ischemic insult. Pretreatment of the cultures with 50 ng/mL of NGF, 18 h prior to OGD insult, conferred 30% of neuroprotection. Time-course experiments showed marked activation of the ERK, JNK, and p-38 MAPK isoforms during the OGD phase, but not during OGD reperfusion. Pretreatment of the cultures with 50 ng/mL of NGF, 18 h prior to OGD insult, resulted in 50% attenuation of OGD-induced activation of JNK 1, and 20% and 50% attenuation of OGD-induced activation of p-38 α and β, respectively. The effect of NGF on gene expression in the PC12 ischemic model using Affymatrix Rat DNA–Microarray technology indicates that only 6% of the genes are differentially regulated (induced/suppressed) by OGD insult and/or NGF. These findings support the notion that pretreatment with NGF confers neuroprotection from OGD insult, a phenomenon coincidentally related to differential inhibition of MAPK stress kinase isoforms and differential gene expression. This ischemic model may be useful to investigate molecular mechanisms of OGD-induced neurotoxicity and NGF-induced neuroprotection, and to generate novel therapeutic concepts for stroke treatment.

KEYWORDS: NGF; PC12; ischemia; neuroprotection; MAPK; gene expression

Address for correspondence: Prof. Philip Lazarovici, Ph.D., Department of Pharmacology and Experimental Therapeutics, School of Pharmacy, Faculty of Medicine, The Hebrew University of Jerusalem, Jerusalem 91120, Israel. Voice: +972-2-6758729, +972-2-6758767; fax: +972-2-6757490.

lazph@md.huji.ac.il; pl57@drexel.edu

**Ann. N.Y. Acad. Sci. 1053: 84–96 (2005). © 2005 New York Academy of Sciences.
doi: 10.1196/annals.1344.008**

STROKE AND ISCHEMIA

Stroke refers to the neurological condition that develops when a part of the whole brain is deprived of oxygen and glucose. In 70–80% of the cases, the precipitating cause is a blood clot that blocks the supply of oxygenated blood to a region of the brain, a situation termed ischemic stroke.

The damage caused to the neurons during ischemia is due to a reduction in oxygen and glucose supply—that is, oxygen and glucose deprivation (OGD).[1,2] Insults to the brain that interrupt its blood supply, as in ischemia, or its oxygen supply, as in hypoxia (>1% O_2) and anoxia (0% O_2), combined with a massive reduction in glucose supply (hypoglycemia), lead to rapid neuronal death.[3,4] The precise mechanism of neuronal cell death is not clear, but it is believed that apoptosis is one of the mechanisms involved in ischemic cell death.[5]

In Vitro *Ischemic Models*

In vitro models of cerebral ischemia may yield information, not possible *in vivo*, at a cellular and molecular level on the pharmacological properties of new drugs. The majority of *in vitro* cellular models, for ischemic investigation, include excitatory neurons. Very few attempts have been made to investigate the effect of ischemia on dopaminergic neurons. This aspect is very important since dopaminergic neurons degenerate during intrauterine embryo asphyxia and in brain substantia nigra, inducing the pathological syndrome named status marmoratus.[6]

PC12 Cells: A Neuronal Dopaminergic In Vitro *Model for Investigating Ischemic Insults*

Pheochromocytoma PC12 cells are a common dopaminergic neuronal model[7] for *in vitro* studies of cell death. PC12 cells are small, round, catecholamine-containing cells, with a doubling time of 48–96 h, that grow in regular serum-supplemented medium (FIG. 1). PC12 cells were cloned from a solid pheochromocytoma tumor passaged subcutaneously in New England Deaconess Hospital Strain white rats.[8]

Upon treatment with nerve growth factor (NGF), PC12 cells stop dividing and initiate the differentiation process expressed by electrical excitability and an increased expression of cholinergic receptors and other differentiation markers.[7] Unlike the adrenal medulla chromaffin cells, in which norepinephrine is the major catecholamine, the PC12 cells contain primarily dopamine (FIG. 1C, orange color). The enzymes required for the synthesis of catecholamines are also abundant in PC12 cells (FIG. 1D, green color).

PC12 cells serve as the prime dopaminergic cellular tool in molecular neuroscience for investigating the NGF mechanism of action,[9] under different insults. PC12 cells have served as cellular models of serum starvation,[10] NGF deprivation,[11,12] excitotoxicity,[13] cytotoxicity,[14] Parkinson's disease,[15] Alzheimer's disease,[16] and ischemia.[17–19] These models are also useful systems for exploring neuroprotective drugs.[20,21]

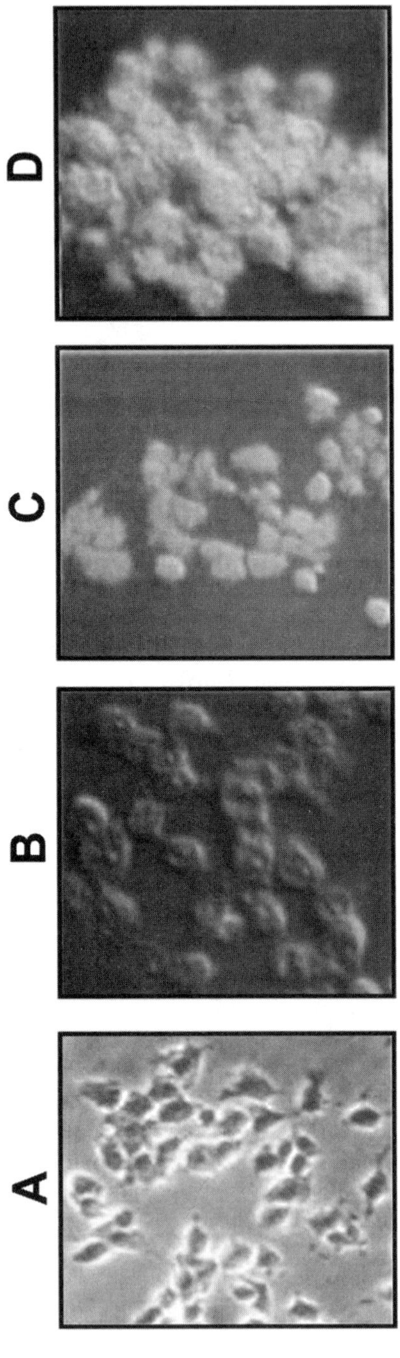

FIGURE 1. Micrographs showing morphological and dopaminergic characteristics of PC12 cells: **(A)** light microscopy (magnification: ×200); **(B)** confocal microscopy (magnification: ×600); **(C)** immunohistochemical staining using antidopamine antibody (confocal view; magnification: ×200); **(D)** immunohistochemical staining using antidopamine hydroxylase antibody (confocal view; magnification: ×600). [Figure reduced to 78%.]

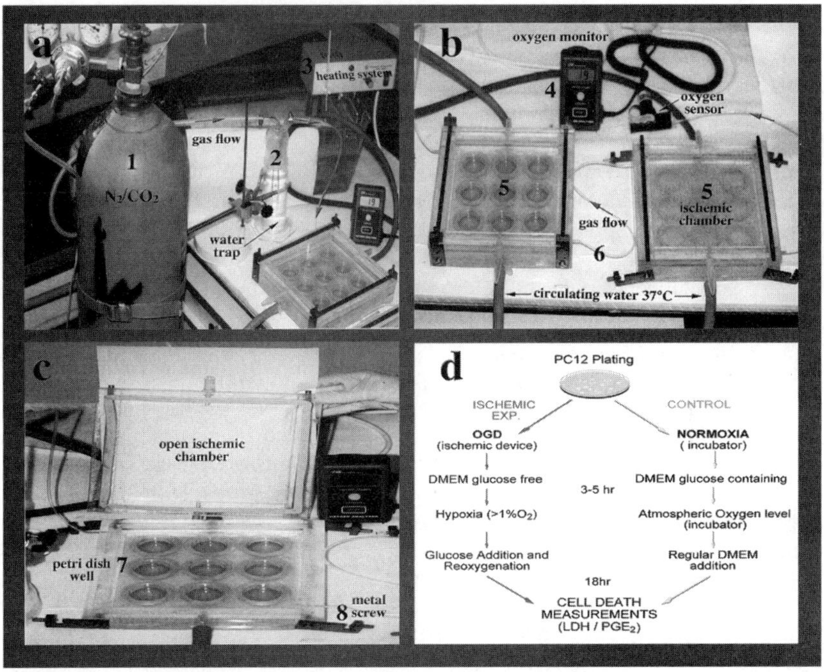

FIGURE 2. Ischemic (oxygen-glucose-deprivation) device and protocol. **(a)** Ischemic system: (1) gas tank (N_2/CO_2 95%:5%); (2) cylinder containing water; (3) water bath with heating system and pump. **(b)** Ischemic chambers and oxygen detection: (4) oxygen monitor and oxygen sensor; (5) ischemic tissue culture chambers; *arrow*: flow of N_2/CO_2 through Teflon tube (6) connecting in series the two chambers of the ischemic device (5). **(c)** Photograph of an open tissue culture ischemic chamber housing the petri dishes containing the PC12 cells (7) and tightly closed by metal screws (8) to seal the chambers. **(d)** Ischemia and normoxia protocols.

PC12 Ischemic Model

Using an ischemic device prepared in our laboratory (FIG. 2) and PC12 cultures, we developed an *in vitro* model based on combined oxygen and glucose deprivation (OGD) insult, followed by reoxygenation, mimicking the pathological conditions of ischemia.[19] In this model, the PC12 cells released large amounts of prostaglandin PGE_2, lowered the ATP level, and underwent cell death, in part by apoptotic mechanism, measured by different cell death parameters.[19,20,22]

NERVE GROWTH FACTOR

NGF is the prototype of the neurotrophin family of growth factor molecules.[23–25] NGF regulates the growth, development, and plasticity of selective neuronal populations in the nervous system.[26–30] It acts through binding and activating specific cell surface receptors named trkA and p-75.[31,32] TrkA is a receptor that stimulates several signal transduction pathways, such as stimulation of phosphatidyl-inositol 3′-kinase, phospholipase C-γ, and mitogen-activated protein kinases (MAPKs).[32]

Neuronal NGF expression *in vivo* is markedly upregulated by seizures, forebrain ischemia, marked hypoglycemia, and tissue injury.[33–35] Studies *in vivo* and *in vitro* indicate that cerebral insults influence NGF gene expression via excitatory amino acid receptors as well as through other pathways.[34] The functional consequences of the increased production of neurotrophic factors following brain insults are not clear, but are supposed to represent intrinsic neuroprotective signals.[35,36] Among its different functions, NGF signaling appears to play important roles in response to injury or disease that subserve neuroprotection and neural repair.[37]

NGF-Induced Neuroprotection in the PC12 Ischemic Model and Implication to Neurodegeneration

NGF-induced neuroprotection, in the OGD-induced PC12 cell death model, is manifested by a decrease in the release of LDH and in caspase-3 activity (FIG. 3). It bears mention that the NGF neuroprotective effect requires 18-h pretreatment.[38] This finding strongly suggests a posttranscriptional effect of NGF and is consistent with the mechanism of action of NGF, which includes early and delayed effects.[7] Results in our laboratory indicate that the OGD-induced PC12 cell death issues in part

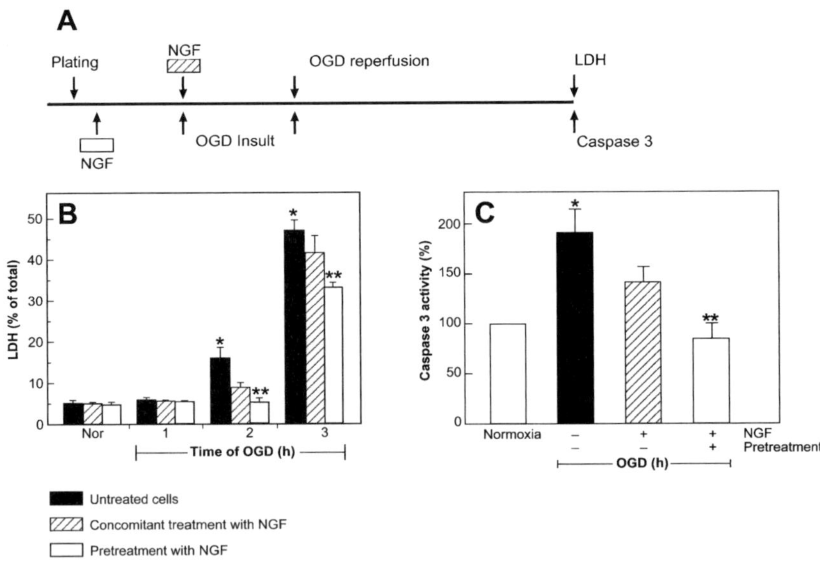

FIGURE 3. The neuroprotective effect of NGF in the PC12 ischemic model. **(A)** The experimental paradigm of the evaluation of NGF's neuroprotective effect: NGF was added to the cultures 18 h prior to the OGD insult (i.e., pretreatment with NGF; *white boxes and bars*) or it was added concomitantly with the exposure to the OGD insult (*hatched boxes and bars*). **(B, C)** Cell death and the neuroprotective effect of NGF were measured by two parameters: the release of lactate dehydrogenase enzyme (LDH) **(B)** and caspase 3 activity **(C)**. Only pretreatment with NGF revealed a significant neuroprotective effect.

due to apoptosis.[22] Therefore, it is tempting to suggest that the neuroprotective effect of NGF is related to a reduction in OGD-induced apoptosis. NGF-induced neuroprotection, in the OGD model, supports the role of NGF as a neuroprotective agent in the nervous system as previously documented in a variety of *in vitro* neuronal insults.[10,17,18,39–45] In recent neurological studies, a correlation was found between depletion and/or reduction in the central nervous system neurotrophin level and the occurrence of neurodegeneration. It has been also shown that, in different neurodegenerative disease models, treatment with neurotrophins like BDNF and NGF may reduce the severity and death of the neurons. Thus, we hypothesize that controlled increase in brain NGF level may be beneficial in ameliorating certain neurodegenerative diseases such as Alzheimer's disease. The fact that NGF's neuroprotective effect requires 18-h pretreatment emphasizes its essential endogenous, maintenance, neuroprotective role in the CNS. Also, we would like to emphasize that, during the ischemic insult, part of the neurons are not dead, but damaged. In our opinion, an early and long exposure of these neurons to NGF treatment may delay or rescue their apoptotic cell death. To date, the major obstacle in therapeutic use of NGF for stroke, Alzheimer's disease, and other neurodegenerative disorders is the inability of recombinant human NGF to permeate through the blood-brain barrier. The development of novel delivery technologies for proteins such as NGF will provide the way for this important neurotrophin to the clinic.

OGD-Induced Activation of MAPK Isoforms in the PC12 Ischemic Model

In view of the critical role of the MAPK pathways in the pathophysiological response of neurons to environmental stress, including ischemic injury,[46,47] we measured MAPK isoform activity during the OGD paradigm. At the end of the 3-h insult, there was a 12- and 25-fold increase in the activation of ERK 1 and ERK 2, respectively,[38] dropping to the control level after 30 min of OGD reperfusion. During the OGD insult, maximal 10-fold and 8-fold JNK 1 and JNK 2 activity, respectively, was observed 3 h from initiation of the insult, declining to a level similar to that under normoxia after an additional 2 h. Similar findings were observed for p-38 enzymes (FIG. 4).

Our study shows that insult-induced activation of MAPKs occurs mainly during the OGD phase. A comparison between the kinetics of OGD-induced cell death[38] and the kinetics of OGD-induced MAPK activation[38] indicates that there is a similar time course, suggesting a coincidental relationship.

These findings support the emerging concept that MAPKs are activated during ischemia, stress, and inflammation,[46] and may be crucial cross points in the neurotoxicity/neuroprotection process.

NGF Attenuation of MAPK Activity during OGD-Induced PC12 Cell Death

The novel finding in our study is that NGF, aside from conferring neuroprotection, also differentially attenuates the phosphorylation of OGD-induced JNK 1, p-38 β, and p-38 α.[38] The neuroprotective effect exerted by NGF after OGD was coincidentally related to 50%, 20%, and 50% inhibition of JNK 1, p-38 α, and p-38 β, respectively. Since JNK and p-38 kinases are considered stress kinases, their inhibition may represent part of the NGF-mediated neuroprotective mechanism against OGD-induced PC12 cell death. Under normoxic, but not OGD conditions, NGF induced ERK phosphorylation.[38] NGF did not have an inhibitory effect on OGD-induced ERK activation (FIG. 4). The most plausible interpretation of the neuroprotective activity of NGF stems from its diametrically opposed effects on MAPKs: on the one hand, prolonged activation of survival kinase ERK; on the other, attenuation of stress kinases JNK and p-38.[48] However, it is possible that inhibition of JNK and p-38,

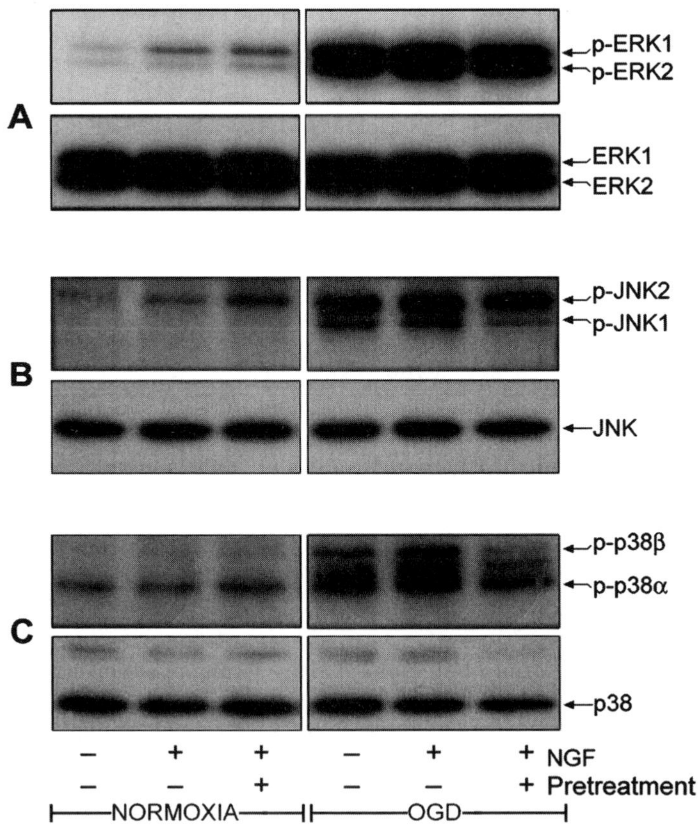

FIGURE 4. Differential effect of NGF on OGD-induced activation of MAPKs in PC12 cells. The experiment was performed using three groups of PC12 cells: (i) untreated cultures (–/–); (ii) cultures treated with 50 ng/mL NGF, added concomitantly with exposure to OGD insult or normoxia (+/–); (iii) cultures pretreated with 50 ng/mL NGF for 18 h prior to and during the OGD insult or normoxia (+/+). Following 3-h exposure to OGD insult, without OGD reperfusion, the cultures were harvested and lysed. Samples of cell extracts were electrophoresed on 12% SDS-PAGE, followed by Western blot, using antibodies specific for the phosphorylated or unphosphorylated MAPK form. **(A)** ERK 1, ERK 2; **(B)** JNK 1, JNK 2; **(C)** p-38 β, p-38 α. The experiment was performed five times (n = 6).

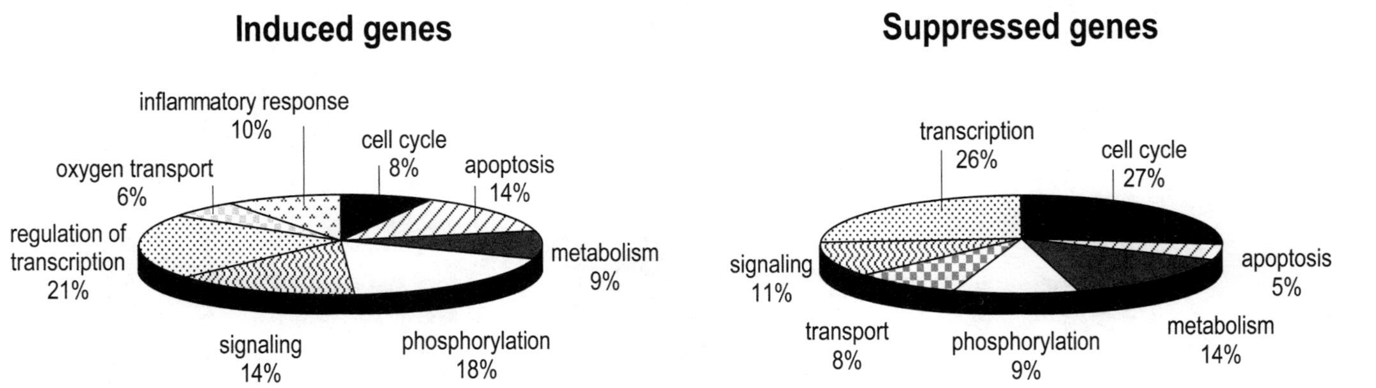

FIGURE 5. Gene expression comparison between OGD and normoxia in the PC12 ischemic model. Out of 1476 genes that were induced and 808 genes that were suppressed, only 365 or 483 genes had a 2-fold induction or suppression, respectively. These genes were analyzed, using David analysis (http://david.niaid.nih.gov/david/ease.htm), and presented in a pie chart according to cellular function.

upon NGF treatment, sustained the OGD-induced activation of ERK 1 and ERK 2 by feedback regulation of the MAPK cascade.[49]

Pretreatment with NGF may be beneficial in neuronal ischemia because of its ability to attenuate stress kinase activity believed to cause OGD-induced cell death.

Gene Expression in the PC12 Ischemic Model

In the present study, we also investigated the effect of OGD insult and the neuroprotective effect of NGF on total gene expression. We evaluated the global gene expression profile using the Affymetrix Gene Chip® Rat, 230-Rat 230A, expression set. A comparison between the cells exposed to the OGD insult and normoxia cells revealed that out of ~16,000 genes tailored on the chip, a 2-fold change (induction or suppression) was observed in less than 6% of the genes (~1248 genes). The most strongly affected genes include those coding for proteins involved in apoptosis, cell cycle, MAPK signaling pathway, and hypoxia-inducible genes (FIG. 5). These findings reinforce the importance and the contribution of apoptotic and MAPK pathways in the OGD-induced, PC12 cell death and neuroprotection, at the level of gene expression. According to Coupled Two-Way Clustering Analysis,[50] a clear difference in gene expression was observed between the 6 experimental groups. As can be seen

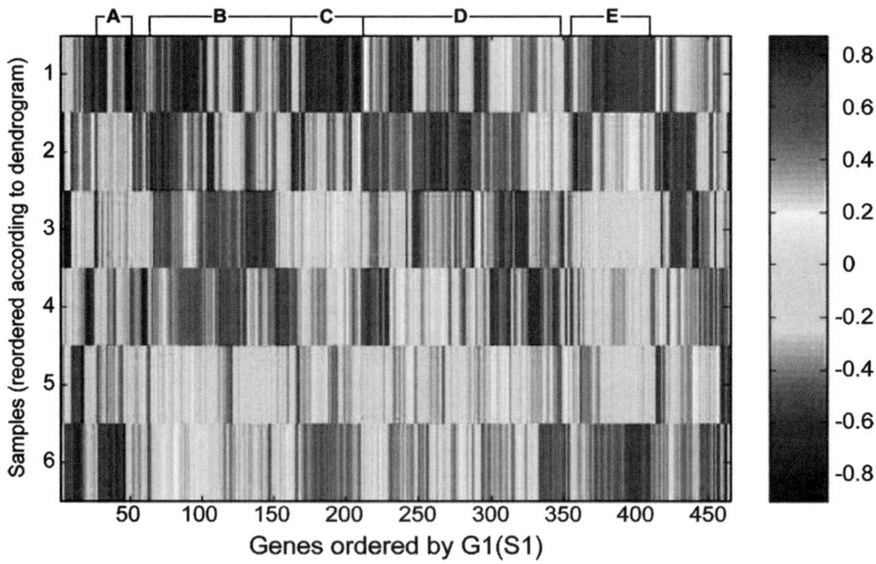

FIGURE 6. Gene expression dendrograms of PC12 cells in the OGD-ischemic model. Analysis of 465 different genes, according to Coupled Two-Way Clustering Analysis, reveals a different pattern of gene expression under various experimental conditions, clearly indicating effects on gene expression of NGF and/or reperfusion process under normoxia or OGD conditions. Groups 1 and 2: normoxia in the absence/presence of NGF, respectively; groups 3 and 4: OGD in the absence/presence of NGF, respectively; groups 5 and 6: OGD followed by reperfusion in the absence/presence of NGF, respectively. **A–E** present the different patterns of gene expression.

in FIGURE 6, analysis of 465 different genes reveals a different pattern of gene expression under various experimental conditions, clearly indicating the effects on gene expression of NGF and/or reperfusion process under normoxia or OGD conditions. Precise identification of the 465 genes is under way. These data will provide novel targets for neuroprotection in the ischemia-reperfusion process and resemble gene expression in the hypocampal neurons exposed to 3-h hypoxia[51] and in the rat occlusion ischemic model.[52]

The Effect of NGF on Gene Expression in the PC12 Ischemic Model

We also examined the effect of NGF on gene expression under different experimental conditions: (i) under normoxic conditions, NGF affected 2284 genes, out of which a 2-fold induction was observed in 365 genes and suppression of 483 genes, compared to nontreated cells; (ii) under OGD insult, NGF affected 2396 genes, out of which a 2-fold induction was observed in 345 genes and suppression of 258 genes, compared to nontreated cells; (iii) under OGD insult followed by reperfusion, NGF affected 1884 genes, out of which a 2-fold induction was observed in 130 genes and suppression of 128 genes, compared to nontreated cells (data not shown). These results indicate a differential effect of NGF on the PC12 transcriptome under normoxia and ischemic conditions. Evaluation of the specific genes and signal transduction pathways affected by ischemic insult may provide a new diagnostic tool for evaluation of the severity of the ischemic damage and may shed light on future therapeutic approaches/targets.

Neuroprotection: A Balanced Process between Cell Death and Cell Survival

In neuronal models such as PC12 cells, the relationship between survival and cell death is determined by the balance between the activated pro- and antiapoptotic signaling proteins (the apoptotic thermostat),[53] regulated in part by neurotrophins such as NGF.[54]

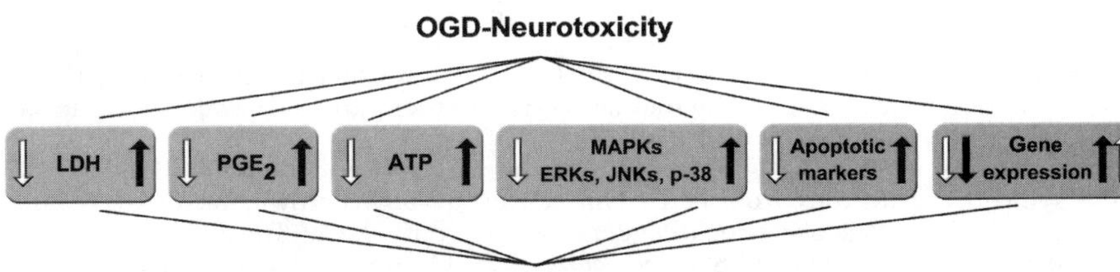

FIGURE 7. OGD-induced neurotoxicity and drug-induced neuroprotection: two antagonistic processes in the PC12 ischemic model. Schematic presentation of the neuroprotection concept as a balanced neuropharmacological process between cell death and cell survival pathways. *White arrows* indicate the neuroprotective processes; *black arrows* indicate OGD-induced neurotoxicity. Addition of neuroprotective compounds such as NGF antagonizes the neurotoxicity process and shifts the balance towards survival of the neurons. There is a dual effect on gene expression under both neurotoxic and neuroprotective processes: part of the genes are being induced, while others are being suppressed.

Our findings support the concept of a fine balance regulation (FIG. 7) between the neuron survival and death pathways: a differential inhibitory effect of NGF on the proapoptotic genes, while upregulating of the antiapoptotic genes (data not shown).

The most plausible interpretation of the neuroprotective activity of NGF stems from its diametrically opposed effects on MAPKs: on the one hand, prolonged activation of survival kinase ERK; on the other, attenuation of stress kinases JNK and p-38.[48] In turn, these kinases, by phosphorylation of their transcription factor substrates, differentially regulate gene expression.[49]

Further investigation of the PC12 cell ischemic model, exploiting the OGD paradigm and specific inhibitors of signal transduction targets coupled with DNA-microarray analysis, may shed light on the differential contribution of the pro- and antiapoptotic proteins during ischemic insult and the neuroprotection conferred by NGF.

REFERENCES

1. SIESJO, B.K. 1992. Pathophysiology and treatment of focal cerebral ischemia. Part I: Pathophysiology. J. Neurosurg. **77:** 169–184.
2. SIESJO, B.K. 1992. Pathophysiology and treatment of focal cerebral ischemia. Part II: Mechanisms of damage and treatment. J. Neurosurg. **77:** 337–354.
3. LUO, X., G.N. LAMBROU, J.A. SAHEL & D. HICKS. 2001. Hypoglycemia induces general neuronal death, whereas hypoxia and glutamate transport blockade lead to selective retinal ganglion cell death *in vitro*. Invest. Ophthalmol. Vis. Sci. **42:** 2695–2705.
4. PEDERSEN, J.Z., G. BERNARDI, D. CENTONZE *et al.* 1998. Hypoglycemia, hypoxia, and ischemia in a corticostriatal slice preparation: electrophysiologic changes and ascorbyl radical formation. J. Cereb. Blood Flow Metab. **18:** 868–875.
5. MATTSON, M.P., W. DUAN, W.A. PEDERSEN & C. CULMSEE. 2001. Neurodegenerative disorders and ischemic brain diseases. Apoptosis **6:** 69–81.
6. BERGER, R. & Y. GARNIER. 2000. Perinatal brain injury. J. Perinat. Med. **28:** 261–285.
7. FUJITA, K., P. LAZAROVICI & G. GUROFF. 1989. Regulation of the differentiation of PC12 pheochromocytoma cells: regulation of differentiation in eukaryotic cells. Environ. Health Perspect. **80:** 127–142.
8. GREENE, L.A. & A.S. TISCHLER. 1976. Establishment of a noradrenergic clonal line of rat adrenal pheochromocytoma cells which respond to nerve growth factor. Proc. Natl. Acad. Sci. USA **73:** 2424–2428.
9. VAUDRY, D., P.J. STORK, P. LAZAROVICI & L.E. EIDEN. 2002. Signaling pathways for PC12 cell differentiation: making the right connections. Science **296:** 1648–1649.
10. RUKENSTEIN, A., R.E. RYDEL & L.A. GREENE. 1991. Multiple agents rescue PC12 cells from serum-free cell death by translation- and transcription-independent mechanisms. J. Neurosci. **11:** 2552–2563.
11. BATISTATOU, A. & L.A. GREENE. 1991. Aurintricarboxylic acid rescues PC12 cells and sympathetic neurons from cell death caused by nerve growth factor deprivation: correlation with suppression of endonuclease activity. J. Cell Biol. **115:** 461–471.
12. PARK, D.S., E.J. MORRIS, L. STEFANIS *et al.* 1998. Multiple pathways of neuronal death induced by DNA-damaging agents, NGF deprivation, and oxidative stress. J. Neurosci. **18:** 830–840.
13. MENEI, P., J.M. PEAN, V. NERRIERE-DAGUIN *et al.* 2000. Intracerebral implantation of NGF-releasing biodegradable microspheres protects striatum against excitotoxic damage. Exp. Neurol. **161:** 259–272.
14. FISCHER, S.J., J.L. PODRATZ & A.J. WINDEBANK. 2001. Nerve growth factor rescue of cisplatin neurotoxicity is mediated through the high affinity receptor: studies in PC12 cells and p75 null mouse dorsal root ganglia. Neurosci. Lett. **308:** 1–4.
15. SHIMOKE, K. & H. CHIBA. 2001. Nerve growth factor prevents 1-methyl-4-phenyl-1,2,3,6-tetrahydropyridine-induced cell death via the Akt pathway by suppressing

caspase-3-like activity using PC12 cells: relevance to therapeutical application for Parkinson's disease. J. Neurosci. Res. **63:** 402–409.
16. TROY, C.M., S.A. RABACCHI, Z. XU *et al.* 2001. Beta-amyloid-induced neuronal apoptosis requires c-Jun N-terminal kinase activation. J. Neurochem. **77:** 157–164.
17. PAN, Z., D. SAMPATH, G. JACKSON *et al.* 1997. Nerve growth factor and oxidative stress in the nervous system. *In* Brain Plasticity, pp. 173–193. Plenum. New York.
18. PAN, Z., D. SAMPATH, G. JACKSON *et al.* 1997. Nerve growth factor and oxidative stress in the nervous system. Adv. Exp. Med. Biol. **429:** 173–193.
19. TABAKMAN, R., P. LAZAROVICI & R. KOHEN. 2002. Neuroprotective effects of carnosine and homocarnosine on pheochromocytoma PC12 cells exposed to ischemia. J. Neurosci. Res. **68:** 463–469.
20. ABU-RAYA, S., V. TREMBOVLER, E. SHOHAMI & P. LAZAROVICI. 1993. A tissue culture ischemic device to study eicosanoid release by pheochromocytoma PC12 cultures. J. Neurosci. Methods **50:** 197–203.
21. ABU-RAYA, S., E. BLAUGRUND, V. TREMBOVLER *et al.* 1999. Rasagiline, a monoamine oxidase-B inhibitor, protects NGF-differentiated PC12 cells against oxygen-glucose deprivation. J. Neurosci. Res. **5:** 456–463.
22. TABAKMAN, R., H. JIANG, R.A. LEVINE *et al.* 2004. Apoptotic characteristics of cell death and the neuroprotective effect of homocarnosine on pheochromocytoma PC12 cells exposed to ischemia. J. Neurosci. Res. **75:** 499–507.
23. BUTTE, M.J., P.K. HWANG, W.C. MOBLEY & R.J. FLETTERICK. 1998. Crystal structure of neurotrophin-3 homodimer shows distinct regions are used to bind its receptors. Biochemistry **37:** 16846–16852.
24. IBANEZ, C.F. 1994. Structure-function relationships in the neurotrophin family. J. Neurobiol. **25:** 1349–1361.
25. ROBINSON, R.C., C. RADZIEJEWSKI, G. SPRAGGON *et al.* 1999. The structures of the neurotrophin 4 homodimer and the brain-derived neurotrophic factor/neurotrophin 4 heterodimer reveal a common Trk-binding site. Protein Sci. **8:** 2589–2597.
26. HUANG, E.J. & L.F. REICHARDT. 2001. Neurotrophins: roles in neuronal development and function. Annu. Rev. Neurosci. **24:** 677–736.
27. REICHARDT, L.F. & I. FARINAS. 1997. Neurotrophic factors and their receptors: roles in neuronal development and function. *In* Molecular and Cellular Approaches to Neuronal Development, pp. 220–263. Oxford University Press. London/New York.
28. SCHINDER, A.F. & M. POO. 2000. The neurotrophin hypothesis for synaptic plasticity. Trends Neurosci. **23:** 639–645.
29. THOENEN, H. 2000. Neurotrophins and activity-dependent plasticity. Prog. Brain Res. **128:** 183–191.
30. TABAKMAN, R., S. LECHT, S. SEPHANOVA *et al.* 2004. Interactions between the cells of the immune and nervous system: neurotrophins as neuroprotection mediators in CNS injury. Prog. Brain Res. **146:** 387–401.
31. BARBACID, M. 1994. The Trk family of neurotrophin receptors. J. Neurobiol. **25:** 1386–1403.
32. KAPLAN, D.R. & F.D. MILLER. 1997. Signal transduction by the neurotrophin receptors. Curr. Opin. Cell Biol. **9:** 213–221.
33. GALL, C.M. & P.J. ISACKSON. 1989. Limbic seizures increase neuronal production of messenger RNA for nerve growth factor. Science **245:** 758–761.
34. LINDVALL, O., Z. KOKAIA, J. BENGZON *et al.* 1994. Neurotrophins and brain insults. Trends Neurosci. **17:** 490–496.
35. ZAFRA, F., E. CASTREN, H. THOENEN & D. LINDHOLM. 1991. Interplay between glutamate and gamma-aminobutyric acid transmitter systems in the physiological regulation of brain derived neurotrophic factor and nerve growth factor synthesis in hippocampal neurons. Proc. Natl. Acad. Sci. USA **88:** 10037–10041.
36. TOKUMINE, J., O. KAKINOHANA, D. CIZKOVA *et al.* 2003. Changes in spinal GDNF, BDNF, and NT-3 expression after transient spinal cord ischemia in the rat. J. Neurosci. Res. **74:** 552–561.
37. SOFRONIEW, M.V., C.L. HOWE & W.C. MOBLEY. 2001. Nerve growth factor signaling, neuroprotection, and neural repair. Annu. Rev. Neurosci. **24:** 1217–1281.

38. TABAKMAN, R., H. JIANG, E. SCHAEFER *et al.* 2004. Nerve growth factor pretreatment attenuates oxygen and glucose deprivation–induced c-Jun amino-terminal kinase 1 and stress-activated kinases p38alpha and p38beta activation and confers neuroprotection in the pheochromocytoma PC12 model. J. Mol. Neurosci. **22:** 237–250.
39. BONIECE, I.R. & J.A. WAGNER. 1995. NGF protects PC12 cells against ischemia by a mechanism that requires the N-kinase. J. Neurosci. Res. **40:** 1–9.
40. HAVIV, R. & R. STEIN. 1999. Nerve growth factor inhibits apoptosis induced by tumor necrosis factor in PC12 cells. J. Neurosci. Res. **55:** 269–277.
41. ENOKIDO, Y. & H. HATANAKA. 1990. High oxygen atmosphere for neuronal cell culture with nerve growth factor. II. Survival and growth of clonal rat pheochromocytoma PC12h cells. Brain Res. **536:** 23–29.
42. SATOH, T., T. YAMAGATA, Y. ISHIKAWA *et al.* 1999. Regulation of reactive oxygen species by nerve growth factor but not Bcl-2 as a novel mechanism of protection of PC12 cells from superoxide anion–induced death. J. Biochem. (Tokyo) **125:** 952–959.
43. DESHMUKH, M. & E.M. JOHNSON. 1997. Programmed cell death in neurons: focus on the pathway of nerve growth factor deprivation–induced death of sympathetic neurons. Mol. Pharmacol. **51:** 897–906.
44. OHYASHIKI, T., E. SATOH, M. OKADA *et al.* 2002. Nerve growth factor protects against aluminum-mediated cell death. Toxicology **176:** 195–207.
45. ITANO, Y., Y. KITAMURA & Y. NOMURA. 1994. 1-Methyl-4-phenylpyridinium (MPP+)–induced cell death in PC12 cells: inhibitory effects of several drugs. Neurochem. Int. **25:** 419–424.
46. KYRIAKIS, J.M. & J. AVRUCH. 2001. Mammalian mitogen-activated protein kinase signal transduction pathways activated by stress and inflammation. Physiol. Rev. **81:** 807–869.
47. IRVING, E.A. & M. BAMFORD. 2002. Role of mitogen- and stress-activated kinases in ischemic injury. J. Cereb. Blood Flow Metab. **22:** 631–647.
48. XIA, Z., M. DICKENS, J. RAINGEAUD *et al.* 1995. Opposing effects of ERK and JNK-p38 MAP kinases on apoptosis. Science **270:** 1326–1331.
49. BRIGHTMAN, F.A. & D.A. FELL. 2000. Differential feedback regulation of the MAPK cascade underlies the quantitative differences in EGF and NGF signalling in PC12 cells. FEBS Lett. **482:** 169–174.
50. GETZ, G., E. LEVINE & E. DOMANY. 2000. Coupled Two-Way Clustering Analysis of gene microarray data. Proc. Natl. Acad. Sci. USA **97:** 12079–12084.
51. JIN, K., X.O. MAO, M.W. ESHOO *et al.* 2002. cDNA microarray analysis of changes in gene expression induced by neuronal hypoxia *in vitro*. Neurochem. Res. **27:** 1105–1112.
52. SORIANO, M.A., M. TESSIER, U. CERTA & R. GILL. 2000. Parallel gene expression monitoring using oligonucleotide probe arrays of multiple transcripts with an animal model of focal ischemia. J. Cereb. Blood Flow Metab. **20:** 1045–1055.
53. CHAUM, E. 2003. Retinal neuroprotection by growth factors: a mechanistic perspective. J. Cell. Biochem. **88:** 57–75.
54. MILLER, F.D. & D.R. KAPLAN. 2001. Neurotrophin signalling pathways regulating neuronal apoptosis. Cell. Mol. Life Sci. **58:** 1045–1053.

Role of Peroxynitrite in Methamphetamine-Induced Dopaminergic Neurodegeneration and Neuroprotection by Antioxidants and Selective NOS Inhibitors

SYED F. ALI,[a] SYED Z. IMAM,[a] AND YOSSEF ITZHAK[b]

[a]*Neurochemistry Laboratory, Division of Neurotoxicology, National Center for Toxicological Research/FDA, Jefferson, Arkansas, USA*

[b]*Department of Psychiatry and Behavioral Sciences, University of Miami School of Medicine, Miami, Florida, USA*

KEYWORDS: peroxynitrite; reactive oxygen species (ROS); reactive nitrogen species (RNS); methamphetamine (METH); 3-nitrotyrosine (3-NT); neuronal nitric oxide synthase (nNOS)

Oxidative stress, reactive oxygen species (ROS), nitrergic stress, and reactive nitrogen species (RNS) have been known to be involved in a multitude of neurodegenerations. Both ROS and RNS have very short half-lives, thereby making their identification very difficult as a specific cause of neurodegeneration. Recently, we have developed a high-performance liquid chromatography/electrochemical detection (HPLC/EC) method to identify 3-nitrotyrosine (3-NT), an *in vivo* biomarker of peroxynitrite production, in brain to evaluate if an agent-driven neurotoxicity is produced by the generation of peroxynitrite. We have shown that a single or multiple injections of methamphetamine (METH) produced a significant increase in the formation of 3-NT in the striatum. This formation of 3-NT correlated with the striatal dopamine depletion caused by METH administration. We have also reported that pretreatment with antioxidants such as selenium and melatonin can completely protect against the formation of 3-NT and depletion of striatal dopamine. We also used two different approaches, pharmacological manipulation and transgenic animal models, in order to further investigate the role of peroxynitrite. We have shown that a selective neuronal nitric oxide synthase (nNOS) inhibitor, 7-nitroindazole (7-NI), significantly protected against the formation of 3-NT as well as striatal dopamine depletion. Similar results were observed with nNOS knockout mouse models. In addition, we have shown that peroxynitrite also played an important role in apoptotic gene expression. METH administration upregulated the protein expression of p53 and downregulated

Address for correspondence: Syed F. Ali, Neurochemistry Laboratory, Division of Neurotoxicology, National Center for Toxicological Research/FDA, Jefferson, AR 72079. sali@nctr.fda.gov

Ann. N.Y. Acad. Sci. 1053: 97–98 (2005).
doi: 10.1196/annals.1344.053

bcl-2 protein expression in the striatum of wild-type mice, but not in the nNOS knockout mice. Together, these data clearly support the hypothesis that the reactive nitrogen species, nitric oxide and peroxynitrite, play a major role in METH-induced dopaminergic neurotoxicity, and selective NOS inhibitors and antioxidants can protect against METH-induced neurotoxicity. These antioxidants and selective NOS inhibitors may have therapeutic potential in the treatment of neurodegenerative diseases.

Questions and Answers

Session II: Mechanisms of Neuroprotection (1)

QUESTIONS FOR NAREN BANIK

From William Slikker, Jr.

Why do some patients with optic neuritis recover completely and others go on to develop MS?

ANSWER: This is still puzzling to clinicians and researchers. It is not known why at least 60% of patients with optic neuritis develop MS. One probably needs to know what triggers optic neuritis, and subsequent factors are involved in the development of MS in some patients.

From Hari Sharma

What is the prospect of calpain inhibitor in spinal cord injury?

ANSWER: The main problem with calpain inhibitors is their solubility. Almost all calpain inhibitors require organic solvent for solubilization. Its therapeutic efficacy in human injury can only be tested after this problem is solved. The lack of solubility is delaying the prospect of its use as a therapeutic agent for SCI.

From Xiaoyang Qi

Very impressive presentation. Two questions: (1) Is the calpain knockout mouse model available? (2) Does calpain affect other neurons (i.e., CNS)?

ANSWER: Thank you. (1) There is no calpain knockout model available because the calpain knockout is embryonically lethal. Maybe one can use siRNA techniques. (2) Yes, calpain affects a variety of neurons, including dopaminergic and cholinergic neurons.

QUESTIONS FOR PHILIP LAZAROVICI

From De-Maw Chuang

You nicely showed that NGF suppressed OGD-induced activation of JNK. What are the upstream mechanisms involved? Does this effect involve a direct action of NGF on JNK or reflect a change in the activity of protein phosphatase of lipase?

ANSWER: The precise mechanisms by which NGF suppresses OGD-induced activation of JNK are not clear. Indeed, we may assume a direct NGF-induced phosphorylation on mixed lineage kinases and/or POSH scaffold of these kinases since it was reported that POSH is activated by NGF deprivation (KUKEKOV & GREENE. 2003.

Ann. N.Y. Acad. Sci. 1053: 99–106 (2005). © 2005 New York Academy of Sciences.
doi: 10.1196/annals.1344.061

EMBO J. **22:** 252). The possibility that we favor is that radical oxygen species (ROS) and NOS are generated during the OGD insult, increasing the redox activity of PC12 cells. This effect is antagonized by NGF by increasing the intracellular level/activity of endogenous antioxidants and eliminating radicals into the peroxisome. Most probably, this effect is achieved by certain kinase/phosphatase signals. In our opinion, OGD-induced activation of phospholipases will also impinge into the ROS/NOS pool and is not related to the neuroprotective effect.

From William Slikker, Jr.

What is the role/effect of NGF-induced differentiation without ischemia and NGF-induced neuroprotection in ischemic PC12 cells?

ANSWER: We assume that the major difference between the two physiological conditions is the signaling of NGF trkA receptor. In normoxic cultures, NGF occupancy of trkA receptor induces activation of rasI MAPKs, as well as PLC-γ/calcium, phosphatidyl inositol 3-kinase/Akt, srcJFAK, and other signals. There are reports that all three members of the MAPK cassette—ERK, JNK, and p38—are activated and required for NGF-induced differentiation. During the ischemic insult, NGF activated trkA to signal mainly survival by amplifying the ERK and Akt activity and inhibiting the stress kinases JNK and p38. The switch mechanism is not yet known.

From Hari Sharma

The effects of NGF are controversial. Did you try some other members of the neurotrophin family in your cell culture model—namely, BDNF or IGF-1? If yes, what is the result of this investigation?

ANSWER: The effects of NGF on OGD models are controversial since many investigators are using nonvalidated models to generate the insult and face difficulties to reproduce neuroprotection because they cannot control the amount of cell death. Our ischemic device and paradigm address these issues. We cannot use BDNF in our experiments since its receptor trkB is not present in PC12 cells; thus, BDNF cannot protect. However, we treated the cells with BDNF because the NGFIBDNF p75 common receptor is present, but no neuroprotective effects were measured, providing indirect evidence on the crucial role of trkA in the NGF neuroprotective effect. We have not investigated the effect of IGF-1 in the OGD model.

From Italo Mocchetti

Why do PC12 cells need 12–15 h of NGF exposure to be protected against OGD? Do you predict that NGF will be neuroprotective against OGD in primary neurons?

ANSWER: In our model, we need 18 h of pretreatment with NGF to induce partial neuroprotection. We attribute this long exposure to the mechanism of NGF action, which involves gene expression followed by protein synthesis, processes requiring a long time. I predict that NGF will also be neuroprotective in primary neurons exposed to OGD if they express trk receptors, and the experiment is performed under stringent conditions using a similar paradigm as we performed.

From Chia Yi Kuan

Have you studied the neuroprotective effects of NGF in cell types other than PC12 cells? Since NGF can induce the differentiation of PC12 cells, I am worried that it may complicate your analysis in applying NGF to PC12 cells.

ANSWER: We have not tried these experiments in other cells since PC12 cells are the prime model to investigate the NGF mechanism of action and because we are interested in the OGD effect on dopaminergic neurons. Your claim is correct, but not the concern. NGF is a pleiotropic factor with multiple signaling pathways. The major goal in our field is to decipher and, if possible, to separate between differentiating and neuroprotective signals. The results obtained with the Affymetrix Gene Chip clearly indicate for the first time a differential effect of NGF on the PC12 cell transcriptome under normoxia and ischemic conditions. We are in the process of identifying selective neuroprotective genes.

From Stephen Skaper

In your PC12 cell model of OGD injury, are MAPKs like ERK, JNK, and p38 activated? Have you tried inhibitors of these kinases for a neuroprotective action?

ANSWER: Yes, these MAPK members are activated during the OGD insult. We have not yet tried commercially available inhibitors of these kinase isoforms due to their toxicity and poor selectivity. However, these experiments are now performed in our laboratory using a selective JNK inhibitor that is under clinical investigation since we measured a direct relationship between JNK inhibition and neuroprotection.

QUESTIONS FOR ANN MARINI

From William Slikker, Jr.

Have you examined the time course of NMDA exposure and/or the time after exposure (washout) in your study design?

ANSWER: We have examined the time course of NMDA and find that 6 h is required to protect the maximum number of neurons against glutamate-mediated excitotoxicity.

From Philip Lazarovici

Since the neuroprotective effect of BDNF has been observed during E20, is this effect limited to a narrow developmental window or may it be extrapolated to the adult hippocampus?

ANSWER: An elegant study was published recently that shows that preconditioning of mice with NMDA protects all vulnerable neurons against kainic acid–induced apoptosis in the hippocampus [OGITA *et al.* 2003. J. Neurochem. **85**(5)**:** 1336–1346]. Whether the preconditioning requires BDNF is unknown. It is known that the induction of BDNF protein by diet restriction protects neurons against hippocampal damage *in vivo* induced by kainic acid *in vivo* [DUAN *et al.* 2001. J. Neurochem.

76(2)**:** 619–626]. However, whether there is a link between these two different paradigms is unknown.

From Steve Skaper

What is the time frame of NF-κB activation by a neuroprotective concentration of NMDA, and would a toxic concentration of NMDA also activate NF-κB? Do you know if a depolarizing stimulus would mimic the neuroprotective effects of NMDA in hippocampal neurons?

ANSWER: A neuroprotective concentration of NMDA activates NF-κB within 40 min. We have not examined whether a toxic concentration of NMDA activates NF-κB, but others have shown that a toxic concentration of glutamate acting on NMDA receptors increases activated NF-κB in the nucleus, and blocking translocation of NF-κB attenuated glutamate-mediated excitotoxicity (GRILLI *et al.* 1996. Science **274:** 1383–1385). This group has shown that NF-κB, p53, and others contribute to glutamate-mediated apoptosis (UBERTI *et al.* 2000. Int. J. Dev. Neurosci. **18:** 447–454). We have not tested whether a depolarizing stimulus would mimic NMDA neuroprotection, but we would expect that depolarization would mimic the effect since depolarization is known to increase BDNF mRNA and the release of BDNF protein.

From Syed Imam

Do you plan to look at P site mutants of CREB or I-κB to assess the neuroprotective role of BDNF or NMDA on glutamate toxicity?

ANSWER: We are very interested in pursuing these lines of experiments. We would expect that dominant negative mutants of CREB and I-κB would attenuate NMDA receptor–mediated neuroprotection.

From De-Maw Chuang

Is it possible that NMDA or low glutamate-induced BDNF expression is mediated by BDNF initially released into the medium? In other words, does BDNF induce BDNF through trkB-mediated mechanisms?

ANSWER: Yes. It has been shown that trkB contributes to the induction of BDNF mRNA (SAARELAINEN *et al.* 2001. Cell. Mol. Neurobiol. **21:** 429–435).

From Sylvain Doré

How long do you let your cells grow in culture before testing and what is the percent of neurons? (Sufficient divisions are recommended for full expression of all submits necessary for the glutamate receptor family members.)

ANSWER: The neurons are cultured for 8 days *in vitro*, at which time an excitotoxic concentration of glutamate is added to the medium. We added an excitotoxic concentration of glutamate to neurons when they are fully susceptible to the excitotoxic actions of glutamate or NMDA, as published by others [MATTSON *et al.* 1995. J. Neurochem. **65:** 1740–1751; GARY & MATTSON. 2002. Neuromol. Med. **2**(3)**:** 261–269; BROWN *et al.* 2003. Neuroscience **117:** 949–955].

QUESTION FOR A. MARINI, S. RUZDIJIC, AND M. YENARI

What is the time course of preconditioning neuroprotection?

ANSWER: Preconditioning of the neurons for 6 h is required for neuroprotection.

QUESTIONS FOR MIDORI YENARI

From Sylvain Doré

Does preconditioning stroke exposure induce HSP70 and could it be a potential mechanism of neuroprotection?

ANSWER: Prior work has shown that HSP70 is upregulated by some preconditioning paradigms and that it is correlated to neuroprotection. However, proof that it is definitely involved is still lacking.

From Hari Sharma

There are three schools of thought regarding HSP expression. According to one, HSP expression is neuroprotective. Others feel that HSP expression indicates cell death. Finally, some believe that HSP represents only activation or nerve cell in glial cells. What is your opinion on the subject?

ANSWER: Using molecular approaches, several groups have shown that overexpression of HSP70 improves cell survival, whereas its deficiency worsens cell death. This notion is separate from the use of HSP as a marker of cell death/stress. While HSP70 is a useful marker of cell death, it also could represent an endogenous cellular response to self-preservation.

From De-Maw Chuang

The expression of Bcl-2 is regulated by the activation of CREB. Thus, have you examined CREB activation as a potential mechanism underlying HSP70-induced Bcl-2 overexpression? Also, have you done comparable studies using HSP90 and HSP27 overexpression to examine for their neuroprotective and anti-inflammatory effects.

ANSWER: These issues has not been studied, but they clearly need to be. We have not studied HSP90 or HSP27, but prior work indicates that HSP90 may bind microglial receptors, leading to their activation. Therefore, HSP90 may have proinflammatory properties.

From Gary Fiskum

Could the robust increase in Bcl-2 expression caused by HSP70 overexpression be due to an increased stress caused by HSP70?

ANSWER: It is possible. However, when we compared transfection with a control vector (lacZ) or a vector expressing glutathione peroxidase, neither upregulated Bcl-2.

From Naren Banik

Since I-κB/NF-κB complex is cleared by both calpain and proteasome, can HSP70 act as a protease inhibitor and block the NF-κB translocation?

ANSWER: It is possible that HSP70 has multiple functions to protect cells. Our data suggest that HSP70 somehow interferes with I-κB phosphorylation, implicating an effect on IKK. However, we have not checked to see if HSP70 has any effects on calpain or the proteasome.

QUESTIONS FOR SABERA RUZDIJIC

From Sylvain Doré

You have shown changes of corticosteroid levels at 12 and not at 18 months. Do you have similar changes of PS and ApoE also at 12 months? Have you confirmed your results by Western blotting (WB) or immunohistochemistry?

ANSWER: Not yet. At this moment, we are finalizing a WB immunohistochemistry study in our project.

From Italo Mocchetti

Did you see any pathological abnormality in animals with increased ApoE mRNA?

ANSWER: No, we did not. ApoE is an important gene carrier of lipids in CNS. In our study, we investigated the effect of food restriction on several genes, as well as ApoE gene expression involved in brain plasticity.

From Philip Lazarovici

During aging, the levels of corticosteroids increase. Have you looked at the effect of dexamethasone in relation to aging on ApoE and/or receptors?

ANSWER: Yes, we have. In our experiments, we also included an acute effect of dexamethasone and demonstrated that the levels of corticosteroids were increased not only during aging, but also during food restriction. Thus, our goal was to study the effects of dexamethasone and food restriction in relation to aging on ApoE gene expression. We have not yet studied the effects of food restriction and dexamethasone on ApoE low-density lipoprotein (LDL) receptor, which plays an important role in plasma lipoprotein metabolism.

From Hari Sharma

What is the rationality of using 4 mg/kg dexamethasone in your experiment? Which route did you choose to administer dexamethasone?

ANSWER: The rationale to use intraperitoneal injection of dexamethasone is the permeability through the blood-brain barrier and the effective transport of synthetic hormone to neurons.

From Steve Skaper

Does dietary restriction differentially affect expression level of ApoE mRNA isoforms?

ANSWER: We did not study the effect of dietary restriction on the expression of ApoE mRNA isoforms. Human ApoE has three major isoforms, ApoE2, ApoE3, and ApoE4, according to amino acid polymorphism. Rat ApoE as well as mouse ApoE are the human ApoE4 type. Therefore, caloric restriction would be most active among ApoE phenotypes in molecular cascades that either promote or prevent the degeneration of neurons.

From Merle Paule

What was the strain of rat used in your studies? What was the control group for the 12-month-old rat study showing increases in ApoE in cortex in ad lib animals?

ANSWER: We are using the Wistar rat strain. The control group for the 12-month-old rat in our study is the 6-month-old animal fed ad libitum.

From De-Maw Chuang

Dr. Mattson's lab at NIH has shown that dietary restriction results in overexpression of BDNF and heat-shock protein. Do you think that these effects are related to your observation that dietary restriction produced a decrease in ApoE and PSI levels in the cortex?

ANSWER: Several mechanisms may be at work in dietary restriction. Different investigations have reported reductions in steady-state oxidative damage to proteins, lipids, and DNA in animals subjected to restricted caloric intake. At the systemic level, dietary restriction lowers glucose, blood insulin, and cholesterol, but also increases corticosteroids and neurotrophic factors. The beneficial effects of BDNF and the other neurotrophic factors were not followed in our study.

QUESTIONS FOR ANDRIUS BASKYS

From William Slikker, Jr.

Postnatal day 7 rat pups are believed to be immature, perhaps reflective of last trimester primate development. Do your studies reflect effects in developmental animals or adults? Could the developmental stage of your studies provide an explanation as to why your results differ from others collected in adult animals?

ANSWER: Organotypic hippocampal cultures prepared from postnatal day 7 (P7) rat pups possess anatomical and functional properties that resemble those of young adults. Specifically, neurons form distinctive layers and glial cells are present; most importantly, unlike in immature tissue, both NMDA and mGluR receptors are present and functional. Electrophysiological properties of these neurons were found to be developmentally equivalent to the properties of neurons in acute slices prepared from P17 rats [DE SIMONI, A., C.B. GRIESINGER & F.A. EDWARDS. 2003. J.

Physiol. **550**(part 1)**:** 135–147] that are most commonly used for studies of synaptic transmission. The main difference between our results and some (but not all) other studies could be best explained by our experimental protocol (DHPG treatment was before the injury in our studies vs. DHPG applied during or after the injury). Of course, until this protocol is tested in adult animals, alternative explanations cannot be entirely ruled out.

From Alan Faden

Your data contrast with considerable data in the literature showing that activation of mGluR1 is neurotoxic and that blockade of mGluR1 is protective in both primary neuronal cultures and *in vivo* models of trauma and ischemia. Can you clarify this?

ANSWER: Agonists for group I mGluRs increased slowly triggered NMDA-induced excitotoxicity [BUISSON, A. & D.W. CHOI. 1995. Neuropharmacology **34**(8)**:** 1081–1087] and facilitated excitotoxic damage when applied either in combination with NMDA or immediately after NMDA [BRUNO, V. *et al.* 1995. Neuropharmacology **34**(8)**:** 1089–1098]. However, DHPG was not toxic when applied on noninjured cultures and only increased cell death when applied after traumatic injury [MUKHIN, A., L. FAN & A.I. FADEN. 1996. J. Neurosci. **16**(19)**:** 6012–6020]. In our experiments, hippocampal cultures were treated with DHPG for 2 h prior to the NMDA-induced injury. The DHPG pretreatment was associated with protection, while post-NMDA treatment was not. Together, these data suggest that the effects of group I mGluR activation (toxicity vs. protection) may depend on the timing of receptor activation. Our explanation of neuroprotection induced by DHPG pretreatment hinges on group I mGluR stimulation of endocytosis protein Rab5b production and on facilitation of internalization of NMDA receptors.

From Naren Banik

How difficult is it to cut slices from spinal cord and have your tried slicing from such tissue using a McIlwain chopper?

ANSWER: We have not tried to culture spinal cord slices.

From Sylvain Doré

Does DHPG pretreatment induce internalization of these receptors and is it sufficient for protection?

ANSWER: Internalization of NMDA receptors appears to be an important factor in DHPG neuroprotection against NMDA-induced injury. In our experiments, inhibition of endocytosis protein Rab5b or blockade of NMDA receptor endocytosis by potassium depletion inhibited or abolished the DHPG protection. However, it is entirely possible that other factors play important roles in neuroprotection as well. Based on the microarray analysis of mGluR activation and some preliminary observations, these factors could include increased GABA-ergic inhibition, reduction of inflammation, or inhibition of apoptosis among others.

Microglial NADPH Oxidase Mediates Leucine Enkephalin Dopaminergic Neuroprotection

LIYA QIN,[a] YUXIN LIU,[a,b] XUN QIAN,[c] JAU-SHYONG HONG,[a]
AND MICHELLE L. BLOCK[a]

[a]*Neuropharmacology Section, Laboratory of Pharmacology and Chemistry, National Institute of Environmental Health Sciences, National Institutes of Health, Research Triangle Park, North Carolina 27709, USA*

[b]*Department of Bioscience and Biotechnology, Dalian University of Technology, Dalian 116024, China*

[c]*Inositol Phosphate Section, Laboratory of Signal Transduction, National Institute of Environmental Health Sciences, National Institutes of Health, Research Triangle Park, North Carolina 27709, USA*

ABSTRACT: Here, we report that leucine enkephalin (LE) is neuroprotective to dopaminergic (DA) neurons at femtomolar concentrations through anti-inflammatory properties. Mesencephalic neuron-glia cultures pretreated with femtomolar concentrations of LE (10^{-15}–10^{-13} M) protected DA neurons from lipopolysaccharide (LPS)–induced DA neurotoxicity, as determined by DA uptake assay and tyrosine hydroxylase (TH) immunocytochemistry (ICC). However, des-tyrosine leucine enkephalin (DTLE), an LE analogue that is missing the tyrosine residue required for binding to the kappa opioid receptor, was also neuroprotective (10^{-15}–10^{-13} M), as determined by DA uptake assay and TH ICC. Both LE and DTLE (10^{-15}–10^{-13} M) reduced LPS-induced superoxide production from microglia-enriched cultures. Further, both LE and DTLE (10^{-14}, 10^{-13} M) reduced the LPS-induced tumor necrosis factor-alpha (TNFα) mRNA and TNFα protein from PHOX$^{+/+}$ microglia, as determined by quantitative real-time RT-PCR and ELISA analysis in mesencephalic neuron-glia cultures, respectively. However, both peptides failed to inhibit TNFα expression in PHOX$^{-/-}$ cultures, which are unable to produce extracellular superoxide in response to LPS. Additionally, LE and DTLE (10^{-14}, 10^{-13} M) failed to show any neuroprotection against LPS in PHOX$^{-/-}$ cultures. Together, these data indicate that LE and DTLE are neuroprotective at femtomolar concentrations through the inhibition of oxidative insult associated with microglial NADPH oxidase and the attenuation of the ROS-mediated amplification of TNFα gene expression in microglia.

KEYWORDS: microglial NADPH oxidase; leucine enkephalin (LE); des-tyrosine leucine enkephalin (DTLE); lipopolysaccharide (LPS); tumor necrosis factor-alpha (TNFα); neuroprotection; neurotoxicity

Address for correspondence: Michelle L. Block, Ph.D., MD F1-01 NIEHS, P. O. Box 12233, Research Triangle Park, NC 27709. Voice: 919-541-5169; fax: 919-541-0841.
block@niehs.nih.gov

Ann. N.Y. Acad. Sci. 1053: 107–120 (2005).
doi: 10.1196/annals.1344.009

INTRODUCTION

Inflammation in the brain has been associated with numerous neurodegenerative diseases such as Alzheimer's disease,[1] Pick's disease,[2] multiple sclerosis,[3] and Parkinson's disease (PD).[4] PD is characterized by the selective and progressive loss of dopaminergic (DA) neurons in the substantia nigra (SN). Microglia are the resident innate immune cells in the brain and release neurotoxic factors, such as reactive oxygen species (ROS), proinflammatory factors (IL-1, TNFα, PGE_2), and reactive nitrogen species upon immunological stimulus.[5] While not all microglia activation is deleterious, the excessive and unregulated activation of microglia has been associated with disastrous neurodegenerative consequences.[6] Several peptides are reported to influence the inflammatory responses from a variety of immune cells. However, there is a dearth of information on how neuropeptides regulate microglia function in the brain to influence neuron survival. Previously, we have reported that dynorphin is neuroprotective at femtomolar concentrations through the inhibition of microglial activation,[7] but the mechanism through which dynorphin exerts its effects was not determined. Recently, we have identified that the smallest neuroprotective peptide fragment of dynorphin is glycine-glycine-phenylalanine (GGF), which is neuroprotective through anti-inflammatory properties.[8] The purpose of the following study was to discern whether the phenomenon of neuroprotective peptides at femtomolar concentrations extended to other opioid peptides known to contain the GGF peptide sequence and to confirm whether these neuroprotective peptides act through the same mechanism.

One potential explanation for the selective DA neurotoxicity seen in PD is that DA neurons are more vulnerable to oxidative and immunological insult when compared to other cell types.[9] For example, DA neurons have low intracellular glutathione.[9] Indeed, several reports have shown that both *in vivo*[10,11] and *in vitro*[11,12] administration of lipopolysaccharide (LPS) results in the selective and progressive loss of DA neurons. Additionally, the SN region contains 4.5 times as many microglia when compared to other regions of the brain,[13] suggesting that, due to regional and cell-type specificity, the DA neurons localized in the SN possess a predisposed vulnerability to microglial activation. Thus, the control of microglial function is likely to be imperative for the survival of DA neurons in the SN. Currently, the homeostatic mechanisms preventing the overactivation of microglia in the SN are unknown.

The list of neuropeptides that are biologically active and neuroprotective at femtomolar concentrations is vast and is steadily increasing. Several studies have indicated the effects of femtomolar concentrations of various peptides on the modulation of immune function, such as chemotaxis,[14,15] antibody production,[16–18] natural killer cell activity,[19] phagocytosis,[20,21] production of proinflammatory factors,[7,22] and neuroprotection.[7,23–25] Recent work from our laboratory has shown that dynorphin is neuroprotective by inhibiting microglial activation[7] through a mechanism independent of the traditional opiate receptors. Currently, the mechanistic details of how femtomolar-acting peptides exert their effects are lacking.

The following study tested the hypothesis that opioid peptides similar to dynorphin, leu-enkephalin (LE), and des-tyrosine leucine enkephalin (DTLE) were neuroprotective and anti-inflammatory at femtomolar concentrations through a mechanism that is independent of the opioid receptors. Further, the following research sought to identify the mechanism through which LE inhibited microglial activation in an effort to elucidate the critical and common factors regulating microglial activation, with the hope of offering novel insight into anti-inflammatory therapy for PD.

MATERIALS AND METHODS

Animals

Adult, timed-pregnant (gestational day 14) female Fischer 344 rats were purchased from Charles River Laboratories (Raleigh, NC). Eight-week-old male (25–30 g) and female (25–30 g) B6.129S6-Cybb^{tm1Din} (PHOX$^{-/-}$) and C57BL/6J 000664 (PHOX$^{+/+}$) mice were purchased from Jackson Laboratories (Bar Harbor, ME) [PHOX = phagocytic oxidase]. B6.129S6-Cybb^{tm1Din} PHOX$^{-/-}$ mice are lacking a functional gp91 protein, the catalytic subunit of the NADPH oxidase complex. NADPH oxidase is an inducible electron transport system in phagocytic cells that is responsible for the generation of the respiratory burst. PHOX$^{-/-}$ mice are unable to generate extracellular superoxide in response to LPS or other immunological stimulus. The PHOX$^{-/-}$ mutation is maintained in the C57BL/6J 000664 background; thus, C57BL/6J 000664 (PHOX$^{+/+}$) mice were used as PHOX$^{-/-}$ control animals. Breeding of the mice was performed to achieve accurate timed-pregnancy within ±0.5 days.

Reagents

LPS (strain O111:B4) was purchased from Calbiochem (San Diego, CA). Cell culture ingredients were obtained from Life Technologies (Grand Island, NY). [^{3}H]-Dopamine (DA; 28 Ci/mmol) was purchased from Perkin Elmer Life Sciences. Monoclonal antibodies against neuron-specific nuclear protein (Neu-N) and against the CR3 complement receptor (OX-42) were obtained from Pharmingen (San Diego, CA). The polyclonal antibody against glial fibrillary acidic protein (GFAP) and antibody diluent came from DAKO (Carpinteria, CA). Rat monoclonal antibody raised against F4/80 antigen was purchased from Serotec (Raleigh, NC). The polyclonal antibody against tyrosine hydroxylase (TH) was a kind gift from D. John Reinhard of GlaxoSmithKline (Research Triangle Park, NC). Tumor necrosis factor-alpha (TNFα) ELISA kits were purchased from R&D Systems (Minneapolis, MN). All other reagents came from Sigma Chemical (St. Louis, MO).

Mesencephalic Neuron-Glia Cultures

Rat and mouse ventral mesencephalic neuron-glia were prepared following a previously described protocol,[26] with modifications. Briefly, ventral mesencephalic tissues dissected from embryonic day 14/15 Fischer 344 rats and 13/14 PHOX$^{+/+}$ and PHOX$^{-/-}$ mice were dissociated by mild mechanical trituration in minimum essential medium (MEM). Cells were plated (5×10^5/well) in 24-well culture plates precoated with poly-D-lysine (20 μg/mL) and cultured using the previously reported procedure.[26] The composition of the mesencephalic neuron-glia cultures was determined by immunocytochemistry (ICC). The mesencephalic neuron-glia cultures contained 10–11% OX-42-IR rat or F4/80-IR mouse microglia, 40% Neu-N-IR neurons, and 1–2% TH-IR DA neurons. The remaining cells were presumed to be astroglia.

Microglia-Enriched Cultures

Primary microglia were prepared from whole brains of 2-day-old rat pups following a previously described protocol.[26] Cells were seeded at 5×10^4/well in 96-well plates for superoxide assay. The purity of microglia was >98%.

Uptake Assay

The ability of cells to take up [^{3}H]-DA was performed using the previously described protocol.[7] Cells were incubated for 20 min at 37°C with 1 μM [^{3}H]-DA in Krebs-Ringer buffer (16 mM NaH_2PO_4, 16 mM Na_2HPO_4, 119 mM NaCl, 4.7 mM KCl, 1.2 mM $MgSO_4$, 1.3 mM EDTA, pH 7.4). Nonspecific uptake was measured in the presence of 10 μM mazindol. After the cells were washed (3×) with ice-cold Krebs-Ringer buffer (1 mL/well) and lysed with 1 N NaOH (0.5 mL/well), the lysate was mixed with 15 mL of scintillation fluid, and radioactivity was determined with a liquid scintillation counter. The specific [^{3}H]-DA was calculated by subtracting the amount of radioactivity obtained in the presence of mazindol from that obtained in the absence of mazindol.

Immunostaining

DA neurons were stained with the polyclonal antibody against TH, and the total number of neurons was determined by staining with the antibody against Neu-N. Rat microglia were stained with OX-42 antibody, and mouse microglia stained with the rat monoclonal antibody raised against the F4/80 antigen. Astroglia were stained with the polyclonal antibody against GFAP. All staining was performed in the manner described previously.[27]

Superoxide Assay

The amount of extracellular superoxide (O_2^-) produced was determined by measuring the superoxide dismutase (SOD)–inhibitable reduction of tetrazolium salt, WST-1.[28–30] Primary rat microglia-enriched cultures were plated at 5×10^4/well in 200 μL culture medium in 96-well plates and incubated for 24 h at 37°C in a humidified atmosphere of 5% CO_2 and 95% air. Cells were washed twice with Hanks' balanced salt solution (HBSS) and pretreated with LE or DTLE for 30 min prior to adding 10 ng/mL of LPS. To each well, 50 μL of peptide (LE or DTLE), 50 μL of HBSS with or without SOD (600 U/mL), 50 μL of vehicle or LPS, and 50 μL of WST-1 (1 mM) in HBSS were added. The cultures were incubated for 30 min at 37°C and 5% CO_2 and 95% air. The absorbance at 450 nm was read with a Spectra Max Plus microtiter plate spectrophotometer (Molecular Devices, Sunnyvale, CA). The amount of SOD-inhibitable superoxide was calculated and expressed as percent of vehicle-treated control cultures.

Real-Time RT-PCR Analysis

The level of TNFα gene expression was quantified using real-time RT-PCR analysis as described by Walker.[31] Briefly, total RNA was isolated from mesencephalic neuron-glia cultures from $PHOX^{+/+}$ mice using Trizol reagent, followed by purification with RNeasy column (QIAGEN, Valencia, CA). Total RNA was reverse transcribed with MuLV reverse transcriptase and random hexamer primers. The following forward and reverse primers for TNFα were designed using Primer Express software (Version 2.0, Applied Biosystems, Foster City, CA)—TNFα forward: 5′-GAC CCT CAC ACT CAG ATC ATC TTC T-3′; TNFα reverse: 5′-CCT CCA CTT GGT GGT TTG CT-3′. The SYBR green DNA PCR kit (Applied Biosystems, Foster City, CA) was used for real-time PCR analysis. The relative differences in expression between groups were expressed using cycle time (Ct) values normalized with β-actin, and relative differences between control and treatment groups were calculated and expressed as relative expression, setting the control as 100%.

TNFα Assay

The release of TNFα was measured with a commercial enzyme-linked immunosorbent assay (ELISA) kit from R&D Systems (Minneapolis, MN), as described previously.[32]

Statistical Analysis

The data are expressed as mean ± SEM and statistical significance was assessed with an analysis of variance followed by Bonferroni's *t* test. A value of $P < 0.05$ was considered statistically significant.

RESULTS

LE and DTLE Protect Dopaminergic Neurons from LPS-Induced Degeneration

The neuroprotective effect of femtomolar concentrations of LE and DTLE was first examined in mesencephalice neuron-glia cultures. Dose response studies showed that LE and DTLE significantly attenuated the LPS-induced loss of DA neuron function at the concentrations of 10^{-15} to 10^{-13} M, as measured by dopamine uptake (FIG. 1A, $P < 0.05$). The ability of DA neurons in mesencephalic neuron-glia cultures to take up [^{3}H]-DA after exposure to 5 ng/mL of LPS was enhanced by approximately 30% with 30-min pretreatment of either LE or DTLE, with the greatest level of protection at the concentration of 10^{-14} M for both peptides. Immunocytochemical staining with an anti–tyrosine hydroxylase antibody (TH), a specific marker for DA neurons, revealed that LE and DTLE pretreatment protected DA neurons against the LPS-induced loss of DA neurons, with the peak protection occurring at 10^{-14} M for both LE and DTLE (FIG. 1B, $P < 0.05$). Morphological analysis further supported that LE and DTLE protected TH-immunoreactive neurons (TH-IR) from LPS-induced cell damage.

The cultures treated with 5 ng/mL of LPS showed loss of dendrites, axon disintegration, and loss of DA neurons when compared to control wells. However, cultures pretreated with 10^{-14} M LE or DTLE prior to the treatment with LPS presented healthy TH-IR neurons, such as extensive dendrites, axon integration (FIG. 1C) and increased number of TH-IR neurons (FIG. 1B) compared with LPS-treated cultures. Taken together, these results indicate that both LE and its analogue DTLE, which is unable to bind conventional opioid receptors, protected DA neurons against LPS-induced neuronal death and loss of function with a similar efficacy and dose

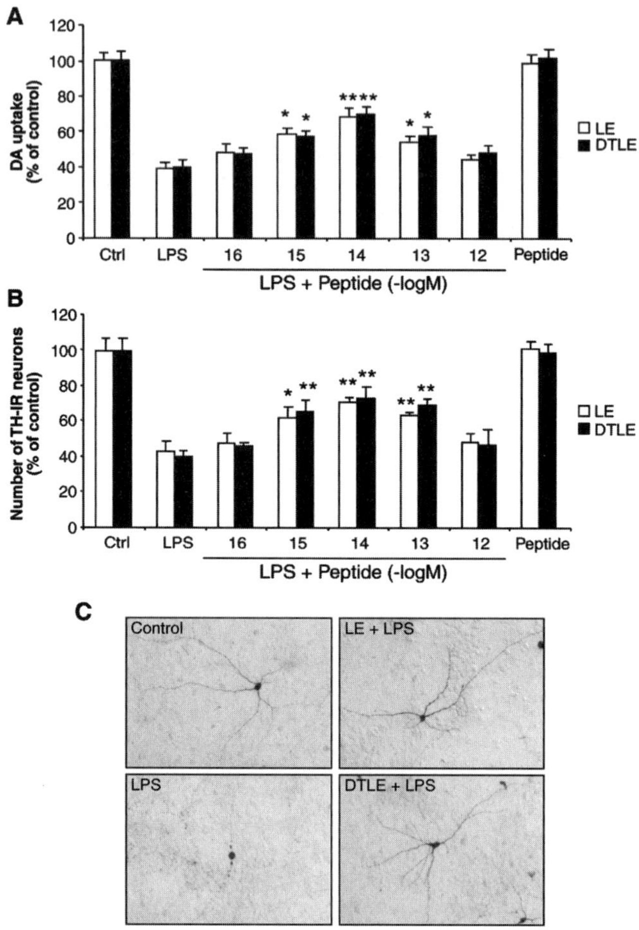

FIGURE 1. Dose response studies with LE and DTLE. See text for details.

response, indicating a common high-affinity site of action and mechanism independent of conventional opioid receptors.

LE and DTLE Reduce LPS-Induced Production of Superoxide in Microglia

It has recently been demonstrated that ROS generated from NADPH oxidase are associated with the production of extracellular superoxide, the early morphological changes in activated microglia, the amplification of microglial proinflammatory factors, and the subsequent death of DA neurons.[27] Recently, we have identified that the dynorphin peptide fragment GGF, naloxone, and dextromethorphan are neuroprotective at femtomolar concentrations through inhibition of NADPH oxidase activation and attenuation of the production of extracellular superoxide.[8,33] To investigate whether LE and DTLE inhibit the microglial production of extracellular superoxide,

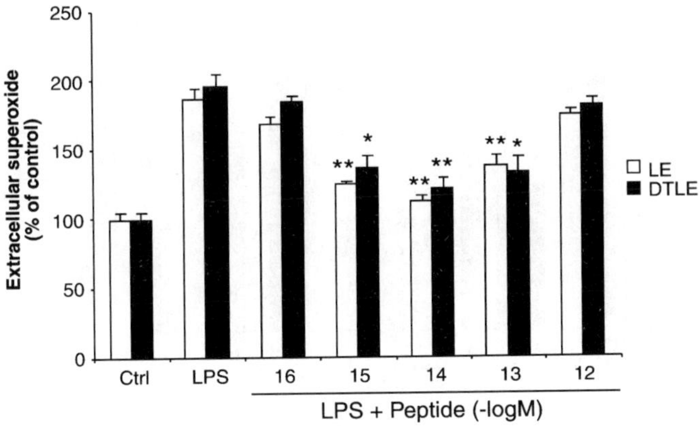

FIGURE 2. Treatment of microglia-enriched cultures with 10 ng/mL of LPS markedly elevated the production of superoxide free radicals ($P < 0.05$). See text for details.

microglia-enriched cultures were pretreated with LE or DTLE over the concentration range of 10^{-16} to 10^{-12} M, exposed to LPS, and extracellular superoxide was then measured. As shown in FIGURE 2, treatment of microglia-enriched cultures with 10 ng/mL of LPS markedly elevated the production of superoxide free radicals ($P < 0.05$). A significant inhibition of the LPS-stimulated superoxide production (50–70%) was observed in the cultures pretreated for 30 min with 10^{-15}–10^{-13} M LE or DTLE ($P < 0.05$). These results demonstrate a similar inhibitory profile and dose response for both peptides (LE and DTLE).

Microglial NADPH Oxidase Is a Critical Component of LE and DTLE Neuroprotection

To determine the role of NADPH oxidase in the neuroprotective effects of LE and DTLE, mixed mesencephalic neuron-glia cultures from $PHOX^{+/+}$ and $PHOX^{-/-}$ mice were first pretreated with LE or DTLE and then exposed to 10 ng/mL of LPS. LE and DTLE significantly protected DA neurons from LPS-induced decrease in DA uptake capacity at 10^{-14} and 10^{-13} M in $PHOX^{+/+}$ cultures (FIG. 3, $P < 0.05$). However, both LE and DTLE failed to show any DA neuroprotective effect in the neuron-glia cultures from $PHOX^{-/-}$ mice (FIG. 3), supporting that NADPH oxidase is one of the primary components contributing to the LPS-induced neurotoxicity. These results suggest that LE and DTLE afford neuroprotection through inactivation of microglial NADPH oxidase. Notably, pretreatment with LE and DTLE in $PHOX^{+/+}$ cultures attenuated the LPS-induced decrease in DA uptake to an approximate 20–30% decline from control, which is comparable to the 25% loss induced by LPS in $PHOX^{-/-}$ cultures, indicating that these low concentrations of peptides inhibit the majority of the NADPH oxidase–induced neurotoxicity.

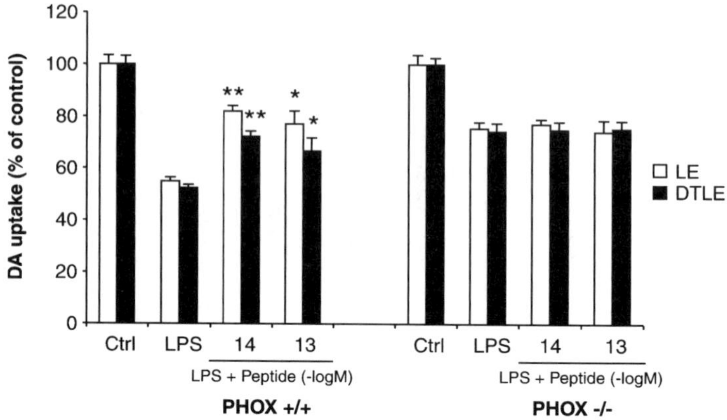

FIGURE 3. LE and DTLE significantly protected DA neurons from LPS-induced decrease in DA uptake capacity at 10^{-14} and 10^{-13} M in PHOX$^{+/+}$ cultures ($P < 0.05$). However, both LE and DTLE failed to show any dopaminergic neuroprotective effect in the neuron-glia cultures from PHOX$^{-/-}$ mice. See text for details.

LE and DTLE Inhibit LPS-Induced TNFα mRNA and Protein Expression through NADPH Oxidase

Inflammation-mediated neurodegeneration involves the participation of proinflammatory and cytotoxic factors produced by activated glia, especially microglia. LPS activates microglia to produce cytokines, such as TNFα, and free radicals, such as superoxide and nitric oxide. These factors act on neurons to induce neurodegeneration.[6] As shown in FIGURES 2 and 3, the inhibition of neurotoxic extracellular superoxide and inactivation of NADPH oxidase are critical components of LE and DTLE neuroprotection at femtomolar concentrations. Earlier reports from our laboratory have shown that NADPH oxidase–derived intracellular ROS are critical components of proinflammatory signaling in microglia.[27] To investigate the effects of LE and DTLE on proinflammatory gene expression and to discern the role of NADPH oxidase on the anti-inflammatory effects of LE and DTLE, LPS-induced TNFα expression was determined in PHOX$^{+/+}$ and PHOX$^{-/-}$ cultures pretreated with LE or DTLE. Mesencephalic neuron-glia cultures from PHOX$^{+/+}$ mice were pretreated with the vehicle or the indicated concentrations of LE or DTLE for 30 min followed by 10 ng/mL of LPS treatment. At 1-h post-LPS treatment, TNFα gene expression was measured by real-time RT-PCR analysis. TNFα gene expression was significantly increased after LPS treatment compared with corresponding vehicle controls ($P < 0.05$). However, the neuron-glia cultures pretreated with LE or DTLE for 30 min showed significant inhibition of TNFα gene expression compared with LPS-treated cultures (FIG. 4A) ($P < 0.05$). To discern the role of NADPH oxidase in LE and DTLE inhibition of TNFα, the secretion of the TNFα protein in the supernatant of mesencephalic neuron-glia cultures from both PHOX$^{+/+}$ and PHOX$^{-/-}$ mice was also measured. Consistent with the real-time RT-PCR analysis, PHOX$^{+/+}$ cultures showed a significant reduction of TNFα with LE and DTLE pretreatment at the concentrations of 10^{-14} and 10^{-13} M ($P < 0.05$). However, PHOX$^{-/-}$ cultures failed

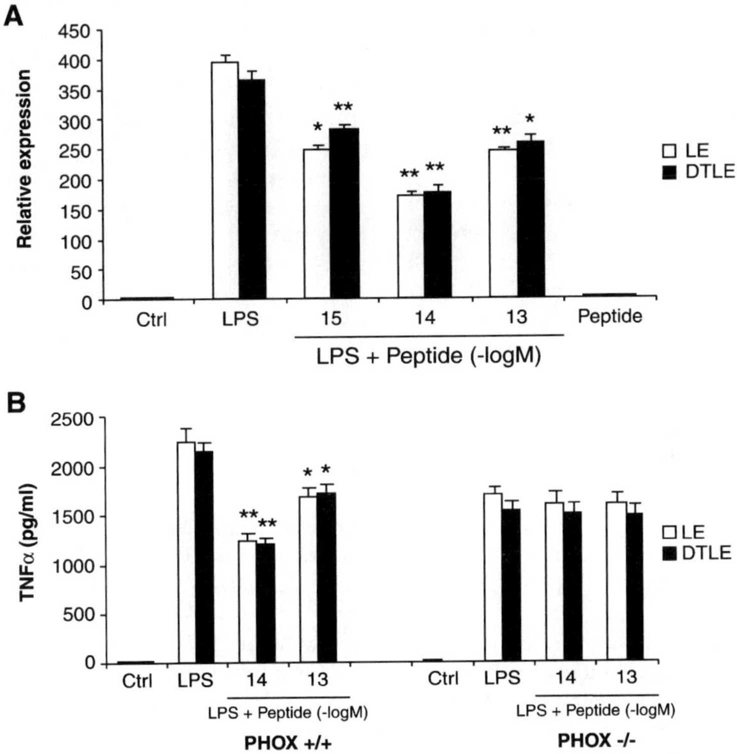

FIGURE 4. Neuron-glia cultures pretreated with LE or DTLE for 30 min showed significant inhibition of TNFα gene expression compared with LPS-treated cultures (**A**). However, $PHOX^{-/-}$ cultures failed to show any TNFα reduction in response to LPS with pretreatment of either neuroprotective peptide (**B**). See text for details.

to show any TNFα reduction in response to LPS with pretreatment of either neuroprotective peptide (FIG. 4B), suggesting that both femtomolar-acting compounds also inhibit the ROS-induced amplification of TNFα expression. In addition, no significant reduction of LPS-stimulated nitrite production was observed with either LE or DTLE treatment (data not shown).

DISCUSSION

The identification of neuroprotective peptides effective at femtomolar concentrations has redefined how cells communicate and has offered great hope for the development of novel therapeutic compounds. Initial research investigating femtomolar-acting neuroprotective agents focused on several related compounds that were reported to both inhibit direct neurotoxicity and possess neurotrophic characteristics.[34–37] Pituitary adenylate cyclase–activating polypeptide (PACAP), vasoactive intestinal peptide (VIP), and activity-dependent neurotrophic factor (ADNF)[38] are a class of interrelated femtomolar-acting regulatory peptides that are effective for ameliorating neurodegeneration. In the current study, we extend this knowledge with the discovery of an additional and unique femtomolar-acting mechanism of neuroprotection, where several related opioid peptides are able to inhibit microglial activation independent of the conventional opioid receptors. Interestingly, similar to LE and its analogue DTLE, the full-length sequence of many of these neuroprotective peptides (VIP, ADNF) do not seem to be required, suggesting a multifaceted homeostatic mechanism in the brain promoting neuroprotection. This finding has wide-reaching implications not only for the development of novel therapeutic compounds, but also because perturbation of these protective peptides may shed much needed insight into the potential pathology of neurodegenerative disease.

We have recently identified that GGF is the minimum dynorphin peptide sequence that is required for neuroprotection at femtomolar concentrations.[8] GGF is missing the tyrosine residue required for binding to the kappa opiate receptor, suggesting the existence of an independent high-affinity site of action. Along with naloxone[8] and dextromethorphan,[33] we have also reported that GGF is neuroprotective at femtomolar concentrations through the inhibition of NADPH oxidase. Interestingly, both LE and DTLE contain the GGF sequence and are neuroprotective through the same mechanism of inhibition of NADPH oxidase. Here, we show that LE and its metabolite join the list of femtomolar-acting compounds that inhibit NADPH oxidase and support the existence of a network of endogenous opiate peptides that regulate microglia activity at femtomolar concentrations.

It is becoming increasingly evident that the inhibition of microglial NADPH oxidase is an ideal therapeutic target for the treatment of neurodegenerative disease. Current treatments for PD are riddled with multiple potential side effects and drug-drug interactions. Recent reports from our laboratory have identified that NADPH oxidase mediates microglia-mediated DA neurotoxicity through two mechanisms. First, activation of NADPH oxidase results in the production of extracellular ROS, which is toxic to DA neurons.[27] In the current study, we show that LE and DTLE inhibit the production of superoxide from microglia and that LE and DTLE have no neuroprotective effect in mice lacking the catalytic subunit of NADPH oxidase. The second mechanism through which PHOX influences DA neurotoxicity occurs because the activation of NADPH oxidase results in an increase in intracellular ROS in microglia. This intracellular ROS increase then amplifies the expression of proinflammatory genes in microglia.[27] In the current study, we show that LE and DTLE inhibit TNFα expression, but have no effect on the LPS-induced TNFα expression in PHOX$^{-/-}$ mice. This suggests that LE and DTLE exert their protective effects solely through their action on NADPH oxidase. FIGURE 5 provides a summary of the protective mechanism through which femtomolar-acting opioid peptides and related femtomolar-acting compounds protect DA neurons through the inhibition of microglial activation.

At this time, the mechanisms through which LE, DTLE, GGF, naloxone, and dextromethorphan are inhibiting NADPH oxidase at femtomolar concentrations are unknown. Currently, we have shown that cells stably transfected with gp91, the membrane-bound catalytic subunit of NADPH oxidase, and p22, the protein that anchors gp91 to the membrane, show an increase in [^{3}H]-naloxone binding, suggesting that naloxone is binding to gp91 (unpublished data). Thus, we speculate that

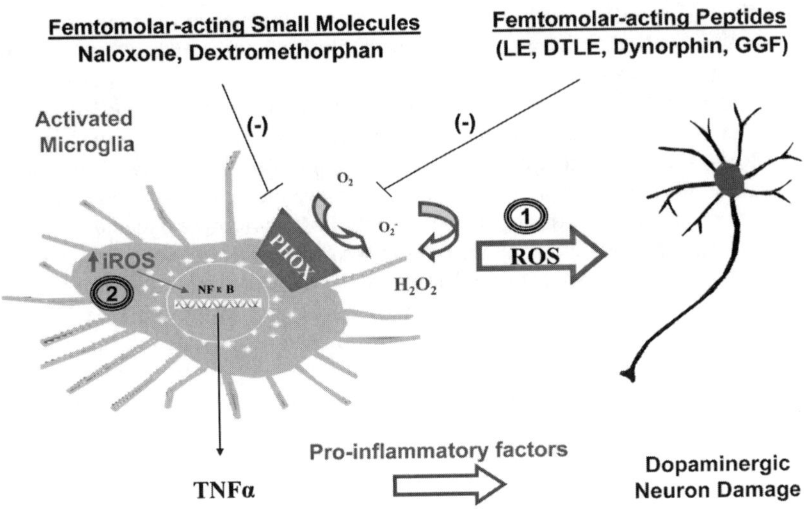

FIGURE 5. Summary of the protective mechanism through which femtomolar-acting opioid peptides and related femtomolar-acting compounds protect DA neurons through the inhibition of microglial activation. See text for details.

these femtomolar-acting compounds may be inhibiting PHOX activity by binding to the catalytic subunit, gp91, to inhibit the enzyme function. Previously, it has been reported that an antibody recognizing a component of gp91 can inhibit superoxide production in a cell-free assay, supporting that the enzyme complex can be inhibited independent of the cytosolic proteins and by binding to the gp91 subunit.[39] Future research in our laboratory is aimed at discerning the binding site on gp91 responsible for the inhibition of NADPH oxidase at femtomolar concentrations.

The bimodal dose response has been reported in several femtomolar-acting neuroprotective compounds tested in our laboratory.[7,8,33] The bimodal dose response is characterized by three unique sections of the dose curve. The physiological effects seen in the higher, micromolar concentrations are often assumed to be the traditional receptor-mediated effects, but this assumption may not be applicable for all cases. For example, GGF is the smallest biologically active fragment of dynorphin and demonstrates a biphasic neuroprotective response,[8] similar to LE and DTLE. However, GGF is unable to bind the kappa opiate receptor, suggesting that the mechanism is independent of the traditional receptors. The femtomolar region of the curve is attributed to an atypical mechanism that is independent of traditional receptor-mediated events, as the effects of the peptide/compound are seen at concentrations that are several orders of magnitude lower than what is expected from opiate receptors and the smallest biologically active fragment (GGF) cannot bind to the kappa receptor. The third component of the neuroprotective bimodal response is the middle portion of the curve (10^{-12}–10^{-10} M), where the neuroprotective response is absent. Presently, there is no clear explanation for the inability of these compounds to show any protective effect in the picomolar range (10^{-12}–10^{-10} M). One interpretation is that there are multiple sites of action for the same peptide/compound, depending upon the dose. In the case of two sites of action, the inhibition seen in the picomolar range may be due to an effect similar to "substrate inhibition", where the site of action for femtomolar concentrations is overwhelmed with increasing dose. Alternatively, a hypothetical third binding site in the picomolar range may mask the effect of these agents at femtomolar concentrations. Further research in our laboratory is focused on identifying the potential sites of action for the femtomolar-acting compounds.

Several reports from our laboratory and others have indicated that NADPH oxidase is critical for microglia-mediated neurotoxicity. Postmortem analyses of PD brains show an increase in gp91 expression, linking NADPH oxidase to neurodegenerative disease in humans.[40] Further, several compounds shown to be selectively toxic to DA neurons, such as paraquat,[41] diesel exhaust particles,[42] β-amyloid,[43] rotenone,[44] and LPS,[27] have a component of neurotoxicity shown to be mediated through NADPH oxidase. Moreover, neurotoxicity associated with the microglial response to MPTP treatment is also reported to be mediated through NADPH oxidase.[45] Given the critical role of this enzyme complex in PD, environmental toxins, and endogenous hallmark proteins associated with neurodegenerative disease, the potential therapeutic utility of inhibition of this enzyme is clear. Thus, the identification of a network of femtomolar-acting peptides that attenuate inflammation-mediated neurodegeneration may both offer valuable insight into the pathogenesis of PD and provide a novel opportunity to design safer compounds with higher therapeutic efficacy.

ACKNOWLEDGMENTS

We would like to thank Sufen Yang for her technical assistance.

REFERENCES

1. McGeer, P.L. & E. McGeer. 2004. Immunotherapy for Alzheimer's disease. Sci. Aging Knowledge Environ. **2004:** PE29.
2. Schofield, E. *et al.* 2003. Severity of gliosis in Pick's disease and frontotemporal lobar degeneration: tau-positive glia differentiate these disorders. Brain **126:** 827–840.
3. Chavarria, A. & J. Alcocer-Varela. 2004. Is damage in central nervous system due to inflammation? Autoimmun. Rev. **3:** 251–260.
4. McGeer, P.L. *et al.* 1988. Reactive microglia are positive for HLA-DR in the substantia nigra of Parkinson's and Alzheimer's disease brains. Neurology **38:** 1285–1291.
5. McGeer, P.L. & E.G. McGeer. 2004. Inflammation and neurodegeneration in Parkinson's disease. Parkinsonism Relat. Disord. **10**(suppl. 1)**:** S3–S7.
6. Liu, B. & J.S. Hong. 2003. Role of microglia in inflammation-mediated neurodegenerative diseases: mechanisms and strategies for therapeutic intervention. J. Pharmacol. Exp. Ther. **304:** 1–7.
7. Liu, B. *et al.* 2001. Femtomolar concentrations of dynorphins protect rat mesencephalic dopaminergic neurons against inflammatory damage. J. Pharmacol. Exp. Ther. **298:** 1133–1141.
8. Qin, L. *et al.* 2005. Microglial NADPH oxidase is a novel target for femtomolar neuroprotection against oxidative stress. FASEB J. **19:** 550–557.
9. Loeffler, D.A. *et al.* 1994. Effects of enhanced striatal dopamine turnover *in vivo* on glutathione oxidation. Clin. Neuropharmacol. **17:** 370–379.
10. Carvey, P.M. *et al.* 2003. Prenatal exposure to the bacteriotoxin lipopolysaccharide leads to long-term losses of dopamine neurons in offspring: a potential, new model of Parkinson's disease. Front. Biosci. **8:** s826–s837.

11. GAO, H.M. *et al.* 2002. Microglial activation–mediated delayed and progressive degeneration of rat nigral dopaminergic neurons: relevance to Parkinson's disease. J. Neurochem. **81:** 1285–1297.
12. GAYLE, D.A. *et al.* 2002. Lipopolysaccharide (LPS)–induced dopamine cell loss in culture: roles of tumor necrosis factor-alpha, interleukin-1beta, and nitric oxide. Brain Res. Dev. Brain Res. **133:** 27–35.
13. KIM, W.G. *et al.* 2000. Regional difference in susceptibility to lipopolysaccharide-induced neurotoxicity in the rat brain: role of microglia. J. Neurosci. **20:** 6309–6316.
14. WIEDERMANN, F.J. *et al.* 2002. Migration of human monocytes in response to procalcitonin. Crit. Care Med. **30:** 1112–1117.
15. GRUBER, B.L., M.J. MARCHESE & R. KEW. 1995. Angiogenic factors stimulate mast-cell migration. Blood **86:** 2488–2493.
16. WILLIAMSON, S.A. *et al.* 1987. Differential effects of beta-endorphin fragments on human natural killing. Brain Behav. Immun. **1:** 329–335.
17. WILLIAMSON, S.A. *et al.* 1988. Effects of beta endorphin on specific immune responses in man. Immunology **65:** 47–51.
18. DAS, K.P. *et al.* 1995. Modulatory effects of [Met5]-enkephalin on interleukin-1 beta secretion from microglia in mixed brain cell cultures. J. Neuroimmunol. **62:** 9–17.
19. FAITH, R.E. *et al.* 1984. Neuroimmunomodulation with enkephalins: enhancement of human natural killer (NK) cell activity *in vitro*. Clin. Immunol. Immunopathol. **31:** 412–418.
20. SOWA, G. *et al.* 1997. Inhibition of swine microglial cell phagocytosis of *Cryptococcus neoformans* by femtomolar concentrations of morphine. Biochem. Pharmacol. **53:** 823–828.
21. GLADYSHEVA, T.B., A.A. KONRADOV & K.A. LEBEDEV. 1989. The dose dependence of various loads using the rosette formation method. Biofizika **34:** 833–834.
22. DELGADO, M. *et al.* 1999. Vasoactive intestinal peptide (VIP) and pituitary adenylate cyclase–activation polypeptide (PACAP) protect mice from lethal endotoxemia through the inhibition of TNF-alpha and IL-6. J. Immunol. **162:** 1200–1205.
23. KONG, L.Y. *et al.* 1999. Reduction of lipopolysaccharide-induced neurotoxicity in mixed cortical neuron/glia cultures by femtomolar concentrations of pituitary adenylate cyclase–activating polypeptide. Neuroscience **91:** 493–500.
24. GOZES, I. *et al.* 1999. A novel signaling molecule for neuropeptide action: activity-dependent neuroprotective protein. Ann. N.Y. Acad. Sci. **897:** 125–135.
25. KONG, L.Y. *et al.* 2000. Reduction of lipopolysaccharide-induced neurotoxicity in mouse mixed cortical neuron/glia cultures by ultralow concentrations of dynorphins. J. Biomed. Sci. **7:** 241–247.
26. LIU, B. *et al.* 2000. Reduction by naloxone of lipopolysaccharide-induced neurotoxicity in mouse cortical neuron-glia co-cultures. Neuroscience **97:** 749–756.
27. QIN, L. *et al.* 2004. NADPH oxidase mediates lipopolysaccharide-induced neurotoxicity and proinflammatory gene expression in activated microglia. J. Biol. Chem. **279:** 1415–1421.
28. PESKIN, A.V. & C.C. WINTERBOURN. 2000. A microtiter plate assay for superoxide dismutase using a water-soluble tetrazolium salt (WST-1). Clin. Chim. Acta **293:** 157–166.
29. LIU, B. & J.S. HONG. 2003. Primary rat mesencephalic neuron-glia, neuron-enriched, microglia-enriched, and astroglia-enriched cultures. Methods Mol. Med. **79:** 387–395.
30. TAN, A.S. & M.V. BERRIDGE. 2000. Superoxide produced by activated neutrophils efficiently reduces the tetrazolium salt, WST-1, to produce a soluble formazan: a simple colorimetric assay for measuring respiratory burst activation and for screening anti-inflammatory agents. J. Immunol. Methods **238:** 59–68.
31. WALKER, N.J. 2001. Real-time and quantitative PCR: applications to mechanism-based toxicology. J. Biochem. Mol. Toxicol. **15:** 121–127.
32. LIU, B., L. DU & J.S. HONG. 2000. Naloxone protects rat dopaminergic neurons against inflammatory damage through inhibition of microglia activation and superoxide generation. J. Pharmacol. Exp. Ther. **293:** 607–617.
33. LI, G. *et al.* 2005. Femtomolar concentrations of dextromethorphan protect mesencephalic dopaminergic neurons from inflammatory damage. FASEB J. **19:** 489–496.

34. Brenneman, D.E. & I. Gozes. 1996. A femtomolar-acting neuroprotective peptide. J. Clin. Invest. **97:** 2299–2307.
35. Gozes, I. & D.E. Brenneman. 1996. Activity-dependent neurotrophic factor (ADNF): an extracellular neuroprotective chaperonin? J. Mol. Neurosci. **7:** 235–244.
36. Gozes, I. *et al.* 1996. Neuroprotective strategy for Alzheimer disease: intranasal administration of a fatty neuropeptide. Proc. Natl. Acad. Sci. USA **93:** 427–432.
37. Arimura, A. *et al.* 1994. PACAP functions as a neurotrophic factor. Ann. N.Y. Acad. Sci. **739:** 228–243.
38. Gozes, I. *et al.* 2000. A novel VIP responsive gene: activity dependent neuroprotective protein. Ann. N.Y. Acad. Sci. **921:** 115–118.
39. Burritt, J.B. *et al.* 2003. Functional epitope on human neutrophil flavocytochrome b558. J. Immunol. **170:** 6082–6089.
40. Wu, D.C. *et al.* 2003. NADPH oxidase mediates oxidative stress in the 1-methyl-4-phenyl-1,2,3,6-tetrahydropyridine model of Parkinson's disease. Proc. Natl. Acad. Sci. USA **100:** 6145–6150.
41. Wu, X. *et al.* 2005. The role of microglia in paraquat-induced dopaminergic neurotoxicity. Antioxid. Redox Signal. **7:** 645–651.
42. Block, M.L. *et al.* 2004. Nanometer size diesel exhaust particles are selectively toxic to dopaminergic neurons: the role of microglia, phagocytosis, and NADPH oxidase. FASEB J. **18:** 1618–1620.
43. Qin, L. *et al.* 2002. Microglia enhance beta-amyloid peptide–induced toxicity in cortical and mesencephalic neurons by producing reactive oxygen species. J. Neurochem. **83:** 973–983.
44. Gao, H.M. *et al.* 2002. Distinct role for microglia in rotenone-induced degeneration of dopaminergic neurons. J. Neurosci. **22:** 782–790.
45. Gao, H.M. *et al.* 2003. Synergistic dopaminergic neurotoxicity of MPTP and inflammogen lipopolysaccharide: relevance to the etiology of Parkinson's disease. FASEB J. **17:** 1957–1959.

Effect of Neuroprotective Drugs on Gene Expression in G93A/SOD1 Mice

SHEILA IGNACIO, DAN H. MOORE, ANDREW P. SMITH, AND NANCY M. LEE

The Forbes Norris ALS Research Center, California Pacific Medical Center Research Institute, San Francisco, California, USA

ABSTRACT: Gene expression analysis is a powerful tool that has been used to define the pathological processes underlying many diseases. Several laboratories, including our own, have used this approach to identify molecular abnormalities in the G93A/SOD1 mouse, an animal model of amyotrophic lateral sclerosis (ALS). Here, we report the results of analysis of an expanded panel of genes throughout the entire lifetime in the spinal cord of these animals. In addition to upregulation of microglia/neuroinflammatory genes identified previously, we observed upregulation of metallothionein-I and -II (MT-I, MT-II). MT-I and MT-II play an important role in disposition of zinc ion, and other studies have also indicated their levels are altered in development of motor neuron disease in these animals. We also analyzed the effect on these expression profiles of several candidate drugs that have been shown to have neuroprotective effects *in vivo* or *in vitro*. That is, we asked whether administration to the G93A/SOD1 mice of any of these drugs could reverse the alterations in gene expression patterns that occur as the animals develop. The mice were given daily doses of these drugs when they were 9–11 weeks old, at a stage early in development of motor neuron disease, continuing for 5 weeks, at which time they were sacrificed. Treatment of the mice with L-carnosine, a dipeptide that scavenges free radicals and chelates zinc, did not affect expression of any of the genes altered in these animals. However, it did upregulate 3 genes unaffected by the presence of the G93A/SOD1 mutation: glial fibrillary acidic protein (GFAP), stroma-derived factor-1 (SDF-1), and excitatory amino acid transporter-2 (EAAT2). In contrast, metallothionein-III (MT-III) was downregulated. Treatment of the animals with baicalein, an herbal extract with anti-inflammatory and numerous other effects, downregulated the microglia markers CD68, CD80, and CD86, all of which were upregulated in untreated mutant animals. Baicalein treatment also downregulated tumor necrosis factor receptor (TNFRp55) and upregulated noninducible nitric oxide synthase (nNOS) and glutamine synthase (GS). These 3 genes were unaffected by the presence of the G93A mutation. We discuss the implication of these results for testing the effects of these and other candidate drugs in mutant SOD1 mice.

KEYWORDS: G93A/SOD1; gene expression; amyotrophic lateral sclerosis (ALS); metallothionein; L-carnosine; baicalein

Address for correspondence: Nancy M. Lee, The Forbes Norris ALS Research Center, California Pacific Medical Center Research Institute, 2324 Sacramento Street, San Francisco, CA 94115. Voice: 415-600-3604; fax: 415-673-5184.

nml@cooper.cpmc.org

**Ann. N.Y. Acad. Sci. 1053: 121–136 (2005). © 2005 New York Academy of Sciences.
doi: 10.1196/annals.1344.010**

INTRODUCTION

Amyotrophic lateral sclerosis (ALS, or Lou Gehrig's disease) is a fatal degenerative disorder of motor neurons. A small portion of the cases are associated with a mutation in the gene Cu/Zn-superoxide dismutase-1 (SOD1), and laboratory mice engineered to carry a human mutant SOD1 gene develop an ALS-like disease. In an attempt to understand the pathological processes that initiate the disease, several groups have carried out gene expression analysis of nervous system tissue from these animals.[1–4] These studies, together with other studies of both mice and humans,[5–9] have provided evidence for the involvement of several different processes, including neurotoxicity, oxidative stress, neuroinflammation, abnormal metal ion regulation, and apoptosis.

While it is now fairly widely accepted that each of these pathological processes may play an important role in at least some cases of ALS, the genesis of the disease remains mysterious. Each of these processes involves a wide-ranging set of metabolic pathways, often overlapping with those of other processes. Moreover, some of these processes, particularly oxidative stress and neuroinflammation, are also involved in many other neurodegenerative diseases, and even in other, nonnervous diseases. What makes ALS distinctive is that these pathologies are confined specifically to motor neurons, although the actions of other types of cells may be involved. This raises the critical question: what are the initial events in motor neurons that result in the cascade of pathological processes?

To address this issue, we have proposed to apply gene expression analysis systematically over a temporal period that encompasses the entire course of disease development, including the presymptomatic period. In this way, we aim to identify the earliest molecular abnormalities associated with disease development, as well as define the entire sequence of processes that follow them. Furthermore, rather than screening for thousands of genes using an approach such as cDNA microarrays, we chose to focus only on a small set of genes representative of the major metabolic pathways implicated in ALS. This allows us to examine the activity of these genes quantitatively over time. Using this approach, we recently reported a gene expression study of G93A/SOD1 mice in which analysis was carried out at 3-week intervals throughout the entire lifetime of the animals.[10] These animals typically begin showing symptoms of motor impairment at 9–12 weeks and die at about 18–20 weeks. The panel of 21 genes analyzed included several representative of neurotoxicity, oxidative stress, neuroinflammation, abnormal metal ion regulation, and apoptosis.

While regulation of genes representative of most of these pathological processes was affected in these animals, alterations of expression at the early, presymptomatic stages were largely confined to genes involved in neuroinflammation and microglia activation, including the cytokine TNF-α, other effector molecules including Gro-α and IL-RA, and the microglia markers CD86 and CD200R. We concluded that abnormal activation of microglia might play a very early role in the development of motor neuron disease in these animals, a conclusion supported by other data.[1–3,11–15]

In the present study, we have expanded this panel with the addition of 13 genes. These include several more genes involved in neuroinflammation, as well as the gene for insulin-like growth factor-1 (IGF1), its receptor (IGFR), and several IGF binding proteins (IGFBPs); and the genes for metallothionein-I, -II, and -III (MT-I, MT-II, and MT-III). Changes in levels of IGF and its binding proteins have been reported in

ALS patients,[16,17] and IGF1 prolongs survival in animals,[18,19] although there was no effect in human trials.[20,21] Metallothioneins chelate Zn^{++} and Cu^{++} ions, which are critical to the activity of SOD1,[22] and deletion of these genes in mutant SOD1 mice has been reported to affect their survival.[23]

The ultimate goal of this research, of course, is to develop new ways to treat ALS. This disease is not only currently incurable, but the one drug approved for its treatment, riluzole, extends the life of patients by a few months at best. Given that gene expression profiling can help identify pathological processes that need to be targeted, it might be useful as a way of screening for candidate drugs that slow down, halt, or reverse these processes, and that therefore might combat the symptoms of the disease. While several studies have tested the effects of drugs on symptom development and/or survival of mutant SOD1 mice,[15,24–30] these studies require that large numbers of animals be closely observed over many weeks. A much faster and simpler approach is offered by certain cell culture models,[31–34] but these may be of limited relevance to ALS.

Here, we report an approach to drug testing that combines the relevance of an *in vivo* model with some of the advantages of a molecular assay. We have tested in G93A/SOD1 mice the effects of several drugs that have previously been shown to have neuroprotective effects either *in vivo* or *in situ* on expression of a panel of genes representative of processes implicated in ALS.

METHODS

Animals

G93A/SOD1 mice were bred in our colony from B6SJLTgN(SOD1-G93A)1Gur mice obtained from Jackson Lab (Bar Harbor, ME). Mice were bred and maintained in microisolators and monitored daily. Hemizygous male mice were bred to B6SJL female wild type from Jackson Lab. Both male and female G93A/SOD1 mice were used in the study, as well as male and female wild-type mice for controls. They were euthanized at various ages, as detailed in RESULTS. G93A/SOD1 mutant mice were matched with their wild-type littermates, and equal numbers of each sex were used in this study. In the drug studies, we used G93A/SOD1 mutant mice, with animals from different litters of comparable age and sex randomly assigned.

Drug Administration

The drugs used in these studies were L-carnosine and baicalein. They were obtained from Sigma-Aldrich (St. Louis, MO). All drugs were dissolved in saline solution and administered once daily to animals at 9–11 weeks of age for 5 weeks. Baicalein was first dissolved in DMSO and diluted with water. The final concentration of DMSO was 10%. Carnosine was given by ip injection, while baicalein was administered in Alzet pumps, sc. Drug doses were as follows—L-carnosine: 2.2 or 11 μmol/kg/day, ip; baicalein: 3.7 or 7.4 nmol/kg/day, sc. At the beginning of this treatment regimen, the animals either showed no symptoms or were slightly weak in one or more limbs. After 5 weeks, the animals had reached the stage of limping or paralysis.

Extraction and Preparation of RNA and Analysis of Gene Expression

These procedures were carried out as previously described.[10] The genes analyzed in this study are listed in TABLE 1. They include the 21 genes that we analyzed in our previous study, as well as 13 new ones. These include several involved in neuroinflammation (ICAM, CX3CR1, COX2, TLR4, and IL-1β); IGF1 and the related genes IGF1R and IGFBP-2, -3, and -5; and MT-I, -II, and -III. Specific primers for these genes were prepared as previously described.[10]

Statistical Analysis

As in our previous study, gene expression was analyzed in groups by multivariate analysis of variance (MANOVA), as well as individually by univariate analysis. These analyses were performed to determine the significance of changes in gene expression in G93A animals vs. wild type at different ages, and also to determine the significance of changes in gene expression in G93A animals treated with various drug-dosing paradigms. To control type 1 error, we first tested all 34 genes (for temporal analysis) to determine whether expression patterns for wild type differed from those for mutant mice with age, as well as strain (wild type vs. G93A) and their interaction as using MANOVA. If the interaction term was statistically significant (at $P < 0.05$), then we performed univariate tests to determine which genes contributed to the significant difference. A significant interaction term indicates that changes in expression over time occurred at different rates in the two strains. All MANOVA tests were based on Wilks' lambda criterion and were carried out on log (base 2) of the expressions since this transformation was required to achieve normal distribution of values.

Finally, to determine the significance of drug treatment on symptom development, we used the log-rank test to compare survival among different groups of animals.

RESULTS

Gene Regulation in Spinal Cord of Mutant G93A/SOD1 Mice

Groups of mutant G93A/SOD1 mice and normal (wild-type) mice were sacrificed at ages 3, 6, 9, 12, 15, and 18 weeks, and spinal cords were removed. Total RNA was prepared, and real-time quantitative RT-PCR used to analyze relative expression of the genes listed in TABLE 1.

TABLE 1 shows the results of MANOVA performed on all 34 genes taken together, analyzed over all the time periods during the range of 3–18 weeks (every 3 weeks and 6 different time intervals in all). A highly significant difference was found between G93A/SOD1 and normal wild-type mice ($P < 0.001$).

As shown in TABLE 1, the 34 genes fall into several subgroups, according to the metabolic processes they are associated with. We next compared G93A and wild-type mice with respect to expression of each individual group of genes, over time. Significant differences were observed for the cell marker group, neuroinflammatory genes, and genes involved in zinc metabolism (TABLE 1).

TABLE 1. Temporal analysis of gene expression in spinal cord of G93A/SOD1 mice

Genes analyzed	Results
Overall	$P < 0.0006$
Cell markers	$P < 0.00001$
CD11B	Upreg (0.01)
CD68	Upreg (0.001)
CD80	Upreg (0.02)
CD86	Upreg (0.01)
CD200	ns
CD200R	Upreg (0.001)
GFAP	Upreg (0.01)
Neuroinflammation	$P < 0.0001$
MIP-2	Upreg (0.001)
IL-1α	Upreg (0.03)
IL-1β	Upreg (0.02)
IL-1RA	Upreg (0.01)
TNF-α	Upreg (0.001)
TNFRp55	Upreg (0.001)
Gro-α	Upreg (0.001)
SDF-1	ns
TLR4	ns
ICAM	Upreg (0.01)
CX3CR1	Upreg (0.02)
Oxidative stress	$P < 0.0001$
nNOS	Downreg (0.02)
iNOS	ns
COX2	ns
Neurotoxicity	ns
EAAT2	ns
GluR1	ns
GS	ns
Apoptosis	$P < 0.0001$
FADD	ns
FAS	ns
Zinc	$P < 0.001$
MT-I	Upreg (0.03)
MT-II	Upreg (0.002)
MT-III	ns

TABLE 1. (*continued*) **Temporal analysis of gene expression in spinal cord of G93A/SOD1 mice**

Genes analyzed	Results
IGF	ns
IGFBP-2	ns
IGFBP-3	ns
IGFBP-5	ns
IGF1	ns
IGF1R	ns

NOTE: Groups of G93A/SOD1 and wild-type mice (n = 10–12 in each group) were sacrificed at 3, 6, 9, 12, 15, and 18 weeks. Spinal cords were removed, total RNA isolated and converted to cDNA, and gene expression analysis carried out as described in METHODS. The first column lists the 34 genes analyzed. The second column summarizes the result of comparing gene expression in G93A/SOD1 vs. wild-type mice. The overall P value is for a multivariate test of whether SOD1 and wild-type expressions are equal across all 34 genes. Individual P values for different subgroups of genes are also shown. The top row shows the overall significance of this comparison. Subsequently, analysis was performed on each of the indicated subgroups of genes, and the significance is shown for each analysis. For subgroups that showed significant differences, the analysis continued on individual genes within that group, and these values are also shown. An "ns" indicates that a univariate two-sided t test of expression difference in SOD1 vs. wild type was not statistically significant at $P < 0.05$. Abbreviations: CD200R, CD200 receptor; GFAP, glial fibrillary acidic protein; MIP-2, macrophage inflammatory protein; IL-1α, interleukin-1α; IL-1β, interleukin-1β; TNF-α, tumor necrosis factor-α; TNFRp55, tumor necrosis factor receptor; Gro-α, growth-related oncogene-1; SDF-1, stroma-derived factor-1; TLR4, toll-like receptor-4; ICAM, intracellular adhesion molecule; nNOS, neuronal nitric oxide synthase; iNOS, inducible nitric oxide synthase; COX-2, cyclooxygenase-2; EAAT2, excitatory amino acid transporter-2; GluR1, glutamate receptor-1; GS, glutamine synthase; MT-I, -II, -III, metallothionein-I, -II, -III; IGF1, insulin-like growth factor-1; IGFBP-2, -3, -5, IGF binding protein-2, -3, -5; IGF1R, IGF1 receptor.

Finally, to determine the relative contribution of individual genes to the global significance, we applied univariate analysis to each gene in the 3 subgroups that showed significant differences, again analyzing across all periods of time. Several individual genes in the G93A animals showed significant differences in expression relative to wild-type mice, including CD68, CD80, CD86, and CD200R. Expression of all of these genes was upregulated and, in agreement with the results of our earlier study,[10] all of these genes are related to neuroinflammation. In addition, expression of 2 of the 13 new genes that we added for this study, MT-I and -II, was also affected. Expression of both was upregulated.

When these individual genes were examined at individual time periods, a further interesting difference was noted (TABLE 1; FIGS. 1 and 2). Upregulation or downregulation of these genes in G93A mice increased with age; thus, the older the animal, the greater the degree of alteration. In wild-type animals, gene expression was more or less constant with age. Hence, the difference between G93A and wild-type mice increased progressively as the animals became older.

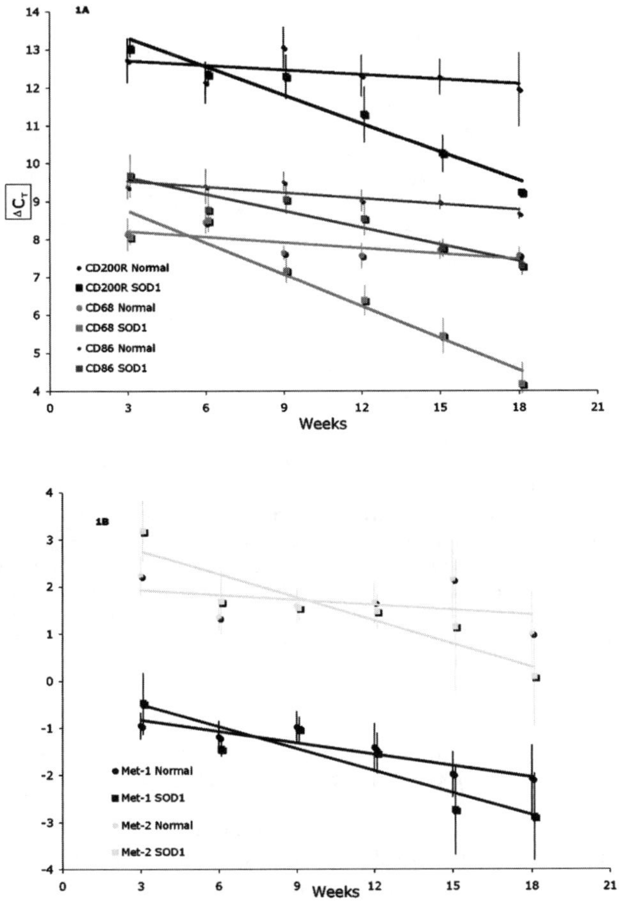

FIGURE 1. Temporal changes in gene expression in G93A/SOD1 mice. Animals were sacrificed at 3, 6, 9, 12, 15, and 18 weeks; spinal cords removed; total RNA isolated; and gene expression analyzed as described in METHODS. The ΔC_T values refer to the number of cycles of PCR required before an arbitrary product detection threshold is reached (normalized by subtracting the cycles of an unaffected housekeeping gene) and are inversely proportional to the base 2 log of the level of expression. Thus, a ΔC_T value of 2 represents a level of expression twice that of a ΔC_T value of 3, and four times that of a ΔC_T of 4. These values are shown at each time period for mutant and control mice, for the indicated genes. The *vertical bars* indicate standard errors. **(A)** Genes CD200R, CD68, and CD86. **(B)** Genes MT-I and MT-II. *Circles* indicate values from nontransgenic wild-type mice; *squares* indicate values for the G93A/SOD1 mice. The *plotted lines* represent the best fits (±) from a linear model, with a term for interaction between each group (G93A/SOD1 or normal wild type) and time.

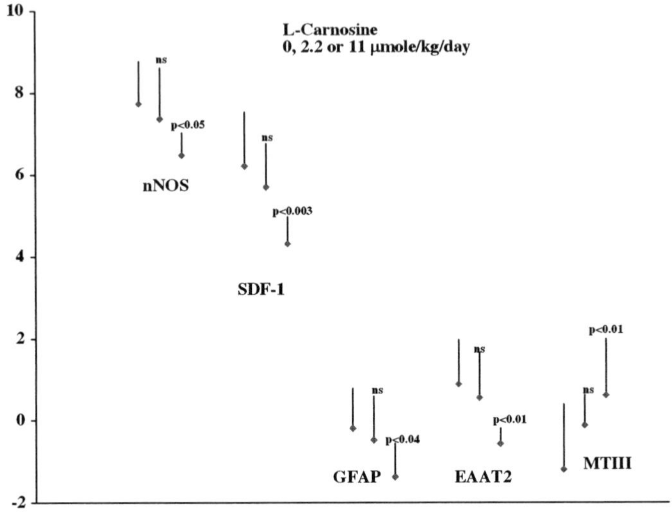

FIGURE 2. Effect of L-carnosine treatment on gene expression in G93A/SOD1 mice. Animals were given daily treatment of the drug beginning at 9–11 weeks of age, and continuing for 5 weeks, after which they were sacrificed and gene expression in spinal cord determined. For each gene are shown three ΔC_T values, which are inversely proportional to the base 2 log of expression of that gene (see legend to FIG. 1). For each gene, the value on the left is for untreated mice; the value in the middle is for mice given the lower dose of L-carnosine (2.2 μmol/kg/day); the value on the right is for mice given the higher dose of L-carnosine (11.0 μmol/kg/day). The values for the different genes are separated horizontally simply for convenience in visualizing. Significant values are shown for each gene and treatment regimen. The *vertical bars* indicate standard errors.

Effect of L-Carnosine Treatment on Gene Expression of Mutant G93A/SOD1 Mice

We next examined the effect of various drug treatments on gene expression in the G93A mice. In particular, we asked whether any of these drugs could prevent or reduce the alterations in expression of specific genes observed in these animals. As described in METHODS, animals began receiving drug when they were 9–11 weeks old, and treatment continued daily for 5 weeks, at which time they were sacrificed and spinal cords removed for gene expression analysis. Mice were given L-carnosine at a dose of 2.2 or 11 μmol/kg/day. We first analyzed all 34 genes together, comparing G93A animals treated with both doses with untreated G93A mice sacrificed at the same age of 14–16 weeks. The difference showed a highly significant effect of L-carnosine ($P < 0.01$; TABLE 2). When the different subgroups were analyzed, significance was found for the following: cell markers, neuroinflammation; neurotoxicity; and zinc regulation.

We next analyzed expression of individual genes in these subgroups, comparing G93A animals treated with either dose of L-carnosine with untreated controls. No significant differences were observed for any genes in the animals treated with the lower dose of L-carnosine (2.2 μmol/kg/day), but expression of 4 individual genes

TABLE 2. Effect of L-carnosine and baicalein on gene expression in spinal cord of G93A/SOD1 mice

	L-Carnosine	Baicalein
Overall	$P < 0.002$	$P < 0.002$
Cell markers	$P < 0.03$	$P < 0.003$
CD11B	ns	ns
CD68	ns	Downreg (0.001)
CD80	ns	Downreg (0.001)
CD86	ns	Downreg (0.01)
CD200	ns	ns
CD200R	ns	ns
GFAP	Upreg (0.02)	nd
Neuroinflammation	$P < 0.0001$	$P < 0.0001$
MIP-2	ns	ns
IL-1α	ns	ns
IL-1β	ns	ns
IL-1RA	ns	ns
TNF-α	ns	ns
TNFRp55	ns	Downreg (0.01)
Gro-α	ns	ns
SDF-1	Upreg (0.001)	ns
TLR4	ns	ns
ICAM	ns	ns
CX3CR1	ns	ns
Oxidative stress	ns	$P < 0.02$
nNOS	ns	Upreg (0.01)
iNOS	ns	ns
COX2	ns	nd
Neurotoxicity	$P < 0.02$	$P < 0.003$
EAAT2	Upreg (0.001)	ns
GluR1	ns	ns
GS	ns	Upreg (0.001)
Apoptosis	ns	ns
FADD	ns	ns
FAS	ns	ns
Zinc	$P < 0.001$	$P < 0.002$
MT-I	ns	ns
MT-II	ns	ns
MT-III	Downreg (0.001)	ns

TABLE 2. (*continued*) Effect of L-carnosine and baicalein on gene expression in spinal cord of G93A/SOD1 mice

	L-Carnosine	Baicalein
IGF	nd	nd
IGFBP-2	nd	nd
IGFBP-3	nd	nd
IGFBP-5	nd	nd
IGF1	nd	nd
IGF1R	nd	nd

NOTE: G93A/SOD1 mice (n = 10–12 each group) at 9–11 weeks of age were administered L-carnosine or baicalein daily for 5 weeks, as described in METHODS. At the end of this period, the animals were sacrificed, spinal cords removed, and gene expression analysis carried out, also as described in METHODS. Treated animals were compared to untreated G93A/SOD1 mice. Initially, analysis was carried out with all genes taken together; P values are shown in the first row. For the L-carnosine studies, all 34 genes were analyzed. For the baicalein studies, only 24 genes were analyzed. This study did not include these genes: GFAP, COX2, and the entire IGF set. Subsequently, analysis was performed on each of the indicated subgroups of genes, and the significance is shown for each analysis. For subgroups that showed significant differences, the analysis continued on individual genes within that group, and these values are also shown; ns, not significant ($P > 0.05$); nd, not determined. Abbreviations of genes are defined in the footnote to TABLE 1.

was significant for the dose of 11 μmol/kg/day of L-carnosine: glial fibrillary acidic protein (GFAP), stroma-derived factor-1 (SDF-1), and excitatory amino acid transporter-2 (EAAT2), all of which were upregulated; and MT-III, expression of which was downregulated (FIG. 2).

Effect of Baicalein Treatment on Gene Expression of Mutant G93A/SOD1 Mice

Another group of G93A animals (9–11 weeks of age) were given daily treatments of baicalein (3.7 or 7.4 nmol/kg) for 5 weeks. Global expression of 27 genes was highly significant when the treated animals were compared with untreated G93A mice ($P < 0.01$; TABLE 2). Analysis of subgroups revealed significant differences for cell markers, neuroinflammation, oxidative stress, neurotoxicity, and zinc regulation. Univariate analysis identified 6 individual genes that were significantly altered in expression (FIG. 3). These included the cell markers CD68, CD80, and CD86, as well as tumor necrosis factor receptor (TNFRp55), noninducible nitric oxide synthase (nNOS), and glutamine synthase (GS). CD68, CD80, CD86 (data not shown), and TNFRp55 were downregulated, and nNOS and GS were upregulated.

Studies of Other Drugs

We also determined the effects of treatment of G93A mice with several other drugs, including andrographolide (3–15 nmol/kg/day), minocycline (0.5–2.0 μmol/kg/day), naloxone (6–60 nmol/kg/day), and dextromethorphan (35 nmol/kg/day). None of these drugs had a significant effect on expression of the 34 genes, analyzed together. Andrographolide treatment (data not shown) resulted in alteration of

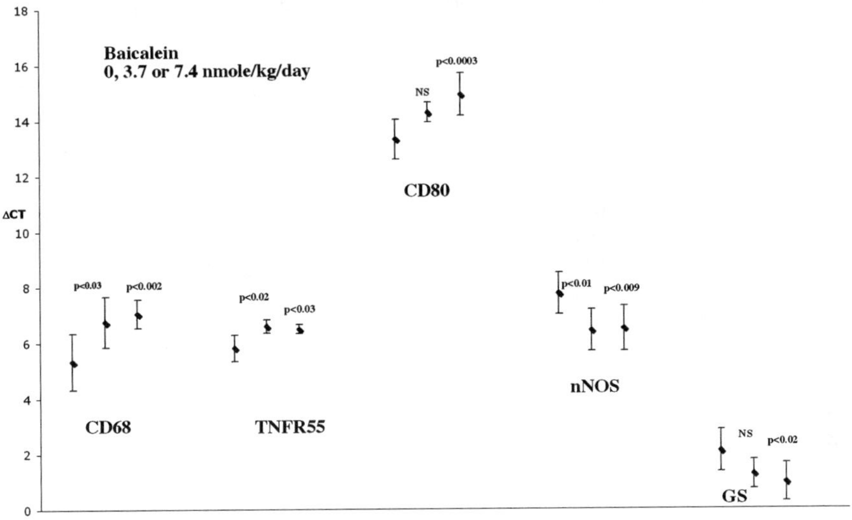

FIGURE 3. Effect of baicalein treatment on gene expression in G93A/SOD1 mice. Animals were given daily treatment of the drug beginning at 9–11 weeks of age, and continuing for 5 weeks, after which they were sacrificed and gene expression in spinal cord determined. For each gene are shown three ΔC_T values, which are inversely proportional to the base 2 log of expression of that gene (see legend to FIG. 1). For each gene, the value on the left is for untreated mice; the value in the middle is for mice given the lower dose of baicalein (3.7 nmol/kg/day); the value on the right is for mice given the higher dose of baicalein (11.0 nmol/kg/day). The values for the different genes are separated horizontally simply for convenience in visualizing. Significant values are shown for each gene and treatment regimen. The *vertical bars* indicate standard errors.

expression of several genes, including TNFRp55, IL-1α, and nNOS, but the effects were not consistent with dose-dependence.

DISCUSSION

In our previous study,[10] we employed a panel of 21 genes representative of several processes implicated in ALS. In this study, we added 13 genes to this original panel, for a total of 34. The new genes (13 in all) included several new inflammation-related genes as well as the metallothioneins, which play an important role in regulating zinc ion, and IGFBPs, levels of which are altered in ALS patients.[16,17] In addition to altered expression of genes related to neuroinflammation in the original panel of 21 that we had identified before,[10] we now found expression of MT-I and MT-II upregulated. MTs play an important role in chelating Zn^{++} and Cu^{++} ions,[35] which are critical to the activity of SOD1,[22] and another group reported upregulation of MT-I and MT-II in mutant SOD1 mice.[36] It has also been reported that G93A animals that lack these genes exhibit an accelerated onset of symptoms and a shorter survival time.[23,37] The upregulation of MT-I and MT-II in G93A animals may therefore be part of a compensatory process in which the organism attempts to stabilize levels of Zn^{++}. Altered levels of this essential ion have been shown to be associated with neurodegeneration.[38,39]

Of additional interest, we found that difference in expression of these genes between G93A and wild-type mice increased with age. While expression of these genes was roughly unchanged with age in the wild-type mice, upregulation became more pronounced in the G93A animals as the animals aged. Thus, differences in gene expression between G93A and wild type became greater as the animals became older. This suggests that expression of these genes is altered at the earliest examined age of the mutant animals, many weeks prior to when detectable symptoms appeared, and that this same trend continued and intensified after symptoms developed. In fact, FIGURES 1 and 2 suggest that the divergence between wild type and G93A occurs at the age of around 9–12 weeks, when the animals develop clear signs of clinical impairment.

Having observed these changes in gene expression in G93A animals, we then used them to test the effects of several drugs on these animals. All of the drugs that we studied have effects on processes that are thought to be involved in ALS, and most of these drugs have been shown to have neuroprotective effects *in vivo* and/or *in vitro*.[27,28,31,33,34,40,41] To our knowledge, though, this is the first study that has investigated the effects of any of these drugs on gene expression patterns in mutant SOD1 mice. This is critically important to understanding how these drugs have their effects on motor neuron disease, as well as to identify which of the altered expression patterns are an essential part of disease development.

We found that L-carnosine and baicalein had significant effects on gene expression, although their effects were markedly different. In the case of L-carnosine, all of the genes affected were different from those altered in G93A animals. That is, the changes in gene expression resulting from the presence of the mutant SOD1 gene were unaffected by L-carnosine treatment. Thus, any beneficial effects that L-carnosine might have on these animals must be mediated not by directly affecting those genes altered by the presence of the mutant SOD1 gene in these animals, but through compensatory processes on other genes.

It is notable that L-carnosine might be expected to alleviate ALS pathology in at least two ways, by chelating zinc and by scavenging free radicals. As noted earlier, Zn^{++} balance is thought to play a critical role in neurodegeneration in general,[38,39] and in ALS in particular,[22,23,37] while the scavenging ability of L-carnosine has been shown to protect against oxidative damage *in vitro* generated by SOD1 mutant protein.[40] Given the evidence that multiple pathological processes are involved in ALS and that multiple drugs may have advantages in delaying symptoms and death,[15] the ability of L-carnosine to target more than one pathological process may enhance its potential as a therapeutic approach. The alteration of MT-III expression by L-carnosine is consistent with some action on Zn^{++} disposition.

Baicalein, an active ingredient from the root *Scutellaria*, has also been reported to have diverse effects. Baicalein has anti-inflammatory activity in such animal models as dextran-induced colitis[42] and rat paw edema,[43] as well as the ability to inhibit lipoxygenase and cyclooxygenase[44] and scavenge free radical species.[45,46] A recent study reported that baicalein blocked lipopolysaccharide(LPS) activation of microglia and protected cultured neurons from degeneration.[41] Zhu *et al.*[47] reported that baicalein, especially its oxidized forms, inhibited the formation of α-synuclein fibrils.

Baicalein altered expression of 6 genes, including 3—the microglia markers CD68, CD80, and CD86—that were among the group altered by the presence of the G93A mutation. Moreover, expression of each of these 3 genes was downregulated by baicalein treatment. Thus, baicalein reduced or antagonized the effect of the G93A mutation, which was to upregulate expression of these genes. Of the 3 remaining genes that were affected by baicalein—TNFRp55, nNOS, and GS—TNFRp55 expression was also downregulated, while expression of nNOS and GS was upregulated. These effects may be compensatory.

We also tested the effect on gene expression of minocycline (0.5–2 μmol/kg/day), naloxone (6–60 nmol/kg/day), dextromethorphan (35 nmol/kg/day), and andrographolide (3–15 nmol/kg/day). The antibiotic minocycline has multiple effects, including inhibition of microglia activation and apoptosis,[48,49] and several studies have reported that it extends survival in these animals.[27,28,48,50] The opioids naloxone and dextromethorphan protect neurons in several tissue models of neurodegenerative diseases.[31,33,34] Crude extracts from *Andrographis* or the purified andrographolide have been shown to exhibit immunostimulatory,[51] antibacterial,[52] hypotensive/antithrombotic,[53,54] and anti-inflammatory[55] activity. Of particular relevance to ALS, andrographolide inhibited nitric oxide production by LPS-activated macrophages.[56]

One explanation for our failure to find changes in gene expression associated with administration of these drugs is that their neuroprotective effects are mediated through other metabolic processes not associated with our panel of genes. It is also possible that we missed the optimum dosages. Another possibility is that their administration must begin earlier, in the presymptomatic period, to have a significant effect on gene expression as well as on behavior.

In conclusion, our studies demonstrate that L-carnosine and baicalein had significant and very different effects on gene expression in G93A/SOD1 mice. Obtaining this kind of information for these drugs, or other candidate drugs, requires less time and fewer animals than most currently used methods, and thus may serve as a prescreening process for these drugs. Compared to other drugs that have been tested on these animals, L-carnosine and baicalein have several potential advantages. Each has multiple effects on processes that are known to be associated with motor neuron disease in these animals. Moreover, our finding that each drug targets a different group of genes suggests that they might be even more effective given together. We have preliminary evidence that L-carnosine given with minocycline also has effects on more genes than L-carnosine alone. A second attractive feature of both of these drugs, particularly L-carnosine, is that they are natural substances that might be ingested regularly and safely. Thus, they could be used by people who are symptom-free, but identified as at risk genetically.

REFERENCES

1. Olsen, M.K. *et al.* 2001. Disease mechanisms revealed by transcription profiling in SOD1-G93A transgenic mouse spinal cord. Ann. Neurol. **50:** 730–740.
2. Yoshihara, T. *et al.* 2002. Differential expression of inflammation- and apoptosis-related genes in spinal cords of a mutant SOD1 transgenic mouse model of familial amyotrophic lateral sclerosis. J. Neurochem. **80:** 158–167.

3. HENSLEY, K. *et al.* 2002. Temporal patterns of cytokine and apoptosis-related gene expression in spinal cords of the G93A-SOD1 mouse model of amyotrophic lateral sclerosis. J. Neurochem. **82:** 365–374.
4. HENSLEY, K. *et al.* 2003. Message and protein-level elevation of tumor necrosis factor α (TNFα) and TNFα-modulating cytokines in spinal cords of the G93A-SOD1 mouse model for amyotrophic lateral sclerosis. Neurobiol. Dis. **14:** 74–80.
5. ROTHSTEIN, J.D. 1995. Excitotoxicity and neurodegeneration in amyotrophic lateral sclerosis. Clin. Neurosci. **3:** 348–359.
6. FERRANTE, R.J. *et al.* 1997. Evidence of increased oxidative damage in both sporadic and familial amyotrophic lateral sclerosis. J. Neurochem. **69:** 2064–2074.
7. GOTO, J.J. *et al.* 2000. Loss of *in vitro* metal ion binding specificity in mutant copper-zinc superoxide dismutases associated with familial amyotrophic lateral sclerosis. J. Biol. Chem. **275:** 1007–1014.
8. MCGEER, P.L. & E.G. MCGEER. 2002. Inflammatory processes in amyotrophic lateral sclerosis. Muscle Nerve **26:** 459–470.
9. RAOUL, C. *et al.* 2002. Motoneuron death triggered by a specific pathway downstream of fas: potentiation by ALS-linked SOD1 mutations. Neuron **35:** 1067–1083.
10. CHEN, L-C. *et al.* 2004. Temporal gene expression patterns in G93A/SOD1 mouse. ALS Other Motor Neuron Disord. **11:** 1–8.
11. KAWAMATA, T. *et al.* 1992. Immunologic reactions in amyotrophic lateral sclerosis brain and spinal cord tissue. Am. J. Pathol. **140:** 691–707.
12. HALL, E.D., J.A. OOSTOVEEN & M.A. GURNEY. 1998. Relationship of microglial and astrocytic activation to disease onset and progression in a transgenic model of familial ALS. Glia **23:** 249–256.
13. POLONI, M. *et al.* 2000. Circulating levels of tumor necrosis factor-α and and its soluble receptors are increased in the blood of patients with amyotrophic lateral sclerosis. Neurosci. Lett. **287:** 211–214.
14. ELLIOTT, J.L. 2001. Cytokine upregulation in a murine model of familial amyotrophic lateral sclerosis. Brain Res. Mol. Brain Res. **95:** 172–178.
15. KRIZ, J., G. GOWING & J-P. JULIEN. 2003. Efficient three-drug cocktail for disease induced by mutant superoxide dismutase. Ann. Neurol. **53:** 429–436.
16. DORE, S. *et al.* 1996. Distribution and levels of insulin-like growth factor (IGF-I and IGF-II) and insulin receptor binding sites in the spinal cords of amyotrophic lateral sclerosis (ALS) patients. Brain Res. Mol. Brain Res. **41:** 128–133.
17. WILCZAK, N., R.A.I. DEVOS & J. DEKEYSER. 2003. Free insulin-like growth factor (IGF)–1 and IGF binding proteins 2, 5, and 6 in spinal motor neurons in amyotrophic lateral sclerosis. Lancet **361:** 1007–1011.
18. LEWIS, M.E. *et al.* 1993. Insulin-like growth factor-I: potential for treatment of motor neuronal disorders. Exp. Neurol. **124:** 73–88.
19. KASPAR, B.K. *et al.* 2003. Retrograde viral delivery of IGF-1 prolongs survival in a mouse ALS model. Science **301:** 839–842.
20. LAI, E.C. *et al.* 1997. Effect of recombinant human insulin-like growth factor-I on progression of ALS: a placebo-controlled study. Neurology **49:** 1621–1630.
21. BORASIO, G.D. *et al.* 1998. A placebo-controlled trial of human insulin-like growth factor-I on amyotrophic lateral sclerosis. Neurology **51:** 583–586.
22. ELLIOTT, J.L. 2001. Zinc and copper in the pathogenesis of amyotrophic lateral sclerosis. Prog. Neuro-Psychopharmacol. Biol. Psychiat. **25:** 1169–1185.
23. PUTTAPARTHI, K. *et al.* 2002. Disease progression in a transgenic model of familial amyotrophic lateral sclerosis is dependent on both neuronal and non-neuronal zinc-binding proteins. J. Neurosci. **22:** 8790–8796.
24. ANDREASSEN, O.A. *et al.* 2000. *N*-Acetyl-L-cysteine improves survival and preserves motor performance in an animal model of familial amyotrophic lateral sclerosis. Neuroreport **11:** 2491–2493.
25. FERRANTE, R.J. *et al.* 2001. Therapeutic efficacy of EGb761 (*Gingko biloba* extract) in a transgenic mouse model of amyotrophic lateral sclerosis. J. Mol. Neurosci. **17:** 89–96.
26. KEEP, M. *et al.* 2001. Intrathecal cyclosporin prolongs survival of late-stage ALS mice. Brain Res. **894:** 327–331.

27. KRIZ, J., M.D. NGUYEN & J.P. JULIEN. 2002. Minocycline slows disease progression in a mouse model of amyotrophic lateral sclerosis. Neurobiol. Dis. **10:** 268–278.
28. VAN DEN BOSCH, L. *et al.* 2002. Minocycline delays disease onset and mortality in a transgenic model of ALS. Neuroreport **13:** 1067–1070.
29. TURNER, B.J., E.C. LOPES & S.S. CHEEMA. 2003. The serotonin precursor 5-hydroxytryptophan delays neuromuscular disease in murine familial amyotrophic lateral sclerosis. ALS Other Motor Neuron Disord. **4:** 171–176.
30. AZZOUZ, M. *et al.* 2004. VEGF delivery with retrogradely transported lentivector prolongs survival in a mouse ALS model. Nature **429:** 413–417.
31. LIU, B., L. DU & J-S. HONG. 2000. Naloxone protects rat dopaminergic neurons against inflammatory damage through inhibition of microglial activation and superoxide generation. J. Pharmacol. Exp. Ther. **293:** 607–617.
32. FLANAGAN, S.W. *et al.* 2002. Overexpression of manganese superoxide dismutase attenuates neuronal death in human cells expressing mutant (G37R) Cu/Zn-superoxide dismutase. J. Neurochem. **81:** 170–177.
33. LIU, Y. *et al.* 2003. Dextromethorphan protects dopaminergic neurons against inflammation-mediated degeneration through inhibition of microglial activation. J. Pharmacol. Exp. Ther. **305:** 212–218.
34. LIU, B. & J-S. HONG. 2003. Role of microgila in inflammation-mediated neurodegenerative diseases; mechanisms and strategies for therapeutic intervention. J. Pharmacol. Exp. Ther. **304:** 1–7.
35. HIDALGO, J. *et al.* 2001. Roles of the metallothionein family of proteins in the central nervous system. Brain Res. Bull. **55:** 133–145.
36. GONG, Y.H. & J.L. ELLIOTT. 2000. Metallothionein expression is altered in a transgenic murine model of familial amyotrophic lateral sclerosis. Exp. Neurol. **162:** 27–36.
37. NAGANO, S. *et al.* 2001. Reduction of metallothioneins promotes the disease expression of familial amyotrophic lateral sclerosis mice in a dose-dependent manner. Eur. J. Neurosci. **13:** 1363–1370.
38. FREDERICKSON, C.J. *et al.* 2000. Importance of zinc in the central nervous system: the zinc-containing neuron. J. Nutr. **130:** 1471S–1483S.
39. DINELEY, K.E., T.V. VOTYAKOVA & I.J. REYNOLDS. 2003. Zinc inhibition of cellular energy production: implications for mitochondria and neurodegeneration. J. Neurochem. **85:** 563–570.
40. KANG, J.H. & W.S. EUM. 2000. Enhanced oxidative damage by the familial amyotrophic lateral sclerosis–associated Cu,Zn-superoxide dismutase mutants. Biochim. Biophys. Acta **1524:** 162–170.
41. LI, F. *et al.* 2003. Inhibition of microglial activation by the herbal flavonoid baicalein attenuates inflammation-mediated degeneration of dopaminergic neurons. J. Neural Transmission **112:** 331–347.
42. HONG, T. *et al.* 2002. Evaluation of the anti-inflammatory effect of baicalein on dextran-sulfate sodium-induced colitis in mice. Planta Med. **68:** 268–271.
43. KUBO, M. *et al.* 1984. Studies on *Scutellaria radix*: VII. Anti-arthritic and anti-inflammatory actions of methanolic extract and flavonoid components from *Scutellaria radix*. Chem. Pharm. Bull. (Tokyo) **32:** 2724–2729.
44. AKIRA, K. *et al.* 1993. Profiling of arachidonic acid metabolites in rabbit platelets by radio gas chromatography. Lipids **28:** 361–364.
45. HAMADA, H. *et al.* 1993. Free radical scavenging action of baicalein. Arch. Biochem. Biophys. **306:** 261–266.
46. SHEN, Y-C. *et al.* 2003. Mechanisms in mediating the anti-inflammatory effects of baicalein and baicalein in human leukocytes. Eur. J. Pharmacol. **465:** 171–181.
47. ZHU, M. *et al.* 2004. The flavonoid baicalein inhibits fibrillation of alpha-synuclein and disaggregates existing fibrils. J. Biol. Chem. **279:** 26846–26857.
48. ZHU, S. *et al.* 2002. Minocycline inhibits cytochrome c release and delays progression of amyotrophic lateral sclerosis. Nature **417:** 74–78.
49. YRJANHEIKKI, J. *et al.* 1998. Tetracyclines inhibit microglia activation and are neuroprotective in global brain ischemia. Proc. Natl. Acad. Sci. USA **95:** 15769–15784.
50. ZHANG, W., M. NARAYANAN & R.M. FRIEDLANDER. 2003. Additive neuroprotective effects of minocycline with creatine in a mouse model of ALS. Ann. Neurol. **53:** 267–270.

51. PANOSSIAN, A. *et al.* 2002. Effect of andrographolide and Kan-Jang fixed combination of extract SHA-10 and extract SHA-3 on proliferation of human lymphocytes, production of cytokines, and immune activation markers in whole blood cells culture. Phytomedicine **9:** 598–605.
52. GABRIELIAN, E.S. *et al.* 2002. A double blind, placebo-controlled study of *Andrographis paniculata* fixed combination Kan Jang in the treatment of acute upper respiratory tract infections including sinusitis. Phytomedicine **9:** 589–597.
53. ZHAO, H.Y. & W.Y. FANG. 1991. Anti-thrombotic effects of *Andrographis paniculata Nees* in preventing myocardial infarction. Chin. Med. J. (Engl. Ed.) **104:** 770–775.
54. ZHANG, C.Y. 1996. Hypotensive activity of aqueous extract of *Andrographis paniculata* in rats. Clin. Exp. Pharmacol. Physiol. **23:** 675–678.
55. DENG, W.L. 1985. Pharmacological studies on thirteen kinds of injections from *Andrographis paniculata*: I. Antipyretic, anti-inflammatory effects, and toxicity. Zhong Yao Tong Bao **10:** 38–42.
56. BATKHUU, J. *et al.* 2002. Suppression of NO production in activated macrophages *in vitro* and *ex vivo* by neoandrographolide isolated from *Andrographis paniculata*. Biol. Pharm. Bull. **25:** 1169–1174.

Brain Response to Injury and Neurodegeneration

Endogenous Neuroprotective Signaling

NICOLAS G. BAZAN, VICTOR L. MARCHESELLI, AND KASIE COLE-EDWARDS

LSU Neuroscience Center and Department of Ophthalmology, Louisiana State University Health Sciences Center School of Medicine, New Orleans, Louisiana 70112, USA

ABSTRACT: Synaptic activity and ischemia/injury promote lipid messenger formation through phospholipase-mediated cleavage of specific phospholipids from membrane reservoirs. Lipid messengers modulate signaling cascades, contributing to development, differentiation, function (e.g., memory), protection, regeneration, and repair of neurons and overall regulation of neuronal, glial, and endothelial cell functional integrity. Oxidative stress disrupts lipid signaling and promotes lipid peroxidation and neurodegeneration. Lipid signaling at the neurovascular unit (neurons, astrocytes, oligodendrocytes, microglia, and cells of the microvasculature) is altered in early cerebrovascular and neurodegenerative disease. We discuss how lipid signaling regulates critical events in neuronal survival. Aberrant synaptic plasticity (e.g., epileptogenesis) is highlighted to show how gene expression may drive synaptic circuitry formation in the "wrong" direction. Docosahexaenoic acid has been implicated in memory, photoreceptor cell biogenesis and function, and neuroprotection. Free docosahexaenoic acid released in the brain during experimental stroke leads to the synthesis of stereospecific messengers through oxygenation pathways. One messenger, 10,17*S*-docosatriene (neuroprotectin D1; NPD1), counteracts leukocyte infiltration and proinflammatory gene expression in brain ischemia-reperfusion. In retina, photoreceptor survival depends on retinal pigment epithelial (RPE) cell integrity. NPD1 is synthesized in RPE cells undergoing oxidative stress, potently counteracts oxidative stress–triggered apoptotic DNA damage in RPE, upregulates antiapoptotic proteins Bcl-2 and Bcl-x_L, and decreases proapoptotic Bax and Bad expression. These findings expand our understanding of how the nervous system counteracts redox disturbances, mitochondrial dysfunction, and proinflammatory conditions. The specificity and potency of NPD1 indicate a potential target for therapeutic intervention for stroke, age-related macular degeneration, spinal cord injury, and other neuroinflammatory or neurodegenerative diseases.

KEYWORDS: docosahexaenoic acid; ischemia-reperfusion; neuroprotectin D1; retinal neuroprotection; oxidative stress

Address for correspondence: Nicolas G. Bazan, LSU Neuroscience Center, 2020 Gravier Street, Suite D, New Orleans, LA 70112. Voice: 504-599-0831; fax: 504-568-5801.
nbazan@lsuhsc.edu

Ann. N.Y. Acad. Sci. 1053: 137–147 (2005).
doi: 10.1196/annals.1344.011

INTRODUCTION

Oxidative stress and proinflammatory signaling are components of numerous neuropathological conditions including neurodegenerative diseases (Alzheimer's disease), amyotropic lateral sclerosis, spinal cord injury, traumatic brain injury, epilepsy, and ischemia-reperfusion (IR).[1–6] The heterogeneity of the root causes of these conditions belies shared prodeath signaling pathways. The purpose of this chapter is to give an overview of how membrane-derived lipids may intervene in these pathways to achieve neuroprotection. Experimental data from our laboratory are presented to illuminate the neuroprotective roles that docosahexaenoic acid (DHA), and derivatives thereof, play in IR injury. As such, special emphasis will be placed on IR injury and its sequelae; however, these findings have implications in how neuroprotective lipids may function in other diseases. Finally, to give a more mechanistic understanding of how lipids may intervene in death signaling at the mitochondrial level, *in vitro* data examining the protective effects of neuroprotectin D1 (NPD1) on retinal pigment epithelial cells exposed to oxidative insults will also be described.

PROINFLAMMATORY SIGNALING AND OXIDATIVE STRESS

Host defense against infection or injury depends upon inflammatory responses to destroy pathogens and stimulate tissue repair. Unresolved inflammatory responses in the brain are associated with many CNS disorders including those mentioned in the INTRODUCTION.[6] Inflammation is marked by multiple, concurrent processes including the activation of microglia and astrocytes, adhesion of leukocytes (T cells, neutrophils, and monocytes/macrophages) to endothelial cells and their subsequent infiltration into the brain parenchyma, as well as release of oxygen- and nitrogen-derived free radicals, cytokines, chemokines, and bioactive lipids by these cells. Leukocyte infiltration, in particular, is an important contributing factor to IR injury due to their release of IL-1β, tumor necrosis factor α (TNFα), myeloperoxidase, and proinflammatory lipid mediators, the prostanoids.[7] Data from experimental models of ischemia suggest that these acute inflammatory processes are injurious. However, the onset of a more delayed inflammation may be reparative. In IR injury, the inflammatory response occurs hours after the actual ischemic insult is sustained.

Oxygen and glucose deprivation resulting from obstructed blood flow initiates a cascade of distinct pathological events stemming from energy depletion, including the collapse of energy-dependent ion transport, nonspecific release of glutamate as well as inhibition of its uptake, intracellular Ca^{2+} overload, and generation of reactive oxygen species (ROS).[8] Generation of ROS after IR injury can be attributed to an overload of Ca^{2+} into mitochondria: reduction of proximal electron carriers in the inner membrane leads to partial reduction of molecular oxygen, forming the superoxide anion and its more toxic derivatives, H_2O_2 and $^{\bullet}OH$. Enzymatic sources of free radical species under these conditions include the cyclooxygenases (COX), lipoxygenases, myeloperoxidase, and nitric oxide synthase. Sudden restoration of blood flow in the reperfusion phase of injury places additional demands on already overwhelmed antioxidant defenses. ROS can modify both free and protein-bound amino acids, leading to alterations in enzyme activity and susceptibility to proteolysis.

Nuclear and mitochondrial DNA are also targeted by ROS, resulting in highly mutagenic base modifications, abasic sites, and strand breaks. Among the most damaging effects of ROS is lipid peroxidation. Hydroxyl radical attack on fatty acid side chains generates carbon-centered radicals and, subsequently, lipoperoxyl radicals capable of attacking adjacent fatty acids and propagating further damage. Of note, the high unsaturated lipid content of neuronal membranes makes neurons excellent at propagating free radical species. Accumulation of lipid hydroperoxides alters membrane permeability and fluidity and oxidizes membrane proteins, leading to alterations in ion transport, notably the intracellular flux of Ca^{2+}.[9]

PHOSPHOLIPID MEMBRANES ARE RESERVOIRS FOR LIPID MESSENGERS: AA AND DHA

Membrane organization has conceptually evolved from the notion of a lipid bilayer with embedded proteins to that of a highly dynamic, heterogeneous patchwork of microdomains containing ion channels, receptors, transporters, and other proteins. In the past, cellular membranes in the nervous system were categorized as being fluid membranes (e.g., those of cells of gray matter) or rigid membranes (e.g., the oligodendrocyte plasma membrane that spirals around the axon to form myelin) based on a higher or lower content of polyunsaturated fatty acids (PUFA) in phospholipids, respectively. We now know that neurons, glia, and endothelial cells of the cerebrovasculature are endowed with phospholipid pools that serve as reservoirs of lipid messengers. Specific lipid messengers are cleaved and released from these reservoir phospholipids by a class of proteins known as the phospholipases in response to signals such as neurotrophic factors, cytokines, membrane depolarization, ion channel activation, and neurotransmitters such as glutamate. These lipid messengers can act intracellularly or in an autocrine and/or paracrine fashion to regulate other signaling cascades, thereby contributing to the development, differentiation, function, protection, and repair of the cells of the nervous system.[10] Our laboratory has devoted considerable effort to sorting out specific signals, mainly those of PUFA and their peroxidation products, generated during IR, and the neuroprotective effects of these compounds.

Phospholipids consist of a glycerol backbone with a hydrophilic phosphate-containing head at *sn3*. Various saturated and unsaturated fatty acids occupy the *sn1* and *sn2* positions, respectively. The latter position is targeted by a family of acylhydrolases known as phospholipase A_2 (PLA_2), which can liberate the PUFA situated here.[10,11] Massive influx of Ca^{2+} during IR triggers PLA_2 activation as reflected by a rapid accumulation of *n*-6 and *n*-3 PUFA, specifically arachidonic acid (AA; 20:4*n*-6) and DHA (22:6*n*-3).[12] PLA_2 activation can also be triggered by the proinflammatory cytokines, IL-1β and TNFα.

AA, an *n*-6 PUFA, is synthesized from dietary sources of linoleic acid, whereas the *n*-3 PUFA (including DHA) are synthesized from α-linoleic acid.[13] Interconversion of linoleic acid and α-linoleic acid is not possible in mammalian tissues; therefore, each is considered to be an essential fatty acid. Linoleic acid is abundant in corn, safflower, sunflower, and soybean oils, while flaxseed oil is the richest source of α-linoleic acid. The former is the main PUFA in human diets; typical diets consist of 20-fold more *n*-6 fats than *n*-3 fats. The same enzymes responsible for the conversion of linoleic acid (18:2n-6) to AA (20:4n-6) mediate conversion of α-linoleic acid (18:3n-3) to eicosapentaenoic acid (EPA) (20:5n-3); thus, substrates in omega-6 and omega-3 pathways are competing for the same enzymes.[13] While AA and its derivatives are potent mediators of inflammation, except lipoxins and other derivatives, omega-3 (n-3) fatty acids such as EPA and its derivative DHA have well-documented anti-inflammatory actions.

AA IS THE PRECURSOR OF PROINFLAMMATORY LIPID MESSENGERS

Unesterified AA is the starting point of a well-defined cascade leading to the production of eicosanoids (prostaglandins, thromboxanes, leukotrienes, and lipoxins). Synthesis of the prostaglandins and thromboxanes, collectively referred to as prostanoids, involves cyclooxygenase (COX or prostaglandin H synthase). COX catalyzes the first committed step of the AA cascade, oxygenating AA to form the short-lived intermediate, prostaglandin H_2 (PGH_2), the precursor to a variety of lipid derivatives.[14] The prostaglandin derivatives are also very short-lived and exert their effects in close proximity to their origin through G-protein-coupled receptors.[15] Prostaglandins have diverse functions that are not well understood and in some cases may antagonize one another. For example, *in vitro* data suggest that PGA_1 and PGE_1 have antiapoptotic effects, whereas PGE_2 is proapoptotic under some conditions. Despite this, their collective synthesis during IR, and other injury paradigms, has unequivocally tied them to proinflammatory processes. Their proinflammatory actions are evinced by the anti-inflammatory effects of traditional nonsteroidal anti-inflammatory drugs (NSAID), which acetylate the COX enzymes, thereby preventing prostanoid production.[16] COX-2, the inducible COX isoform present almost exclusively in neurons, is upregulated during IR and contributes to neuronal death.[17] This is best illustrated by the protection afforded to neurons derived from COX-2 gene–deleted animals after IR.[18] The AA-COX-2-PG cascade is deleterious to neurons during IR. However, the question remains: are there any bioactive lipids derived from PUFA during oxidative injury that are neuroprotective?

EPA AND DHA HAVE ANTI-INFLAMMATORY ACTIONS

As mentioned earlier, in contrast to AA, the omega-3 fatty acids have anti-inflammatory actions. Fish oil is the major source of the omega-3 fatty acids, EPA (20:5n-3) and DHA (22:6n-3). In the absence of fish oil, α-linoleic acid is the precursor to EPA and DHA. Increased consumption of oily fish increases EPA- and DHA-containing phospholipids at the expense of decreased AA incorporation into phospholipids.[13] Dietary supplementation of EPA and DHA has beneficial effects in many diverse disorders including asthma, heart disease, rheumatoid arthritis, cancer, mental depression, and transplant rejection.[19–24] In some of these conditions, such as cardiovascular disease, the benefits of fish oil have been attributed solely to DHA. For many years, the positive effects of DHA were attributed to its ability to antagonize the production of AA and its derivatives, the prostanoids.[13] However, whether these effects are due to specific lipid products derived from DHA was unknown.

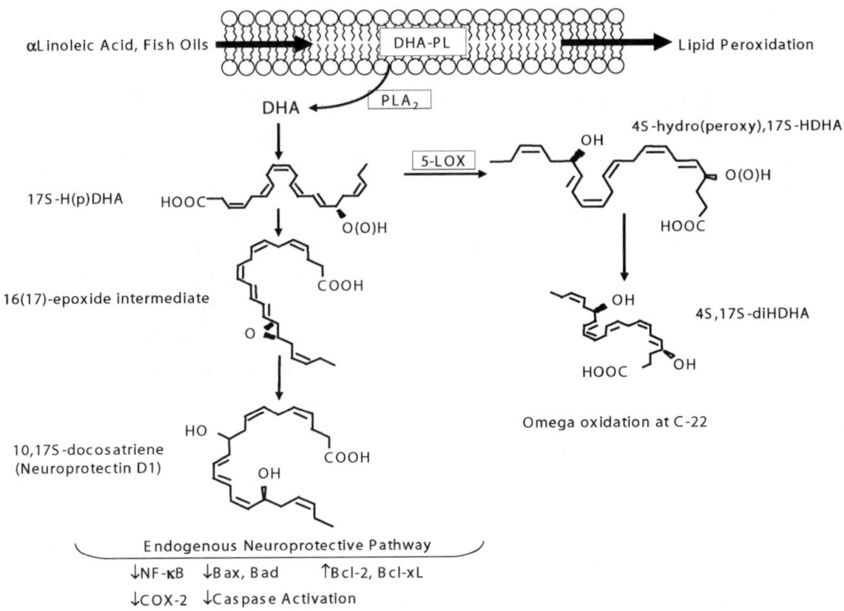

FIGURE 1. Proposed biosynthetic pathways for 10,17*S*-docosatriene. In brain tissue from mice exposed to IR injury, stereospecific DHA-oxygenation pathways lead to the formation of novel messengers. Endogenous lipid signaling pathways after IR injury involve the synthesis of 10,17*S*-docosatriene, which we have named neuroprotectin D1 (NPD1). After PLA_2 releases DHA from the membrane, a lipoxygenase-like enzyme catalyzes the synthesis of 17*S*-H(p)DHA, which in turn is converted to a 16(17)-epoxide that is enzymatically converted to NPD1. Addition of exogenous NPD1 markedly attenuates death after IR. This is associated with decreased PMN infiltration, NF-κB activation, and COX-2 upregulation. NPD1 also affects levels of the Bcl-2 family proteins and inhibits caspase activation when exogenous NPD1 is applied to ARPE-19 cells injured with $TNF\alpha/H_2O_2$. Dietary intake of DHA or its precursor, α-linoleic acid, leads to NPD1 uptake by the liver and then distribution to other organs through blood lipoproteins. Membrane DHA content is lost from membrane phospholipids through PLA_2 activation and lipid peroxidation.

DHA-DERIVED DOCOSATRIENES ARE ANTI-INFLAMMATORY SIGNALS

DHA is enriched in the CNS and in retinal synapses, and it is required for the proper development of the brain and retina. It is also implicated in excitable membrane function, memory, photoreceptor biogenesis, and neuroprotection.[25–33] We have very recently identified stereospecific DHA derivatives that are synthesized by an enzyme-catalyzed DHA-oxygenation pathway after middle cerebral artery occlusion (MCAO), a model of transient focal cerebral ischemia.[12] Two DHA-oxygenation pathways give rise, on the one hand, to 10,17*S*-docosatriene (NPD1) and, on the other, to the synthesis of resolvin-type messengers (17*R*-DHA; FIG. 1). Both of these oxygenation pathways generate messengers that act as counter-proinflammatory signals.

NPD1

Anti-inflammatory and Neuroprotective Actions of NPD1 in IR Injury

Free DHA generated from membrane phospholipids following reperfusion was met with the appearance of a novel stereospecific DHA-derived messenger, 10,17*S*-docosatriene or NPD1. This docosatriene was also recently described as being present in human blood, glial cells, and mouse brain.[34] NPD1 attenuates classical features of inflammation, namely, PMN infiltration and proinflammatory gene signaling. Administration of exogenous NPD1 inhibits PMN infiltration induced by peritonitis. Likewise, continuous infusion of either DHA or NPD1 into the third ventricle during the initial two days of reperfusion inhibits PMN infiltration into the hippocampus (one of the most vulnerable regions to ischemic injury) and the neocortex. IR-induced increases in NF-κB binding activity and upregulation of COX-2 mRNA were also attenuated by DHA and NPD1 infusion. These results were mirrored in cultured human neural progenitor cells treated with the proinflammatory cytokine, IL-1β; this cytokine was chosen since it increases during IR as a result of PMN infiltration. The significance of NPD1's anti-inflammatory effects is underscored by its ability to reduce the infarct volume by approximately half, demonstrating the considerable neuroprotective effects of this DHA-derived lipid after IR injury. Of note, NPD1 levels were bolstered by exogenous administration of DHA, and infusion of either DHA or NPD1 led to indistinguishable outcomes in the PMN infiltration and proinflammatory signaling measures described above. This implies that exogenous DHA is used as a precursor for NPD1 synthesis under these conditions and points to NPD1 as a possible mediator of DHA's observed anti-inflammatory effects in other conditions. That brain responses to IR injury, including synthesis of DHA-derived messengers such as NPD1, were not successful in preventing death suggests that they were counterbalanced by prodeath signals, lipid-derived and otherwise. Depending on its magnitude, injury-induced protective lipid-signaling responses may be overwhelmed. We know that DHA is susceptible to oxidation and yields neuroprostanes during IR.[35] Therefore, given its propensity for peroxidation, formation of neuroprotective, DHA-derived messengers such as NPD1 may be thwarted under conditions of severe oxidative stress.

Given the anti-inflammatory effects of DHA and DHA-derived lipids, the arguments for a diet rich in α-linoleic acid or DHA-containing fish oils are apparent. However, altering phospholipid content in the brain may not be so easy. Due to the very high content of brain DHA and due to its tenacious retention, it is difficult to modify brain content by simple dietary manipulation. In addition, there seems to be a specific liver-to-brain (and retina) DHA-supply system that provides DHA for the biogenesis and repair of membranes. It has been postulated that when ischemia removes free DHA from brain, its replenishment may be met through DHA-carrying blood proteins. What blood proteins may perform this function is unclear, but albumin is a possible candidate. Albumin has been shown to induce mobilization of *n*-3 PUFA and is thought to replenish these PUFA lost from the membrane after ischemia.[36] In addition, human serum albumin, when systemically injected, does cross the blood-brain barrier, reaching even intraneuronal sites, and elicits neuroprotection in IR in experimental animals. In any case, identification of proteins involved in maintenance and replenishment of DHA-containing PUFA in the brain may prove to be useful targets for therapeutic interventions following ischemia.

Mitochondrial Apoptotic Pathways Are an NPD1 Target

Oxidative injury, depending on its magnitude, can lead to varied forms of cell death. Necrosis refers to the immediate, uncontrolled cellular disintegration resulting from an acute injury such as would occur in the ischemic core. This type of death elicits an inflammatory response that involves leukocyte invasion and edema with damage to surrounding tissues. Areas surrounding the core, also known as the penumbra, are vulnerable to a more delayed death that retains features of apoptosis, a programmed cell death exemplified by the developing nervous system. Neuronal apoptosis is regarded to be a major cause of loss of function associated with not only brain ischemia, but also aging, Alzheimer's disease, amyotropic lateral sclerosis, traumatic brain injury, and spinal cord injury. Apoptosis is characterized by cytoplasmic condensation, cell shrinkage, and membrane blebbing. It is consistently associated with fragmentation of nuclear DNA into 120–200 base pair fragments, or multiples thereof, also known as oligonucleosomal fragments, and it is considered by some to be one of the hallmarks of apoptosis. Programmed cell death pathways are initiated through engagement of receptors at the surface of the cell, or through the mitochondria, with the latter pathway serving as a feed-forward mechanism for the receptor pathways.[37] A family of cysteine proteases known as the caspases (cysteine aspartic acid–specific proteases) orchestrate the orderly breakdown of cells during apoptosis, and the mitochondrial pathway of caspase activation is triggered in response to a variety of cellular stresses such as growth factor withdrawal, heat shock, DNA damage, and oxidative stress.[37] TNFα/H_2O_2 injury of ARPE-19 cells (spontaneously transformed human retinal pigment epithelial cells [RPE]) is a well-established model of apoptosis triggered through the mitochondrial pathway.[38] Accordingly, we used this model to investigate NPD1 by examining its effects on apoptotic mediators (caspases) and regulators (Bcl-2 protein family).

Before discussing findings related to NPD1 and mitochondrial pathways of apoptosis, a discussion of the clinical significance of oxidative stress–induced RPE death is in order. RPE cells are derived from neuroectoderm and form a monolayer above tips of the photoreceptor outer segments. RPE cells perform functions vital to photoreceptor survival, including the transport and reisomerization of bleached visual pigments, the maintenance of the blood–outer retinal barrier, and the recycling of rod outer segments. Photoreceptor outer segments contain rhodopsin and the highest content of DHA of any cell type.[32,39] In a daily cycle, RPE cells engulf and phagocytize the distal tips of photoreceptor outer segments. This process is tightly regulated so that photoreceptor length and phospholipid composition are maintained.[27,40,41] Thus, given photoreceptors' high DHA content, RPE cells are particularly pertinent to this discussion since they are strategically positioned to be targets of DHA-derived messengers. Importantly, oxidative stress–induced apoptosis of RPE cells compromises photoreceptor survival and impairs vision. These processes are clinically applicable to age-related macular degeneration and Stargardt disease.[42,43]

Experiments examining the effect of NPD1 on apoptosis in ARPE-19 cells revealed that inclusion of this lipid at nanomolar concentrations inhibits apoptosis induced by TNFα/H_2O_2 injury as measured by decreased nuclear condensation and

DNA fragmentation.[38] This protective effect was accompanied by an attenuation of caspase-3 activation. Next, NPD1's effects on levels of the proapoptotic Bcl-2 family members (Bad and Bax), as well as on those of antiapoptotic members (Bcl-2 and Bcl-x_L), were examined. Bcl-2 family proteins participate in the initiation and amplification of premitochondrial events in the apoptotic cascade, primarily through their ability to regulate cytochrome c release from the mitochondrial intermembrane space, which triggers caspase activation. Levels of the antiapoptotic protein Bcl-x_L increased in response to TNFα/H_2O_2, but those of Bcl-2 did not. Inclusion of NPD1 enhanced levels of both proteins after injury. The proapoptotic proteins, Bax and Bad, were upregulated by TNFα/H_2O_2, and this upregulation was lessened by the inclusion of NPD1. NPD1 was also capable of inhibiting increased promoter activity of the COX-2 gene in ARPE-19 cells treated with IL-1β. NPD1's ability to act upstream of caspase activation by influencing expression of the Bcl-2 proteins suggests that it is part of an immediate, early response to injury that targets premitochondrial events. It is possible that NPD1 modulates signaling at the transcription factor level and regulates promoters of the genes encoding death repressors and effectors of the Bcl-2 family of proteins. This is a plausible explanation given that many of the Bcl-2 family members contain NF-κB consensus sequences in their promoters.[44] Alternatively, translational or posttranslational events may integrate a concerted response to counteract oxidative stress. This newly uncovered "NPD1 regulatory pathway" may aid our understanding of the effects of other neuroprotective mediators in retinal degeneration. For example, a connection between NPD1 and certain growth factors important to photoreceptor survival should be explored. In any case, the effects of NPD1 on RPE survival-signaling pathways have several implications in the understanding of how NPD1, endogenously synthesized in the brain, modulates IR injury responses.

As discussed earlier, the primary insult arising from IR is oxidative in nature (combined with an excitotoxic component), with a secondary wave of inflammatory processes providing additional injury. As such, our findings related to TNFα/H_2O_2 injury of ARPE-19 can be extended to IR injury. That is, NPD1-mediated coordinate regulation of Bcl-2 family members and inhibition of caspase activation may be occurring during IR as well. That NPD1 negatively regulates NF-κB activity and, as a consequence, leads to downregulation of proinflammatory gene expression in IR is consistent with the *in vitro* findings regarding COX-2 promoter activity and suggests that NPD1 acts at or above the level of transcription factor regulation. Other transcription factors, such as AP-1 and p53, have been implicated in IR injury, and NPD1's protective effects may also be explained, at least in part, by its ability to regulate their activity. In the same way, NPD1 may have positive effects on prosurvival signaling pathways such as those involving protein kinase B (Akt). Like other bioactive lipids, such as PAF (1-*O*-alkyl-2-acetyl-glycero-3-phosphocholine), NPD1 may achieve its gene-regulatory effects through an intracellular and/or extracellular receptor. The identification of any such receptor(s) will be essential from a therapeutic standpoint and awaits further characterization. Also, given the short-lived nature of lipid signals, another important aspect of NPD1 function worthy of investigation is its spatial distribution, both intra- and intercellular, after oxidative injury. Release of NPD1 may elicit or amplify survival signaling by the same cell in an autocrine fashion and/or it may act on neighboring cells, counteracting their production of proinflammatory gene expression. Regulation of the signals that control NPD1 synthesis and degradation will also yield insights necessary to take advantage of the therapeutic potential of NPD1.

CONCLUSIONS

To summarize, our findings demonstrate that NPD1 exerts counterregulatory actions on cellular and molecular signaling that promote brain injury after IR and oxidative stress–induced retinal injury. Thus, we now know that DHA's neuroprotective effects are due at least in part to the synthesis of specific lipid messengers, resolvins and NPD1. Moreover, it is probable that the neuroprotective effects of DHA in other neuropathologic conditions can be explained, at least in part, by these DHA-derived messengers, especially NPD1. Our findings also highlight a fundamental principle in brain injury: that is, the brain responds to injury with a plethora of signals, some harmful and some protective, and the preponderance of signals in either direction influences the overall outcome (neuronal survival or death). Such is the case with inflammatory and counterinflammatory lipid messengers. Therapeutic strategies targeting synthesis and degradation of DHA-derived messengers will tip the balance in favor of neuroprotection in IR injury and possibly other CNS disorders with a neuroinflammatory component. The potent bioactivity of NPD1 makes it a particularly important target for therapeutic, neuroprotective interventions in these diseases. Finally, other as yet uncharacterized bioactive lipids with neuroprotective actions undoubtedly exist. Their discovery will improve our understanding of the therapeutic possibilities for neuroinflammatory diseases.

REFERENCES

1. Bazan, N.G., V. Colangelo & W.J. Lukiw. 2002. Prostaglandins and other lipid mediators in Alzheimer's disease. Prostaglandins Other Lipid Mediat. **68/69:** 197–210.
2. Danton, G.H. & W.D. Dietrich. 2003. Inflammatory mechanisms after ischemia and stroke. J. Neuropathol. Exp. Neurol. **62:** 127–136.
3. Dirnagl, U., R.P. Simon & J.M. Hallenbeck. 2003. Ischemic tolerance and endogenous neuroprotection. Trends Neurosci. **26:** 248–254.
4. Lo, E.H., T. Dalkara & M.A. Moskowitz. 2003. Mechanisms, challenges, and opportunities in stroke. Nat. Rev. Neurosci. **4:** 399–415.
5. Iadecola, C. 2004. Neurovascular regulation in the normal brain and in Alzheimer's disease. Nat. Rev. Neurosci. **5:** 347–360.
6. Minghetti, L. 2004. Cyclooxygenase-2 (COX-2) in inflammatory and degenerative brain diseases. J. Neuropathol. Exp. Neurol. **63:** 901–910.
7. Basu, A., J.K. Krady & S.W. Levison. 2004. Interleukin-1: a master regulator of neuroinflammation. J. Neurosci. Res. **78:** 151–156.
8. Choi, D.W. & S.M. Rothman. 1990. The role of glutamate neurotoxicity in hypoxic-ischemic neuronal death. Annu. Rev. Neurosci. **13:** 171–182.
9. Mattson, M.P. 1998. Modification of ion homeostasis by lipid peroxidation: roles in neuronal degeneration and adaptive plasticity. Trends Neurosci. **21:** 53–57.
10. Bazan, N.G. 2003. Synaptic lipid signaling: significance of polyunsaturated fatty acids and platelet-activating factor. J. Lipid Res. **44:** 2221–2233.
11. Horrocks, L.A. & A.A. Farooqui. 1994. NMDA receptor–stimulated release of arachidonic acid: mechanisms for the Bazan effect. *In* Cell Signal Transduction, Second Messengers, and Protein Phosphorylation in Health and Disease, pp. 113–128. Plenum. New York.

12. MARCHESELLI, V.L., S. HONG, W.J. LUKIW *et al.* 2003. Novel docosanoids inhibit brain ischemia-reperfusion-mediated leukocyte infiltration and pro-inflammatory gene expression. J. Biol. Chem. **278:** 43807–43817.
13. CAPPER, E.A. & L.A. MARSHALL. 2001. Mammalian phospholipases A(2): mediators of inflammation, proliferation, and apoptosis. Prog. Lipid Res. **40:** 167–197.
14. SMITH, W.L. & L.J. MARNETT. 1991. Prostaglandin endoperoxide synthase: structure and catalysis. Biochim. Biophys. Acta **1083:** 1–17.
15. HATA, A.N. & R.M. BREYER. 2004. Pharmacology and signaling of prostaglandin receptors: multiple roles in inflammation and immune modulation. Pharmacol. Ther. **103:** 147–166.
16. SIMMONS, D.L., R.M. BOTTING & T. HLA. 2004. Cyclooxygenase isozymes: the biology of prostaglandin synthesis and inhibition. Pharmacol. Rev. **56:** 387–437.
17. BAZAN, N.G. & G. ALLAN. 1996. Platelet-activating factor in the modulation of excitatory amino acid neurotransmitter release and of gene expression. J. Lipid Mediat. Cell Signal. **14:** 321–330.
18. IADECOLA, C., K. NIWA, S. NOGAWA *et al.* 2001. Reduced susceptibility to ischemic brain injury and *N*-methyl-D-aspartate-mediated neurotoxicity in cyclooxygenase-2-deficient mice. Proc. Natl. Acad. Sci. USA **98:** 1294–1299.
19. RAPP, J.H., W.E. CONNOR, D.S. LIN & J.M. PORTER. 1991. Dietary eicosapentaenoic acid and docosahexaenoic acid from fish oil: their incorporation into advanced human atherosclerotic plaques. Arterioscler. Thromb. **11:** 903–911.
20. MCLENNAN, P., P. HOWE, M. ABEYWARDENA *et al.* 1996. The cardiovascular protective role of docosahexaenoic acid. Eur. J. Pharmacol. **300:** 83–89.
21. HIBBELN, J.R. 1998. Fish consumption and major depression. Lancet **351:** 1213.
22. BILLMAN, G.E., J.X. KANG & A. LEAF. 1999. Prevention of sudden cardiac death by dietary pure omega-3 polyunsaturated fatty acids in dogs. Circulation **99:** 2452–2457.
23. MARCHIOLI, R. 1999. Results of GISSI Prevenzione: diet, drugs, and cardiovascular risk—researchers of GISSI Prevenzione. Cardiologia **44**(suppl. 1)**:** 745–746.
24. STEPHENSEN, C.B. 2004. Fish oil and inflammatory disease: is asthma the next target for *n*-3 fatty acid supplements? Nutr. Rev. **62:** 486–489.
25. WHEELER, T.G., R.M. BENOLKEN & R.E. ANDERSON. 1975. Visual membranes: specificity of fatty acid precursors for the electrical response to illumination. Science **188:** 1312–1314.
26. DE CALDIRONI, M.I. & N.G. BAZAN. 1977. Acyl groups, molecular species, and labeling by ^{14}C-glycerol and ^{3}H-arachidonic acid of vertebrate retina glycerolipids. Adv. Exp. Med. Biol. **83:** 397–404.
27. STINSON, A.M., R.D. WIEGAND & R.E. ANDERSON. 1991. Recycling of docosahexaenoic acid in rat retinas during *n*-3 fatty acid deficiency. J. Lipid Res. **32:** 2009–2017.
28. ORGANISCIAK, D.T., R.M. DARROW, Y.L. JIANG & J.C. BLANKS. 1996. Retinal light damage in rats with altered levels of rod outer segment docosahexaenoate. Invest. Ophthalmol. Vis. Sci. **37:** 2243–2257.
29. KIM, H.Y., M. AKBAR, A. LAU & L. EDSALL. 2000. Inhibition of neuronal apoptosis by docosahexaenoic acid (22:6*n*-3): role of phosphatidylserine in antiapoptotic effect. J. Biol. Chem. **275:** 35215–35223.
30. ANDERSON, R.E., M.B. MAUDE & D. BOK. 2001. Low docosahexaenoic acid levels in rod outer segment membranes of mice with rds/peripherin and P216L peripherin mutations. Invest. Ophthalmol. Vis. Sci. **42:** 1715–1720.
31. LITMAN, B.J., S.L. NIU, A. POLOZOVA & D.C. MITCHELL. 2001. The role of docosahexaenoic acid containing phospholipids in modulating G protein–coupled signaling pathways: visual transduction. J. Mol. Neurosci. **16:** 237–242.
32. ANDERSON, R.E., M.B. MAUDE, M. MCCLELLAN *et al.* 2002. Low docosahexaenoic acid levels in rod outer segments of rats with P23H and S334ter rhodopsin mutations. Mol. Vis. **8:** 351–358.
33. BICKNELL, I.R., R. DARROW, L. BARSALOU *et al.* 2002. Alterations in retinal rod outer segment fatty acids and light-damage susceptibility in P23H rats. Mol. Vis. **8:** 333–340.
34. HONG, S., K. GRONERT, P.R. DEVCHAND *et al.* 2003. Novel docosatrienes and 17*S*-resolvins generated from docosahexaenoic acid in murine brain, human blood, and glial cells: autacoids in anti-inflammation. J. Biol. Chem. **278:** 14677–14687.

35. ROBERTS, L.J., T.J. MONTINE, W.R. MARKESBERY *et al.* 1998. Formation of isoprostane-like compounds (neuroprostanes) *in vivo* from docosahexaenoic acid. J. Biol. Chem. **273:** 13605–13612.
36. BELAYEV, L., V.L. MARCHESELLI, L. KHOUTOROVA *et al.* 2005. Docosahexaenoic acid complexed to albumin elicits high-grade ischemic neuroprotection. Stroke **36:** 118–123.
37. CREAGH, E.M., H. CONROY & S.J. MARTIN. 2003. Caspase-activation pathways in apoptosis and immunity. Immunol. Rev. **193:** 10–21.
38. MUKHERJEE, P.K., V.L. MARCHESELLI, C.N. SERHAN & N.G. BAZAN. 2004. Neuroprotectin D1: a docosahexaenoic acid–derived docosatriene protects human retinal pigment epithelial cells from oxidative stress. Proc. Natl. Acad. Sci. USA **101:** 8491–8496.
39. BAZAN, N.G. 1990. Supply of *n*-3 polyunsaturated fatty acids and their significance in the central nervous system. *In* Nutrition and the Brain, pp. 1–24. Raven Press. New York.
40. BAZAN, N.G., T.S. REDDY, T.M. REDMOND *et al.* 1985. Endogenous fatty acids are covalently and noncovalently bound to interphotoreceptor retinoid-binding protein in the monkey retina. J. Biol. Chem. **260:** 13677–13680.
41. GORDON, W.C., E.B. RODRIGUEZ DE TURCO & N.G. BAZAN. 1992. Retinal pigment epithelial cells play a central role in the conservation of docosahexaenoic acid by photoreceptor cells after shedding and phagocytosis. Curr. Eye Res. **11:** 73–83.
42. SIEVING, P.A., P. CHAUDHRY, M. KONDO *et al.* 2001. Inhibition of the visual cycle *in vivo* by 13-*cis* retinoic acid protects from light damage and provides a mechanism for night blindness in isotretinoin therapy. Proc. Natl. Acad. Sci. USA **98:** 1835–1840.
43. SPARROW, J.R., H.R. VOLLMER-SNARR, J. ZHOU *et al.* 2003. A2E-epoxides damage DNA in retinal pigment epithelial cells: vitamin E and other antioxidants inhibit A2E-epoxide formation. J. Biol. Chem. **278:** 18207–18213.
44. GLASGOW, J.N., J. QIU, D. RASSIN *et al.* 2001. Transcriptional regulation of the BCL-X gene by NF-kappaB is an element of hypoxic responses in the rat brain. Neurochem. Res. **26:** 647–659.

Early Effects of Modulating Nuclear Factor-κB Activation on Traumatic Spinal Cord Injury in Rats

OCTAVIO JIMÉNEZ-GARZA,[a] JAVIER CAMACHO,[a] ANTONIO IBARRA,[b,c] ANGELINA MARTÍNEZ,[c] AND GABRIEL GUÍZAR-SAHAGÚN[b,c]

[a]*Pharmacology Section, CINVESTAV-IPN, México City 07360, México*

[b]*Research Unit for Neurological Diseases, IMSS, México City 14050, México*

[c]*Proyecto Camina A. C., México City 14050, México*

ABSTRACT: Genes regulated by NF-κB play an important role on secondary damage and repair after spinal cord injury (SCI). To assess the early effects of the pharmacological inhibition and overactivation of NF-κB, pyrrolidine dithiocarbamate (PDTC) or lipopolysaccharide were given to rats before or after SC contusion. The amount of spared SC tissue was higher ($P < 0.05$) at 24 h postinjury in rats posttreated with PDTC; both PDTC-treated rats showed no significant trend to decrease polymorphonuclear infiltrate. p65 subunit was present in inflammatory cells, neurons, and astrocytes at the injury site. These data support further investigation on functional effects of NF-κB inhibition in acute SCI.

KEYWORDS: pyrrolidine dithiocarbamate; lipopolysaccharide; inflammation; nuclear factor-κB (NF-κB); spared tissue; spinal cord injury (SCI)

Gene expression after spinal cord injury (SCI) is associated with both destructive and reparative processes.[1] Nuclear factor-κB (NF-κB) is activated after SCI[2] and regulates the transcription of many genes associated, among others, with inflammation and apoptosis.[3] Previous studies have demonstrated that, following brain injury, activation of NF-κB in neurons induces production of antiapoptotic gene products and proteins involved in modulating synaptic plasticity, while activation in astrocytes and microglia results in production of proinflammatory cytokines, potentially neurotoxic reactive oxygen species, and excitotoxins.[3] Also, NF-κB activation in neuronal tissue has been proapoptotic as well as antiapoptotic in different models.[4]

Our objective was to identify early effects of inhibiting or overactivating NF-κB activation before and immediately after an experimental SCI.

Anesthetized adult rats were subjected to SCI at the T9 level by dropping onto the exposed dura (through laminectomy) a rod weighing 10 g from a height of 25 mm using the well-characterized NYU impactor device. Pyrrolidine dithiocarbamate

Address for correspondence: Gabriel Guízar-Sahagún, IMSS–Proyecto Camina, Tlalpan 4430, México City 14050, México. Voice: +52-(55)-5573-0029; fax: +52-(55)-5573-5545. guizarg@prodigy.net.mx

Ann. N.Y. Acad. Sci. 1053: 148–150 (2005). © 2005 New York Academy of Sciences. doi: 10.1196/annals.1344.012

(PDTC, 100 mg/kg, ip), a specific NF-κB inhibitor, or a potent activator, lipopolysaccharide (LPS, 100 μg/kg, ip), were given as a single dose before (1 h) or after (5 min) injury ($n = 6$). Control rats were vehicle-treated. Twenty-four hours after injury, rats were anesthetized and perfused intracardially with normal saline solution followed by 4% paraformaldehyde. One cm of spinal cord, with the injured area in the center, was routinely processed and embedded in paraffin. Sections were obtained in the sagittal plane from the central portion, taking as reference the presence of ependyma, and were stained with eosin/hematoxylin for morphometry. Infarction area and spared tissue were delimited and the latter measured in mm^2. The numbers of polymorphonuclear (PMN) cells were counted in 15 consecutive fields (at ×100) in the zone of infarction and expressed for each rat as the mean. Using additional sections, we performed double-immunostaining for confocal colocalization of the p65 subunit (NF-κB activated form) with neurofilament 160 for neurons, GFAP for astrocytes, and propidium iodide for inflammatory cell nuclei. Differences were assessed using ANOVA followed by Dunnett's test.

Rats treated with PDTC after injury had a greater amount of SC spared tissue compared with controls ($P < 0.05$, FIG. 1A). Although not significant, the amount of PMN cells showed a trend to decrease in rats pre- and posttreated with PDTC (FIG. 1B). p65 subunit was found in neurons, astrocytes, and inflammatory cells at the infarction and neighboring areas, while absent in uninjured controls.

Taking into account that NF-κB is involved in both destructive and protective processes following central nervous system damage,[3] we here manipulated its activation to observe early effects of this modulation in a model of SCI. In this preliminary study, NF-κB inhibition, but not overactivation, was better in preserving SC tissue at the site of injury. Interestingly, only PDTC treatment given after injury was favorable, suggesting that the very early NF-κB-dependent gene expression could be beneficial as part of self-protection. In accordance with literature about the possible

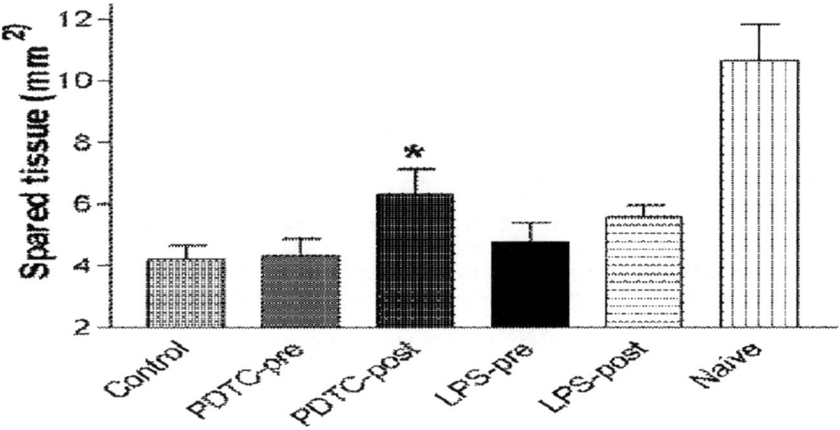

FIGURE 1A. Effect of PDTC and LPS on spared tissue at 24 h after injury. The naïve group is shown only as a reference. *$P < 0.05$.

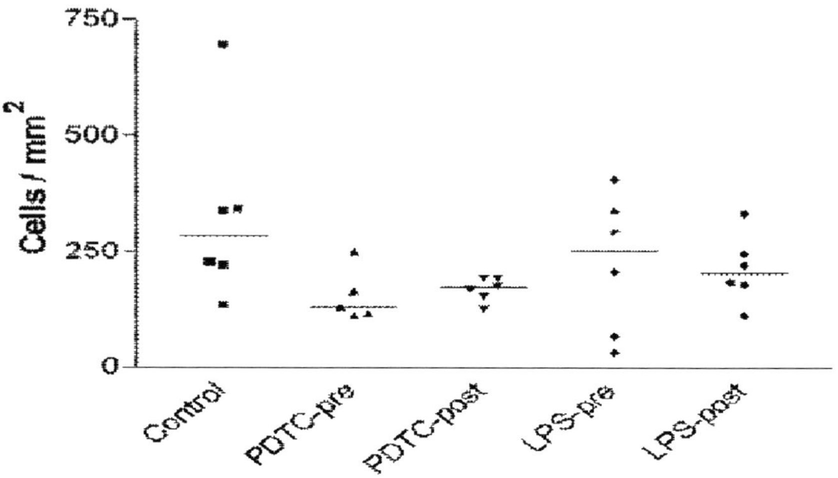

FIGURE 1B. Effect of PDTC and LPS on PMN infiltrate at 24 h after injury. Although not significant, the groups treated with PDTC showed a trend to decrease PMN number at the infarction area.

effects of NF-κB activation in CNS damage, where it is proposed that NF-κB gene expression in glia is detrimental for neurons,[3] we attribute the beneficial effects observed to a reduction in the production of cytotoxic agents.

Our results support the idea that the final balance achieved by inhibition (instead of overactivation) of NF-κB in SCI could be protective. Further research on functional outcome after manipulation of NF-κB activation as a strategy for gene expression control after injury to improve restorative events is desirable.

REFERENCES

1. VELARDO, M.J., C. BURGER, P. WILLIAMS *et al.* 2004. Patterns of gene expression reveal a temporally orchestrated wound healing response in the injured spinal cord. J. Neurosci. **24**(39)**:** 8562–8576.
2. BETHEA, J., M. CASTRO, R.W. KEANE *et al.* 1998. Traumatic spinal cord injury induces nuclear factor-κB activation. J. Neurosci. **18**(9)**:** 3251–3260.
3. MATTSON, M. & S. CAMANDOLA. 2001. NF-κB in neuronal plasticity and neurodegenerative disorders. J. Clin. Invest. **107**(3)**:** 247–254.
4. MATTSON, M., C. CULMSEE, Z. YU & S. CAMANDOLA. 2000. Roles of nuclear factor-κB in neuronal survival and plasticity. J. Neurochem. **74:** 443–456.

Role of Inflammation in the Pathogenesis of Parkinson's Disease

Models, Mechanisms, and Therapeutic Interventions

JAU-SHYONG HONG

Neuropharmacology Section, Laboratory of Pharmacology and Chemistry, NIEHS/NIH, Research Triangle Park, North Carolina 27709, USA

KEYWORDS: Parkinson's disease (PD); inflammation; neurodegeneration; microglia; therapy

The theme of this paper is first to describe newly created rodent Parkinson's disease (PD) models that mimic the progressive disease development in PD patients. With these models, we have elucidated the novel mechanisms of microglial activation that lead to inflammation-mediated neurodegeneration. These insights have then led us to develop innovative anti-inflammatory therapy for PD.

CREATION OF INFLAMMATION-MEDIATED RODENT PD MODELS

In an effort to evaluate the role of inflammation in the pathogenesis of PD, we first developed new PD animal models and primary midbrain neuron-glia cultures. The salient features of these models are (a) prominent inflammation in the process of producing neuronal death; and (b) delayed, progressive, and selective nature of dopaminergic (DA) neuronal death, both *in vivo* and *in vitro*. These models were the first to mimic the delayed and progressive nature of the disease symptoms in PD patients. These unique features are absent from existing PD models, such as 1-methyl-4-phenyl-1,2,3,6-tetrahydropyridine (MPTP), because this toxin kills DA neurons rapidly after injections.

MECHANISM OF INFLAMMATION-MEDIATED DEGENERATION: ROLE OF MICROGLIA

We have demonstrated that microglia are the major player in mediating the inflammation-related neurodegeneration of DA neurons, triggered by a variety of environmental toxins. These findings are critical to the novel concept that microglia

Address for correspondence: Jau-Shyong Hong, Ph.D., Neuropharmacology Section, Laboratory of Pharmacology and Chemistry, NIEHS/NIH, P. O. Box 12233, Research Triangle Park, NC 27709. Voice: 919-541-2358; fax: 919-541-0841.
hong3@niehs.nih.gov

Ann. N.Y. Acad. Sci. 1053: 151–152 (2005). © 2005 New York Academy of Sciences.
doi: 10.1196/annals.1344.054

do not merely serve a passive role as scavengers. Instead, microglia play an active role in the pathogenesis of PD and other neurodegenerative diseases. We have identified a series of proinflammatory factors released from activated microglia, which mediate toxin-induced neuronal damage. Moreover, we have elucidated the molecular mechanisms underlying the regulation of expression for these proinflammatory genes.

DEVELOPMENT OF NOVEL ANTI-INFLAMMATORY THERAPY FOR PD

Information generated from the above studies has provided insights for us to develop a series of novel anti-inflammatory and neuroprotective agents. Unique from the conventional strategies for developing anti-inflammatory drugs, which often target a specific proinflammatory factor, our approach is to prevent the over-production of the majority of proinflammatory factors through the inhibition of the overactivation of microglia, which would prevent the subsequent inflammatory process. Furthermore, we have discovered several small molecules, including peptides and alkaloids, which are both anti-inflammatory and neuroprotective at femtomolar concentrations. In addition to their potential therapeutic benefits, the discovery of femtomolar-acting peptides also offers valuable insight to the potential physiological mechanisms governing microglial activation and DA neuron survival in the substantia nigra.

Mechanisms of Ischemic Neuroprotection by Acetyl-L-carnitine

SANTINA A. ZANELLI,[a] NINA J. SOLENSKI,[b] ROBERT E. ROSENTHAL,[c] AND GARY FISKUM[d]

[a]*Department of Pediatrics,* [b]*Department of Neurology, University of Virginia School of Medicine, Charlottesville, Virginia 22908, USA*

[c]*Department of Surgery, Program in Trauma,* [d]*Department of Anesthesiology, University of Maryland School of Medicine, Baltimore, Maryland 21201, USA*

ABSTRACT: Acetyl-L-carnitine is a naturally occurring substance that, when administered at supraphysiologic concentrations, is neuroprotective in several animal models of global and focal cerebral ischemia. Three primary mechanisms of action are supported by neurochemical outcome measures performed with these models and with *in vitro* models of acute neuronal cell death. The metabolic hypothesis is based on the oxidative metabolism of the acetyl component of acetyl-L-carnitine and is a simple explanation for the reduction in postischemic brain lactate levels and elevation of ATP seen with drug administration. The antioxidant mechanism is supported by reduction of oxidative stress markers, for example, protein oxidation, in both brain tissue and cerebrospinal fluid. The relatively uncharacterized mechanism of inhibiting excitotoxicity could be extremely important in both acute brain injury and chronic neurodegenerative disorders. New experiments performed with primary cultures of rat cortical neurons indicate that the presence of acetyl-L-carnitine significantly inhibits both acute and delayed cell death following exposure to NMDA, an excitotoxic glutamate antagonist. Finally, several other mechanisms of action are possible, including a neurotrophic effect of acetyl-L-carnitine and inhibition of mitochondrial permeability transition. While the multiple potential mechanisms of neuroprotection by acetyl-L-carnitine limit an accurate designation of the most important mode of action, they are compatible with the concept that several brain injury pathways must be inhibited to optimize therapeutic efficacy.

KEYWORDS: metabolism; mitochondria; oxidative stress; excitotoxicity; cardiac arrest; stroke

INTRODUCTION

Ischemic and hypoxic brain injury caused by stroke, cardiac arrest, and perinatal asphyxia leads to neurologic morbidity or mortality in over one million individuals in the United States alone each year. At this juncture, the only neuroprotective inter-

Address for correspondence: Dr. Gary Fiskum, Department of Anesthesiology, University of Maryland School of Medicine, 685 West Baltimore Street, MSTF 5.34, Baltimore, MD 21201. Voice: 410-706-3418; fax: 410-706-2550.
gfisk001@umaryland.edu

Ann. N.Y. Acad. Sci. 1053: 153–161 (2005).
doi: 10.1196/annals.1344.013

ventions demonstrated to be efficacious in large, multicenter clinical trials include administration of tissue plasminogen factor (TPA) to improve cerebral blood flow in a small subset of thromboembolic stroke victims, or of mild systemic hypothermia following cardiac arrest and resuscitation. The quest for a neuroprotective drug effective in humans has been elusive and a complete failure. One possible reason why many of these trials were unsuccessful is that the drug dosage was severely limited by dangerous side effects. Many investigators have thus turned their attention to compounds that are normally present in humans and can be administered at relatively high doses without evidence of toxicity. Examples of such compounds that have been or soon will be tested clinically for various neurologic disorders include creatine, coenzyme Q, and acetyl-L-carnitine (ALCAR). We have focused on the use of ALCAR in animal models of both global and focal cerebral ischemia. Our results and those of other laboratories indicate that ALCAR is neuroprotective in both small and large animal models of global cerebral ischemia and in a rat model of permanent focal ischemia.[1–3] Studies are in progress to determine if ALCAR is also therapeutically effective in a neonatal rat model of hypoxia/ischemia and in a rat model of traumatic brain injury.

STIMULATION OF AEROBIC CEREBRAL ENERGY METABOLISM

Three separate studies using a clinically relevant canine cardiac arrest and resuscitation model have demonstrated neuroprotection by postischemic intravenous administration of ALCAR.[1,4,5] Most importantly, ALCAR administration significantly improves neurologic outcome 23 h following cardiac arrest.[1] In this study, ALCAR (100 mg/kg) was administered immediately following resuscitation after 10 min of normothermic cardiac arrest, and 50-mg/kg doses were administered at 6, 12, and 18 h. Animals were randomized to drug- and vehicle-treated groups and neurologic examinations were performed by examiners blinded to the treatment protocol. This same investigation documented a decrease in the brain lactate level and lactate/pyruvate ratio in animals sacrificed at 2-h reperfusion. Similar results were obtained with immediate postischemic ALCAR administration using a rat 4-vessel occlusion model of global cerebral ischemia and reperfusion. ^{1}H- and ^{31}P-NMR spectroscopy of brain tissue obtained at various reperfusion times indicated that ALCAR significantly reduces levels of lactate and inorganic phosphate and elevates ATP and creatine-phosphate, as compared to vehicle-treated animals.[6] Collectively, these effects of ALCAR on levels of cerebral energy metabolites are consistent with the hypothesis that the acetyl component of ALCAR is metabolized in the brain, thereby promoting oxidative cerebral energy production and minimizing anaerobic glycolysis and lactic acidosis (FIG. 1). As peri-ischemic cerebral acidosis is generally considered to promote neuronal cell death by several different mechanisms, the metabolic mechanism of neuroprotection by ALCAR is the simplest explanation for its primary activity. This mechanism of action is particularly attractive in light of the finding by several laboratories that a profound reperfusion-dependent inhibition of the activity of the enzyme pyruvate dehydrogenase occurs in selectively vulnerable brain regions.[5,7,8] This enzyme catalyzes the conversion of pyruvate to acetyl-CoA and represents the sole bridge between anaerobic and aerobic cerebral energy metabolism (FIG. 1). Indirect evidence in support of ALCAR metabolism as a mechanism of neuroprotec-

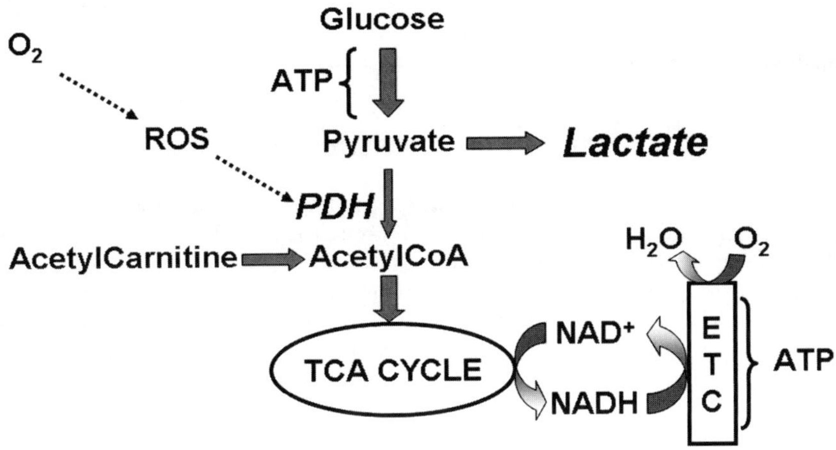

FIGURE 1. Possible metabolism of acetyl-L-carnitine (ALCAR) after cerebral ischemia. ALCAR may serve as an exogenous, alternative source of acetyl-CoA, thereby promoting aerobic energy metabolism via the electron transport chain (ETC), reducing tissue acidosis, and improving neurologic outcome after cerebral ischemia due to cardiac arrest or stroke. The pyruvate dehydrogenase complex (PDH) is a target of reactive oxygen species (ROS) and is inhibited following cerebral ischemia. Such inhibition may be responsible for chronically elevated brain lactate levels following ischemic episodes as this enzyme constitutes the bridge between aerobic and anaerobic cerebral energy metabolism.

tion is that neuroprotection is not observed in animals treated with free carnitine plus acetate.[9] Nevertheless, pretreatment with free carnitine is neuroprotective in other animal models of neurodegeneration, including the 3-nitropropionic acid neurotoxicity model of Huntington's disease.[10] It remains to be seen if carnitine or ALCAR pretreatment is neuroprotective for ischemic brain injury. Studies are in progress using NMR spectroscopy of brain tissue samples following infusion of ^{13}C-ALCAR in sham-operated animals and in dogs following cardiac arrest to determine if the acetyl moiety of ALCAR is indeed metabolized to intermediates of aerobic energy metabolism in the adult brain and if its metabolism is accelerated in response to the metabolic roadblock created by postischemic inhibition of pyruvate dehydrogenase.

One observation suggesting that the metabolic effects of ALCAR may not be exclusively responsible for its postischemic neuroprotection is that, when administration of ALCAR to dogs following cardiac arrest is delayed by 30 min after resuscitation, no neuroprotection is observed, despite normalization of cerebral cortex lactate levels at 2-h reperfusion.[11] In addition to questioning the validity of the metabolic hypothesis, this finding and other results obtained with a rat global cerebral ischemia model indicate that, as with most other neuroprotective agents, there is a limited window of therapeutic opportunity for administration of ALCAR.[12] A limited window of opportunity has severely restricted effective treatment of ischemic stroke patients since the majority of patients are diagnosed several hours following the onset of the ischemic event. In contrast, cardiac arrest patients can potentially be treated almost immediately, as most successful resuscitations occur in the hands of paramedics in the field or of physicians at hospitals. Considering the outstanding safety and tolerance profile of ALCAR, this agent may prove to be an exceptional candidate for neuroprotection clinical trials after cardiac arrest.

PROTECTION AGAINST OXIDATIVE STRESS

One study using the canine cardiac arrest model found that ALCAR treatment significantly reduces the level of protein carbonyl groups in the brains of dogs both at 2- and 24-h reperfusion after 10-min cardiac arrest.[4] Protein carbonyl groups are a marker of oxidative tissue injury and increase significantly during ischemia/ reperfusion. ALCAR likely protects against oxidative stress indirectly through its amelioration of tissue lactic acidosis, a condition that promotes the formation of

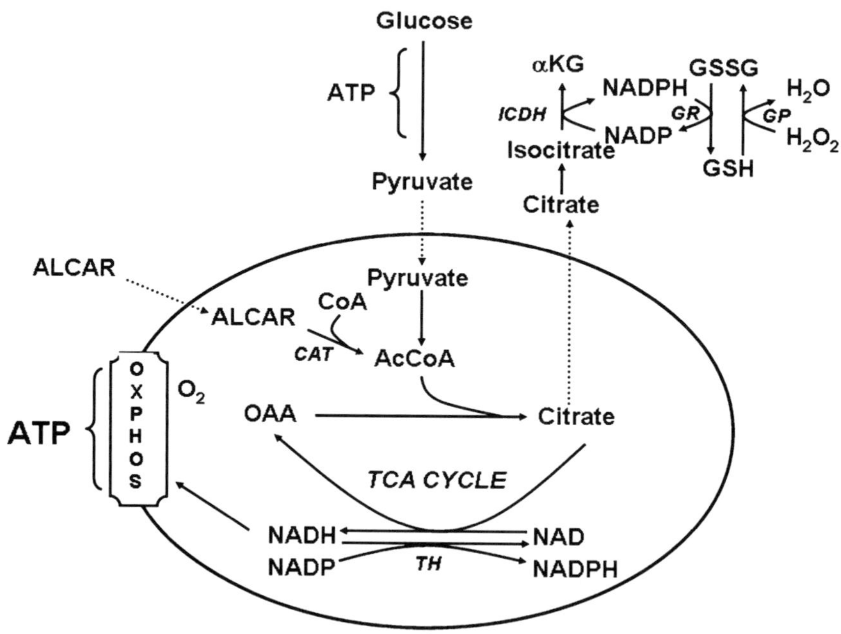

FIGURE 2. Possible shift in cellular redox state caused by ALCAR metabolism. ALCAR can be metabolized to acetyl-CoA by the carnitine acetyltransferase (CAT) reaction. Metabolism of acetyl-CoA by the tricarboxylic acid (TCA) cycle provides NADH that is then used for oxidative phosphorylation (OXPHOS) and for reducing intramitochondrial NADP to form NADPH via the transhydrogenase (TH) reaction. Elevation of intramitochondrial citrate results in transport out to the cytosol, where it is converted to isocitrate. The cytosolic isocitrate dehydrogenase (ICDH) reaction oxidizes isocitrate to form α-ketoglutarate (αKG) and NADPH. NADPH provides the reducing power for converting oxidized glutathione (GSSG) to reduced glutathione (GSH) via the glutathione reductase (GR) reaction. Reduced glutathione provides the reducing power for detoxifying H_2O_2 and organic peroxides via the glutathione peroxidase (GP) reaction. Intramitochondrial NADPH is also used to detoxify peroxides by an intramitochondrial glutathione reductase/peroxidase system (not shown).

reactive oxygen species. It is also possible that metabolism of ALCAR can cause a reduced shift in both the mitochondrial and cytosolic redox state, thus increasing the reducing power necessary for detoxification of reactive oxygen species, for example, H_2O_2, via the glutathione peroxidase/reductase system, and for maintaining the normal redox state of protein sulfhydryl groups via the thioredoxin/thioredoxin reductase system (FIG. 2).

Another report established a strong trend toward improved levels of brain pyruvate dehydrogenase enzyme activity at 30-min and 24-h reperfusion in post–cardiac arrest animals treated with ALCAR compared to the drug vehicle.[5] As evidence suggests that the loss of pyruvate dehydrogenase activity during reperfusion is due to oxidative stress, this finding can be interpreted as reflecting the indirect effects of ALCAR on brain protein oxidation. These results present the intriguing possibility that oxidative inactivation of pyruvate dehydrogenase occurs very rapidly during reperfusion, but that the inhibition is reversible upon administration of reducing power, for example, that potentially provided by metabolism of ALCAR.

ALCAR may also exert an indirect antioxidant activity through induction of one or more antioxidant genes. Primary rat cortical astrocyte cultures treated with ALCAR exhibit increased expression of the antioxidant enzyme heme oxygenase-1 and are protected against mitochondrial alterations and cell death caused by inflammatory cytokines.[13] The effect of ALCAR on heme oxygenase expression is apparently mediated by increased expression of Nrf2, a transcriptional activating factor that can stimulate the expression of a wide array of antioxidant genes and even indirectly stimulates transcription of genes located on the mitochondrial genome.

ALCAR is also effective at inhibiting the oxidative stress and death caused by exposure of neural cells to A-beta-amyloid, a neurotoxic peptide that accumulates in the brain of Alzheimer's patients and is strongly implicated in the etiology of neurodegeneration.[14,15] Treatment of multiple sclerosis with oral ALCAR for 6 months reduces several markers of oxidative stress that are typically elevated in the CSF of these patients.[16]

PROTECTION AGAINST EXCITOTOXICITY

ALCAR was reported in the mid-1990s to inhibit hippocampal neuronal cell death in response to glutamate exposure.[17] Like many excitotoxicity experiments, conditions were used to maximize glutamate excitotoxicity. These conditions include the omission of magnesium and the inclusion of the coagonist glycine in the medium. We recently performed experiments with primary cultures of rat cortical neurons to determine if ALCAR is cytoprotective in the absence of added glycine and in the presence of magnesium, a physiological divalent cation normally present in the brain interstitium at ~1 mM concentration. The results of these experiments are shown in FIGURES 3 and 4. Exposure of cortical neurons at 10–14 days *in vitro* to the ionotropic glutamate receptor agonist *N*-methyl-D-aspartate (NMDA) at a concentration of 100 μM for 30 min resulted in significant cell death compared to control cells subjected to a change of media, but not exposed to NMDA (FIG. 3). When 1 mM ALCAR was present together with NMDA, no significant cell death was observed. To test for the possibility that ALCAR only delayed the onset of cell death, a separate set of experiments was conducted where cell death was measured 24 h after the 30-min

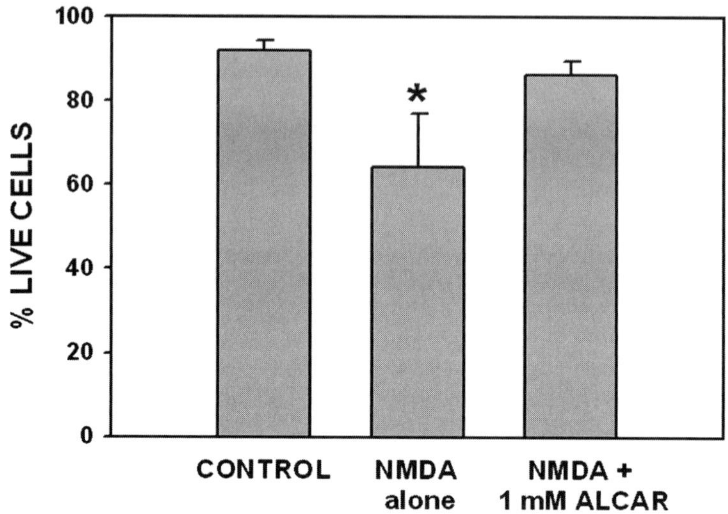

FIGURE 3. Protection by ALCAR against NMDA-induced acute neuronal death. Cultured cortical neurons (DIV 10–14) were exposed to 100 μM NMDA for 30 min and immediately examined for cell death using the calcein-AM/PI ratio (live/dead). Exposure to NMDA resulted in significant neuronal cell death as compared to controls: 64.3±12.9% live cells in the NMDA group vs. 91.8±2.4% live cells in the control group (*P = 0.007 vs. control). In the presence of 1 mM ALCAR, cell death after exposure to NMDA was not significant: 86.2±3.4% live cells (P = 0.5 vs. control). Differences between the mean were determined by ANOVA, and a Holm-Sidak test was applied for pairwise multiple comparisons. Results are shown as the mean ± SEM for n = 3 experiments.

exposure to NMDA in the absence and presence of 1 mM ALCAR both during and after the NMDA treatment. The results described in FIGURE 4 indicate that, while significant cell death was also present at 24 h postinjury in the absence of ALCAR, no significant death was observed in its presence. The death observed with the live/dead assay reflects the additional cell death that ensues after NMDA is removed from the medium. These results confirm the results reported earlier for hippocampal neurons and extend them by demonstrating neuroprotection in the presence of magnesium and in the absence of glycine. Our findings also indicate that neuroprotection is observed with cortical as well as hippocampal neurons, two populations that are sensitive to cell death *in vivo* in response to insults (e.g., stroke) that involve excitotoxicity. Moreover, ALCAR cytoprotection is observed both during the acute phase of excitotoxicity and during the delayed phase after transient exposure to NMDA. Further studies are thus needed to determine if the antiexcitotoxic activity of ALCAR contributes to its neuroprotection in animal models of acute ischemic and traumatic brain injury.

Protection by ALCAR against excitotoxic cell death could be due to direct antagonism of glutamate receptors, to activation of gamma-aminobutyric acid (GABA) receptors that cause neuronal hyperpolarization and therefore resistance to NMDA receptor activation, or to inhibition of secondary events.[17] These secondary events could include activation of the mitochondrial permeability transition that can cause

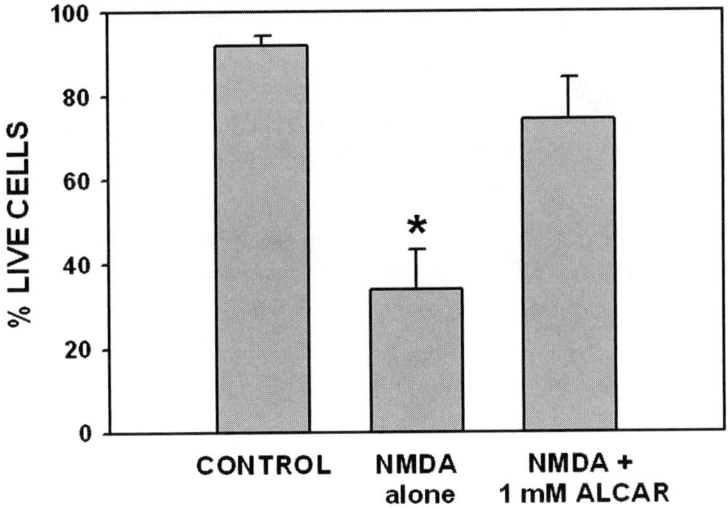

FIGURE 4. Protection by ALCAR against NMDA-induced delayed neuronal death. Cultured cortical neurons (DIV 10–14) were exposed to 100 μM NMDA for 30 min and examined for cell death at 24 h postinjury using the calcein-AM/PI ratio (live/dead). Exposure to NMDA for 30 min followed by a 24-h recovery period resulted in significant neuronal cell death as compared to controls: 33.7±9.6% live cells in the NMDA group vs. 91.8±12.9% live cells in the control group (*$P = 0.005$ vs. control). In neurons treated with ALCAR during NMDA exposure and during the recovery period, cell death was not significantly different than controls (74.4±9.9% live cells; $P = 0.09$ vs. control) and significantly less than with NMDA in the absence of ALCAR (*$P = 0.006$ vs. NMDA). Differences between the mean were determined by ANOVA, and a Holm-Sidak test was applied for pairwise multiple comparisons. Results are shown as the mean ± SEM for $n = 3$ experiments.

release of mitochondrial cytochrome c and stimulation of mitochondrial ROS production,[18] and delayed neuronal calcium deregulation caused by opening of plasma membrane transient receptor potential (Trp) cation channels in response to the oxidative stress.[19] Studies are in progress to test for these different possible effects of ALCAR.

OTHER MECHANISMS OF NEUROPROTECTION

Several other potential mechanisms of ALCAR neuroprotection are implicated based on studies performed both *in vitro* and *in vivo* with models other than acute neuronal cell death due to ischemia and excitotoxicity. For instance, exposure of cultured neural cells to ALCAR inhibits apoptosis caused by deprivation of serum or neurotrophic factors, suggesting that ALCAR may have an as yet undefined neurotrophic activity.[20,21] Apoptosis that occurs following acute brain injury results either from initial intracellular alterations (e.g., elevated calcium or oxidative stress) or from the response to extracellular factors (e.g., inflammatory cytokines and “cell death ligands", such as Fas).[22] Treatment of rats with carnitine and carnitine esters significantly lowers circulating levels of TNFα and interleukins using a lipopolysaccharide (endotoxin)–induced systemic inflammatory response.[23] It is thus possible that ALCAR may also reduce the inflammatory reactions in the brain following acute injury. Finally, it is also very likely that at least the carnitine component of ALCAR can "buffer" the toxic intracellular free fatty acids that are released by enzymes such as calcium-dependent phospholipase 2 during cerebral ischemia and trauma. The reduction in free fatty acids due to formation of fatty acyl carnitine esters inhibits their ability to induce the mitochondrial permeability transition[24] and appears responsible for the protection against anoxic death of hepatocytes afforded by carnitine.[25] While the multiple potential mechanisms of neuroprotection by ALCAR limit an accurate designation of the most important mode of action, they are compatible with the concept that several brain injury pathways must be inhibited to optimize therapeutic efficacy.

ACKNOWLEDGMENTS

This work was supported by NIH Grant No. P01 HD16596 and by Sigma-Tau Research Inc.

REFERENCES

1. ROSENTHAL, R.E., R. WILLIAMS, Y.E. BOGAERT *et al.* 1992. Prevention of postischemic canine neurological injury through potentiation of brain energy metabolism by acetyl-L-carnitine. Stroke **23:** 1312–1318.
2. LOLIC, M.M., G. FISKUM & R.E. ROSENTHAL. 1997. Neuroprotective effects of acetyl-L-carnitine after stroke in rats. Ann. Emerg. Med. **29**(6)**:** 758–765.
3. SHUAIB, A., T. WAQAAR, T. WISHART *et al.* 1995. Acetyl-L-carnitine attenuates neuronal damage in gerbils with transient forebrain ischemia only when given before the insult. Neurochem. Res. **20**(9)**:** 1021–1025.
4. LIU, Y., R.E. ROSENTHAL, P. STARKE-REED *et al.* 1993. Inhibition of post–cardiac arrest brain protein oxidation by acetyl-L-carnitine. Free Rad. Biol. Med. **15:** 667–670.
5. BOGAERT, Y.E., R.E. ROSENTHAL & G. FISKUM. 1994. Post-ischemic inhibition of cerebral cortex pyruvate dehydrogenase. Free Rad. Biol. Med. **16:** 811–820.
6. AURELI, T., A. MICCHELI & M.E. DI COCCO. 1994. Effect of acetyl-L-carnitine on recovery of brain phosphorus metabolites and lactic acid level during reperfusion after cerebral ischemia in the rat—study by 31P- and 1H-NMR spectroscopy. Brain Res. **643**(1/2)**:** 92–99.
7. BOGAERT, Y.E., K.F. REX-SHEU, P.R. HOF *et al.* 2000. Neuronal subclass-selective loss of pyruvate dehydrogenase immunoreactivity following canine cardiac arrest and resuscitation. Exp. Neurol. **161:** 115–125.
8. ZAIDAN, E., K.F. SHEU & N.R. SIMS. 1998. The pyruvate dehydrogenase complex is partially inactivated during early recirculation following short-term forebrain ischemia in rats. J. Neurochem. **70**(1)**:** 233–241.
9. MARTIN, E., R.E. ROSENTHAL & G. FISKUM. 2005. Pyruvate dehydrogenase complex: metabolic link to ischemic brain injury and target of oxidative stress. J. Neurosci. Res. **79:** 240–247.
10. BINIENDA, Z., A. VIRMANI, B. PRZYBYLA-ZAWISLAK *et al.* 2004. Neuroprotective effect of L-carnitine in the 3-nitropropionic acid (3-NPA)–evoked neurotoxicity in rats. Neurosci. Lett. **367:** 264–267.
11. ROSENTHAL, R.E., Y.E. BOGAERT & G. FISKUM. 2005. Delayed therapy of experimental global cerebral ischemia with acetyl-L-carnitine in dogs. Neurosci. Lett. **378**(2)**:** 82–87.

12. SHUAIB, A., T. WAQAAR, T. WISHART *et al.* 1995. Acetyl-L-carnitine attenuates neuronal damage in gerbils with transient forebrain ischemia only when given before the insult. Neurochem. Res. **20**(9)**:** 1021–1025.
13. CALABRESE, V., A. RAVAGNA, C. COLOMBRITA *et al.* 2005. Acetylcarnitine induces heme oxygenase in rat astrocytes and protects against oxidative stress: involvement of the transcription factor Nrf2. J. Neurosci Res. **79**(4)**:** 509–521.
14. DHITAVAT, S., D. ORTIZ, T.B. SHEA *et al.* 2002. Acetyl-L-carnitine protects against amyloid-beta neurotoxicity: roles of oxidative buffering and ATP levels. Neurochem. Res. **27**(6)**:** 501–505.
15. VIRMANI, M.A., V. CASO, A. SPADONI *et al.* 2001. The action of acetyl-L-carnitine on the neurotoxicity evoked by amyloid fragments and peroxide on primary rat cortical neurons. Ann. N.Y. Acad. Sci. **939:** 162–178.
16. CALABRESE, V., G. SCAPAGNINI, A. RAVAGNA *et al.* 2003. Disruption of thiol homeostasis and nitrosative stress in the cerebrospinal fluid of patients with active multiple sclerosis: evidence for a protective role of acetylcarnitine. Neurochem. Res. **28**(9)**:** 1321–1328.
17. FORLONI, G., N. ANGERETTI & S. SMIROLDO. 1994. Neuroprotective activity of acetyl-L-carnitine: studies *in vitro*. J. Neurosci. Res. **37**(1)**:** 92–96.
18. STARKOV, A.A., B.M. POLSTER & G. FISKUM. 2002. Regulation of mitochondrial reactive oxygen species generation by calcium and Bax. J. Neurochem. **83:** 220–228.
19. CHINOPOULOS, C., A.A. GERENCSER, J. DOCZI *et al.* 2004. Inhibition of glutamate-induced delayed calcium deregulation by 2-APB and Li^{3+} in cultured cortical neurons. J. Neurochem. **91:** 471–483.
20. ISHII, T., Y. SHIMPO, Y. MATSUOKA *et al.* 2000. Anti-apoptotic effect of acetyl-L-carnitine and L-carnitine in primary cultured neurons. Jpn. J. Pharmacol. **83**(2)**:** 119–124.
21. BIGINI, P., S. LARINI, C. PASQUALI *et al.* 2002. Acetyl-L-carnitine shows neuroprotective and neurotrophic activity in primary culture of rat embryo motoneurons. Neurosci. Lett. **329**(3)**:** 334–338.
22. POLSTER, B.M. & G. FISKUM. 2004. Mitochondrial mechanisms of neural cell apoptosis. J. Neurochem. **90:** 1281–1289.
23. WINTER, B.K., G. FISKUM & L.L. GALLO. 1995. Effects of L-carnitine on serum triglyceride and cytokine levels in rat models of cachexia and septic shock. Br. J. Cancer **72**(5)**:** 1173–1179.
24. STARKOV, A.A., O.V. MARKOVA, E.N. MOKHOVA *et al.* 1994. Fatty acid–induced Ca(2+)-dependent uncoupling and activation of external pathway of NADH oxidation are coupled to cyclosporin A–sensitive mitochondrial permeability transition. Biochem. Mol. Biol. Int. **32**(6)**:** 1147–1155.
25. PASTORINO, J.G., J.W. SNYDER, A. SERRONI *et al.* 1993. Cyclosporin and carnitine prevent the anoxic death of cultured hepatocytes by inhibiting the mitochondrial permeability transition. J. Biol. Chem. **268**(19)**:** 13791–13798.

Identification of Rat Hippocampal mRNAs Altered by the Mitochondrial Toxicant, 3-NPA

BEATA D. PRZYBYLA-ZAWISLAK,[a,b] BRETT T. THORN,[c] SYED F. ALI,[a] RICHARD A. DENNIS,[b] ANTONINO AMATO,[d] ASHRAF VIRMANI,[e] AND ZBIGNIEW K. BINIENDA[a]

[a]*Division of Neurotoxicology, National Center for Toxicological Research, Food and Drug Administration, Jefferson, Arkansas, USA*

[b]*Department of Geriatrics, University of Arkansas for Medical Sciences, Little Rock, Arkansas, USA*

[c]*Z-Tech Incorporated, Jefferson, Arkansas, USA*

[d]*Sigma-Tau Research, Incorporated, Gaithersburg, Maryland, USA*

[e]*Sigma-Tau Health Science, S.p.A., Roma, Italy*

ABSTRACT: 3-Nitropropionic acid (3-NPA) is a model mitochondrial inhibitor that causes selective neurodegeneration in brain. 3-NPA-induced neurodegeneration occurs via a secondary neurotoxicity, caused initially by ATP depletion and redox changes in the cell. It is known that the hippocampal degeneration caused by mitochondrial dysfunction affects learning and memory, cognitive functions commonly disturbed in neurodegenerative diseases. The 3-NPA-treated animal model can be used to study molecular mechanisms underlying selective degeneration in the brain. In this study, a microarray approach was utilized to define changes in the expression of 530 genes in the rat hippocampus after acute exposure to 3-NPA at 30 mg/kg, sc. The microarray data were collected at 30 min, 2 h, and 4 h post-3-NPA. Statistical modeling using an ANOVA mixed model applied to Van der Waerden scores of rank-transformed intensity data was used to assign statistical significance to 44 transcripts. These transcripts represent genes associated with energy metabolism, calcium homeostasis, the cytoskeleton, neurotransmitter metabolism, and other cellular functions. Changes in the transcripts of genes encoding 2 transporters [blood-brain specific anion transporter (*Slco1c1*) and sodium-dependent inorganic phosphate cotransporter (*Slc17a7*)] were confirmed by real-time RT-PCR. In conclusion, this study identified 2 new potential targets for enhancement of neuroprotection or inhibition of neurodegeneration associated with ATP depletion in the hippocampus.

KEYWORDS: microarrays; RT-PCR; hippocampus; gene expression; *Slco1c1*; *Slc17a7*; glutamate vesicular transporter; 3-nitropropionic acid (3-NPA); rat

Address for correspondence: Dr. Beata Przybyla-Zawislak, Division of Neurotoxicology, HFT-132, FDA/NCTR, Jefferson, AR 72079-9502. Voice: 870-543-7053; fax: 870-543-7745. bzawislak@nctr.fda.gov

Ann. N.Y. Acad. Sci. 1053: 162–173 (2005).
doi: 10.1196/annals.1344.014

INTRODUCTION

The hippocampus is one of several brain regions vulnerable to neurotoxic damage caused by 3-nitropropionic acid (3-NPA).[1–3] 3-NPA irreversibly inhibits succinate dehydrogenase (SDH), one of the critical enzymes of the TCA cycle and oxidative phosphorylation.[4] The inhibition of SDH causes a decrease in ATP production, which leads to an excitotoxic cascade and damage in brain regions rich in excitatory circuits. The ATP-dependent accumulation of the excitatory neurotransmitter, glutamate, overactivates glutamate receptors, leading to a release of calcium from intracellular stores. This alteration of calcium homeostasis leads directly to the activation of mitochondrial permeability pores and cell death. Details of these excitotoxic processes are reviewed elsewhere.[5–7] Each step in the excitotoxic cascade can be aggravated by an increase in endogenously produced free radicals that are produced during declines in oxidative phosphorylation.

Nerve degeneration in the hippocampus, caused by either endogenous or exogenous toxic factors, is of special interest because the subgranular zone of the dentate gyrus in the hippocampus is a unique area in the adult brain where the highest number of new neurons is generated throughout life.[8–10] In addition, the hippocampus is important for learning and memory, cognitive functions commonly disturbed in neurodegenerative diseases. Impairment of learning and memory with age can be related to a decline in metabolism associated with reduced mitochondrial function in the hippocampus.[11,12] The molecular mechanisms underlying hippocampal degeneration caused by defects in energy production have not been defined yet. In this study, deciphering gene expression changes over time is used to address this issue. The 3-NPA model of energetically compromised mitochondria was used to identify genes related to energy depletion–related neurotoxic damage in the hippocampus. A time-course microarray experiment was carried out to monitor early (1–4 h) mRNA responses in the rat hippocampus to an acute dose of 3-NPA (30 mg/kg). An ANOVA mixed model was applied in the analysis of the microarray data.[13–15] The 44 transcripts identified by these analyses primarily represent genes related to energy metabolism, the cytoskeleton, and calcium homeostasis, as well as to neurotransmitter turnover. A "spot check" of 5 genes identified by our microarray results using real-time RT-PCR confirmed transcript changes of 2 genes encoding blood-brain specific anion transporter (NM_053441) and sodium-dependent inorganic phosphate co-transporter (NM_053859). The potential role of these transporters in the mediation of 3-NPA-evoked neurotoxicity in the hippocampus is discussed.

MATERIALS AND METHODS

Animals

Twenty-one adult male, Sprague-Dawley rats, obtained from the NCTR breeding colony, were housed under controlled environmental conditions (temperature 22°C, relative humidity 45–55%, 12-h light:dark cycle with lights off at 1800 h). Animals had free access to food and tap water. All animal care and procedures were in accordance with the NIH Guide for the Care and Use of Laboratory Animals and were approved by the NCTR/FDA Institutional Animal Care and Use Committee.

Treatment

Rats were injected subcutaneously with 3-NPA dissolved in 0.1 M phosphate buffer (pH 7.4) at 30 mg/kg. The dose of 30 mg/kg was found previously to cause a 50% decrease in ATP, to increase ROS scavengers in the brain,[16] and to induce neurotoxicity (overt brain lesions, activation of biomarkers). Five control rats were injected with the buffer vehicle. Animals were sacrificed by decapitation at 30, 120, and 240 min after the injection.

RNA Isolation

Hippocampi were dissected from each rat onto ice, immediately frozen in liquid nitrogen, and stored at –80°C. Total RNA was isolated using Tri Reagent (Molecular Research Center, Cincinnati, OH) and RNeasy Kit (Qiagen, Valencia, CA). Samples were treated with DNase (RNase-free DNase set, Qiagen, Valencia, CA) when still bound to Qiagen columns. The integrity and purity of RNA were determined using the RNA 6000 LabChip kit and Agilent 2100 Bioanalyzer (Agilent Technologies, Wilmington, DE). The RNA concentrations were verified using a NanoDrop ND-1000 Spectrophotometer (NanoDrop Technologies, Wilmington, DE). The average yield of RNA isolated from total rat hippocampus (200 mg) was 150 μg.

cDNA Preparation and Labeling

Forty grams of total RNA in 18 μL of RNase-free water was mixed with 4 μL of Oligo-dT,[12–18] at a concentration of 0.5 ng/μL (Invitrogen, Carlsbad, CA), and incubated at 65°C for 10 min, at 25°C for 5 min, and finally at 4°C for 5 min. Eighteen μL of Superscript II reagents (Invitrogen, Carlsbad, CA) was added to attain a final volume of 40 μL. The dNTP mix contained 10 mM aa-dUTP (Ambion, Austin, TX). Reverse transcription was carried out at 42°C for 2 h and terminated with 1 M NaOH at 65°C (15 min). The reaction was neutralized by adding 10 μL of 1 M HCl and 24 μL of 1 M HEPES (pH 7.5). The cDNAs were purified using Microcon YM30 concentrators (Millipore, Billerica, MA). The cDNAs were evaporated almost to dryness in a speed-vac and stored overnight at –20°C. The next day, each of two fluorescent dyes, cy3 and cy5, from CyDye postlabeling reactive dye pack (Amersham, Carlsbad, CA), was resuspended in 15 μL of 0.1 M $NaHCO_3$ (pH 9.0) buffer. Each cDNA sample volume was brought to 15 μL with RNase-free water and divided in half. One half (7.5 μL) of cDNA was mixed with 7.5 μL of cy3 dye, and the other half was mixed with the cy5 dye (dye swapping experiment). The labeling reaction lasted 1 h at room temperature in the dark. Unincorporated dye was quenched with 5 μL of 4 M hydroxylamine-HCl. Labeled probes were purified using QIAquick columns (Qiagen, Valencia, CA).

Hybridization

Samples were diluted in 120 μL of salt-based hybridization buffer (MWG, Greensboro, NC), prewarmed to 42°C, and kept for 3 min at 95°C. The hybridization mixture was set on ice for 3 min, spun down briefly, and applied to a slide with an attached slide frame. A polyester coverslip was placed over the gene frame on the slide, and then the slide was transferred to a wet hybridization chamber for incubation at 42°C for 20 h. On the next day, the slides were washed for 5 min at 30°C with agitation in each of the following filter-sterilized solutions: 2× SSC + 0.1%SDS, 1× SSC, and 0.5× SSC. Slides were dried by centrifugation in 50-mL conical tubes for 5 min at 500*g* and immediately scanned.

Scanning

Slides were scanned with an arrayWoRx[e] Biochip Reader (Applied Precision, Issaquah, WA) at 10-µm pixel size. For each slide, two TIF (16-bit) files were obtained, one each for cy3 and cy5. These TIF files were analyzed using the softWoRx™ Tracker Microarray Experiment Management and Analysis Software (Applied Precision, Issaquah, WA).

Microarrays

Slides containing 530 genes selected from the Pan Rat 10K oligonucleotides were printed by MWG-Biotech (Greensboro, NC). The MWG-Biotech arrays use 50-mer oligonucleotides within the defined coding regions. All oligonucleotides are matched in GC content and Tm, are free from secondary structures, and are self-annealing. The majority of selected genes were related to mitochondrial function, cell protection, and neurotransmitter function.

Statistical Analysis of Microarray Data

Design

The dye-swap reference design was applied (FIG. 1). The reference design is optimal in time-course studies where further collection of samples at other time points is planned.[17,18]

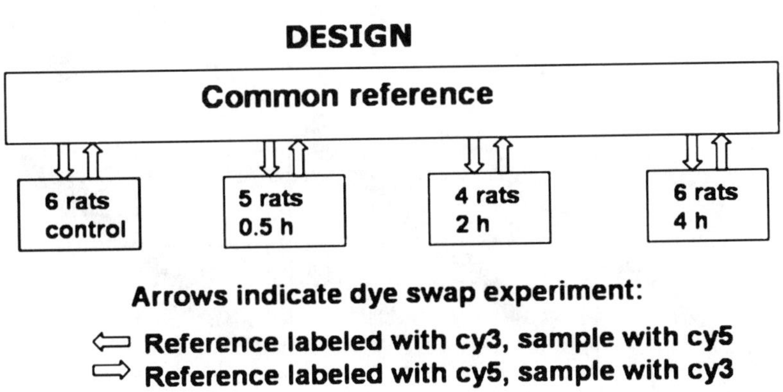

FIGURE 1. Experimental design: 21 rats were divided into 4 treatment groups. cDNA prepared from hippocampus of each animal was labeled twice: with cy3 and cy5.

Transformation

Raw intensity data were rank-transformed for each dye, and Van der Waerden (VDW) scores were calculated using nonparametric SAS procedures. VDW scores are approximations of the normal scores, which are obtained by applying a probit transformation, Φ^{-1}, to the order statistics of the original data.[19] Computationally, the score for observation X_i is

$$S_i = \Phi^{-1}[r_i/(n+1)]$$

where r_i is the rank of observation X_i.

Quality of Intensity Data Evaluation

In order to detect erroneous data, the VDW scores were analyzed using an Array Group Correlations method available in SAS Microarray Solution v1.01 Software (SAS Institute, Cary, NC). An example of such an analysis is shown in FIGURE 2.

ANOVA Analysis and Statistical Inference

The VDW score for each gene was analyzed using a mixed model analysis of variance (Mixed Model Analysis method in SAS Microarray Solution v1.01, SAS

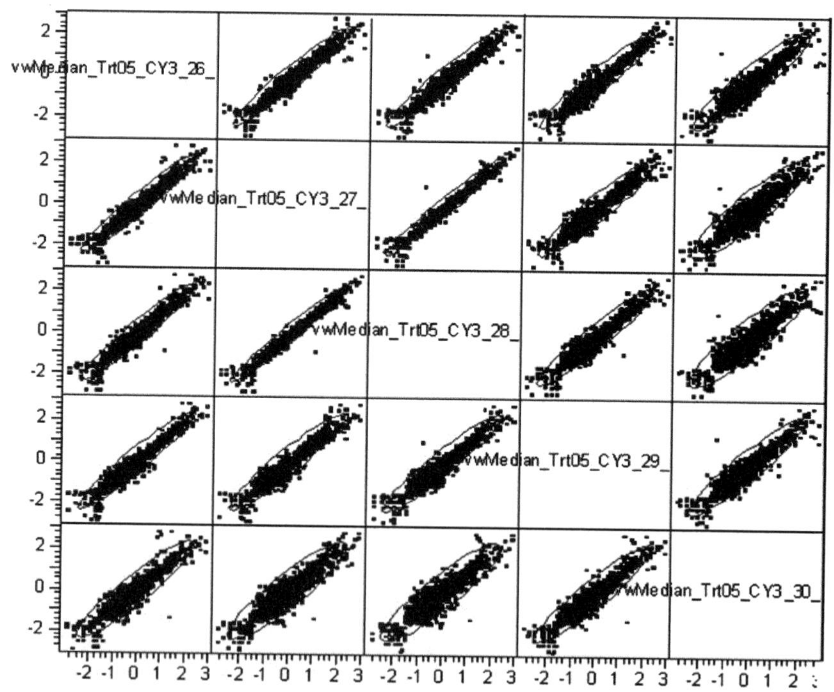

FIGURE 2. An example of Array Group Correlations analysis. Here, correlations are calculated between transformed intensity data of animals from the 30-min treatment group labeled with cy3.

Institute, Cary, NC). In this model, the scores are considered to be a function of fixed effects (treatment, dye, treatment-dye interactions) and random effects (animal). Contrasts were formed to compare various treatments, dyes, etc., including a linear trend contrast with treatment. The *P* values were corrected for multiple comparisons using the false-discovery-rate (FDR) method.[20]

RT-PCR

Real-Time RT-PCR Procedure

Two μg of total RNA was reverse-transcribed using an iScriptcDNA Synthesis Kit (Bio-Rad Laboratories, Hercules, CA). iQ SYBR Green Supermix (Bio-Rad) was used for PCR reactions. The same RNA samples were used for the microarray experiments. Primers, listed in TABLE 1, were designed with Beacon Designer (Premier, Biosoft International, Palo Alto, CA). The AB PRISM 7700 Sequence Detector was used (Applied Biosystems, Foster City, CA). A standard curve was prepared for each target gene and for the endogenous reference (18S ribosomal RNA). To construct the standard curve, equal amounts of all cDNA samples were mixed and serially diluted in fourfold dilutions. The PCR parameters for the thermocycler were 10 min at 95°C followed by a total of 45 two-temperature cycles (15 s at 95°C and 1 min at 60°C). Fluorescent data for the dissociation curve were collected for 20 min after completion of PCR during ramping of the temperature from 60°C to 95°C.

Statistical Analysis of RT-PCR Data

Unpaired *t*-test analyses of RT-PCR data were carried out using Sigma Stat Software (SPSS, Inc.). The differences found between treated and control animals were considered statistically significant when $P \leq 0.05$.

TABLE 1. Primer sequences for seven rat genes used in RT-PCR

GenBank	Gene no.	Primer 5′-3′
NM_031510	8	GTGGAACTGGATCTGCATAGCT ACTTGACGCCGACGTTGTATT
NM_053311	12	ATGACATTGTGAAGACGGTGATTG CCGGTGACGACATCGTTCTC
U52950	23	CTGTCGCACCGCTTCCTAGA CCTCAGGTGCTCTTCGGTCA
NM_053441	26	GCAAATGTTCAGACTCAAAATGGG ATATAATGTTCTTTCCACTCCGGC
NM_053859	27	CCAATGTGCGAAAGCTGATGAA ACGCCCTTGGAGTGTGAGTA
NM_017122	45	CGAGCATGTCTTCCGCACTT CTCAGAGCGATGATGAACTCCC
X62145	(18S)	TTSGAACGTCTGCCCTATCAA ATGGTAGGCACGGCGACTA

NOTE: cDNA sequences were retrieved from the GenBank database (NCBI). Gene number matches that used in TABLE 2.

TABLE 2. List of significant genes

No.	rtR	Trend	0.5 h	2 h	4 h	GenBank	Gene description
							Energy metabolism
1		LT	–	↑	↑	NM_022215	Glycerol 3-phosphate dehydrogenase
2		–	–	↓	–	NM_013098	Glucose-6-phosphatase catalytic subunit
3		–	↓	↓	–	NM_053716	Fructose biphosphatase 2
4		LT	–	↓	↓	M19044	F1-ATPase beta subunit
5		LT	–	↑	↑	M17091	*R*-Pyruvate kinase
6		–	–	↓	–	NM_053291	Phosphoglycerate kinase 1
7	X	LT	–	↓	↓	NM_031510	Cytosolic NADP-dependent isocitrate dehydrogenase
8		–	↓	↓	↓	NM_053922	Acetyl-coenzyme A carboxylase beta
9		LT	↑	–	↓	X59737	Ubiquitous mitochondrial creatine kinase
10		–	↑	↓	–	NM_053290	Phosphoglycerate mutase 1
							Calcium regulation/signaling
11	X	–	↑	↓	–	NM_053311	ATPase, calcium transporting plasma membrane
12		LT	↑	–	↑	NM_017290	ATPase, calcium transporting sarcoplasmic reticulum
13		LT	↑	–	↑	NM_012920	Calcium/calmodulin-dependent protein kinase 2 alpha
14		–	↑	↑	↑	NM_021584	Calcium/calmodulin-dependent kinase-related peptide
15		–	–	↓	↑	NM_024366	Neuronal calcium sensor
16		–	↑	–	–	AF203698	T-calcium channel subunit
17		LT	↓	–	↑	NM_013049	TNF receptor superfamily, member 4
							Cytoskeleton
18		–	–	↓	–	X03369	Beta-tubulin
19		–	–	↓	–	NM_022298	Alpha-tubulin
20		–	↓	↓	–	M84156	Big tau tau
21		LT	–	↓	↓	NM_017024	Microtubule-associated protein 6
22	X	LT	–	↑	↑	U52950	Microtubule-associated protein 1b
23		LT	–	–	↓	NM_017029	Neurofilament protein
							Transporters
24		–	↓	↓	–	M22063	Glucose transporter
25		–	–	↑	↑	NM_030834	Putative monocarboxylate transporter
26	X	LT	↑	↓	↓	NM_053441	Blood-brain specific anion transporter
27	X	LT	↑	–	↑	NM_053859	Sodium-dependent inorganic phosphate cotransporter
28		–	–	↓	–	NM_053502	ABC-transporter (ATP-binding cassette)

TABLE 2. (*continued*) List of significant genes

No.	rtR	Trend	0.5 h	2 h	4 h	GenBank	Gene description
							Neurotransmitter metabolism and regulation
29		–	–	↑	–	D50671	GABA receptor rho-3 subunit precursor
30		–	–	↑	–	NM_017263	Glutamate receptor, ionotropic
31		–	↑	↑	↑	NM_01377	Glutamate oxaloacetate transaminase 2
32		–	↑	–	↑	NM_019225	Glutamate transporter
33		–	↑	–	↑	NM_017007	Glutamate decarboxylase
							Glia-specific proteins
34		–	↑	–	↑	AJ243949	Astrocytic protein PEA-15
35		–	–	↓	–	NM_031032	Glia maturation factor
							Oxidative stress
36		LT	–	↓	↑	NM_012806	Stress-activated protein kinase beta
37		–	↓	–	↓	U41853	150-kDa oxygen-regulated protein
38		LT	↓	↓	–	AJ249546	Endothelial nitric oxide synthase 3
							DNA synthesis/degradation
39		LT	–	↑	↑	D64059	Helicase 2
40		LT	–	–	↓	NM_024134	DNA-damage-induced transcript 3
							Translation
41		LT	–	–	↑	NM_019356	Eukaryotic translation initiation factor 2
							Miscellaneous
42		–	↑	↑	↑	NM_022395	Mitochondrial processing peptidase beta subunit
43		–	–	↓	–	NM_031062	Mevalonate pyrophosphate decarboxylase
44		LT	↓	–	–	NM_030861	*N*-Acetylglucosaminyltransferase
45	X	–	↑	↑	↑	NM_017122	Neuron-specific calcium binding protein p23k

NOTE: LT marks statistically significant linear trend. The up and down arrows correspond to an increase and decrease of mRNA levels, respectively. The "–" marks an absence of statistically significant changes. rtR: real-time RT-PCR.

RESULTS

TABLE 2 summarizes the results of the microarray analyses. The presence of statistically significant linear trends (LT) was detected in 19 genes. The genes numbered from 1 to 44 in TABLE 2 showed a significant effect of treatment at least in one of three time points: 30 min, 2 h, and 4 h. The change in gene no. 45 was found to be statistically significant using nonparametric ANOVA analysis (unpublished data). The genes in TABLE 2 are organized into several functional groups representing energy metabolism, calcium homeostasis, cytoskeleton, transporters, neurotransmitter

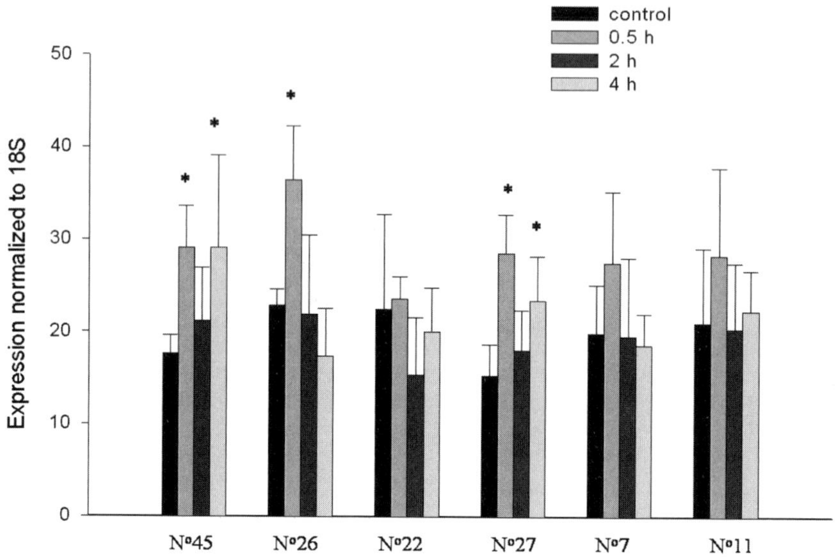

FIGURE 3. Real-time RT-PCR of 6 genes from TABLE 2. The transcripts represent the following genes: neuron-specific calcium binding protein p23k (no. 45), blood-brain specific anion transporter *Slco1c1* (no. 26), microtubule-associated protein 1b (no. 22), sodium-dependent inorganic phosphate cotransporter *Slc17a7* (no. 27), cytosolic NADP-dependent isocitrate dehydrogenase (no. 7), and calcium transporting plasma membrane ATP-ase (no. 11).

metabolism and regulation, glial specific proteins, oxidative stress, DNA synthesis/degradation, translation, and miscellaneous. The transporters may have roles in all listed functional groups. They are listed in TABLE 2 as a separate group to emphasize that regulation of small molecule trafficking may be an important factor in early cellular responses to declines in energy metabolism.

The transcript changes varied from about 100% below to 100% above the level of those observed in untreated animals (data not shown). The 0.5-h change in transcript of gene no. 26 as well as the 0.5-h and 4-h transcript changes for gene no. 27 were confirmed using the real-time RT-PCR analysis (FIG. 3). This initial real-time RT-PCR analysis was performed for 6 genes from TABLE 2, including gene no. 45. The genes listed as no. 26 and no. 27 encode the blood-brain barrier (BBB) specific anion transporter (*Slco1c1*) and sodium-dependent inorganic phosphate cotransporter (*Slc17a7*), respectively.

DISCUSSION

In this study, the effect of 3-NPA on the mRNA levels of 530 genes in the rat hippocampus was measured. Forty-four statistically significant transcript changes were found using an ANOVA mixed model and FDR criteria. The genes identified using this microarray analysis highlight processes that are known to be associated with excitotoxicity[21] and hippocampal damage.[22] Changes were found in transcripts related to glutamate processing and transport. Glutamate transport, in turn, relies on energy provided by mitochondria. The cytoskeleton (e.g., microtubules) is also recognized as a sensor of calcium changes. Changes in calcium homeostasis trigger toxic intracellular events by affecting protein kinase C, calcium/calmodulin-dependent protein kinase II, phospholipases, proteases, phosphatases, nitric oxide synthases, endonucleases, and others.[23] The stimulation of these enzymes can result in damage to cellular membranes, the cytoskeleton, and the DNA. Our microarray results indicate that changes in the level of calcium/calmodulin-dependent protein kinase II and nitric oxide synthase can be detected in the hippocampus within 4 h after exposure to 3-NPA.

The changes in mRNA levels noted at early time points are more likely to result from changes in an existing mRNA turnover rather than from new transcription. Initiation of new transcription is energy-costly and time-consuming. Cells might first alter usage of existing proteins (posttranslational modification) or existing transcripts (alternative splicing).[24] Such factors should be considered in interpretation of mRNA changes obtained using microarray techniques. The ANOVA and FDR analyses are very powerful approaches in microarray analyses.[25] They allow for the identification of more candidate genes than other methods. On the other hand, the flexibility and less-stringent selection criteria used by this approach can introduce false-positive and false-negative results. Thus, the validation of results with other methods of measurement of mRNA levels such as real-time RT-PCR and/or *in situ* hybridization is vital for verification of the outcome of analysis. An example of a false negative is gene no. 45 (TABLE 2). This gene was found using another analysis (nonparametric ANOVA, unpublished data) to be significantly altered, and this was validated by real-time RT-PCR. (Examples of false positives have not been confirmed yet by the real-time RT-PCR.) Additional real-time analysis of genes from TABLE 2 will allow us to define other genetic markers of early responses to a decline in cellular energy production. The microarray results presented in this report identified 2 transporters as potential mediators of 3-NPA-evoked neurotoxicity. The *Slco1c1* gene encodes organic anion polypeptide localized in brain endothelial capillary cells, which is involved in the elimination of harmful substances from the brain.[26,27] Under metabolic stress, the brain would increase efflux of toxic waste into the capillary. Our finding suggests, for the first time, a protective role for a BBB transporter during energy decline–induced neurotoxicity. Previous research has shown that leakage of the BBB can contribute to 3-NPA-evoked neurotoxicity.[28–30] Further functional study of *Slco1c1* may clarify the neuroprotective role of this BBB transporter. Another identified transporter, encoded by *Slc17a7*, is a sodium-dependent inorganic phosphate cotransporter.[31] This transporter regulates the intraneural concentration of inorganic phosphate, which is important for both synthesis of ATP and maintaining the phosphorylation potential of the cell. It is only expressed in certain populations of neurons. This cotransporter has been recently identified as a vesicular glutamate transporter, critical for Ca^{2+}-dependent release of glutamate from astrocytes.[31] Under metabolic stress, astrocyte-neuron communication may be critical for neuroprotective responses.

In summary, the microarray data presented in this report provide evidence that transporters in the BBB and astrocytes may play roles in neuroprotection against energy depletion in the brain.

REFERENCES

1. Hamilton, B.F. & D.H. Gould. 1987. Nature and distribution of brain lesions in rats intoxicated with 3-nitropropionic acid: a type of hypoxic (energy deficient) brain damage. Acta Neuropathol. **72:** 286–297.
2. Binienda, Z. *et al.* 1995. The effects of perinatal hypoxia on the behavioral, neurochemical, and neurohistological toxicity of the metabolic inhibitor 3-nitropropionic acid. Metab. Brain Dis. **10:** 269–282.
3. Noer, H. *et al.* 2002. 3-Nitropropionic acid neurotoxicity in hippocampal slice cultures: developmental and regional vulnerability and dependency on glucose. Exp. Neurol. **176:** 237–246.
4. Alston, T.A., L. Mela & H.J. Bright. 1977. 3-Nitropropionate, the toxic substance of *Indigofera*, is a suicide inactivator of succinate dehydrogenase. Proc. Natl. Acad. Sci. USA **74:** 3767–3771.
5. Novelli, A. *et al.* 1988. Glutamate becomes neurotoxic via the *N*-methyl-D-aspartate receptor when intracellular energy levels are reduced. Brain Res. **451:** 205–212.
6. Atlante, A. *et al.* 1996. Rapid uncoupling of oxidative phosphorylation accompanied glutamate toxicity in rat cerebellar granule cells. Neuroreport **7:** 2519–2523.
7. Ikonomidou, C. & L. Turski. 1996. Neurodegenerative disorders: clues from glutamate and energy metabolism. Crit. Rev. Neurobiol. **10:** 239–263.
8. Gould, E. & C.G. Gross. 2002. Neurogenesis in adult mammals: some progress and problems. J. Neurosci. **22:** 619–623.
9. Bruel-Jungerman, E., S. Laroche & C. Rampon. 2005. New neurons in the dentate gyrus are involved in the expression of enhanced long-term memory following environmental enrichment. Eur. J. Neurosci. **21:** 513–521.
10. Snyder, J. *et al.* 2005. A role for adult neurogenesis in spatial long-term memory. Neuroscience **130:** 843–852.
11. Lu, T. *et al.* 2004. Gene regulation and DNA damage in the ageing human brain. Nature **429:** 883–891.
12. Li, Y. *et al.* 2004. Behavioral and neurochemical effects of the intrahippocampal co-injection of beta-amyloid protein 1–40 and ibotenic acid in rats. Int. J. Neurosci. **114:** 1521–1531.
13. Kerr, K.M., M. Martin & G.A. Churchill. 2000. Analysis of variance for gene expression microarray data. J. Computat. Biol. **7:** 819–837.
14. Wolfinger, R.D. *et al.* 2001. Assessing gene significance from cDNA microarray expression data via mixed models. J. Computat. Biol. **8:** 625–637.
15. Yang, Y. *et al.* 2003. Statistical methods for analyzing microarray feature data with replications. J. Computat. Biol. **10:** 157–169.
16. Binienda, Z. *et al.* 1998. Effect of acute exposure to 3-nitropropionic acid on activities of endogenous antioxidants in the rat brain. Neurosci. Lett. **251:** 173–176.
17. Yang, Y.H. & T. Speed. 2002. Design issues for cDNA microarray experiments. Nat. Rev. Genet. **3:** 579–588.
18. Dobbin, K., J. Shih & R. Simon. 2003. Statistical design of reverse dye microarrays. Bioinformatics **19:** 803–810.
19. Hollander, M. & D. Wolfe. 1999. Nonparametric Statistical Methods. Wiley. New York.
20. Benjamini, Y. & Y. Hochberg. 1995. Controlling the false discovery rate: a practical and powerful approach to multiple testing. J. R. Stat. Soc. **B57:** 289–300.
21. Nicholls, D.G. & S.L. Budd. 1998. Mitochondria and neuronal glutamate excitotoxicity. Biochim. Biophys. Acta **1366:** 97–112.
22. Geddes, J.W., Z. Pang & D.H. Wiley. 1996. Hippocampal damage and cytoskeletal disruption resulting from impaired energy metabolism: implications for Alzheimer disease. Mol. Chem. Neuropathol. **28:** 65–74.
23. Sola, C. *et al.* 1999. The Ca^{2+}/calmodulin signaling system in the neural response to excitability: involvement of neuronal and glial cells. Prog. Neurobiol. **58:** 207–232.
24. Munch, C. *et al.* 2003. Differential regulation of 5′ splice variants of the glutamate transporter EAAT2 in an *in vitro* model of chemical hypoxia induced by 3-nitropropionic acid. J. Neurosci. Res. **71:** 819–825.

25. CUI, X. & G.A. CHURCHILL. 2003. Statistical tests for differential expression in cDNA microarray experiments. Genome Biol. **4:** 210.
26. LI, J., R. BOADO & W. PARDRIDGE. 2001. Blood-brain barrier genomics. J. Cereb. Flow Metab. **21:** 61–68.
27. SUGIYAMA, D. *et al.* 2003. Functional characterization of rat brain-specific organic anion transporter (Oatp14) at the blood-brain barrier. J. Biol. Chem. **278:** 43489–43495.
28. KIM, G.W. *et al.* 2003. Neurogeneration in striatum induced by the mitochondrial toxin 3-nitropropionic acid: role of matrix metalloproteinase-9 in early blood-brain barrier disruption? J. Neurosci. **24:** 8733–8742.
29. NISHINO, H. *et al.* 1995. Hypothalamic neurons are resistant to the intoxication with 3-nitropropionic acid that induces lesions in the striatum and hippocampus via the damage in the blood-brain barrier. Neurobiology **3:** 257–267.
30. NISHINO, H. *et al.* 2000. The striatum is the most vulnerable region in the brain to mitochondrial energy compromise: a hypothesis to explain its specific vulnerability. J. Neurotrauma **17:** 251–260.
31. MONTANA, V. *et al.* 2004. Vesicular glutamate transporter–dependent glutamate release from astrocytes. J. Neurosci. **24:** 2633–2642.

L-Carnitine and Neuroprotection in the Animal Model of Mitochondrial Dysfunction

ZBIGNIEW BINIENDA,[a] BEATA PRZYBYLA-ZAWISLAK,[a] ASHRAF VIRMANI,[b] AND LARRY SCHMUED[a]

[a]*Division of Neurotoxicology, National Center for Toxicological Research, Food and Drug Administration, Jefferson, Arkansas 72079, USA*

[b]*Research and Development, Sigma-Tau Health Science, Pomezia 00040, Italy*

ABSTRACT: We have shown previously that pretreatment with L-carnitine (LC) prior to 3-nitropropionic acid (3-NPA) exposure, while not significantly attenuating succinate dehydrogenase (SDH) inhibition, prevented hypothermia and oxidative stress. The plant and fungal toxin, 3-NPA, acts as an inhibitor of mitochondrial function via irreversible inactivation of the mitochondrial inner membrane enzyme, SDH. Inhibition of SDH disturbs electron transport, leading to cellular energy deficits and oxidative stress–related neuronal injury. In the study presented here, a neurohistological method was applied to examine the mitochondriotropic effect of LC pretreatment against 3-NPA-induced neurotoxicity. Twenty adult male Sprague-Dawley rats randomly divided into two groups (n = 10/group) were injected twice with 3-NPA at 30 mg/kg sc, at 2 days apart, or received LC pretreatment at 100 mg/kg, at 30–40 min before 3-NPA administration. Rats in both groups were perfused 7 days later and their brains harvested. Degenerating neurons were identified and localized via the fluorescent marker Fluoro-Jade B. Data analysis showed that LC was protective against 3-NPA-induced toxicity, as reflected by both reduced mortality and significantly reduced neuronal degeneration.

KEYWORDS: 3-nitropropionic acid; carnitine; mitochondria; striatum; neuroprotection

MITOCHONDRIAL DYSFUNCTION

In normoxic conditions, the mitochondrial oxidative phosphorylation system is responsible for the maximum cellular output of energy in the form of adenosine triphosphate (ATP). The ATP is generated by formation of pyruvate in the last reaction of glycolysis catalyzed by pyruvate kinase, but far more energy is generated by oxidation of NADH and $FADH_2$ supplied by the tricarboxylic acid cycle (TCA) and β-oxidation of fatty acids. This pathway is initiated by conversion of acetyl coenzyme A (acetyl- CoA) from pyruvate by oxidation via the pyruvate dehydrogenase complex in the mitochondrial matrix. The energy released by a transfer of electrons to O_2 through the electron transport chain complexes I–IV is used by ATP synthase

Address for correspondence: Dr. Zbigniew K. Binienda, Division of Neurotoxicology, HFT-132, FDA/NCTR, Jefferson, AR 72079-9502. Voice: 870-543-7920; fax: 870-543-7745. zbinienda@nctr.fda.gov

Ann. N.Y. Acad. Sci. 1053: 174–182 (2005). © 2005 New York Academy of Sciences. doi: 10.1196/annals.1344.015

(complex V) to condense ADP and orthophosphate (Pi) into ATP. The disruption of mitochondrial ATP production is particularly harmful to organs of high metabolic rate such as brain, heart, and kidneys, as well as skeletal muscles and the endocrine system.[1] Chronic mitochondrial energy deficit in the brain is postulated to underlie aging and neurodegenerative disorders such as Kearns-Sayre myopathy, Parkinson's disease, Alzheimer's disease, and Huntington's chorea.[2,3]

Metabolic stress leads to direct or indirect excitotoxicity via either an increase of glutamate or loss of the voltage-gated Mg^{2+} block of the NMDA receptor channel that lowers threshold to unaltered levels of glutamate.[4] Additionally, mitochondrial dysfunction and decreased ATP production result in increased formation of reactive oxygen species (ROS), toxic by-products of mitochondrial energy metabolism. The ROS level is controlled by free radical scavenging enzymes such as mitochondrial manganese superoxide dismutase (Mn-SOD), catalase, or glutathione peroxidase. Overproduction of ROS alters the level of antioxidant enzymes, followed by activation of mitochondrial permeability transition pores (mtPTP), leakage of macromolecules, increase influx of Ca^{2+}, and consequently initiation of apoptosis–programmed cell death.

ANIMAL MODEL OF MITOCHONDRIAL DYSFUNCTION

Mitochondrial energy disruption is a frequently observed effect of neurotoxicants, including inhibitors of the mitochondrial electron transport chain such as MPTP (as MPP^+; complex I), 3-nitropropionic acid (3-NPA; complex II), antimycin A (complex III), and cyanide (complex IV). In our research, we focused on 3-NPA, a model inhibitor of succinate dehydrogenase (SDH), a component of mitochondrial complex II.[5] Although the 3-NPA toxicity leads to potential neurogeneration in multiple brain regions,[6,7] selective striatal lesions can be induced by adjusting the dosage and time course of systemic 3-NPA injections.[8,9] In fact, 3-NPA neurotoxicity has been studied by many investigators in an attempt to find the most suitable animal model for Huntington's disease in which severe neuronal degeneration in the striatum is observed.[10] The goal of our study was to define physiological and biochemical endpoints of compromised mitochondrial function *in vivo* and to establish an animal model that would allow detection of toxicants that target the respiratory chain.

Adult, male Sprague-Dawley rats from the FDA/NCTR breeding colony were used in this research effort. Animals were kept under controlled environmental conditions (temperature 22°C, relative humidity 45–55%, 12-h light/dark cycle) and housed individually with food and water supplied *ad libitum*. Animal care and use procedures followed along the guidelines of the Association for Assessment and Accreditation of Laboratory Animal Care International (AAALAC) and were approved by the Institutional Animal Care and Use Committee (IACUC).

Several endpoints associated with 3-NPA-evoked mitochondrial inhibition have been identified. They include increased free fatty acids (FFA) in all brain regions,[11] an alteration of endogenous antioxidants,[12] a decrease in body temperature correlated with a decreased brain temperature,[13,14] and a decline in the electrocerebral activity monitored via electroencephalography recording.[15]

Neuroprotective Effects of L-Carnitine

L-Carnitine (LC) (4-*N*-trimethylammonium-3-hydroxybutyric acid) and its acetylated form, acetyl-L-carnitine (ALC), play an important role in metabolism of long-chain FFA, facilitating transport of the FFA across the mitochondrial membrane for β-oxidation. Carnitine controls the acetyl-CoA/CoA ratio, stimulating the activity of the pyruvate dehydrogenase complex and the supply of NADH for the respiratory electron transport chain. Thus, carnitine actions affect not only FFA, but also glucose metabolism.[16] Transfer of acyl moieties from mitochondria into the cytoplasm provides a substrate for acetylcholine production as well.

Neuroprotective effects of carnitine were shown in several studies.[16,17] Administration of LC promotes formation of ALC and the reacylation of phospholipids important in cellular membrane repair.[18] Neuroprotective effects of LC are obtained through its action against oxidative stress and lipid peroxidation.[19] LC attenuated 3-NPA-induced rat cortical cell damage *in vitro*.[20] In our animal model, pretreatment with LC prevented the increase in endogenous free radical scavenging enzymes, including catalase and superoxide dismutase, observed when 3-NPA was administered alone.[21]

Temperature

While rats treated with 3-NPA experienced a progressive hypothermia within 3 h after injection,[13] a normoxia after 3-NPA injection was maintained when LC was injected 30 min before 3-NPA.[14] The normoxic effects of LC were not linked with a direct LC interaction with 3-NPA because the SDH remained significantly inhibited by 3-NPA in the presence of LC.[22]

Electroencephalography (EEG)

Studies have shown that energy failure after intrastriatal 3-NPA exposure led to a significant loss of DA, but not GABA neurons.[23] Whether this effect may contribute to a depression of motor activity and somnolence in the initial stage of 3-NPA-induced neurotoxicity is unknown. However, interference with GABAergic neurotransmission may increase excitability and lower the threshold for inducing seizures observed at later stages of exposure to 3-NPA.

The effect of 3-NPA alone vs. 3-NPA with LC pretreatment on the electrocerebral activity was assessed in our animal model using the EEG (FIG. 1). The ECoG was recorded via bipolar, epidural electrodes implanted at the level of the somatosensory cortex. Following baseline recording (vehicle injection), rats were administered 3-NPA sc at 30 mg/kg or pretreated with LC administered 30 min prior to 3-NPA ip at 100 mg/kg. The power spectra obtained by use of fast Fourier transformations were divided into 1.25–4.50 Hz (delta), 4.75–6.75 Hz (theta), 7.00–9.50 Hz (alpha-1), 9.75–12.50 Hz (alpha-2), 12.75–18.50 Hz (beta-1), and 18.75–35.00 Hz (beta-2). Treatment with 3-NPA was associated with a trend toward a power decrease in the EEG frequency band (FIGS. 2 and 3). Power was elevated in all frequency bands in rats pretreated with LC prior to 3-NPA. Data indicated the dominance of inhibitory neurotransmission during acute 3-NPA exposure and the stimulatory effects of LC administration toward electrical activity of the brain despite the 3-NPA treatment.

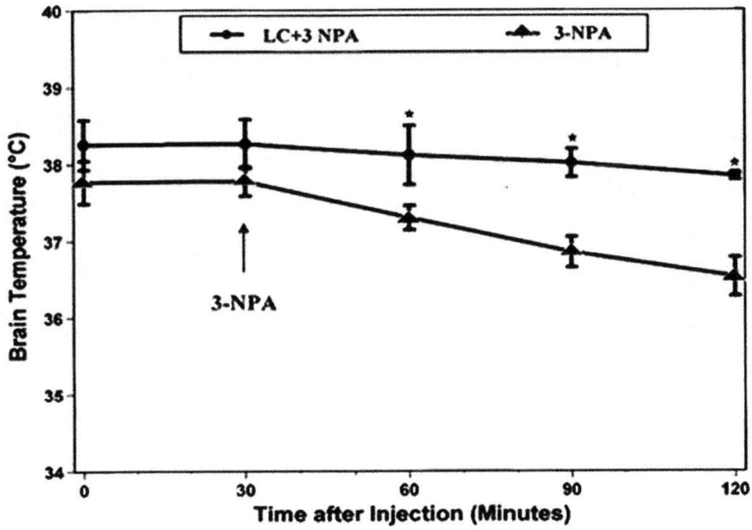

FIGURE 1. The effects of 3-nitropropionic acid administration (3-NPA) at 30 mg/kg sc and after pretreatment with L-carnitine (LC + 3-NPA) at 100 mg/kg ip on the intracranial temperature within the first 2 h of exposure. Vehicle (0.1 M phosphate buffer) or LC were injected at time zero. ↑: 3-NPA injected at time 30 min. Mean ± SEM.

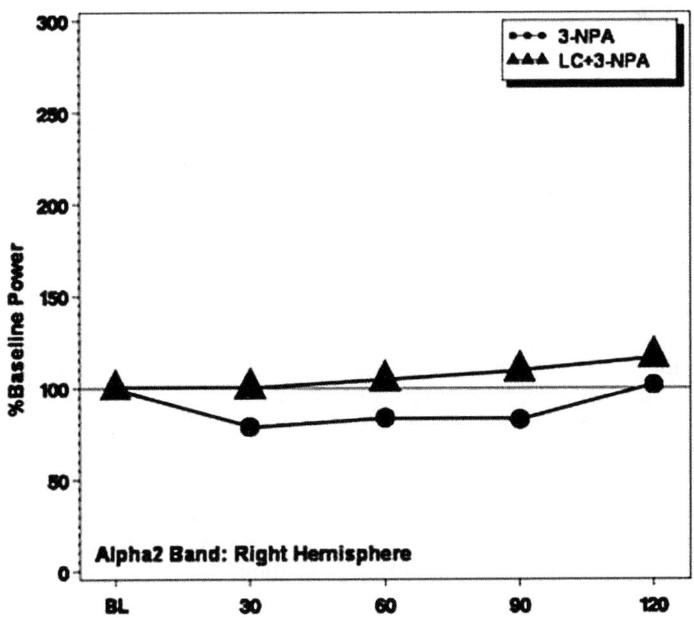

FIGURE 2. Delineation of time-course effects produced by 3-NPA administration at 30 mg/kg sc on α_2 power spectrum (9.75–12.50 Hz). Power values calculated as percent of the 30-min baseline power (assigned a value of 100%). BL: baseline.

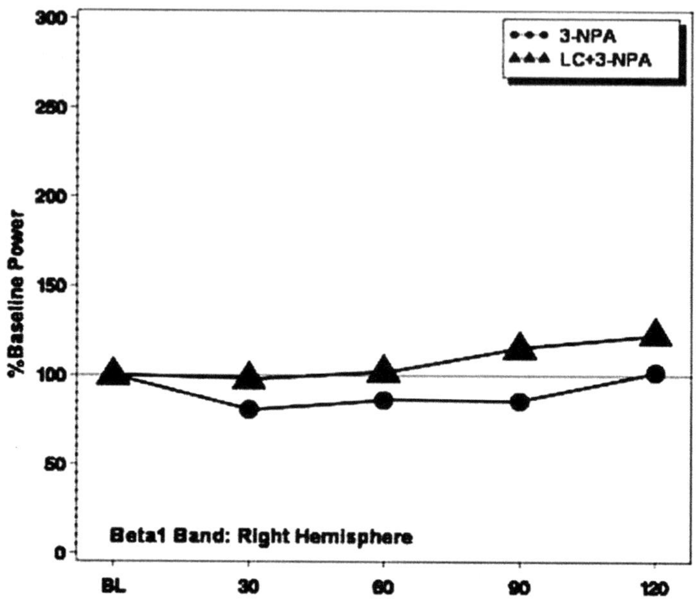

FIGURE 3. Delineation of time-course (up to 120 min) effects produced by 3-NPA administration at 30 mg/kg sc on β_1 power spectrum (12.75–18.50 Hz). Power values calculated as percent of the 30-min baseline power (assigned a value of 100%). BL: baseline.

Neurohistology

The protection of LC against the 3-NPA-induced toxicity observed in previous experiments required confirmation in evaluating overt brain damage using a histochemical method. Rats were randomly divided into two 3-NPA and LC/3-NPA groups (n = 10/group). Animals in the 3-NPA group received two subcutaneous (sc) injections, over a 2-day interval, of a vehicle (0.1 M phosphate buffer, pH 7.4) and 3-NPA in a phosphate buffer solution at 30 mg/kg. Rats in the LC/3-NPA group were injected intraperitoneally (ip) with LC solution at 100 mg/kg, and 30–40 min later with a solution of 3-NPA at 30 mg/kg sc. Seven days after the first injection of 3-NPA, animals were anesthetized with an ip injection of 20% chloral hydrate and perfused with 300 mL of 0.1 M neutral phosphate-buffered 10% formalin via the ascending aorta. The brains were postfixed for the next 2–4 days in the same fixative solution plus 20% sucrose. Brain tissue was cut on a freezing sliding microtome at a thickness of 25 μm, and sections were collected in 0.1 M phosphate buffer. The sections were then mounted on 1% gelatin-coated slides and air-dried. The slides were stained with Fluoro-Jade B (Histo-Chem Inc., Jefferson, AR), an anionic fluorescein derivative useful for detecting neuronal degeneration.[24] The tissue was then examined using an epifluorescent microscope with blue (450–490 nm) excitation light. We found that LC pretreatment was associated with diminished mortality and a significant decrease in neuronal degeneration observed following the 3-NPA treatment (see FIGS. 4 and 5).

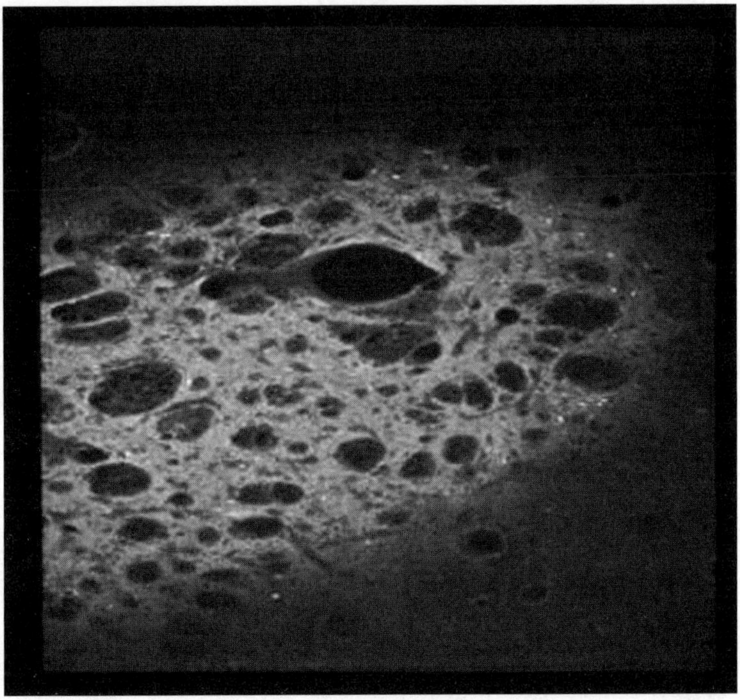

FIGURE 4. Extensive Fluoro-Jade B labeling of degenerating neuronal cells in the rat striatum after 3-NPA administration (30 mg/kg sc, twice over a 2-day interval). Magnification: ×100.

In the 3 animals that survived 3-NPA dosing, 1 exhibited no pathology, 1 exhibited moderate unilateral damage to the striatum, and 1 exhibited extensive bilateral neuronal degeneration in multiple forebrain regions. In the 7 surviving animals that received LC prior to 3-NPA insult, 6 exhibited no lesions, while 1 exhibited a modest unilateral lesion in the striatum. When death or brain damage, regardless of the extent, was considered as "a negative" outcome and no changes as "a positive", the compared difference between outcomes analyzed with Barnard's unconditional test reached a statistical significance at the $P < 0.05$ level ($P = 0.027$).

DISCUSSION AND CONCLUSIONS

Data gathered in our studies indicate neuroprotection achieved by LC pretreatment against 3-NPA-induced neurotoxicity *in vivo*. The carnitine-driven metabolic enhancement and possible increase in cerebral blood flow both may underlie the increasing electrical brain activity observed in our study. Alterations in ECoG may be related to alterations in metabolic activity in the frontal cortex. It was shown that regional cerebral blood flow increased in acute exposure to ALC in human studies.[25]

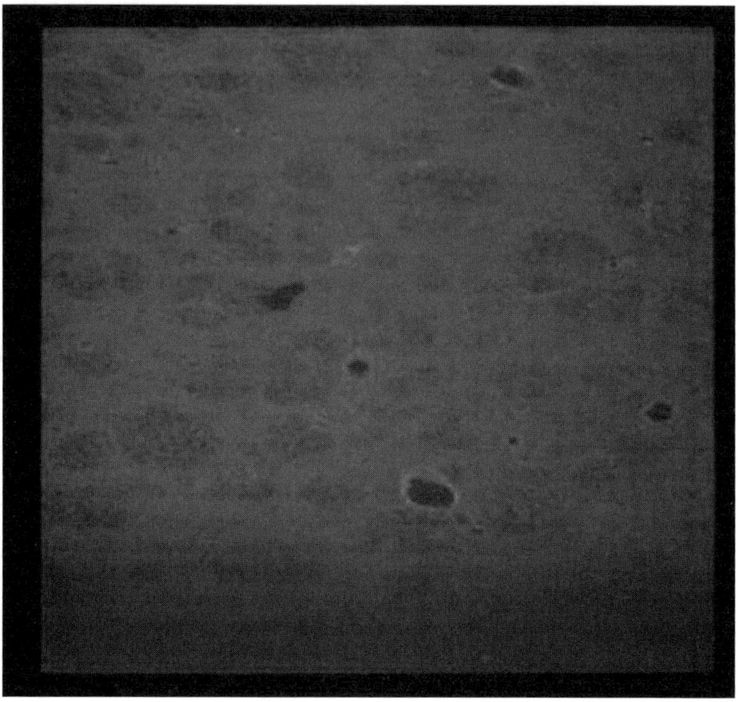

FIGURE 5. Lack of neuronal degeneration in the rat striatum. LC administered ip at 100 mg/kg prior to each 3-NPA injection at 30 mg/kg sc, twice over a 2-day interval. Magnification: ×100.

The inhibition of mitochondrial function and biochemical alterations detrimental to cell energy metabolism following exposure to the 3-NPA are comparable to those seen in hypoxia/ischemia. The accumulation of FFA observed in both conditions leads to accumulation of long-chain acyl-CoA and affects the activity of the cell transport system and permeability.[26] The inhibition of SDH by 3-NPA triggers both the fast pathway of cell death, that is, necrosis through activation of glutamate NMDA receptors, and programmed cell death, that is, apoptosis.[27] The role of LC in attenuating mitochondrial membrane permeability transition pore (MPT) opening and the suppression of apoptosis, as well as its actions toward the oxidation of carbohydrates, may greatly contribute to the neuroprotective effects of LC.

Mitochondria control apoptosis via release of cytochrome c into the cytosol through the MPT and activation of the caspase cascade activity. Long-chain acyl-CoA (LCACoA) has been shown to be a promoter of MPT opening.[28] LC administration leads to a shift from LCACoA to long-chain acyl-carnitine, preventing induction of MPT and apoptosis.[29]

Stimulation of the pyruvate dehydrogenase complex and a direct enhancement of oxidative phosphorylation may underlie LC's protective actions against 3-NPA-evoked energy decline, membrane depolarization, excitatory activation of NMDA receptors, and cell necrosis. It appears that the neuroprotection observed in our studies comes from the mitochondriotropic effects of LC related to energy metabolism combined with its antiapoptotic and membrane-stabilizing actions.

REFERENCES

1. WALLACE, D.C. 1999. Mitochondrial diseases in man and mouse. Science **283:** 1482–1488.
2. LINNANE, A.W., S. MARZUKI, T. OZAWA *et al.* 1989. Mitochondrial DNA mutations as an important contributor to ageing and degenerative diseases. Lancet **1:** 642–645.
3. BEAL, M.F. 2003. Mitochondria, oxidative damage, and inflammation in Parkinson's disease. Ann. N.Y. Acad. Sci. **991:** 120–131.
4. ZEEVALK, G.D., E. DERR-YELLIN & W.J. NICKLAS. 1995. Relative vulnerability of dopamine and GABA neurons in mesencephalic culture to inhibition of succinate dehydrogenase by malonate and 3-nitropropionic acid and protection by NMDA receptor blockade. J. Pharmacol. Exp. Ther. **275:** 1124–1130.
5. ALSTON, T.A., L. MELA & H.J. BRIGHT. 1977. 3-Nitropropionate, the toxic substance of *Indigofera*, is a suicide inactivator of succinate dehydrogenase. Proc. Natl. Acad. Sci. USA **74:** 3767–3771.
6. HAMILTON, B.F. & D.H. GOULD. 1987. Nature and distribution of brain lesions in rats intoxicated with 3-nitropropionic acid: a type of hypoxic (energy deficient) brain damage. Acta Neuropathol. **72:** 286–297.
7. BINIENDA, Z., D.L. FREDERICK, S.A. FERGUSON *et al.* 1995. The effects of perinatal hypoxia on the behavioral, neurochemical, and neurohistological toxicity of the metabolic inhibitor 3-nitropropionic acid. Metab. Brain Dis. **10:** 269–282.
8. LUDOLPH, A., M. SEELING, A. LUDOLPH *et al.* 1992. 3-Nitropropionic acid—exogenous animal neurotoxin and possible human striatal toxin. Can. J. Neurol. Sci. **18:** 492–498.
9. BORLONGAN, C.V., T.K. KOUTOUZIS, T.B. FREEMAN *et al.* 1996. Behavioral pathology induced by repeated systemic injections of 3-nitropropionic acid mimics the motoric symptoms of Huntington's disease. Brain Res. **697:** 254–257.
10. BORLONGAN, C., T. SHIMIZU & P.R. SANBERG. 2000. Comparative study on 3-nitropropionic acid neurotoxicity. *In* Mitochondrial and Neurodegenerative Disorders, pp. 93–106. Humana Press. Totowa, NJ.
11. BINIENDA, Z. & C.S. KIM. 1997. Increase in levels of total free fatty acids in rat brain regions following 3-nitropropionic acid administration. Neurosci. Lett. **230:** 199–201.
12. BINIENDA, Z., C. SIMMONS, S. HUSSAIN *et al.* 1998. Effect of acute exposure to 3-nitropropionic acid on activities of endogenous antioxidants in the rat brain. Neurosci. Lett. **251:** 173–176.
13. NONY, P.A., A.C. SCALLET, R.L. ROUNTREE *et al.* 1999. 3-Nitropropionic acid (3-NPA) produces hypothermia and inhibits histochemical labelling of succinate dehydrogenase (SDH) in rat brain. Metab. Brain Dis. **14:** 83–94.
14. BINIENDA, Z. 2003. Neuroprotective effects of L-carnitine in induced mitochondrial dysfunction. Ann. N.Y. Acad. Sci. **993:** 289–295.
15. BINIENDA, Z., B. PRZYBYLA-ZAWISLAK, J. SUMMAGE *et al.* 2003. Soc. Neurosci. Abstr. no. 539.9.
16. DI LISA, F. 2002. Biochemical and pharmacological relevance of carnitine. Riv. Ital. Nutr. Parent. Enter. **20:** 1–10.
17. VIRMANI, A. & Z. BINIENDA. 2004. Role of carnitine esters in brain neuropathology. Mol. Asp. Med. **25:** 533–549.
18. ARDUINI, A., N. DENISOVA, M.A. VIRMANI *et al.* 1994. Evidence for the involvement of carnitine-dependent long-chain acyltransferases in neuronal triacylglycerol and phospholipid fatty acid turnover. J. Neurochem. **62:** 1530–1538.
19. KUMARAN, S., B. DEEPAK, B. NAVEEN *et al.* 2003. Effects of levocarnitine on mitochondrial antioxidant systems and oxidative stress in aged rats. Drugs RD **4:** 141–147.
20. VIRMANI, A., R. BISELLI, A. SPADONI *et al.* 1995. Protective actions of L-carnitine and acetyl-L-carnitine on the neurotoxicity evoked by mitochondrial uncoupling or inhibitors. Pharmacol. Res. **32:** 383–389.

21. BINIENDA, Z., J.R. JOHNSON, A.A. TYLER-HASHEMI *et al.* 1999. Protective effect of L-carnitine in the neurotoxicity induced by the mitochondrial inhibitor 3-nitropropionic acid (3-NPA). Ann. N.Y. Acad. Sci. **890:** 173–178.
22. BINIENDA, Z. & S.F. ALI. 2001. Neuroprotective role of L-carnitine in the 3-nitropropionic acid induced neurotoxicity. Tox. Lett. **125:** 67–73.
23. BROUILLET, E., B.G. JENKINS, B.T. HYMAN *et al.* 1993. Age-dependent vulnerability of the striatum to the mitochondrial toxin 3-nitropropionic acid. J. Neurochem. **60:** 356–359.
24. SCHMUED, L.C. & K.J. HOPKINS. 2000. Fluoro-Jade B: a high affinity fluorescent marker for the localization of neuronal degeneration. Brain Res. **874:** 123–130.
25. ROSADINI, G., S. MARENCO, F. NOBILI *et al.* 1990. Acute effects of acetyl-L-carnitine on regional cerebral blood flow in patients with brain ischaemia. Int. J. Clin. Pharmacol. Res. **10:** 123–128.
26. BRECHER, P. 1983. The interaction of long chain acyl CoA with membranes. Mol. Cell Biochem. **139:** S115–S119.
27. PANG, Z. & J.W. GEDDES. 1997. Mechanisms of cell death induced by the mitochondrial toxin 3-nitropropionic acid: acute excitotoxic necrosis and delayed apoptosis. J. Neurosci. **17:** 3064–3073.
28. WIECKOWSKI, M.R., D. BRDICZKA & L. WOJTCZAK. 2000. Long-chain fatty acids promote opening of the reconstituted mitochondrial permeability transition pore. FEBS Lett. **484:** 61–64.
29. KASHIWAGI, A., T. KANNO, K. ARITA *et al.* 2001. Suppression of T_3- and fatty acid–induced membrane permeability transition by L-carnitine. Comp. Biochem. Physiol. **B130:** 411–418.

Effects of Metabolic Modifiers Such as Carnitines, Coenzyme Q10, and PUFAs against Different Forms of Neurotoxic Insults: Metabolic Inhibitors, MPTP, and Methamphetamine

ASHRAF VIRMANI,[a] FRANCO GAETANI,[a] AND ZBIGNIEW BINIENDA[b]

[a]*Research and Development, Sigma-Tau Health Science, Pomezia 00040, Italy*

[b]*Neurophysiology Laboratory, Division of Neurotoxicology, National Center for Toxicological Research, Food and Drug Administration, Jefferson, Arkansas 72079, USA*

ABSTRACT: A number of strategies using the nutritional approach are emerging for the protection of the brain from damage caused by metabolic toxins, age, or disease. Neural dysfunction and metabolic imbalances underlie many diseases, and the inclusion of metabolic modifiers may provide an alternative and early intervention approach that may prevent further damage. Various models have been developed to study the impact of metabolism on brain function. These have also proven useful in expanding our understanding of neurodegeneration processes. For example, the metabolic compromise induced by inhibitors such as 3-nitropropionic acid (3-NPA), rotenone, and 1-methyl-4-phenylpyridinium (MPP^+) can cause neurodegeneration in animal models and these models are thought to simulate the processes that may lead to diseases such as Huntington's and Parkinson's diseases. These inhibitors of metabolism are thought to selectively kill neurons by inhibiting various mitochondrial enzymes. However, the eventual cell death is attributed to oxidative stress damage of selectively vulnerable cells, especially highly differentiated neurons. Various studies indicate that the neurotoxicity resulting from these types of metabolic compromise is related to mitochondrial dysfunction and may be ameliorated by metabolic modifiers such as L-carnitine (L-C), creatine, and coenzyme Q10, as well as by antioxidants such as lipoic acid, vitamin E, and resveratrol. Mitochondrial function and cellular metabolism are also affected by the dietary intake of essential polyunsaturated fatty acids (PUFAs), which may regulate membrane composition and influence cellular processes, especially the inflammatory pathways. Cellular metabolic function may also be ameliorated by caloric restriction diets. L-C is a naturally occurring quaternary ammonium compound that is a vital cofactor for the mitochondrial entry and oxidation of fatty acids. Any factors affecting L-C levels may also affect ATP levels. This endogenous compound, L-C, together with its acetyl ester, acetyl-L-carnitine (ALC), also participates in the control of the mitochondrial acyl-CoA/CoA ratio, peroxisomal oxidation of fatty acids, and production of ketone bodies. A deficiency of

Address for correspondence: Dr. Ashraf Virmani, Sigma-Tau Health Science, Via Treviso 4, Pomezia 00040, Italy. Voice: +(39)-06-916-19721; fax: +(39)-06-916-12631.
ashraf.virmani@st-hs.it

Ann. N.Y. Acad. Sci. 1053: 183–191 (2005). © 2005 New York Academy of Sciences.
doi: 10.1196/annals.1344.016

carnitine is known to have major deleterious effects on the CNS. We have examined L-C and its acetylated derivative, ALC, as potential neuroprotective compounds using various known metabolic inhibitors, as well as against drugs of abuse such as methamphetamine.

Keywords: L-carnitine; acetyl-L-carnitine; mitochondria; methamphetamine; MPTP; 1-methyl-4-phenylpyridinium (MPP^+); Parkinson's disease; apoptosis; metabolic compromise; metabolic modifier; oxidative phosphorylation; respiratory chain; glycolysis; free radicals; reactive oxygen species (ROS); aging; rotenone; cyanide; 3-NPA; coenzyme Q10; creatine; PUFA; lipoic acid; brain developmental disorders

INTRODUCTION

There are a number of risk factors in brain developmental disorders, including nutritional deficiency (TABLE 1). The pathways by which nutritional deficiencies affect the brain are related mainly to metabolic compromise. It has become evident that the nutritional status determines cellular and mitochondrial function as well as possible susceptibility to cellular damage. It is the antioxidant status, the level of pro-/anti-inflammatory agents, as well as the metabolic cofactors and substrates that determine cellular health and its resistance to damaging insults. Various models have been developed to study the impact of this factor on brain function and have also proven useful in expanding our understanding of the neurodegenerative process.[1,2] For example, the metabolic compromise by inhibitors such as 3-nitropropionic acid (3-NPA), rotenone, and 1-methyl-4-phenylpyridinium (MPP^+), causes neurodegeneration *in vitro* as well as in animal models, and this is thought to simulate what may be occurring at the biochemical-level processes that may underlie diseases such as Huntington's and Parkinson's diseases.[3,4] These inhibitors of metabolism are thought to selectively damage or kill neurons by inhibiting various mitochondrial enzymes. However, the eventual cell death is attributed to the oxidative stress damage of selectively vulnerable cells, especially highly differentiated neurons. MPP^+ is known to inhibit energy metabolism, causing inhibition of the enzymatic activity of NADH-dehydrogenase of the mitochondrial complex.[5–7] Further, it may affect complexes I, III, and IV, and this effect was shown to be much greater in aged animals.[8] Indeed, recent studies suggested that MPP^+ toxicity, at least during its initial stages, was primarily due to the decrease in ATP synthesis by mitochondria and not to free radical formation.[9,10] However, it is also known that the mitochondrial superoxide

TABLE 1. Risk factors for brain developmental disorders

- Environmental toxins (PCB, dioxan, estrogens, 3-NPA, rotenone), alcohol, drugs
- Infectious disease (prions, viruses, bacteria)
- Nutritional deficiencies and intolerances
- Traumatic events (pregnancy complication, head injury)
- Genetic vulnerability
- Age (↓ anabolic hormone)
- Poverty

formation resulting from disturbed electron transfer within the respiratory chain can affect the activities of respiratory chain complexes I, II, III, IV, and V and underlie some CNS pathologies. Various studies indicate that the neurotoxicity resulting from these types of mitochondrial dysfunction may be ameliorated by metabolic modifiers such as L-carnitine (L-C), creatine, and coenzyme Q10.[2,11,12]

THE LETHAL TRIPLET

It is energy impairment, excitotoxicity, and oxidative stress that together form the triplet of cooperative pathways that trigger neurodegeneration, and may explain in part the regional selectivity of neurotoxicity by the various inhibitors.[13] Regional differences may also depend upon the differences in mitochondrial type, level of antioxidant defenses, and substrate preferences, as well as the differences in substrate transporters and their susceptibilities to inhibition. For example, the high-affinity uptake of L-C in placental choriocarcinoma (BeWo) cells was inhibited by amphetamines, and this may affect brain development.[14] Since the formation of ATP in the mitochondria depends on the entry of substrates, and L-C is a naturally occurring quaternary ammonium compound that is a vital cofactor for the mitochondrial entry and oxidation of fatty acids, any factors affecting L-C levels will affect ATP levels. This endogenous compound, L-C, together with its acetyl ester, acetyl-L-carnitine (ALC), also participates in the control of the mitochondrial acyl-CoA/CoA ratio, peroxisomal oxidation of fatty acids, and production of ketone bodies. A deficiency of carnitine is known to have major deleterious effects on the CNS. Several syndromes of secondary carnitine deficiency have been described that may result from defects in intermediary metabolism and alterations principally involved in mitochondrial oxidative pathways.[12,15] Primary carnitine deficiency leads to hepatic encephalopathy (Reye-like syndrome) and is often accompanied by hypoglycemia and hypoketonemia. Other symptoms may include failure to thrive, weakness, episodes of coma, seizures, and neuropathy. We have examined L-C and its acetylated derivative, ALC, as potential neuroprotective compounds using various known metabolic inhibitors, as well as against drugs of abuse such as methamphetamine.

PROTECTION AGAINST EFFECTS OF METABOLIC INHIBITORS BY L-CARNITINE

Previously, we demonstrated that neurotoxicity to a specific mitochondrial complex I inhibitor, rotenone, using *in vitro* primary cultured rat cortical neurons was, in part, attenuated by the coincubation of the cells with 1 mM L-C or ALC.[3] The cell death induced by rotenone is related to its inhibition of mitochondrial complex I in the respiratory chain, and rotenone has been shown to cause parkinsonism in animals.[16]

Similarly, the toxicity due to inhibition of succinate dehydrogenase (SDH) complex II by 3-NPA was attenuated by 5 mM ALC, and that due to cyanide (NaCN)–evoked inhibition of complex IV by 5 mM L-C. The toxicity of the mitochondrial uncoupler, *p*-(trifluoromethoxy)phenylhydrazone (FCCP), was also significantly reduced by 5 mM L-C or ALC.

3-NPA is used in animal models to create a progressive and localized striatal neurodegeneration mimicking many of the pathological features of Huntington's disease and other forms of metabolic compromise such as cerebral ischemia, carbon monoxide poisoning, and hypoglycemia.[17,18]

PROTECTION AGAINST EFFECTS OF MPTP BY L-CARNITINE

MPP^+ affects energy metabolism by inhibition of the enzymatic activity of NADH-dehydrogenase of mitochondrial complex I, and studies suggest that MPP^+ toxicity, at least during its initial stages, is primarily due to a decrease in ATP synthesis by mitochondria and not to free radical formation. We have results showing that ALC attenuated toxicity of MPP^+ in PC12 cells, as measured by the MTT response.[19] The effect of MPP^+ on dopamine content in the PC12 cells was not altered by the presence of 1 mM ALC. However, a significant increase in the XTT response indicative of neuroprotection was noted. Similar protection by ALC against MPP^+ has also been reported in other cell types, including murine brain neuroblastoma cells, as well as *in vivo* in rats and primates.[20–22]

PROTECTION AGAINST EFFECTS OF METHAMPHETAMINE (METH) BY L-CARNITINE

We have previously shown that the toxicity of METH was attenuated *in vivo* in rats by administration of L-C.[5] METH toxicity can also be reduced by antioxidants such as selenium, melatonin, and the selective nNOS inhibitor, 7-nitroindazole, suggesting a role of nitrosative stress. Part of the mechanism of METH toxicity may be related to the inhibition of L-C uptake by its specific organic cation transporter (OCTN-2) since, in a recent study with choriocarcinoma (BeWo) cells, the uptake of L-C was inhibited by METH and other amphetamine derivatives.[14]

ROLE OF GLUCOSE AND FATTY ACID METABOLISM IN NEURODEGENERATION

Although fatty acids are utilized as an energy substrate in all tissues, their role in brain under normal conditions is not thought to be important, and glucose is the main energetic substrate in adult brain.[23] However, recently, it was shown that fatty acids are used by brain as an energy substrate as well, and the oxidation of ^{13}C-octanoate in brain contributes to nearly 20% of the total oxidative energy production.[24]

Astrocytes are more resistant to nitrosative stress than neurons, possibly due to differences in key regulatory steps of glucose metabolism, that is, upregulation of high-affinity glucose transporter, stimulation of glycolysis at 6-phosphofructo-1-kinase, and activation of the pentose-phosphate pathway at glucose-6-phosphate dehydrogenase.[25] The stimulation of glucose-metabolizing pathways by nitric oxide could be a mechanism to compensate for the impaired energy status and the oxidized glutathione, which would increase the chances of survival.

The carnitines may stimulate pyruvate dehydrogenase complex (PDH) activity and enhance nonoxidative glucose metabolism by increasing mitochondrial acetyl-carnitine efflux in the absence of exogenous fatty acids. The PDH complex, the key irreversible rate-limiting step in carbohydrate oxidation, is modulated by the intra-mitochondrial ratio of acetyl-CoA/CoA. An increased ratio results in the inhibition of PDH activity. A decreased ratio can relieve the inhibition of PDH as shown by the transfer of acetyl groups from acetyl-CoA to carnitine, forming acetylcarnitine, a reaction catalyzed by carnitine acetyltransferase. This activity of L-C would modulate the intramitochondrial acetyl-CoA/CoA ratio and thereby may affect glucose oxidation.[12,26] This may explain the partial protection that we find with L-C and ALC against the various metabolic inhibitors. However, further studies are necessary to clarify the neuroprotective mechanism.

It is also possible to boost the cognitive performance of the older rats by giving them glucose injections.[27] Similarly, supplementation with metabolic substrates such as carbohydrates, proteins, and fats may also augment cellular energy and play a vital role in the pathogenesis of chronic conditions such as Parkinson's disease. A further strategy may be to augment the metabolic cofactors and antioxidant defenses to improve the actual metabolic machinery.[28,29] It is possible, for example, to specifically target the major cell-energy-producing organelle, the mitochondria, improving their function and thereby restoring cellular energy levels to normal and limiting production of reactive oxygen species (ROS). The effectiveness of diet and dietary supplements in Parkinson's disease would impact upon mitochondrial energy function as well as antioxidant status.[30]

PROTECTIVE EFFECTS OF Q10 VIA EFFECT ON CELLULAR ENERGY

Coenzyme Q10 is necessary for function of the mitochondrial respiratory chain and transfers electrons from complexes I and II to III. It has antioxidant properties and has been shown to prevent peroxidation of membrane lipids. It also protects mitochondrial DNA (mtDNA) from free oxygen radicals. Low levels of coenzyme Q10 are associated with impaired antioxidant protection in various diseases (cardiomyopathy, encephalopathy). In Parkinson's disease, there is reduced activity of complex I of the electron transport chain in brain and platelets. Platelet mitochondria from parkinsonian patients were found to have lower levels of coenzyme Q10 than mitochondria from age/sex-matched controls.[31] In clinical studies, coenzyme Q10 appears to slow the progressive deterioration of function in Parkinson's disease.[32] Coenzyme Q10 also attenuated MPTP-induced loss of striatal dopamine and dopaminergic axons in aged mice.[33] This neuroprotective ability of Q10 may be due to antiapoptotic action that may vary depending on cell type and mode of cell death induction.[34]

Further, the protective effects of Q10 seemed to be enhanced by the presence of the metabolic substrate, nicotinamide.[35] This has led to the proposal of novel dietary strategy designed to lower the risk of Parkinson's disease as well as other neurodegenerative disorders. This includes a nutritionally balanced diet containing adequate amounts of fruits and vegetables, along with adequate dietary supplementation of *S*-adenosyl-L-methionine; vitamins C, B6, and B12; and folate.[30]

PROTECTIVE EFFECTS OF POLYUNSATURATED FATTY ACIDS (PUFAs) VIA EFFECTS ON INFLAMMATION

Another strategy in neuroprotection is to reduce the overproduction of inflammatory factors. The role of dietary omega-3 fatty acids in the development of the central nervous and visual systems is well known since they are necessary for neural membrane structure and function. However, these macronutrients also play an important anti-inflammatory role.[36] Omega-3 fatty acids cannot be synthesized by the body; thus, they must be obtained from external sources through diet or supplements. The most important omega-3 fatty acids are two essential PUFAs, eicosapentaenoic acid C20:5 (EPA) and docosahexaenoic acid C22:6 (DHA). EPA is required for the proper functioning of many body tissues and is a precursor of biologically active eicosanoid hormones. DHA is essential for optimum brain and eye function. Low levels have been correlated with memory loss, changes in visual function, and other neurological conditions. DHA synthesis in the mitochondria depends on adequate L-C levels, and factors affecting L-C will affect its synthesis.[37] Both DHA and EPA are powerful inhibitors of inflammation. PUFAs have been shown to have neuroprotective actions, possibly by reducing the proinflammatory cytokines and also by opening of background K(+) channels, like TREK-1 and TRAAK, which are located both pre- and postsynaptically.[38]

A recent clinical study showed that PUFAs in combination with coenzyme Q10 and ALC was able to stop and even reverse the damage to the retinal epithelium that otherwise could lead to age-related macular degeneration.[39]

OXIDATIVE STRESS AND THE ROLE OF ANTIOXIDANTS

An adequate intake of antioxidant micronutrients (e.g., vitamins C and E) as well as the intrinsic cellular defenses protect the brain against the damage caused by oxidative stress. The effectiveness of neuroprotective agents such as ALC has been shown to be improved in combination with antioxidants such as lipoic acid.[40] Lipoic acid is a potent antioxidant, which regenerates through redox cycling other antioxidants like vitamins C and E, and also raises intracellular glutathione levels. Dietary administration to aged rats with ALC and lipoic acid significantly reduced the extent of oxidized RNAs and reversed hippocampal age-associated mitochondrial structural decay, possibly by lowering oxidative damage.

ROLE OF CALORIC RESTRICTION IN THE NEUROPROTECTION STRATEGY

There are a number of animal studies showing the neuroprotective action of caloric restriction diet.[41] A recent study demonstrated that a low-calorie diet could lessen the severity of neurochemical deficits and motor dysfunction in a primate model of Parkinson's disease.[42] The adult male rhesus monkeys were maintained for 6 months on a reduced calorie diet [30% caloric restriction (CR)] or an *ad libitum* control diet followed by administration of a neurotoxin to produce a hemiparkinson condition. After neurotoxin treatment, CR monkeys exhibited significantly higher levels of locomotor activity compared with control monkeys, as well as higher levels of dopamine (DA) and DA metabolites in the striatal region. The beneficial effects of dietary restriction may be related in part to reduced formation of ROS and also to increased production of neurotrophic factors and cytoprotective protein chaperones in neurons. Conversely, other studies suggest that caloric restriction in the aging brain may be preserving DNA repair enzymes in their intact form and/or upregulating specific antiapoptotic proteins involved in neuronal cell death.[42]

CONCLUSIONS

A number of strategies using the nutritional approach are emerging for the protection of the brain from damage caused by metabolic toxins, age, or disease. Neural dysfunction and metabolic imbalances underlie many diseases, and the inclusion of metabolic modifiers may provide an alternative and early intervention approach that may limit further damage. The neuroprotective potential of L-C, ALC, coenzyme Q10, lipoic acid, PUFAs, and a growing list of compounds needs to be studied further. Their mechanism of action on cellular processes in the central and peripheral nervous system is still not completely clear, but the neuroprotective actions could be related to stabilization of mitochondria and enhancement of β-oxidation/glycolysis, as well as protection against free radicals. Further experiments are needed to try combinations of these compounds, as well as to test the effectiveness in combination with the caloric restriction diet.

REFERENCES

1. VanItallie, T.B. & T.H. Nufert. 2003. Ketones: metabolism's ugly duckling. Nutr. Rev. **61:** 327–341.
2. Beal, M.F. 2003. Bioenergetic approaches for neuroprotection in Parkinson's disease. Ann. Neurol. **53:** S39–S47.
3. Koller, W.C. & M.G. Cersosimo. 2004. Neuroprotection in Parkinson's disease: an elusive goal. Curr. Neurol. Neurosci. Rep. **4:** 277–283.
4. Orth, M. & S.J. Tabrizi. 2003. Models of Parkinson's disease. Mov. Disord. **18:** 729–737.
5. Fiskum, G., A. Starkov, B.M. Polster & C. Chinopoulos. 2003. Mitochondrial mechanisms of neural cell death and neuroprotective interventions in Parkinson's disease. Ann. N.Y. Acad. Sci. **991:** 111–119.
6. Adams, J.D., Jr., M.L. Chang & L. Klaidman. 2001. Parkinson's disease–redox mechanisms. Curr. Med. Chem. **8:** 809–814.
7. Beal, M.F. 2003. Mitochondria, oxidative damage, and inflammation in Parkinson's disease. Ann. N.Y. Acad. Sci. **991:** 120–131.
8. Greenamyre, J.T., T.B. Sherer, R. Betarbet & A.V. Panov. 2001. Complex I and Parkinson's disease. IUBMB Life **52:** 135–141.
9. Desai, V.G., R.J. Feuers, R.W. Hart & S.F. Ali. 1996. MPP^+-induced neurotoxicity in mouse is age-dependent: evidenced by the selective inhibition of complexes of electron transport. Brain Res. **715:** 1–8.
10. Fonck, C. & M. Baudry. 2003. Rapid reduction of ATP synthesis and lack of free radical formation by MPP^+ in rat brain synaptosomes and mitochondria. Brain Res. **975:** 214–221.
11. Gonzalez-Polo, R.A., G. Soler, J.C. Alonso *et al.* 2003. MPP(+) causes inhibition of cellular energy supply in cerebellar granule cells. Neurotoxicology **24:** 219–225.
12. Virmani, A. & Z. Binienda. 2004. Role of carnitine esters in brain neuropathology. Mol. Aspects Med. **25:** 533–549.

13. Alexi, T., P.E. Hughes, R.L. Faull & C.E. Williams. 1998. 3-Nitropropionic acid's lethal triplet: cooperative pathways of neurodegeneration. Neuroreport **9:** R57–R64.
14. Rytting, E. & K.L Audus. 2005. Novel organic cation transporter 2–mediated carnitine uptake in placental choriocarcinoma (BeWo) cells. J. Pharmacol. Exp. Ther. **312:** 192–198.
15. Binienda, Z. & A. Virmani. 2003. The mitochondriotropic effects of L-carnitine and its esters in the central nervous system. Med. Chem. CMC-CNSA **3:** 275–282.
16. Kotake, Y. & S. Ohta. 2003. MPP^+ analogs acting on mitochondria and inducing neuro-degeneration. Curr. Med. Chem. **10:** 2507–2516.
17. Binienda, Z., D.L. Frederick, S.A. Ferguson *et al.* 1995. The effects of perinatal hypoxia on the behavioral, neurochemical, and neurohistological toxicity of the metabolic inhibitor 3-nitropropionic acid. Metab. Brain. Dis. **10:** 269–282.
18. Roberts, T.J. 2005. 3-Nitropropionic acid model of metabolic stress: assessment by magnetic resonance imaging. Methods Mol. Med. **104:** 203–220.
19. Virmani, A., F. Gaetani, Z. Binienda *et al.* 2004. Role of mitochondrial dysfunction in neurotoxicity of MPP^+: partial protection of PC12 cells by acetyl-L-carnitine. Ann. N.Y. Acad. Sci. **1025:** 267–273.
20. Bodis-Wollner, I., E. Chung, M.F. Ghilardi *et al.* 1991. Acetyl-levo-carnitine protects against MPTP-induced parkinsonism in primates. J. Neural Transm. Parkinson's Dis. Dementia Sect. **3:** 63–72.
21. Mazzio, E., K.J. Yoon & K.F. Soliman. 2003. Acetyl-L-carnitine cytoprotection against 1-methyl-4-phenylpyridinium toxicity in neuroblastoma cells. Biochem. Pharmacol. **66:** 297–306.
22. Steffen, V., M. Santiago, C.P. de la Cruz *et al.* 1995. Effect of intraventricular injection of 1-methyl-4-phenylpyridinium: protection by acetyl-L-carnitine. Hum. Exp. Toxicol. **14:** 865–871.
23. Heininger, K. 2002. The cerebral glucose–fatty acid cycle: evolutionary roots, regulation, and (patho)physiological importance. Int. Rev. Neurobiol. **51:** 103–158.
24. Ebert, D., R.G. Haller & M.E. Walton. 2003. Energy contribution of octanoate to intact rat brain metabolism measured by ^{13}C nuclear magnetic resonance spectroscopy. J. Neurosci. **23:** 5928–5935.
25. Bolanos, J.P., P. Cidad, P. Garcia-Nogales *et al.* 2004. Regulation of glucose metabolism by nitrosative stress in neural cells. Mol. Aspects Med. **25:** 61–73.
26. Rosenthal, R.E., R. Williams, Y.E. Bogaert *et al.* 1992. Prevention of postischemic canine neurological injury through potentiation of brain energy metabolism by acetyl-L-carnitine. Stroke **23:** 1312–1317.
27. McNay, E.C., R.C. McCarty & P.E Gold. 2001. Fluctuations in brain glucose concentration during behavioral testing: dissociations between brain areas and between brain and blood. Neurobiol. Learn. Mem. **75:** 325–337.
28. Beal, M.F. 2004. Mitochondrial dysfunction and oxidative damage in Alzheimer's and Parkinson's diseases and coenzyme Q10 as a potential treatment. J. Bioenerg. Biomembr. **36:** 381–386.
29. Virmani, A., F. Gaetani, S. Imam *et al.* 2002. The protective role of L-carnitine against neurotoxicity evoked by drug of abuse, methamphetamine, could be related to mitochondrial dysfunction. Ann. N.Y. Acad. Sci. **965:** 225–232.
30. Zhu, B.T. 2004. CNS dopamine oxidation and catechol-*O*-methyltransferase: importance in the etiology, pharmacotherapy, and dietary prevention of Parkinson's disease. Int. J. Mol. Med. **13:** 343–353.
31. Shults, C.W., R.H. Haas & M.F. Beal. 1999. A possible role of coenzyme Q10 in the etiology and treatment of Parkinson's disease. Biofactors **9:** 267–272.
32. Shults, C.W. *et al.* 2002. Effects of coenzyme Q10 in early Parkinson disease: evidence of slowing of the functional decline. Arch. Neurol. **59:** 1541–1550.
33. Beal, M.F., R.T. Matthews, A. Tieleman & C.W. Shults. 1998. Coenzyme Q10 attenuates the 1-methyl-4-phenyl-1,2,3-tetrahydropyridine (MPTP) induced loss of striatal dopamine and dopaminergic axons in aged mice. Brain Res. **783:** 109–114.
34. Kagan, T., C. Davis, L. Lin & Z. Zakeri. 1999. Coenzyme Q10 can in some circumstances block apoptosis, and this effect is mediated through mitochondria. Ann. N.Y. Acad. Sci. **887:** 31–47.

35. SCHULZ, J.B. *et al.* 1995. Coenzyme Q10 and nicotinamide and a free radical spin trap protect against MPTP neurotoxicity. Exp. Neurol. **132:** 279–283.
36. SINGH, R.B., D. PELLA, V. MECHIROVA & K. OTSUKA. 2004. Can brain dysfunction be a predisposing factor for metabolic syndrome? Biomed. Pharmacother. **58:** S56–S68.
37. VIRMANI, A. & Z. BINIENDA. 2004. Role of carnitine esters in brain neuropathology. Mol. Aspects Med. **25:** 533–549.
38. LAURITZEN, I. *et al.* 2000. Polyunsaturated fatty acids are potent neuroprotectors. EMBO J. **19:** 1784–1793.
39. FEHER, J. *et al.* 2003. Mitotropic compounds for the treatment of age-related macular degeneration: the metabolic approach and a pilot study. Ophthalmologica **217:** 351–357.
40. LIU, J., H. ATAMNA, H. KURATSUNE & B.N. AMES. 2002. Delaying brain mitochondrial decay and aging with mitochondrial antioxidants and metabolites. Ann. N.Y. Acad. Sci. **959:** 133–166.
41. MASWOOD, N. *et al.* 2004. Caloric restriction increases neurotrophic factor levels and attenuates neurochemical and behavioral deficits in a primate model of Parkinson's disease. Proc. Natl. Acad. Sci. USA **101:** 18171–18176.
42. LOVE, R. 2005. Calorie restriction may be neuroprotective in AD and PD. Lancet Neurol. **4:** 84.

Questions and Answers

Session IV: Role of Carnitines and Other Agents in Neuroprotection

QUESTIONS FOR GARY FISKUM

From William Slikker, Jr.

Why are the levels of lactate so slow to recover after reperfusion injury (and low brain pH)?

ANSWER: Our current working hypothesis for the chronic brain lactic acidosis that is observed in our cardiac arrest and resuscitation model is that oxidative stress during reperfusion impairs the activity of pyruvate dehydrogenase and thus limits aerobic cerebral energy metabolism. Anaerobic glycolysis accelerates in an attempt to generate the ATP that would normally be generated primarily by oxidative phosphorylation.

From Philip Lazarovici

The mechanism of acetyl-L-carnitine neuroprotective effect was explained as an antioxidant indirect effect. How will it be reconciled with the high brain endogenous antioxidant activity? Lactate dehydrogenase is also sensitive to free radicals. What is the contribution of LDH inhibition to the acetyl-L-carnitive effect?

ANSWER: While the brain may have relatively high antioxidant activities compared to some other tissues, oxidative stress still contributes significantly to both acute brain injury and neurodegenerative diseases. We believe that the antioxidant effects of acetyl-L-carnitine are indirect due to its effects on energy metabolism and possibly on cellular redox state. While virtually all enzymes can be inhibited when exposed to enough oxidative stress, we found that pyruvate dehydrogenase is far more sensitive to inactivation by the hydroxyl radical than is lactate dehydrogenase. We also found that ischemia/reperfusion results in a >50% loss of pyruvate dehydrogenase activity under conditions where no loss of lactate dehydrogenase activity occurs (see BOGAERT, Y.E. *et al.* 1994. Free Radical Biol. Med. **16:** 811–820).

From Kenneth Maynard

Have you ever measured how acetyl-L-carnitine affects energy metabolism during cardiac arrest?

ANSWER: We have not tested the effects of acetyl-L-carnitine when administered prior to cardiac arrest since our primary goal is to develop a neuroprotective intervention practical for use following cardiac arrest. However, as up to 20% of patients

Ann. N.Y. Acad. Sci. 1053: 192–194 (2005). © 2005 New York Academy of Sciences.
doi: 10.1196/annals.1344.063

that undergo surgical procedures involving cardiac arrest experience some form of brain injury, preadministration could potentially be beneficial for these patients.

From Zbigniew Binienda

Is the negative effect of L-carnitine and acetate administered in combination in your study related to the timing of this treatment? After cardiac arrest, the activity of carnitine acetyltransferase is compromised. If so, L-carnitine may not be esterified to acetyl-L-carnitine. What is your opinion?

ANSWER: If carnitine acetyltransferase is inhibited to an extent that limits acetyl-carnitine formation from carnitine and acetate, this inhibition should also limit the oxidative metabolism of exogenously administered acetylcarnitine. It is possible that the protective effects of acetyl-L-carnitine are due to a mechanism other than its metabolism, in which case the inhibition of its synthesis from carnitine and acetate would be important.

From Hari Sharma

You have shown us a very nice improvement in the neurological outcome after the drug treatment in dogs. Normally, functional outcome does not always correlate in the cell and tissue injury. What is the outcome of cell and tissue injury in your model after this drug treatment?

ANSWER: We have some unpublished results indicating that acetyl-L-carnitine protects against the death of cerebellar Purkinje neurons after 10-min cardiac arrest and 24-h reperfusion, but more rigorous quantitative histopathology in the cerebellum, cortex, and hippocampus is needed. However, in a rat irreversible focal ischemia (stroke) model, we found that acetyl-L-carnitine improved neurologic outcome and reduced weight loss without having a significant effect on brain infarct volume. I therefore agree that functional outcome can at times be affected by interventions that do not demonstrate significant effects on neuronal cell death.

QUESTIONS FOR JOHN HONG

From William Slikker, Jr.

Have there been epidemiology studies that have followed subjects with episodes of inflammation to determine if they are more susceptible to PD or AD?

ANSWER: Yes, there were epidemiology studies documenting higher PD incidence for the people suffering from encephalitis.

From Italo Mocchetti

Based on the anti-inflammatory effect of IL-10 and its ability to block LPS-induced toxicity, did you try to compare IL-10 activity versus DM?

ANSWER: No, we have not performed this experiment. It is an interesting suggestion, and we plan to compare these two compounds.

From Philip Lazarovici

How do you exclude the possibility that neuroprotection measured by ^{3}H-DA uptake in the presence of naloxone analogues is not induced by increased number and/or affinity of DA transporters? What is the experimental evidence excluding the involvement of astroglia opiate receptors in naloxone analogue neuroprotection?

ANSWER: The ^{3}H-DA uptake studies were always compared with the cell count based on immunocytochemical analysis of TH staining. The results are very comparable. We use both (−) and (+) isomers of naloxone, and the results showed that they are equipotent. This experiment strongly indicates that the effect of naloxone is mediated through the conventional opiate receptors.

QUESTIONS FOR WEI ZHANG

From Kenneth Maynard

Have you looked at the effect of 3-HM in a postinsult treatment paradigm and, if so, have you measured clinical behavioral scores and shown a protective effect?

ANSWER: No, we have not done this experiment yet.

From Karl Sanzenbacher

Dextromethorphan is available off the shelf and has been used in status migraine. The rationale was its action on the mu opiate receptor. These patients are in a phase of migraine with an inflammatory component. Maybe we were attracting the inflammatory component. What was the dose you used in the PD patient?

ANSWER: The dose used in the PD patient was 30–60 mg/day.

QUESTIONS FOR SYED ALI

From Sylvain Doré

In light of recent results with nNOS-1 females, do you expect similar changes as you reported in males to be present in nNOS-1 females?

ANSWER: Currently, we do not have the data from nNOS-1 female mice, but I expect the same results.

From Naren Banik

You showed very interesting data on neuroprotection by melatonin on the methamphetamine model *in vivo*. Melatonin seems to exert a protective effect in spinal cord injury. Have you looked at the activity and expression of calpain and caspase-3 activity in your model?

ANSWER: No, but we are in the process of exploring the role of caspase-3 in METH-induced neurotoxicity and hopefully we will have some data by the next meeting.

The Antiapoptotic Actions of Mood Stabilizers

Molecular Mechanisms and Therapeutic Potentials

DE-MAW CHUANG

Molecular Neurobiology Section, Biological Psychiatry Branch, Mood and Anxiety Disorders Program, National Institute of Mental Health, National Institutes of Health, Bethesda, Maryland 20892-1363, USA

ABSTRACT: Two primary drugs used to treat bipolar mood disorder are lithium and valproate. Emerging evidence supports the notion that both mood stabilizers have neuroprotective effects. In primary cultures of rat cerebellar granule cells and cortical neurons, lithium and valproate robustly and potently protect against glutamate-induced, *N*-methyl-D-aspartate (NMDA) receptor–mediated excitotoxicity. The neuroprotective mechanisms involve inactivation of NMDA receptors through inhibition of NR2B tyrosine phosphorylation, activation of cell survival factors such as the PI 3-kinase/Akt signaling pathway, and induction of neurotrophic/neuroprotective proteins, including brain-derived neurotrophic factor, heat-shock protein (HSP), and Bcl-2. Both drugs are also effective against other forms of insults such as ER stress in neurally related cell types. The molecular targets likely involve glycogen synthase kinase-3 (GSK-3) and histone deacetylase (HDAC) for lithium and valproate, respectively. In a rat cerebral artery occlusion model of stroke, postinsult treatment with lithium or valproate reduces ischemia-induced brain infarction, caspase-3 activation, and neurological deficits, and these neuroprotective effects are associated with HSP70 upregulation and, in the case of valproate, HDAC inhibition. In a rat excitotoxic model of Huntington's disease in which an excitotoxin is infused into the striatum to activate NMDA receptors, short-term lithium pretreatment is sufficient to protect against DNA damage, caspase activation, and apoptosis of striatal neurons, and this neuroprotection is concurrent with Bcl-2 induction. Moreover, lithium treatment increases cell proliferation near the site of striatal injury, and some newborn cells have phenotypes of neurons and astroglia. Thus, lithium and valproate are potential drugs for treating some forms of neurodegenerative diseases.

KEYWORDS: BDNF; Bcl-2; excitotoxicity; heat-shock protein; lithium; neurodegeneration; neurogenesis; neuroprotection; valproate

Lithium and valproate are two of the most prominent drugs approved by the United States Federal Food and Drug Administration (FDA) used in the treatment of bipolar mood disorder. This mental illness, which includes symptomatology of alternating depression and mania, is recognized by the World Health Organization as a leading debilitating neuropsychiatric disorder that affects about 1.3% of both sexes globally.[1]

Address for correspondence: De-Maw Chuang, Ph.D., Molecular Neurobiology Section, National Institute of Mental Health, National Institutes of Health, Building 10, Room 4C-206, 10 Center Drive, MSC 1363, Bethesda, MD 20892-1363. Voice: 301-496-4915; fax: 301-480-9290.
chuang@mail.nih.gov

Ann. N.Y. Acad. Sci. 1053: 195–204 (2005).
doi: 10.1196/annals.1344.018

Over 50 years ago, lithium was discovered to be efficacious in the control of acute mania. Additional findings showed it to be prophylactic against recurrent manic and depressive episodes, and to be augmentative of the activity of classical antidepressants in some depressive patients. Recent evidence has supported that certain anticonvulsants, for example, valproate, carbamazepine, and lamotrigine, also have clinical efficacy in the treatment of bipolar disorder (for review, see refs. 2 and 3). Valproate is effective, like lithium, in preventing manic episodes; however, as with lithium, it is also less beneficial in the prevention of depression. Research continues to focus on the underlying mechanisms of lithium and valproate, which still remain uncharacterized, and current studies have led to an appreciation of the complexity of bipolar disorder etiology and that the effects of mood stabilizing drugs may result from multiple routes of action (for review, see ref. 4). Since mood stabilizers require chronic treatment for their beneficial effects, it has been hypothesized that alterations of signaling pathways and gene expression may be involved. Hence, great interest has been raised in the investigation of lithium and other mood stabilizing agents on gene expression and cellular signaling in both basic and preclinical laboratories.

Our pioneering studies have shown that chronic exposure of cultured rat cerebellar granule cells with therapeutic concentrations of lithium increases m_3-muscarinic acetylcholine receptor–mediated second messenger production as well as c-fos and m_3-receptor expression.[5] Lithium at therapeutic doses increases the activities of two prominent transcription factors, AP-1 and CREB (cyclic AMP–response element binding protein), in cultured cerebellar granule cells and in distinct brain areas (e.g., frontal cortex, amygdala, hippocampus, and cerebellum) in rats treated by diet for 2 or 4 weeks.[6] A growing body of evidence suggests that m_3-muscarinic receptors and the DNA binding activities of AP-1 and CREB have prominent roles in the regulation of cell viability. Accordingly, we proposed that mood stabilizers have neuroprotective and neurotrophic actions.

Glutamate-induced excitotoxicity in discrete brain areas has been linked to a variety of neurodegenerative diseases such as stroke, Huntington's disease, ALS, brain trauma, cerebellar degeneration, spinal cord injury, and possibly Alzheimer's disease and Parkinson's disease (for review, see refs. 7–9). Therefore, we investigated the effects of lithium on glutamate-induced excitotoxicity using primary cultures of cerebellar granule cells (CGCs) as a model. We found that chronic lithium treatment robustly reduces glutamate-induced excitotoxicity and this can be completely blocked by *N*-methyl-D-aspartate (NMDA) receptor antagonists.[10] This neuroprotection is long-lasting, occurs at therapeutically relevant concentrations ($EC_{50} \approx 1$ mM), and requires 6–7 days of pretreatment for maximal effects. The action is also unrelated to lithium's inhibition of inositol monophosphatases in that coaddition with excessive myoinositol fails to reverse lithium's neuroprotective effects. The neuroprotection by lithium involves blockade of the apoptotic component of glutamate excitotoxicity and is due, in part, to a reduction in NMDA receptor–mediated intracellular calcium increase. Because long-term pretreatment is necessary to elicit these neuroprotective effects, gene expression is likely involved. In support of this notion, we found that treatment with lithium induces the cytoprotective Bcl-2 protein, but downregulates the proapoptotic proteins such as p53 and Bax.[11] Conversely, glutamate treatment downregulates Bcl-2, but upregulates p53 and Bax, and these actions of glutamate are reversed by lithium pretreatment. It has also been reported that chronic lithium and VPA treatments upregulate Bcl-2 in the brain of rats.[12]

Lithium also exerts its effects on the cell survival factor, Akt, which is a downstream kinase of phosphatidylinositol 3-kinase (PI 3-kinase). Lithium treatment of rat CGCs was found to rapidly activate PI 3-kinase, resulting in increased phosphorylation of Akt at Ser473 and enhanced Akt activity.[13] Additionally, induced Akt activation by lithium is associated with enhanced phosphorylation levels at Ser21 of glycogen synthase kinase-3α (GSK-3α), previously thought to be directly inhibited by lithium[14] and a known phosphorylation substrate of Akt. The presence of a PI 3-kinase inhibitor, LY 294002, abolishes lithium-induced phosphorylation of GSK-3α and GSK-3β, further suggesting the involvement of the PI 3-kinase/Akt signaling pathway. In contrast, glutamate treatment causes a rapid, but reversible loss of Akt (Ser473) phosphorylation and activity apparently through protein phosphatase activation,[13] and these effects are also prevented by lithium.

CREB is a downstream signaling target of the mitogen-activated protein kinase (MAP kinase) system that, upon phosphorylation, has a major role in mediating adaptive responses at glutamatergic synapses and cell survival by promoting the expression of cell-protective proteins such as BDNF and Bcl-2 (for review, see ref. 15). In CGCs, we showed that toxic concentrations ($\geq$50 μM) of glutamate induce an NMDA receptor–dependent decrease in CREB phosphorylation at Ser133 (and hence CREB inactivation),[16] and that chronic lithium treatment, concurrent with the neuroprotective effects, suppresses glutamate-induced loss of phosphorylated CREB (p-CREB). Studies using selective inhibitors demonstrate that protein phosphatase 1 predominantly regulates glutamate-induced decrease in p-CREB levels. The MEK/ERK MAP kinases are upstream of CREB and known to be involved in cytoprotection (for review, see ref. 15). Treatment with glutamate induces a rapid increase in MEK activity in CGCs and this is potentiated by long-term lithium pretreatment, an effect blocked by the MEK inhibitor, PD 98059.[16] Our results suggest that long-term lithium exposure is necessary to maintain higher activated CREB levels in CGCs subjected to glutamate excitotoxicity and that this may be the result of the inhibition of protein phosphatase 1 as well as promotion of the activities of MEK/ERK by itself.

c-Jun N-terminal kinase (JNK) and p38 kinase, another member of the MAP kinase family, are activated by site-specific phosphorylation in response to a variety of apoptotic insults (for review, see ref. 17). The p38 kinase and JNK often act synergistically to enhance AP-1 binding activity. Using rat CGC cultures, we tested the hypothesis that AP-1 binding activation is involved in glutamate excitotoxicity and is a target of lithium as part of lithium-induced neuroprotection. We found that glutamate, through NMDA receptor activation, causes a rapid activation of JNK and p38 kinase, which then phosphorylate c-Jun (at Ser63) and p53 (at Ser15), leading to a robust increase in AP-1 binding that precedes apoptotic death.[18] Long-term lithium pretreatment can block these glutamate-induced apoptotic effects; moreover, SB 203580, a p38 kinase inhibitor, selectively prevents glutamate-induced p38 activation, p53 phosphorylation, and AP-1 binding activation, and shows neuroprotection. Curcumin, a potent inhibitor of AP-1 activity, inhibits glutamate-induced AP-1 binding and protects CGCs from glutamate excitotoxicity. Our results suggest that NMDA receptor–mediated apoptotic death requires both the actions of JNK and p38 to enhance AP-1 binding and p53 phosphorylation (and hence p53 stabilization). Moreover, suppression of receptor-mediated activation of the JNK/p38 MAP kinase pathway and subsequent AP-1 activation play a role in lithium neuroprotection.

CGCs have also been used to test the neuroprotective effects of another mood stabilizer, valproate, against excitotoxicity. Treatment of CGCs with SYM-2081 [(2*S*,4*R*)-4-methylglutamate], an inhibitor of excitatory amino-acid transporters and an agonist of low-affinity kainate receptors, induces apoptotic cell death.[19] The SYM-2081-induced excitotoxicity is blocked by an NMDA receptor antagonist and associated with a rapid and robust nuclear translocation of glyceraldehyde-3-phosphate dehydrogenase (GAPDH), a housekeeping gene previously shown to be proapoptotic (for review, see ref. 20). Recent studies identified histone deacetylase (HDAC) as a direct target of valproate.[21,22] We found that pretreatment of CGCs with valproate or other HDAC inhibitors such as butyrate and trichostatin A induces a time- and concentration-dependent neuroprotection against SYM-2081 excitotoxicity.[19] Moreover, the valproate neuroprotection is associated with suppression of SYM-2081-induced nuclear accumulation of GAPDH, which is associated with hyperacetylated histone H3, including Lys9-acetylated histone.

Primary cultures of rat cerebral cortical neurons have also been used in our studies because abnormalities in volume, cell density, and neuronal size have been found in the cerebral cortex of bipolar patients (for review, see refs. 23 and 24). Rat cortical neurons are highly vulnerable to glutamate excitotoxicity, with an LD_{50} of only 8–10 μM. This form of toxicity is also NMDA receptor–mediated in this cell type.[25] Protracted lithium pretreatment for 5–6 days is necessary for complete protection against glutamate excitotoxicity, and significantly less lithium is required compared to CGC cultures.[25] Thus, neuroprotective effects of lithium are observed in the subtherapeutic and therapeutic concentrations of 0.2–1.6 mM, with an optimal dose at 1 mM. Additionally, the neuroprotection is specific for lithium since other monovalent ions (Rb and Cs) and classical antidepressants (imipramine, desipramine, clomipramine, and fluoxetine) are ineffective.

In cultured cortical neurons, lithium neuroprotection is also associated with an attenuation of NMDA receptor–mediated calcium influx.[25] Concomitant with this inhibition, lithium induces a time-dependent selective decrease in phosphorylation of Tyr1472 of the NR2B receptor subtype. Mutation studies have shown that phosphorylation of NR2B at Tyr1472 is crucial in mediating NMDA receptor channel activity.[26] Thus, lithium-induced decrease of NR2B Tyr1472 phosphorylation likely plays a role in the observed reduction of NMDA receptor–mediated Ca^{2+} influx. Tyrosine phosphorylation of NR2B (and NR2A) is mediated by the Src family kinases, which bind to scaffolding proteins in the NMDA receptor complex. Levels of phosphorylated Src kinase at Tyr416, an index of Src activation, were found to be reduced after long-term treatment with LiCl (1 mM).[27] Moreover, an Src kinase inhibitor, SU-6656, and an NR2B antagonist, ifenprodil, partially block glutamate excitotoxicity. Together, these data are suggestive that the inactivation of Src kinase and resulting NR2B NMDA receptor inhibition is a mechanism by which lithium confers neuroprotection against glutamate toxicity.

We next studied the neuroprotective roles of BDNF, a neurotrophin that is essential for neuronal survival, synaptic plasticity, and cortical development, and likely plays a role in the actions of antidepressants (for review, see refs. 15 and 24). We hypothesized a critical role of BDNF/TrkB in the mediation of lithium neuroprotection against glutamate excitotoxicity in rat cortical neurons and diverse signaling pathways mediated by mood stabilizers.[28] Results showed that a Trk tyrosine kinase inhibitor, K252a, and a BDNF-neutralizing antibody can suppress lithium-induced neuroprotection against excitotoxicity, which suggests the involvement of BDNF/TrkB activation. Evidence supporting this hypothesis comes from our findings in cortical neurons that lithium transiently increases intracellular BDNF followed by an increase in levels of phosphorylated TrkB (at Tyr490). Thus, long-term lithium enhances BDNF expression, secretion, and subsequent activation of TrkB receptors. In addition, we found in cortical neurons that exon III mRNA levels of BDNF and promoter III activity of the BDNF gene are increased by lithium treatment.[29] It is important to note that lithium does not protect cortical neurons derived from either heterozygous (+/–) or homozygous (–/–) BDNF knockout mice from glutamate excitotoxic death, while it completely protects cultures derived from wild-type mice littermates.[28] Altogether, our results suggest that in cortical neurons lithium causes elevation of BDNF to a critical level, which is essential for this drug to exert its protective effects against excitotoxicity, and that the BDNF/TrkB signal pathway likely mediates many of the reported downstream effectors. It is also noteworthy that valproate similarly protects against glutamate excitotoxicity in cortical neuronal cultures[25] and substantially increases neuronal culture life spans.[30] The latter protective effect is mimicked by HDAC inhibitors and associated with histone hyperacetylation and induction of heat-shock protein 70.[30]

In addition to glutamate excitotoxicity, lithium can also protect against other forms of insults in CNS neurons and neurally related cell lines. Our studies revealed that lithium rescues rat CGC cultures from apoptosis induced by potassium deprivation, supratherapeutic concentrations of anticonvulsants (phenytoin and carbamazepine), and spontaneous death.[31] Lithium also protects pheochromocytoma PC 12 cells from apoptosis induced by thapsigargin, an inhibitor of Ca^{2+}-ATPase on the endoplasmic reticulum (ER) and an inducer of Ca^{2+} release from the ER.[32] This protection is concomitant with suppression of thapsigargin-triggered intracellular calcium release from the ER, and induction of Bcl-2 and Grp 78 (glucose-regulated protein 78). The protection against ER stress in PC 12 cells is also induced by valproate pretreatment.[32] Moreover, treatment of PC 12 cells or CGCs with beta-amyloid peptide (1–42) for 24 h induces a decrease in cellular redox activity, which is accompanied by cell death, and this effect is markedly attenuated by long-term (7 days) lithium pretreatment.[33] The neuroprotective effects in beta-amyloid-treated cells are temporally correlated with upregulation of Bcl-2 protein levels. Accordingly, we have proposed that lithium's use in the treatment of Alzheimer's disease should be reexamined.[33] This notion is strengthened by the recent report that inhibition of GSK-3 by lithium results in the suppression of beta-amyloid production from its precursor protein.[34] Indeed, mounting evidence from various laboratories further supports the view that lithium can be neuroprotective against diverse forms of death insults, suggesting that it is a multifunctional neuroprotectant (for review, see refs. 24 and 35–38).

Based on the findings that both lithium and valproate are protective against glutamate excitotoxicity and other insults in CNS neurons, we hypothesized that these two mood stabilizers may have beneficial effects in multiple forms of neurodegenerative diseases, particularly those linked to excitotoxicity. Stroke is one neurodegenerative disease with a glutamate excitotoxicity component, and is a major cause of mortality and morbidity worldwide. Following brain ischemia, a substantial excess release of glutamate occurs and the resulting overstimulation of glutamate receptors leads to brain damage. With this as background, we investigated the effects of mood stabilizing drugs in a rodent model of stroke.

Our pilot studies employed a permanent middle cerebral artery occlusion (MCAO) stroke model in rats in which a nylon suture was inserted via the left external carotid artery into the left internal carotid artery to occlude the origin of the left middle cerebral artery, which results within 24 h in a massive brain infarct of the middle cerebral artery territory, including the cerebral cortex and the lateral segment of the caudate nucleus.[39] By pretreating rats for 16 days with subcutaneous injections of LiCl at therapeutic concentrations, we observed a >50% reduction in infarct volume. Moreover, the MCAO-induced neurological deficits such as hemiplegia and posture abnormality were also significantly suppressed.[39] Furthermore, our laboratory showed that lithium treatment markedly increases the number and intensity of neurons expressing Bcl-2 in brain areas vulnerable to ischemic insult.[40,41] As best as can be determined, this is the first demonstration of lithium protection against brain injury in an animal model of stroke, and these neuroprotective effects of long-term lithium treatment have been confirmed by others.[42]

The next rational step was to investigate whether postinsult treatment with lithium is neuroprotective in the MCAO model, which would support the use of this mood stabilizer as a potential therapy for acute stroke. We used a transient ischemia model in which rats were subjected to MCAO for 1 h followed by reperfusion, a model likely more related to the pathophysiology of acute stroke in humans. LiCl (0.5–3.0 mEq/kg) administered by subcutaneous injection immediately after MCAO was found to reduce infarct volume measured 24 h later.[43] The effective dose range used maintains plasma lithium concentrations at the therapeutic to subtherapeutic level at 12 and 24 h after injection. Similar drug treatments administered every 24 h cause a dose-dependently reduced neurological deficit score as measured by motor, sensory, and reflex tests over a period of 1 week or longer. Infarct volume and neurological deficit reductions were observed at therapeutic doses (0.5 and 1.0 mEq/kg) of lithium and even when injected (1.0 mEq/kg) at least up to 3 h after MCAO induction.[43] Suppression of MCAO/reperfusion-induced caspase-3 activation and DNA damage in neurons additionally supports the use of lithium as a neuroprotective agent.

Heat-shock protein 70 (HSP70) is known to play a major cytoprotective part in apoptosis and is induced in the ischemic penumbra where neuronal recovery is predominantly found (for review, see ref. 43). Moreover, transgenic mice overexpressing rat HSP70 showed reduced brain infarction in a permanent focal ischemia model.[44] We therefore investigated the role that heat-shock response may play in lithium neuroprotection, especially in light of a recent report that lithium inhibition of GSK-3 is associated with activation of heat-shock factor-1 (HSF-1),[45] a transcription factor for HSP70. Immunohistochemistry and Western blotting showed that lithium time-dependently superinduces HSP70 in the ischemic brain.[43] Moreover, EMSA showed that this HSP70 induction is preceded by a marked increase in the DNA binding activity of HSF-1 to the heat-shock element. Collectively, our research has demonstrated that postinsult lithium administration robustly protects neurons in the rat MCAO/reperfusion stroke model and that this lithium treatment may upregulate heat-shock response as part of the neuroprotective mechanisms.

Recently, we investigated the neuroprotective efficacy of valproate using the same MCAO/reperfusion paradigm in rats. Valproate (300 mg/kg) injected subcutaneously after ischemic induction, followed by injections every 12 h, significantly reduces infarct size and neurological deficits observed 48 h later,[46] and also markedly suppresses MCAO-induced caspase-3 activation in the cortex. Additionally, VPA increases acetylated histone H3 levels in a time-dependent manner in cortex and striatum of both ipsilateral and contralateral hemispheres, suggesting that HDAC activity is inhibited *in vivo*. Furthermore, valproate neuroprotection is associated with a robust increase in HSP70 levels in both ipsilateral and contralateral cortical and striatal areas.[46] Thus, similar to the *in vitro* results, valproate-induced HSP70 upregulation could be triggered by HDAC inhibition and participates in the neuroprotection against cerebral ischemia.

Huntington's disease (HD) is a devastating neurodegenerative disorder involving a selective loss of neurons in the brain, notably in the striatum and, to a lesser extent, in the cortex, and is characterized by involuntary hyperkinetic movement, impaired cognition, and psychiatric syndromes, especially depression.[8,47] It is widely believed that an expansion of CAG repeats in the exon I region of the gene encoding huntingtin[48] is the mutation responsible for HD; however, the direct link between the mutation and neurodegeneration found clinically remains obscure. In the investigation of HD, a frequently used animal model utilizes the infusion of quinolinic acid (QA), as a neuronal excitotoxin, into the striatum (for review, see ref. 49). Striatal QA infusion causes the death of medium-sized spiny neurons via activation of NMDA receptors and produces many of the neuroanatomical changes found in HD. In initial experiments, we pretreated rats with subcutaneous injections of therapeutic doses of LiCl for 16 days prior to unilateral infusion with QA. Results showed that lithium pretreatment markedly reduces the sizes of QA-induced striatal lesions,[40] and detailed analysis showed the number and intensity of DNA-damaged striatal neurons near the QA infusion site to be markedly decreased when compared to controls. Moreover, an increase in Bcl-2 immunostaining in medium-sized projection neurons and large interneurons in the striatum as well as in the frontal cortex is correlated with long-term lithium-induced neuroprotection. These early QA excitotoxicity HD studies were expanded by investigating the neuroprotective effects of short-term lithium pretreatment, characterizing specific striatal cell populations that could be protected, and investigating possible underlying mechanisms. Our results showed that subcutaneous LiCl injections given 24 h before and 1 h after unilateral infusion of QA into the striatum reduce the number of neurons showing caspase-3 activation and DNA damage, and decrease the loss of neurons immunostained by NeuN (a neuronal marker). However, this acute treatment fails to prevent the loss of NADPH-diaphorase-positive striatal interneurons.[41] Additionally, 24-h lithium pretreatment also upregulates Bcl-2 protein levels in the striatal tissue and increases the number and density of Bcl-2-immunostained striatal neurons.

Because lithium has the ability to increase neurogenesis in the rat hippocampus *in vivo*[50] and to stimulate neuroblast proliferation in rat neuronal cultures,[51] we investigated the effects of lithium on striatal cell proliferation in the rat QA model. One week after QA infusion of rats not treated with lithium, we found very few BrdU-labeled (or replicating) cells in the injured striatum near the QA injection site,[41] but densely packed BrdU-positive cells located in the subventricular zone (SVZ) of both ipsilateral (QA-infused) and contralateral (intact) striata. Of interest, in rats pretreated with lithium, we found a large number of BrdU-labeled cells near the QA-infused site, and this increase in the injured striatum is accompanied by a reduction in BrdU-labeled cells in the SVZ. Moreover, although the majority of proliferating cells were found to be neither mature neurons nor astrocytes, a small population of NeuN-stained cells with strong BrdU-labeling and some GFAP-expressing cells with weak labeling were observed. Thus, it appears that lithium can induce the migration of progenitor cells from the SVZ to the area damaged by QA infusion and/or can stimulate localized proliferation of neuronal and astroglial progenitor cells in the injured striatum. Both this cell-proliferating effect of lithium as well as its antiapoptotic property may underlie the neuroprotection observed in the QA-induced excitotoxicity model.

In conclusion, accumulating evidence strongly supports that the mood stabilizers, lithium and valproate, exert multiple effects that lead to neuroprotection against glutamate excitotoxicity and other insults in cultured CNS neurons and neurally related cell types. In rodent models of stroke, postinsult treatments with lithium and valproate reduce infarct volume and improve functional outcome. In the QA model of HD, both short- and long-term lithium pretreatments reduce the excitotoxin-induced loss of striatal spiny neurons. *In vitro* studies show that induction of BDNF is a prerequisite for inducing the multiple actions and resultant protective effects. Lithium also has the ability to enhance cell proliferation in neuronal cultures as well as in the vicinity of a brain injury, and this particular action may contribute to its observed neuroprotective effect. In light of the recent evidence showing the loss of neurons and glial cells in discrete brain areas of unipolar and bipolar patients and the possible involvement of glutamate in stress-induced depression, the neuroprotective effects of lithium may be the mechanisms that give clinical relevance to the use of this drug in the treatment of bipolar patients. Moreover, in view of the role that glutamate excitotoxicity plays in the pathophysiology of several neurodegenerative diseases, lithium, valproate, and perhaps other mood stabilizers may be found to have an expanded use in the suppression or prevention of neurodegeneration, in addition to their mainstay use to treat bipolar disorder.

REFERENCES

1. World Health Organization. 2003. World Health Report 2003. WHO. Geneva.
2. Manji, H.K., W.C. Drevets & D.S. Charney. 2001. The cellular neurobiology of depression. Nat. Med. **7:** 541–547.
3. Post, R.M., A.M. Speer, G.V. Obvocea & G.S. Leverich. 2002. Acute and prophylactic effects of anticonvulsants in bipolar depression. Clin. Neurosci. Res. **2:** 228–251.
4. Jope, R.S. 1999. Anti-bipolar therapy: mechanism of action of lithium. Mol. Psychiatry **4:** 117–128.
5. Gao, X-M., F. Fukamauchi & D-M. Chuang. 1993. Long-term biphasic effects of lithium treatment on phospholipase C–coupled m_3-muscarinic acetylcholine receptors in cultured cerebellar granule cells. Neurochem. Int. **22:** 395–403.
6. Ozaki, N. & D-M. Chuang. 1997. Lithium increases transcription factor binding to AP-1 and cyclic AMP response element in cultured neurons and rat brain. J. Neurochem. **69:** 2336–2344.
7. Yuan, J. & B.A. Yankner. 2000. Apoptosis in the nervous system. Nature **407:** 802–829.
8. Friedlander, R.M. 2003. Apoptosis and caspases in neurodegenerative diseases. N. Engl. J. Med. **348:** 1365–1375.
9. Mattson, M.P. & G. Kroemer. 2003. Mitochondria in cell death: novel targets for neuroprotection and cardioprotection. Trends Mol. Med. **9:** 196–205.
10. Nonaka, S., C. Hough & D-M. Chuang. 1998. Chronic lithium treatment robustly protects CNS neurons against excitotoxicity by inhibiting NMDA receptor–mediated calcium influx. Proc. Natl. Acad. Sci. USA **95:** 2642–2647.
11. Chen, R-W. & D-M. Chuang. 1999. Long term lithium treatment suppresses p53 and Bax expression, but increases Bcl-2 expression: a prominent role in neuroprotection against excitotoxicity. J. Biol. Chem. **274:** 6039–6042.

12. CHEN, G., W-Z. ZENG, P-X. YUAN *et al.* 1999. The mood-stabilizing agents lithium and valproate robustly increase the levels of the neuroprotective protein bcl-2 in the CNS. J. Neurochem. **72:** 879–882.
13. CHALECKA-FRANASZEK, E. & D-M. CHUANG. 1999. Lithium activates the serine/threonine kinase Akt-1 and suppresses glutamate-induced inhibition of Akt-1 activity in neurons. Proc. Natl. Acad. Sci. USA **96:** 8745–8750.
14. KLEIN, P.S. & D.A. MELTON. 1996. A molecular mechanism for the effect of lithium on development. Proc. Natl. Acad. Sci. USA **93:** 8455–8459.
15. FINKBEINER, S. 2000. CREB couples neurotrophin signals to survival messages. Neuron **25:** 11–14.
16. KOPNISKY, K.L., E. CHALECKA-FRANASZEK, M. GONZALEZ-ZULUETA & D-M. CHUANG. 2003. Chronic lithium treatment antagonizes glutamine-induced decrease of phosphorylated CREB in neurons by reducing PP1 and increasing MEK activities. Neuroscience **116:** 425–435.
17. MIELKE, K. & T. HERDEGEN. 2000. JNK and p38 stress kinases—degenerative effectors of signal-transduction-cascades in the nervous system. Prog. Neurobiol. **61:** 45–60.
18. CHEN, R-W., Z-H. QIN, M. REN *et al.* 2003. Regulation of c-Jun N-terminal kinase, p38 kinase, and AP-1 DNA binding in cultured brain neurons: roles in glutamate excitation and lithium neuroprotection. J. Neurochem. **84:** 566–575.
19. KANAI, H., A. SAWA, R-W. CHEN *et al.* 2004. Valproic acid inhibits histone deacetylase activity and suppresses excitotoxicity-induced GAPDH nuclear accumulation and apoptotic death in neurons. Pharmacogen. J. **4:** 336–344.
20. CHUANG, D-M., C. HOUGH & V.V. SENATOROV. 2005. Glyceraldehyde-3-phosphate dehydrogenase, apoptosis, and neurodegenerative diseases. Annu. Rev. Pharmacol. Toxicol. **45:** 269–290.
21. PHIEL, C.J., F. ZHANG, E.Y. HUANG *et al.* 2001. Histone deacetylase is a direct target of valproic acid, a potent anticonvulsant, mood stabilizer, and teratogen. J. Biol. Chem. **276:** 36734–36741.
22. GÖTTLICHER, M., S. MINUCCI, P. ZHU *et al.* 2001. Valproic acid defines a novel class of HDAC inhibitors inducing differentiation of transformed cells. EMBO J. **20:** 6969–6978.
23. DREVETS, W.C. 2001. Neuroimaging and neuropathological studies of depression: implications for the cognitive-emotional features of mood disorders. Curr. Opin. Neurobiol. **11:** 240–249.
24. MANJI, H.K., J.A. QUIROZ, J. SPORN *et al.* 2003. Enhancing neuronal plasticity and cellular resilience to develop novel, improved therapeutics for difficult-to-treat depression. Biol. Psychiatry **53:** 707–742.
25. HASHIMOTO, R., C. HOUGH, T. NAKAZAWA *et al.* 2002. Lithium protection against glutamate excitotoxicity in rat cerebral cortical neurons: involvement of NMDA receptor inhibition possibly by decreasing NR2B tyrosine phosphorylation. J. Neurochem. **80:** 589–597.
26. TAKASU, M.A., M.B. DALVA, R.E. ZIGMOND & M.E. GREENBERG. 2002. Modulation of NMDA receptor–dependent calcium influx and gene expression through EphB receptors. Science **295:** 491–495.
27. HASHIMOTO, R., K. FUJIMAKI, M-R. JEONG & D-M. CHUANG. 2003. Lithium-induced inhibition of Src tyrosine kinase in rat cerebral cortical neurons: a role in neuroprotection against *N*-methyl-D-aspartate receptor–mediated excitotoxicity. FEBS Lett. **538:** 145–148.
28. HASHIMOTO, R., N. TAKEI, K. SHIMAZU *et al.* 2002. Lithium induces brain-derived neurotrophic factor and activates TrkB in rodent cortical neurons: an essential step for neuroprotection against glutamate excitotoxicity. Neuropharmacology **43:** 1173–1179.
29. YASUDA, S. & D-M. CHUANG. 2003. Lithium activates promoter III of brain-derived neurotrophic factor (BDNF) gene in rat cortical neurons. Abstract no. 458.2. Thirty-third Annual Meeting: Society for Neuroscience.
30. JEONG, M.R., R. HASHIMOTO, V.V. SENATOROV *et al.* 2003. Valproic acid, a mood stabilizer and anticonvulsant, protects rat cerebral cortical neurons from spontaneous cell death: a role of histone deacetylase inhibition. FEBS Lett. **542:** 74–78.

31. NONAKA, S., N. KATSUBE & D-M. CHUANG. 1998. Lithium protects rat cerebellar granule cells against apoptosis induced by anticonvulsants, phenytoin and carbamazepine. J. Pharmacol. Exp. Ther. **286:** 539–547.
32. HIROI, T., H. WEI, C. HOUGH *et al.* 2005. Protracted lithium treatment protects against the ER stress elicited by thapsigargin in rat PC12 cells: roles of intracellular calcium, GRP78, and Bcl-2. Pharmacogen. J. **5:** 102–111.
33. WEI, H., P.R. LEEDS, Y. QIAN *et al.* 2000. β-Amyloid peptide–induced death of PC 12 cells and cerebellar granule cell neurons is inhibited by long-term lithium treatment. Eur. J. Pharm. **392:** 117–123.
34. PHIEL, C.J., C.A. WILSON, V.M.Y. LEE & P.S. KLEIN. 2003. GSK-3 alpha regulates production of Alzheimer's disease amyloid-beta peptides. Nature **423:** 435–439.
35. CHUANG, D-M. & C. HOUGH. 2003. Neuroprotection against apoptosis: what has it got to do with the mood stabilizer lithium? *In* Molecular Mechanisms of Programmed Cell Death, pp. 145–154. Kluwer Academic/Plenum. New York.
36. JOPE, R.S. & G.N. BIJUR. 2002. Mood stabilizers, glycogen synthase kinase-3 beta, and cell survival. Mol. Psychiatry **7**(suppl. 1): S35–S45.
37. LENOX, R.H. & L. WANG. 2003. Molecular basis of lithium action: integration of lithium-responsive signaling and gene expression networks. Mol. Psychiatry **8:** 135–144.
38. ROWE, M. & D-M. CHUANG. 2004. Lithium neuroprotection: molecular mechanisms and clinical implications. Exp. Rev. Mol. Med. **6:** 1–18.
39. NONAKA, S. & D-M. CHUANG. 1998. Neuroprotective effects of chronic lithium on focal cerebral ischemia in rats. NeuroReport **9:** 2081–2084.
40. WEI, H., Z-H. QIN, V. SENATOROV *et al.* 2001. Lithium suppresses excitotoxicity-induced striatal lesions in a rat model of Huntington's disease. Neuroscience **106:** 603–612.
41. SENATOROV, V.V., M. REN, H. KANAI *et al.* 2004. Short-term lithium treatment promotes neuronal survival and proliferation in rat striatum infused with quinolinic acid, an excitotoxic model of Huntington's disease. Mol. Psychiatry **9:** 371–385.
42. XU, J.H., J. CULMAN, A. BLUME *et al.* 2003. Chronic treatment with a low dose of lithium protects the brain against ischemic injury by reducing apoptotic death. Stroke **34:** 1287–1292.
43. REN, M., V.V. SENATOROV, R-W. CHEN & D-M. CHUANG. 2003. Post-insult treatment with lithium reduces brain damage and facilitates neurological recovery in a rat ischemia/reperfusion model. Proc. Natl. Acad. Sci. USA **100:** 6210–6215.
44. RAJDEV, S., K. HARA, Y. KOKUBO *et al.* 2000. Mice overexpressing rat heat shock protein 70 are protected against cerebral infarction. Ann. Neurol. **47:** 782–791.
45. BIJUR, G.N. & R.S. JOPE. 2000. Opposing actions of phosphatidylinositol 3-kinase and glycogen synthase kinase-3 in the regulation of HSF-1 activity. J. Neurochem. **75:** 2401–2408.
46. REN, M., Y. LENG, M.R. JEONG *et al.* 2004. Valproic acid reduces brain damage induced by transient focal cerebral ischemia in rats: potential roles of histone deacetylase inhibition and heat shock protein induction. J. Neurochem. **89:** 1358–1367.
47. HICKEY, M.A. & M.F. CHESSELET. 2003. Apoptosis in Huntington's disease. Prog. Neuro-Psychopharm. Biol. Psychiatry **27:** 255–265.
48. CATTANEO, E., D. RIGAMONTI, D. GOFFREDO *et al.* 2001. Loss of normal huntingtin function: new developments in Huntington's disease research. Trends Neurosci. **24:** 182–188.
49. SCHWARCZ, R. & R. PELLICCIARI. 2002. Manipulation of brain kynurenines: glial targets, neuronal effects, and clinical opportunities. J. Pharmacol. Exp. Ther. **303:** 1–10.
50. CHEN, G., G. RAJKOWSKA, F. DU *et al.* 2000. Enhancement of hippocampal neurogenesis by lithium. J. Neurochem. **75:** 1729–1734.
51. HASHIMOTO, R., V.V. SENATOROV, H. KANAI *et al.* 2003. Lithium stimulates progenitor proliferation in cultured brain neurons. Neuroscience **117:** 55–61.

Circulatory Arrest as a Model for Studies of Global Ischemic Injury and Neuroprotection

LARS WIKLUND,[a] HARI SHANKER SHARMA,[a] AND SAMAR BASU[b]

[a]*Department of Surgical Sciences/Anesthesiology and Intensive Care Medicine,*
[b]*Department of Public Health and Caring Sciences/Geriatrics/Clinical Nutrition,*
Uppsala University Hospital, SE-751 85 Uppsala, Sweden

ABSTRACT: Despite many programs aimed at better immediate care of cardiac arrest victims, the subsequent mortality rate is high, with myocardial and central nervous system (CNS) injuries as the most common causes of death. Preclinical research is badly needed to produce a sound base for future clinical trials and possible improvements in clinical outcome. In our laboratory, we use piglets weighing approximately 25 kg. Ventricular fibrillation is produced by an AC current and left without treatment for 8–12 min, after which cardiopulmonary resuscitation according to current human guidelines is undertaken. The heart is then defibrillated and restoration of spontaneous circulation induced. During the procedure, blood pressure and flow measurements are obtained in the systemic, pulmonary, and cerebral circulation. Peroxidation and inflammation are monitored by systemic and cerebral venous plasma concentrations of isoprostane (8-iso-$PGF_{2\alpha}$), an indicator of oxidative damage, and prostaglandin $F_{2\alpha}$ metabolite (15-keto-dihydro-$PGF_{2\alpha}$), an indicator of cyclooxygenase-2 activity, respectively. Neurocellular damage is monitored by the jugular plasma concentration of protein S-100β. Neurological outcome is assessed at >24 h after the incident. Our results show that plasma concentrations of 8-iso-$PGF_{2\alpha}$ are greater after more extended periods of ischemia. PBN (α-phenyl-*N*-tert-butyl nitrone), a so-called spin-trap scavenger, has a neuroprotective effect since neurological outcome is enhanced, and the 8-iso-$PGF_{2\alpha}$ concentration is decreased during reperfusion. Use of water-soluble sulfonated PBN (S-PBN) results in better autoregulation of cerebral cortical blood flow and less peroxidation of CNS lipids during reperfusion. These observations suggest that our model can be used to explore neuroprotective effects of potential therapeutic agents.

KEYWORDS: cardiac arrest; cerebral protection; neurological deficit; neurological pathology; oxidative stress; inflammation

INTRODUCTION

Cardiovascular disease is one of the major causes of death in the Western world and afflicts approximately 100 per 100,000 inhabitants annually. In Sweden, with a

Address for correspondence: Lars Wiklund, M.D., Ph.D., Professor of Anesthesiology and Intensive Care Medicine, Department of Surgical Sciences/Anesthesiology and Intensive Care Medicine, Uppsala University Hospital, SE-751 85 Uppsala, Sweden. Voice: +46-18-6114851; fax: +46-18-559357.
lars.wiklund@surgsci.uu.se

Ann. N.Y. Acad. Sci. 1053: 205–219 (2005). © 2005 New York Academy of Sciences.
doi: 10.1196/annals.1344.019

population of 9 million inhabitants, approximately 15,000 persons die each year due to cardiovascular disease, two-thirds of whom suffer cardiac arrest outside of a hospital. About 2000 of these out-of-hospital patients undergo cardiopulmonary resuscitation (CPR) by ambulance staff when they arrive on the scene. Upon arrival at the hospital, 15–50% of these patients are still alive, but only 5% are alive at 1 month after their cardiac arrest.[1,2] In spite of major efforts to improve these results, little has happened during the past 25 years. It is commonly agreed that the human brain cannot survive much more than 5 min of normothermic untreated circulatory arrest. Recent statistics from Sweden[2] reveal that the median time from witnessed arrest to alarm is 3–4 min, and there is a median time of 4–10 min from arrest to ambulance arrival and 6–10 min from alarm to defibrillation, indicating that only a minority of out-of-hospital patients are within reach of effective treatment. Twenty-five percent of cardiac arrests strike patients between 20 and 60 years of age. Similar data are available from most Western countries, necessitating improvements in care such as through pharmacological augmentation of central nervous system (CNS) tolerance for anoxia and its consequences.

The aim of our investigations was to use the porcine cardiac arrest model to study CNS effects of global ischemia, the pathophysiology leading to neurological damage, and possibilities for enhancing neurological function after cardiac arrest and subsequent CPR.

OUTLINE OF THE METHODOLOGY

In the experimental investigations described, piglets of approximately 25 kg body weight and 10 weeks of age were used after approval from the local Institutional Review Board. They were anesthetized by intramuscular injection of 6 mg/kg of Zoletil® and 2 mg/kg of Rompun® in combination with an intravenous (iv) injection of 7 mg/kg of thiopental supplemented by iv injection of 100 mg of morphine. Anesthesia was maintained by iv continuous administration of 4 mg/kg/h of pentobarbital. During preparation, nitrous oxide was used. Where applicable, catheters were inserted in a small branch of the carotid artery, the external jugular vein, the pulmonary artery, the internal jugular vein, and a superior sagittal vein. Pressures were registered in the arterial, pulmonary arterial, right atrial, sinus sagittal, and intracranial compartments. Blood flow in the aorta, carotid, and pulmonary arteries was measured by ultrasonic flowmetry. Cerebral cortical blood flow was determined by laser-Doppler flowmetry. Acid-base status and blood gases were determined in arterial, internal jugular, sagittal sinus, and mixed venous blood. Cerebral tissue pH and PCO_2 were also determined. Ventilation was adjusted to maintain a normal $PaCO_2$. After preparation and discontinuation of nitrous oxide and a resting period of 1 h, control measurements were performed. Thereafter, ventricular fibrillation, that is, circulatory arrest defined as a typical EKG with loss of systolic blood pressure, was induced by a transthoracic alternating current of 40–60 volts. This circulatory arrest received no treatment for a period of 2 to 15 min, according to the protocol in the specific investigation. Thereafter, ventilation with 100% oxygen and thoracic compressions were administered using a mechanical hand-driven compressor (Rentsch Cardiac Press Device) (80 compressions/min) or, later, an automatic pneumatic compressor (Lucas®) (100 compressions/min) for 8–15 min according to the specific study protocol. The pigs were ventilated with pure oxygen during CPR and during the early reperfusion phase, after which the oxygen concentration was reduced to 30%. After the scheduled circulatory arrest, the heart was defibrillated. A maximum of 5 min was allowed for regaining spontaneous circulation. Restoration of spontaneous circulation (ROSC) was defined as a pulsatile cardiac rhythm with a systolic

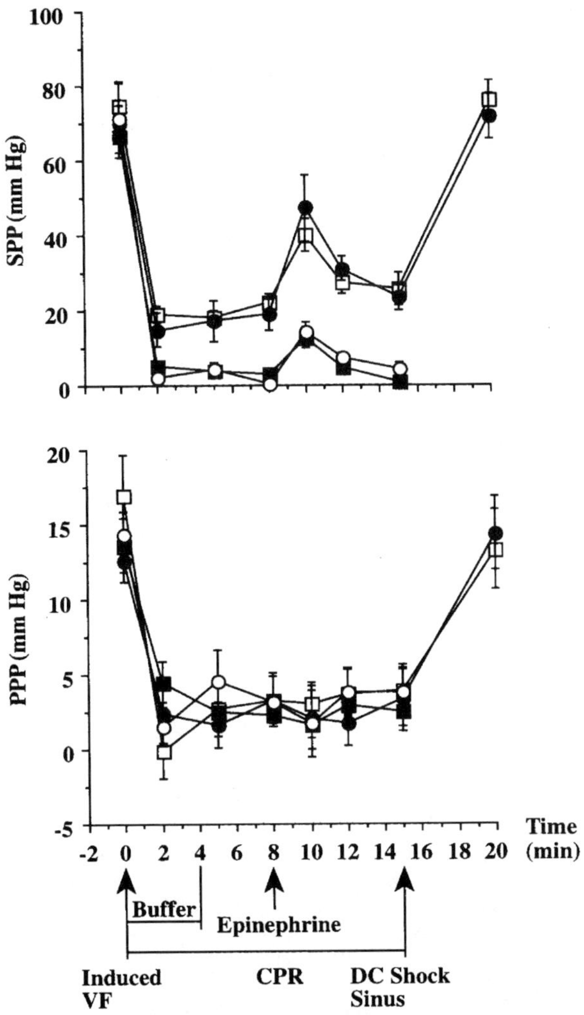

FIGURE 1. Systemic perfusion pressure (SPP) (*top*) and pulmonary perfusion pressure (PPP) (*bottom*) before, during, and after cardiopulmonary resuscitation (CPR) expressed as mean values ± SEM in the open-chest CPR groups (*open squares* and *solid circles*) and in the closed-chest CPR groups (*solid squares* and *open circles*). SPP was significantly higher during open-chest CPR. There was no statistical difference in PPP between the groups. VF, ventricular fibrillation; DC, direct current. Courtesy of ref. 7.

blood pressure of at least 60 mmHg. The follow-up time after ROSC varied from 4 to 30 h. Neurological outcome was determined by the neurological deficit score and the overall performance categorization[3] at 24 h after the incident, where applicable.

At the end of the experiment, after termination of the experimental protocol and after potassium chloride–induced circulatory arrest, Evans blue dye was administered, the skull was opened, and the brain taken out. The brains were immersed in 4% buffered formalin and stored at room temperature for 1 week. Coronal sections (3 to 5 mm thick) of the pig brain (one cerebral hemisphere) were made and photographed. Small tissue pieces ($<3 \times 5$ mm) from the parietal, temporal, occipital, and pyriform cortices were dissected out. In addition, portions of thalamus (median thalamus) and brain stem were also taken out. These tissue pieces were dehydrated in a graded series of alcohol, rinsed in xylene, and embedded in low-temperature paraffin (56–58°C) according to standard protocol.[4] About 3- to 5-µm-thick multiple sections (6 to 8) were cut from each tissue block and collected on glass slides. After deparaffinization, duplicate sections were stained with either Nissl (cresyl violet) or hematoxylin and eosin stain using a commercial protocol.[4]

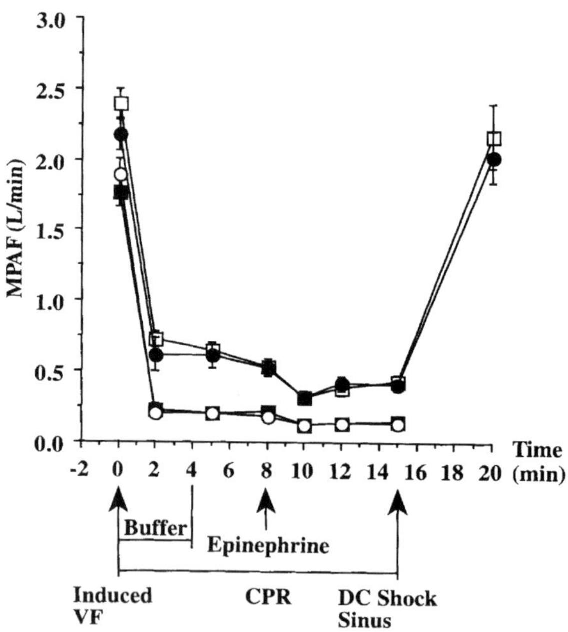

FIGURE 2. Mean pulmonary arterial blood flow (cardiac output) (MPAF) before, during, and after cardiopulmonary resuscitation (CPR) expressed as mean values ± SEM in the open-chest CPR groups (*open squares* and *solid circles*) and in the closed-chest CPR groups (*solid squares* and *open circles*). MPAF was significantly higher during open-chest CPR. VF, ventricular fibrillation; DC, direct current. Courtesy of ref. 7.

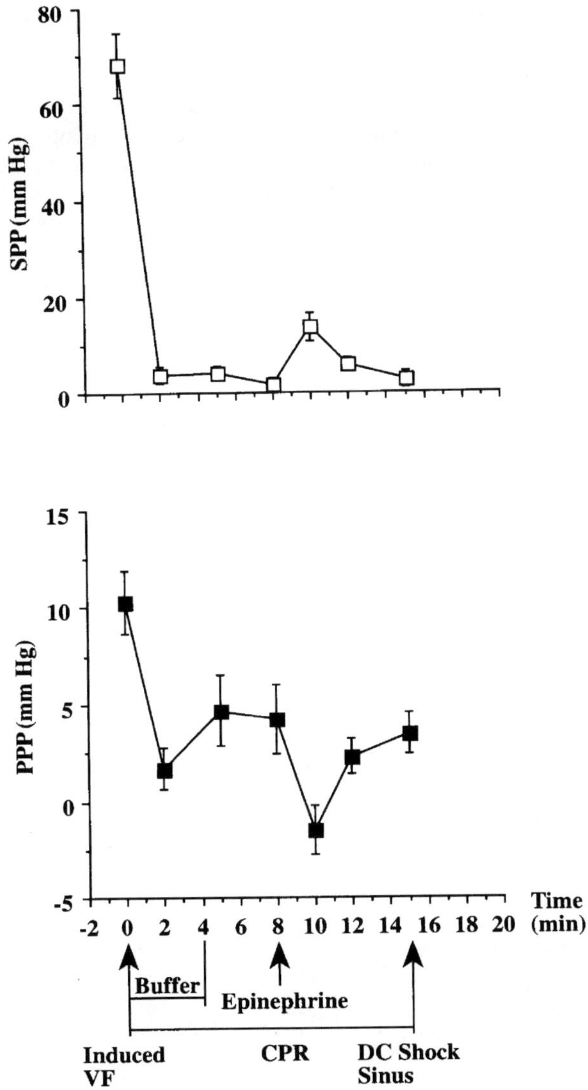

FIGURE 3. Systemic perfusion pressure (SPP) (*open squares*) (*top*) and pulmonary perfusion pressure (PPP) (*solid squares*) (*bottom*) before and during cardiopulmonary resuscitation (CPR). Values are expressed as mean ± SEM. Two min after the administration of epinephrine, SPP significantly increased, while PPP decreased. VF, ventricular fibrillation; DC, direct current. Courtesy of ref. 7.

RESULTS AND COMMENTS

As it has been demonstrated that human brain function is dependent upon its nutrient blood flow, delivery of oxygen, and elimination of carbon dioxide, much of the effort to improve neurological outcome after cardiac arrest has focused on the possibilities of increasing systemic and cerebral blood flow (CBF) during CPR.[5,6] Thus, the magnitude and mechanism for generation of the blood flow have been of considerable interest. Through comparison of open-chest and closed-chest CPR, it was demonstrated[7] that the systemic perfusion pressure during open-chest CPR was considerably greater than that during closed-chest CPR, and in both cases this perfusion pressure was increased by administration of epinephrine (FIG. 1). In contrast, the pulmonary arterial blood flow, that is, the cardiac output, during CPR as well as the pulmonary perfusion pressure were decreased by epinephrine administration (FIGS. 2 and 3). This seems to be an adequate explanation as to why open-chest cardiac resuscitation, for example, during cardiac surgery, results in so much better survival than closed-chest CPR. Arterial carbon dioxide (CO_2) elimination was shown to correlate well with cardiac output.[8] The need for effective reperfusion after ROSC has received even more emphasis,[5] and we were therefore surprised to find that large or repeated dosages of epinephrine actually decreased the cerebral cortical blood flow in the period before as well as after ROSC.[9] Thus, alternatives to epinephrine could be less harmful. Occlusion of the abdominal aorta by means of an aortic occlusion catheter, thereby increasing myocardial and carotid blood flow, proved to be such a method.[10,11] This method in combination with aortic adminis-

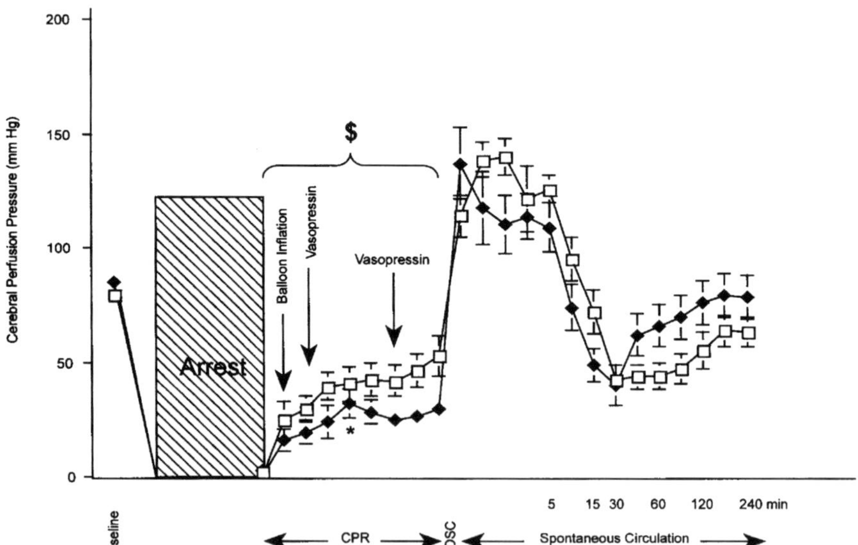

FIGURE 4. Cerebral perfusion pressure (mmHg) at baseline, during closed-chest CPR, and after restoration of spontaneous circulation (ROSC). All values expressed as mean ± SEM. ◆ = group given intravenous vasopressin; □ = group given intra-aortic vasopressin above abdominal aortic occlusion; $ = significant difference between the groups. Courtesy of ref. 20.

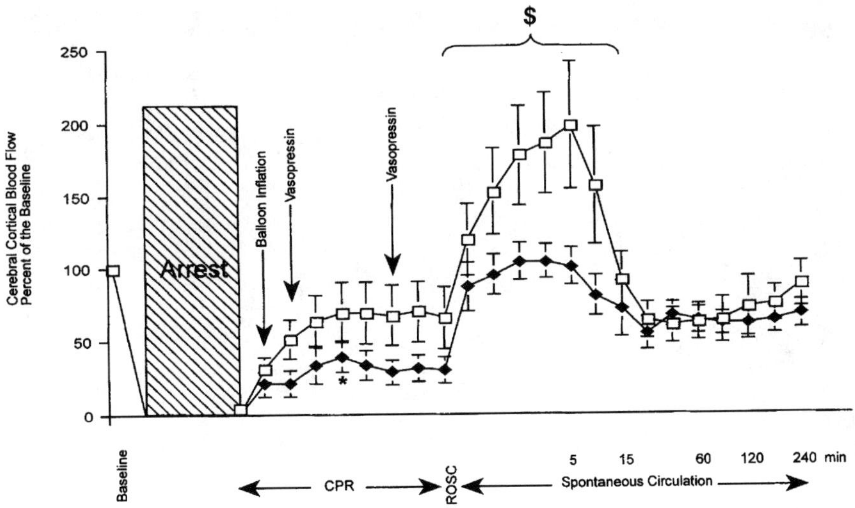

FIGURE 5. Cerebral cortical blood flow as a fraction of the steady-state baseline level. All values expressed as mean ± SEM. ◆ = group given intravenous vasopressin; □ = group given intra-aortic vasopressin above abdominal aortic occlusion; $ = significant difference between the groups. Courtesy of ref. 20.

tration of vasopressin enhanced not only the cerebral perfusion pressure, but also the cerebral cortical blood flow and the cerebral elimination of CO_2 (FIGS. 4 and 5), especially during the reperfusion phase subsequent to cardiac arrest.[11] Vasopressin administered intravenously had previously been proven to exert a hypertensive effect similar to that of epinephrine,[12,13] though with a longer duration,[14] in experimental models, but in a subsequent multicenter clinical trial it resulted in only marginally better survival.[15] However, we consider these results to be due to shortcomings in this particular trial, which also included unwitnessed arrests, regarding the way in which CPR was delivered.[16,17] Maximization of CBF as well as its distribution[18] are still desirable goals, and expansion of the plasma volume has thus been tried with some success, especially with respect to CBF.[19,20] Further enhancement of CBF can be achieved by the use of automatic mechanical compression of the thoracic cage.[21–23]

Pigs subjected to a 5-min survival after cardiac arrest showed a mild to moderate degree of nerve cell damage in the cortical regions that also exhibited extravasation of Evans blue dye (FIG. 6a). Moderate to severe nerve cell damage was also present in the subcortical regions, for example, the mid-thalamic nuclei and the brain stem reticular formation. The magnitude of nerve cell damage was most pronounced in the brain stem region. In the cortex, sporadic nerve cell damage was observed in cortical cell layers III to IV. The other cellular layers in the same cortical region contained normal nerve cells (FIG. 6b).

The pathological studies of ischemic damage can encompass possibilities of determining how this injury arises. In most reviews of this field, the effects of the reactive oxygen and nitrogen species are considered of importance. During the reperfusion phase in particular, the action of these compounds is regarded as crucial. However, a difficulty related to assessing the pathophysiology of reperfusion injury

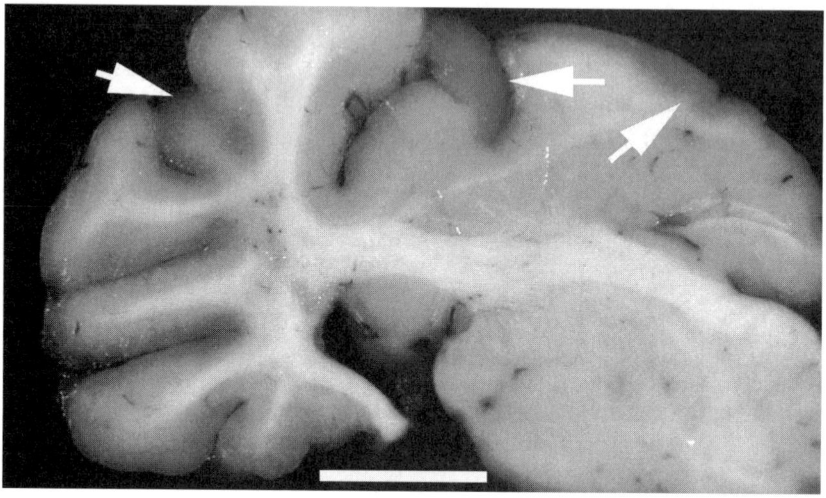

FIGURE 6a. Coronal section of the pig brain passing through parietal cerebral cortex shows extravasation of Evans blue in some parts of the cortex (*arrows*). The animal was allowed to survive 5 min after the cardiac arrest. Bar: 3 mm.

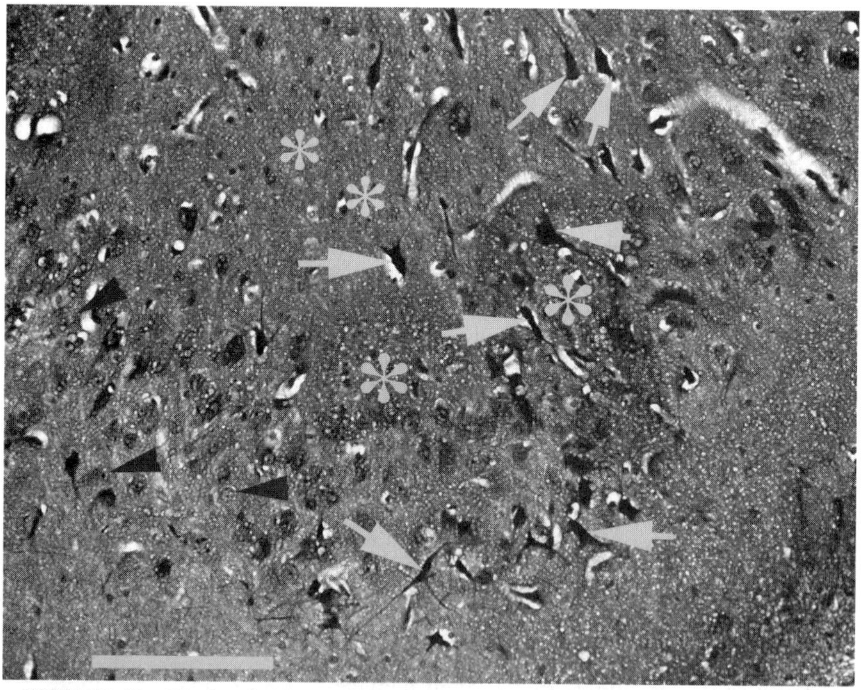

FIGURE 6b. Nissl-stained, paraffin section (3 μm thick) from pig brain obtained from the parietal cerebral cortex region in the vicinity of Evans blue extravasation. Many dark and distorted nerve cells (*arrows*) are seen in deeper layers of the cortex. Some normal nerve cells (*arrowheads*) are also seen in the periphery. Sponginess and edema (*) are clearly evident. Bar: 50 μm.

has been the great limitations in the current practice of *in vivo* measurements of free radical concentrations or the generation of stable end products after free radical oxidation of CNS lipids. In order to circumvent this problem, we have developed methods for determination of nonenzymatic free radicals and enzymatic (cyclooxygenase catalyzed) products of lipid peroxidation (8-iso-PGF$_{2\alpha}$ and 15-keto-dihydro-PGF$_{2\alpha}$, respectively).[24] We were able to demonstrate that both these processes were more active in the CNS than in the rest of the body (FIGS. 7 and 8).[24]

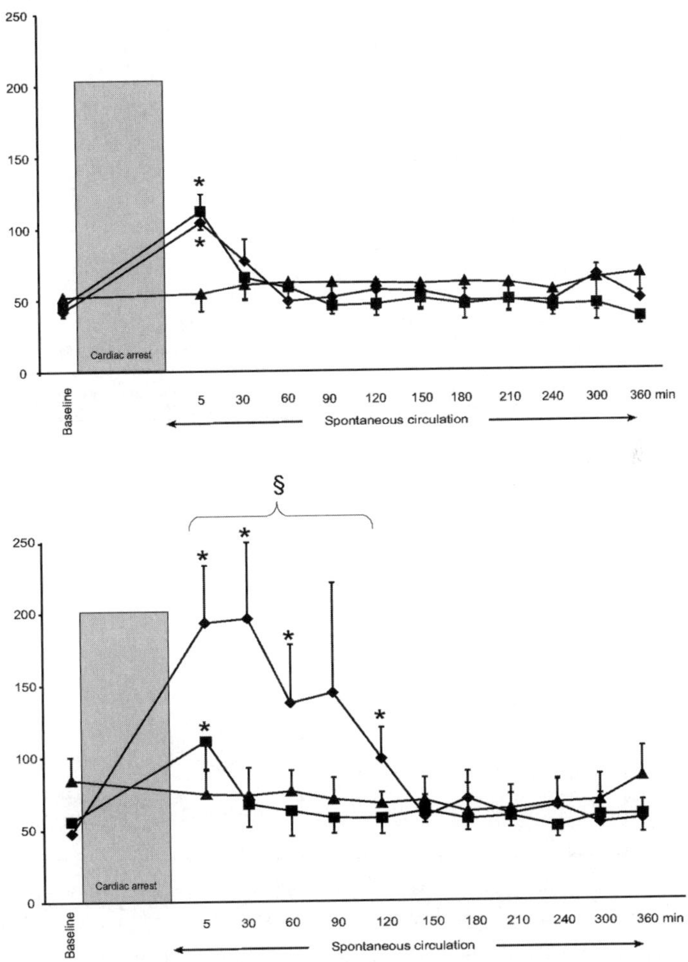

FIGURE 7. Mixed venous plasma levels of 8-iso-PGF$_{2\alpha}$ at baseline (before induction of cardiac arrest) and after ROSC (*upper panel*). Jugular bulb plasma levels of 8-iso-PGF$_{2\alpha}$ at baseline and after ROSC (*lower panel*). ◆ = group subjected to 5-min cardiac arrest; ■ = group subjected to 2-min cardiac arrest; ▲ = control group not subjected to cardiac arrest; *, significant difference vs. baseline; §, significant difference between group subjected to 5-min cardiac arrest versus other groups. Values expressed as mean ± SEM. Courtesy of ref. 24.

As already stated, it has been claimed that the efficacy of reperfusion is of paramount importance regarding the possibility of mitigating neurological damage after a circulatory arrest.[5,25,26] We therefore undertook a series of experiments where we compared piglets in which reperfusion had been maximized, but where, in addition, one group had received vasopressin instead of epinephrine and PBN (α-phenyl-*N*-

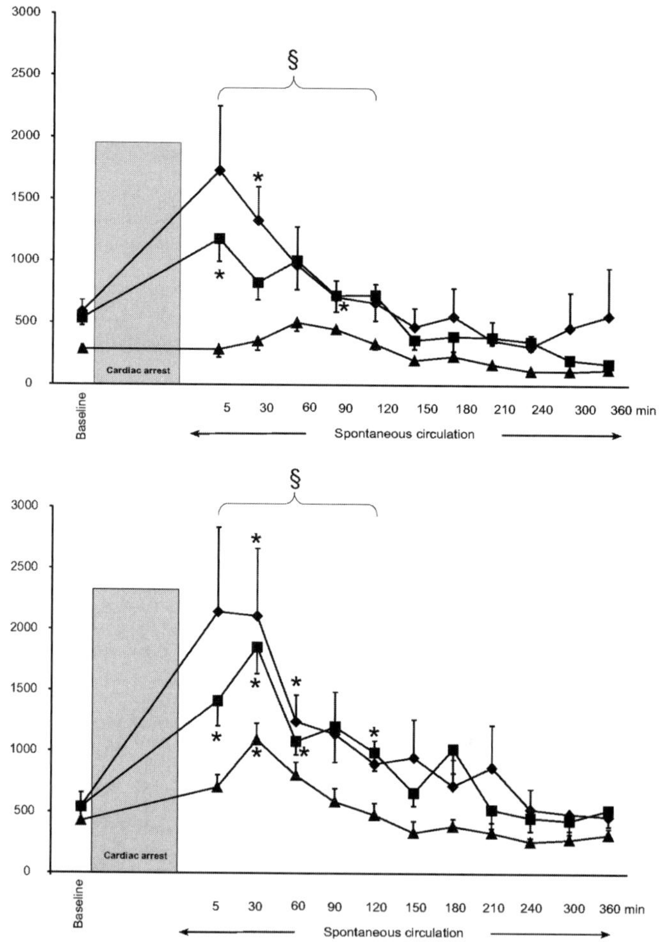

FIGURE 8. Mixed venous plasma levels of 15-keto-dihydro-$PGF_{2\alpha}$ at baseline (before induction of cardiac arrest) and after ROSC (*upper panel*). Jugular bulb plasma levels of 15-keto-dihydro-$PGF_{2\alpha}$ at baseline and after ROSC (*lower panel*). ◆ = group subjected to 5-min cardiac arrest; ■ = group subjected to 2-min cardiac arrest; ▲ = control group not subjected to cardiac arrest; *, significant difference vs. baseline; §, significant difference between group subjected to 5-min cardiac arrest versus other groups. Values expressed as mean ± SEM. Courtesy of ref. 24.

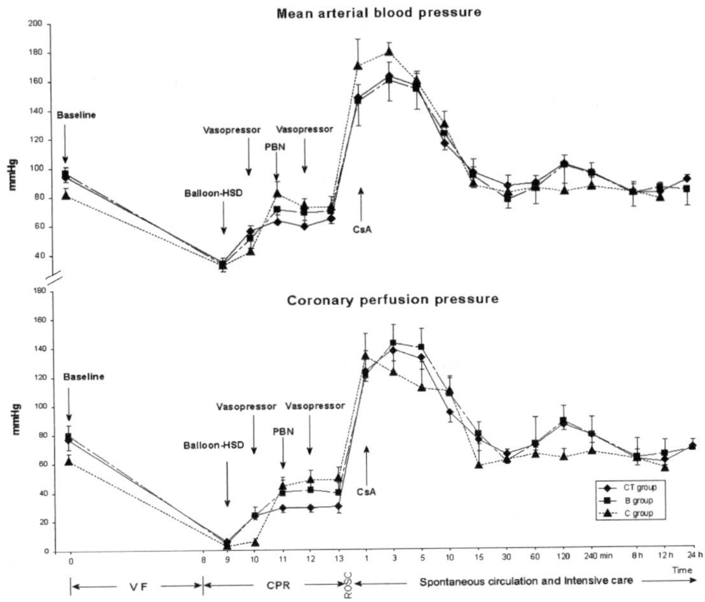

FIGURE 9. Mean arterial blood pressure (mmHg) and coronary perfusion pressure (mmHg) before, during, and after experimental CPR. Results expressed as mean ± SEM. ◆ = group treated with CPR including aortic balloon occlusion, vasopressin, and PBN; ■ = group treated with CPR including aortic balloon occlusion; ▲ = group treated with standard CPR only. Courtesy of ref. 25.

tert-butyl nitrone), a scavenger of the so-called spin-trap type.[25,27] The animals were studied for 24 h after the incident. At that time point, the neurological deficit score was significantly less in those that had received PBN and vasopressin, in spite of equal perfusion pressure in the two groups (FIGS. 9 and 10). In fact, the neurological deficit was somewhat greater in the piglets where reperfusion had been maximized without use of vasopressin and PBN, and worse than that registered in a control group where reperfusion had not been maximized.[25] The mode of action of PBN was elucidated in a subsequent study where the water-soluble and sulfonated derivative of PBN (S-PBN) was administered. It was demonstrated that autoregulation during the reperfusion phase was better preserved when S-PBN was administered than in a group given a weak vasodilator,[27] where autoregulation of cerebral cortical blood flow was not functioning during early reperfusion after ROSC. Thus, our results imply that the jugular bulb plasma concentration of 8-iso-$PGF_{2\alpha}$ (indicating free radical–mediated lipid peroxidation) is proportional to both the duration of ischemia[28] (FIGS. 11 and 12) and the resulting neurological deficit after experimental cardiac arrest and CPR[25] (FIG. 13).

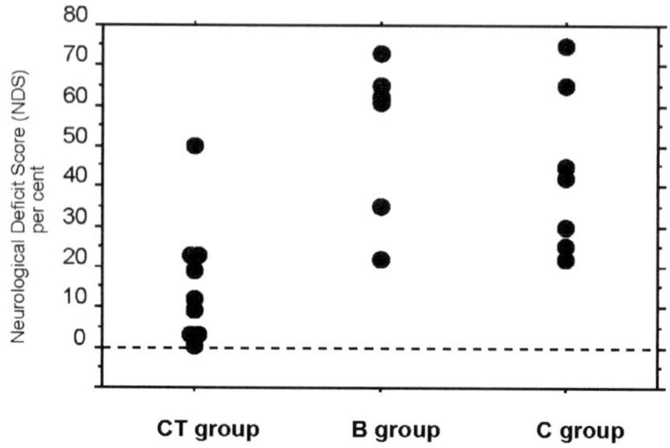

n	9	6	7
Mean	16	53	43
SD	5	8	7
Median	12	61.5	42

FIGURE 10. Neurological deficit score in each of the surviving animals. CT group: group treated with CPR including aortic balloon occlusion, vasopressin, and PBN; B group: group treated with CPR including aortic balloon occlusion; C group: group receiving standard CPR only. Courtesy of ref. 25.

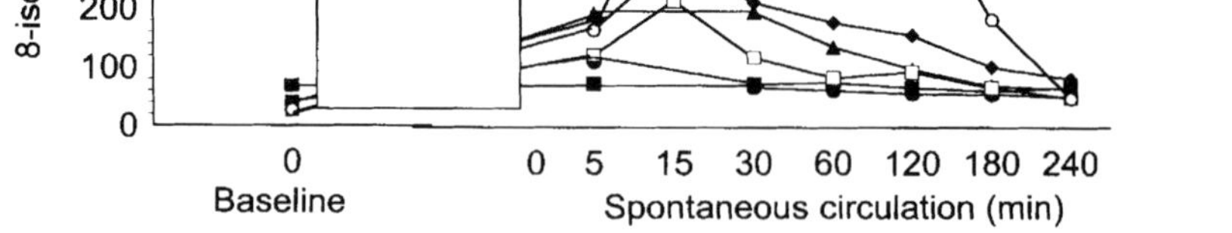

FIGURE 11. Mean jugular bulb plasma levels of 8-iso-PGF$_{2\alpha}$ at baseline and after restoration of spontaneous circulation with various durations of circulatory arrest (VF) and in control animals as defined in the upper right corner. VF2, ventricular fibrillation of 2 min; VF5, ventricular fibrillation of 5 min; VF8, ventricular fibrillation of 8 min; VF10, ventricular fibrillation of 10 min; VF12, ventricular fibrillation of 12 min. Values in animals not subjected to cardiac arrest are described as controls. Courtesy of ref. 28.

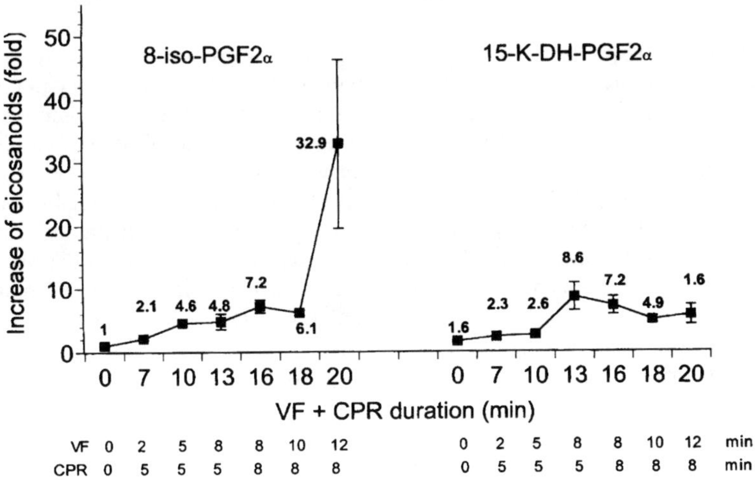

FIGURE 12. Levels of maximum increase (in fold) of plasma eicosanoids compared to baseline (8-iso-PGF$_{2\alpha}$ in *left panel*; 15-keto-dihydro-PGF$_{2\alpha}$ in *right panel*) and the various durations of ventricular fibrillation (VF) and cardiopulmonary resuscitation (CPR). Values in animals not subjected to cardiac arrest (control animals = 0) are set to 1-fold. Actual values of fold-increase are also mentioned adjacent to and together with separate experiments. The y-axis represents the maximum increase of eicosanoids in fold compared to the baseline in various duration groups of VF and CPR. Courtesy of ref. 28.

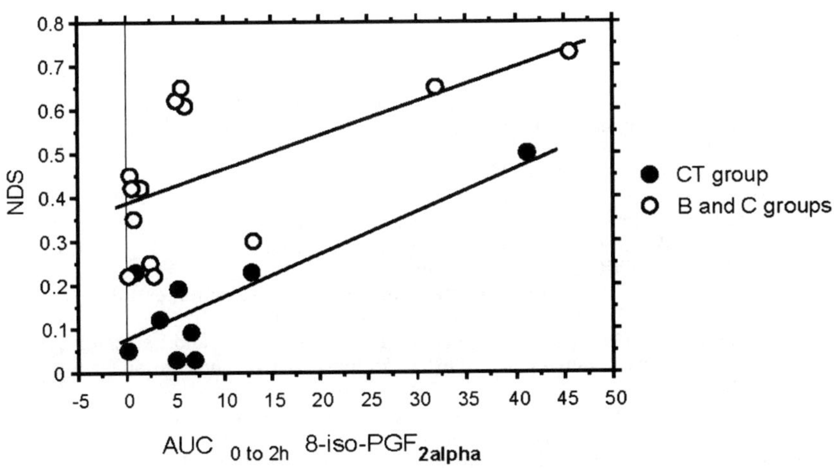

FIGURE 13. Linear correlation between neurologic outcome and 8-iso-PGF$_{2\alpha}$ (AUC) at 0 to 2 h after return of spontaneous circulation (ROSC). ● = group treated with CPR including aortic balloon occlusion, vasopressin, and PBN; ○ = group treated with CPR including aortic balloon occlusion or receiving standard CPR only. Courtesy of ref. 25.

CONCLUSIONS

Restoration of spontaneous circulation (ROSC) can frequently be achieved after up to 15 min or more of normothermic circulatory arrest. Ischemic injury in the porcine brain is observed after 5 min of normothermic circulatory arrest, and 8 min of circulatory arrest results in very pronounced neurological dysfunction and deficit. Maximization of CBF during cardiopulmonary resuscitation and after ROSC does not ameliorate the neurological deficit as observed 24 h after ROSC. In contrast, treatment with PBN seems to reduce the neurological damage considerably, even if administered after the incident. Global cerebral anoxia induced by circulatory arrest in a porcine model seems to be able to produce neuronal damage and severe neurological dysfunction after only 5–8 min of circulatory arrest. This experimental model has also proved to be a sensitive tool for detection and evaluation of therapeutic effects of neuroprotective pharmaceutical agents in general.

ACKNOWLEDGMENTS

We are indebted to all the researchers in the Uppsala CPR group: Sten Rubertsson, Rolf Gedeborg, Erik Edgren, Ala Nozari, Xiaoli Liu, Gunnel Bjerneroth, Adriana Miclescu, Jakob Johansson, Erik Mörtberg, and Johanna Nordmark. Continued financial support over the years from the Laerdal Foundation for Acute Medicine is also gratefully acknowledged.

REFERENCES

1. Fredriksson, M., J. Herlitz & J. Engdahl. 2003. Nineteen years' experience of out-of-hospital cardiac arrest in Gothenburg—reported in Utstein style. Resuscitation **58:** 37–47.
2. Herlitz, J.H.S. 2004. Nationellt register för hjärtstopp utanför sjukhus [National register on cardiac arrests occurring outside hospitals].
3. Bircher, N. & P. Safar. 1985. Cerebral preservation during cardiopulmonary resuscitation. Crit. Care Med. **13:** 185–190.
4. Sharma, H.S. & J. Cervos-Navarro. 1990. Brain oedema and cellular changes induced by acute heat stress in young rats. Acta Neurochir. Suppl. (Wien) **51:** 383–386.
5. Hossmann, K.A. 1988. Resuscitation potentials after prolonged global cerebral ischemia in cats. Crit. Care Med. **16:** 964–971.
6. Hossmann, K.A. 1999. The hypoxic brain: insights from ischemia research. Adv. Exp. Med. Biol. **474:** 155–169.
7. Rubertsson, S., A. Grenvik & L. Wiklund. 1995. Blood flow and perfusion pressure during open-chest versus closed-chest cardiopulmonary resuscitation in pigs. Crit. Care Med. **23:** 715–725.
8. Wiklund, L., D. Soderberg, S. Henneberg *et al.* 1986. Kinetics of carbon dioxide during cardiopulmonary resuscitation. Crit. Care Med. **14:** 1015–1022.
9. Gedeborg, R., H.C. Silander, E. Ronne-Engstrom *et al.* 2000. Adverse effects of high-dose epinephrine on cerebral blood flow during experimental cardiopulmonary resuscitation. Crit. Care Med. **28:** 1423–1430.
10. Gedeborg, R., S. Rubertsson & L. Wiklund. 1999. Improved haemodynamics and restoration of spontaneous circulation with constant aortic occlusion during experimental cardiopulmonary resuscitation. Resuscitation **40:** 171–180.

11. GEDEBORG, R., C.S.H. SILANDER, S. RUBERTSSON *et al.* 2001. Cerebral ischemia in experimental cardiopulmonary resuscitation—comparison of epinephrine and aortic occlusion. Resuscitation **49:** 319–329.
12. LINDNER, K.H., A. BRINKMANN, E.G. PFENNINGER *et al.* 1993. Effect of vasopressin on hemodynamic variables, organ blood flow, and acid-base status in a pig model of cardiopulmonary resuscitation. Anesth. Analg. **77:** 427–435.
13. LINDNER, K.H., B. DIRKS, H.U. STROHMENGER *et al.* 1997. Randomised comparison of epinephrine and vasopressin in patients with out-of-hospital ventricular fibrillation. Lancet **349:** 535–537.
14. NOZARI, A., S. RUBERTSSON & L. WIKLUND. 2001. Differences in the pharmacodynamics of epinephrine and vasopressin during and after experimental cardiopulmonary resuscitation. Resuscitation **49:** 59–72.
15. WENZEL, V., A.C. KRISMER, H.R. ARNTZ *et al.* 2004. A comparison of vasopressin and epinephrine for out-of-hospital cardiopulmonary resuscitation. N. Engl. J. Med. **350:** 105–113.
16. WIK, L., J.O. KRAMER-JOHANSEN, H. MYKLEBUST *et al.* 2005. Quality of cardiopulmonary resuscitation (CPR) performance by ambulance personnel. In press.
17. SUNDE, K., L. WIK & P.A. STEEN. 1997. Quality of mechanical, manual standard, and active compression-decompression CPR on the arrest site and during transport in a manikin model. Resuscitation **34:** 235–242.
18. HOSSMANN, K.A. 1997. Reperfusion of the brain after global ischemia: hemodynamic disturbances. Shock **8:** 95–101 [discussion, pp. 102–103].
19. FISCHER, M., A. DAHMEN, J. STANDOP *et al.* 2002. Effects of hypertonic saline on myocardial blood flow in a porcine model of prolonged cardiac arrest. Resuscitation **54:** 269–280.
20. NOZARI, A., S. RUBERTSSON & L. WIKLUND. 2000. Improved cerebral blood supply and oxygenation by aortic balloon occlusion combined with intra-aortic vasopressin administration during experimental cardiopulmonary resuscitation. Acta Anaesthesiol. Scand. **44:** 1209–1219.
21. WARD, K.R., J.J. MENEGAZZI, R.R. ZELENAK *et al.* 1993. A comparison of chest compressions between mechanical and manual CPR by monitoring end-tidal PCO_2 during human cardiac arrest. Ann. Emerg. Med. **22**(4)**:** 669–674.
22. RUBERTSSON, S.K.R. 2005. Increased cortical cerebral blood flow with LUCAS; a new device for mechanical chest compressions as compared to standard external compressions during experimental cardiopulmonary resuscitation. Resuscitation. In press.
23. STEEN, S., Q. LIAO, L. PIERRE *et al.* 2002. Evaluation of LUCAS, a new device for automatic mechanical compression and active decompression resuscitation. Resuscitation **55:** 285–299.
24. BASU, S., A. NOZARI, X.L. LIU *et al.* 2000. Development of a novel biomarker of free radical damage in reperfusion injury after cardiac arrest. FEBS Lett. **470:** 1–6.
25. LIU, X.L., A. NOZARI, S. BASU *et al.* 2002. Neurological outcome after experimental cardiopulmonary resuscitation: a result of delayed and potentially treatable neuronal injury? Acta Anaesthesiol. Scand. **46:** 537–546.
26. NOZARI, A., S. RUBERTSSON, R. GEDEBORG *et al.* 1999. Maximisation of cerebral blood flow during experimental cardiopulmonary resuscitation does not ameliorate post-resuscitation hypoperfusion. Resuscitation **40:** 27–35.
27. LIU, X.L., L. WIKLUND, A. NOZARI *et al.* 2003. Differences in cerebral reperfusion and oxidative injury after cardiac arrest in pigs. Acta Anaesthesiol. Scand. **47:** 958–967.
28. BASU, S., X. LIU, A. NOZARI *et al.* 2003. Evidence for time-dependent maximum increase of free radical damage and eicosanoid formation in the brain as related to duration of cardiac arrest and cardio-pulmonary resuscitation. Free Radical Res. **37:** 251–256.

Possible Neuroprotective Mechanism of Human Neuroglobin

KEISUKE WAKASUGI,[a,b] CHIHIRO KITATSUJI,[a] AND ISAO MORISHIMA[a]

[a]*Department of Molecular Engineering, Graduate School of Engineering, Kyoto University, Kyoto 615-8510, Japan*

[b]*Precursory Research for Embryonic Science and Technology (PRESTO), Japan Science and Technology Agency (JST), Saitama 332-0012, Japan*

ABSTRACT: Neuroglobin (Ngb) is a newly discovered hexacoordinate globin that is expressed in vertebrate brain and can reversibly bind oxygen. Expression of Ngb increases in response to oxygen deprivation and protects neurons from hypoxia *in vitro* and *in vivo*. Recent work on human Ngb has shed light on the mechanism of this neuroprotection by human Ngb, as discussed in this review. Human ferric Ngb has been found to act as a guanine nucleotide dissociation inhibitor for the α subunit of heterotrimeric G proteins. Moreover, other Ngb-binding proteins also have been identified. These findings suggest that human Ngb may function as a regulator of signal transduction in the brain.

KEYWORDS: neuroglobin (Ngb); protein-protein interaction; oxidative stress; neuroprotection

INTRODUCTION

Neuroglobin (Ngb) is a recently discovered monomeric globin found in the vertebrate brain that has a high affinity for oxygen (O_2).[1,2] Globins are iron porphyrin complex (heme)–containing proteins that bind reversibly to O_2 and, as such, play an important role in respiratory function. The two principal globins that have been described in vertebrates are hemoglobin (Hb) and myoglobin (Mb). Hb is present in red blood cells, where it is responsible for transporting O_2 from the lungs to the tissues, whereas Mb is a monomeric intracellular globin that stores O_2 in muscle tissue and facilitates its diffusion from the periphery of the cell to mitochondria. Although Ngb shares only 21–25% sequence identity with Hb and Mb, the key amino acid residues that are required for Mb and Hb function are conserved.[1] Like Hb and Mb, Ngb can reversibly bind O_2.[1,3,4] The iron atom in the heme prosthetic group of each globin normally exists in either the ferrous (Fe^{2+}) or ferric (Fe^{3+}) redox state. In the absence of exogenous ligands, Hb and Mb are normally pentacoordinated in the ferrous form, leaving the sixth position empty and available to bind exogenous ligands such as O_2, and hexacoordinated in the ferric state, with a water molecule coordinated to the ferric

Address for correspondence: Keisuke Wakasugi, Department of Molecular Engineering, Graduate School of Engineering, Kyoto University, Kyoto 615-8510, Japan. Voice: +81-75-383-2537; fax: +81-75-383-2541.
kei@wakasugi.mbox.media.kyoto-u.ac.jp

**Ann. N.Y. Acad. Sci. 1053: 220–230 (2005). © 2005 New York Academy of Sciences.
doi: 10.1196/annals.1344.020**

iron. By contrast, both the ferric and ferrous forms of Ngb are hexacoordinated to their endogenous protein ligands, namely, proximal His96 and distal His64 residues, and O_2 can displace the distal His64 residue of ferrous Ngb to produce ferrous-O_2 Ngb.[3]

The mammalian brain can consume up to 20% of the total O_2 supply available, even though it constitutes only 2% of total body weight, and it is the most sensitive organ to the effects of tissue hypoxia.[5] Ngb is widely expressed in neurons of the cerebral cortex, hippocampus, thalamus, hypothalamus, cerebellum, and retina, and in the endocrine pancreatic islets of Langerhans.[1,6–8] Recently, it has been suggested that Ngb plays a role in the neuronal response to hypoxia and ischemia.[9,10] Expression of Ngb has been reported to increase in response to neuronal hypoxia *in vitro* and focal cerebral ischemia *in vivo*.[9,10] Neuronal survival after hypoxia was found to be reduced by inhibiting Ngb expression with an antisense oligodeoxynucleotide and enhanced by overexpression of Ngb, supporting the notion that Ngb protects neurons from hypoxic-ischemic insults.[9] Moreover, Ngb has been found to protect the brain from experimentally induced stroke *in vivo*.[10]

Ngb is present in high amounts in the retina.[7] The estimated concentration of Ngb is about 100-fold higher in the retina than in the brain and is in the same range as that of Mb in the muscle.[7] O_2 affinities for Ngb are similar to those observed for Mb and Hb. Therefore, it is possible that Ngb functions as an O_2 carrier in the retina in a manner similar to the way that Mb acts in muscle cells. However, the low concentration (in the micromolar range) of Ngb in other brain tissues perhaps argues against a role for Ngb in storing and carrying significant amounts of O_2. These findings led us to investigate the mechanism by which Ngb affords neuroprotection under oxidative stress conditions such as ischemia and reperfusion. In this review, we summarize recent findings on the novel functions of Ngb.

HUMAN FERRIC NGB AS A NOVEL Gα PROTEIN GUANINE NUCLEOTIDE DISSOCIATION INHIBITOR

Heterotrimeric G Proteins and Their Regulators

To search for homologous proteins with human Ngb, online BLAST searches were performed via the Web site of the National Center for Biotechnology Information. These analyses revealed that human Ngb shares 25–35% amino acid sequence homology with regulators of G protein signaling (RGS) and RGS domains of G protein–coupled receptor kinases (GRKs). Both RGS and GRK proteins are modulators of heterotrimeric G proteins.[11,12] Heterotrimeric G proteins consist of an α subunit (Gα) with GTPase activity and a βγ dimer (Gβγ), and belong to a family of proteins whose signal transduction function depends on the binding of guanine nucleotides.[13–15]

Ligand- or signal-activated G protein–coupled receptors (GPCRs) induce the release of GDP from a Gα subunit, which is followed by the binding of GTP. Binding of GTP to Gα causes conformational changes that result in dissociation of the GTP-bound Gα from both the receptor and the Gβγ dimer. The GTP-bound Gα and Gβγ subunits regulate the activities of different downstream effectors and remain activated until the intrinsic GTPase activity of Gα hydrolyzes GTP to GDP.

Three groups of protein modulators control this cycle of G protein signaling: guanine nucleotide exchange factors (GEFs), which stimulate GDP dissociation and subsequent GTP binding; guanine nucleotide dissociation inhibitors (GDIs), which inhibit GDP dissociation; and GTPase-activating proteins (GAPs), which enhance GTP hydrolysis.[12–17] GPCRs play a role as functional analogues of GEFs,[13–15] whereas RGS proteins act as GAPs for $G\alpha_i$ and $G\alpha_o$ ($G\alpha_{i/o}$).[12]

Human Ferric Ngb Binds to GDP-Bound Gα and Acts as a GDI

Glutathione S-transferase (GST) pull-down assays clarified that human ferric Ngb, which is generated spontaneously as a result of rapid autoxidation, interacts with $G\alpha_{i/o}$, but not with small G proteins such as Ras and Rab3A (FIGS. 1A and 1B). Moreover, the interaction between Ngb and $G\alpha_{i/o}$ has been examined by surface plasmon resonance (SPR) measurements.[18] Human ferric Ngb, but not ferric Mb, was found to bind specifically to immobilized $G\alpha_{i/o}$, whereas ferrous ligand-bound Ngb under normoxia did not bind to $G\alpha_{i/o}$.[18] Coupled with Mg^{2+}, aluminum tetrafluoride (AlF_4^-) can interact with $G\alpha_{i/o}$-bound GDP and mimic GTP, thereby activating $G\alpha_{i/o}$.[13–15] In the presence of Mg^{2+}, GDP, and AlF_4^-, human ferric Ngb

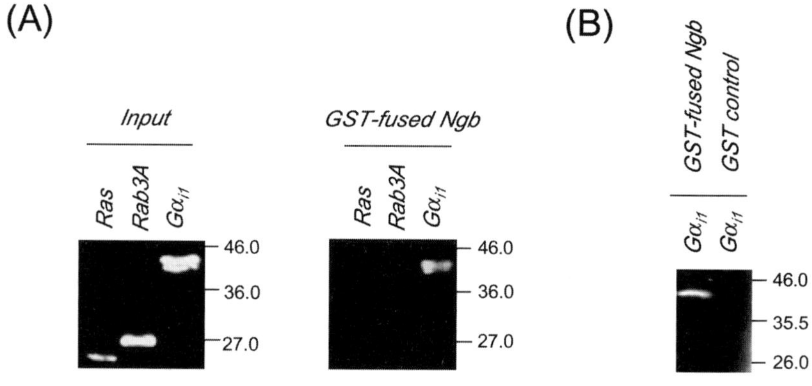

FIGURE 1. Human ferric Ngb interacts with $G\alpha_{i1}$, but not with Ras and Rab3A. Glutathione S-transferase (GST) and a fusion protein of GST and human Ngb were prepared as described previously.[41,49] Rat myristoylated $G\alpha_{i1}$ (Calbiochem, San Diego, CA), human Ras (Calbiochem), or human Rab3A (BIOMOL, Plymouth Meeting, PA) was incubated with either GST alone or GST-fused ferric Ngb immobilized on glutathione sepharose 4B beads (Amersham Biosciences, Buckinghamshire, England) for 1 h at 4°C. The beads were washed extensively three times with buffer (10 mM Hepes, 150 mM NaCl, 0.1% Tween 20, pH 7.4), and the samples were then resuspended in Laemmli sample buffer, heated for 5 min at 95°C, and separated by 12.5% SDS-polyacrylamide gel electrophoresis. For Western blot analyses, the proteins were transferred onto Sequi-Blot™ PVDF membranes (Bio-Rad, Hercules, CA) and incubated with the following primary antibodies: anti-$G\alpha_{i1}$ mouse monoclonal antibody (NeoMarkers, Fremont, CA); anti-Ras mouse monoclonal antibody (Oncogene, San Diego, CA); anti-Rab3A rabbit polyclonal antibody (Calbiochem). After being washed, the membranes were incubated with HRP-linked $F(ab')_2$ fragments of sheep anti-mouse and donkey anti-rabbit Ig (Amersham Biosciences). ECL™ Mini-Camera (Amersham Biosciences) was used. **(A)** GST pull-down assays of $G\alpha_{i1}$, Rab3A, or Ras by using GST-fused ferric Ngb. Western blot analyses of the input samples used for the GST pull-down assays were also performed. Molecular size markers (in kDa) are shown on the right. **(B)** GST pull-down assays of $G\alpha_{i1}$ by using either GST or GST-fused ferric Ngb. Molecular size markers (in kDa) are shown on the right.

did not bind to the activated $G\alpha_{i/o}$,[18] whereas ferric Ngb was found to bind to GDP-bound $G\alpha_{i/o}$.[18] Thus, human ferric Ngb clearly interacts exclusively with the inactive form of $G\alpha_{i/o}$.

Although human ferrous ligand-bound Ngb had no effect on the binding of GTPγS (a nonhydrolyzable analogue of GTP) to $G\alpha_{i/o}$, ferric Ngb inhibited the binding of this analogue.[18] Moreover, in the presence of an excess amount of unlabeled GTP, [^{3}H]GDP release from [^{3}H]GDP-bound $G\alpha_{i/o}$ was inhibited by ferric Ngb.[18] The inhibition of GDP dissociation by ferric Ngb suggests that ferric Ngb diminishes the rates of spontaneous GTPγS binding to $G\alpha_{i/o}$ by blocking the release of GDP. In other words, ferric Ngb functions as a GDI for $G\alpha_{i/o}$. Because human Ngb does not contain the GoLoco motif that is conserved among GDIs for heterotrimeric G proteins, Ngb represents a previously unknown type of GDI for $G\alpha_{i/o}$.

Ngb May Function as an Oxidative Stress–Responsive Sensor for Signal Transduction in the Brain

During ischemia and reperfusion, nitric oxide (NO) is overproduced due to the induction of NO synthetase expression.[19] Reactive oxygen species (ROS), which have been identified as central mediators in certain signaling events, are also generated.[20] The reaction of ferrous-O_2 Hb or Mb with NO and/or ROS converts these proteins to their ferric forms.[21–23] Thus, ferrous-O_2 Ngb may be converted to ferric Ngb during ischemia and reperfusion. In fact, a recent histochemical study has suggested that the Ngb transcript is expressed in brain areas important for adaptive responses to stressful events and that Ngb and NO synthetase are coexpressed.[24]

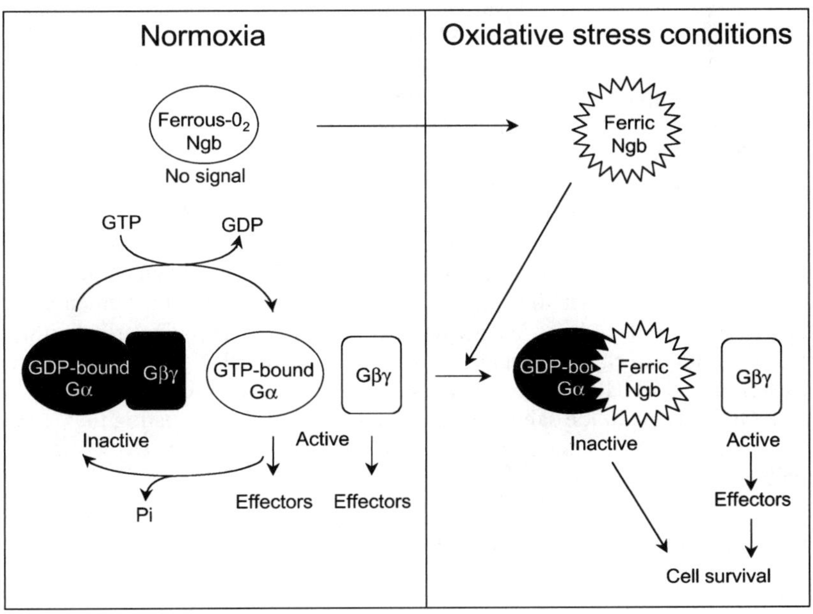

FIGURE 2. Human Ngb as an oxidative stress–responsive sensor for signal transduction in the brain.

$G\alpha_{i/o}$ proteins have been reported to be direct target proteins of ROS generated during ischemia and reperfusion, and to be activated in the absence of GPCR-mediated signaling.[25,26] ROS have been found to modify two cysteine residues of $G\alpha_{i/o}$.[26] The modification of $G\alpha_{i/o}$ by ROS accelerates the release of GDP from $G\alpha_{i/o}$ and increases formation of the GTP-bound form of $G\alpha_{i/o}$ without GPCR activation.[25,26] Moreover, this modification of $G\alpha_{i/o}$ prevents $G\beta\gamma$ from reassociating with the $G\alpha$ subunit and thus leads to enhanced $G\beta\gamma$-dependent signaling. The intracellular signal transduction pathways induced by $G\beta\gamma$ protect cells against oxidative stress:[28–30] for example, $G\beta\gamma$ stimulates proliferation via mitogen-activated protein kinase pathways and promotes cell survival by the activation of phosphatidylinositol-3-kinase.

Our preliminary experiments suggested that human ferric Ngb binds to modified $G\alpha$ as well as to unmodified $G\alpha$, and acts as a GDI that keeps $G\alpha_{i/o}$ in its inactive state. Because inactivation of $G\alpha_{i/o}$ protects neuronal cells against oxidative stress,[27] the function of human Ngb as a GDI for $G\alpha_{i/o}$ will provide an important neuroprotective role. Taking these findings together, human Ngb may function as a novel oxidative stress–responsive regulator for signal transduction in the brain (FIG. 2).

MECHANISM OF Gα REGULATION BY NGB

Investigation of Gα-Binding Sites in Ngb by Exon Swapping

Although Ngb was originally identified in mammalian species, it is also present in nonmammalian vertebrates, including the puffer fish *Tetraodon nigroviridis* and the zebra fish *Danio rerio*.[2,31] Mammalian and fish Ngb proteins share about 50% amino acid sequence identity. Fish Ngb proteins are also hexacoordinated globins with similar oxygen-binding kinetics.[31] The genes of human and zebra fish Ngb are made up of four exons interrupted by three introns, and the exons 1, 2, 3, and 4 correspond to compact structural units, "modules", termed M1, M2, M3, and M4, respectively (FIG. 3).[1,31,32] Recently, we found that zebra fish ferric Ngb does not exhibit GDI activity for $G\alpha_i$.[33]

On the basis of the results of homology searches, the modules M2–M4, but not module M1, of human Ngb share 25–35% amino acid sequence homology with RGS domains.[18] As we have previously shown that module substitution is very useful for designing and producing novel functional proteins,[34–36] we used an exon swapping technique to narrow down the regions that are important in the human-specific contacts between Ngb and $G\alpha$. We prepared a chimeric ZHHH Ngb variant, in which module M1 of human Ngb was replaced with that of zebra fish Ngb, and demonstrated that this chimeric ZHHH Ngb forms almost the same structure as human Ngb and acts as a GDI for $G\alpha$ in the same manner as human Ngb,[33] suggesting that residues in modules M2–M4 of human Ngb are essential for the GDI activity specific to human Ngb.

Investigation of Binding Sites of Ngb with Gα by Site-Directed Mutagenesis

X-ray structural analyses of globins have shown that the CD-D region of human ferric Ngb protrudes from the protein core and exhibits conformational flexibility.[37] In addition, the CD-D region connecting helices C and E of *Vitreoscilla* Hb, which

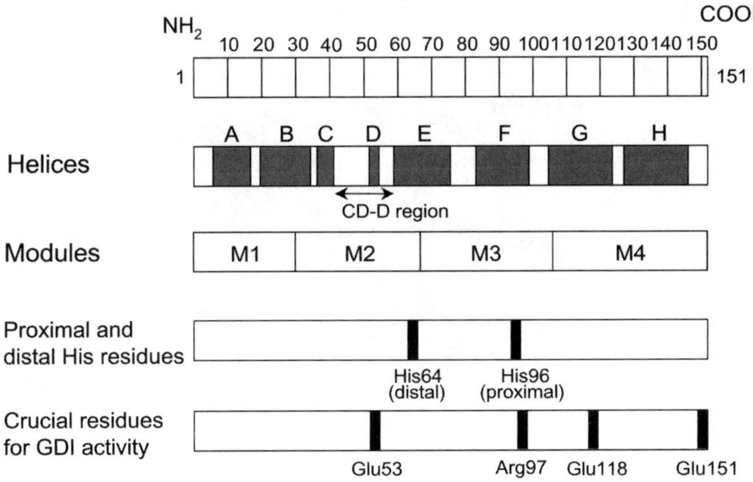

FIGURE 3. Schematic representation of human Ngb. The positions of helices,[37] modules, proximal and distal histidine residues, and crucial residues for its GDI activity[33] are shown. The numbers denote amino acid sequence positions.

is synthesized under hypoxic conditions, is also disordered in the crystal structure.[38] Mutagenesis experiments on this protein have shown that a negatively charged glutamic acid residue in the CD-D region is involved in *Vitreoscilla* Hb binding to a flavin domain of 2,4-dinitrotoluene dioxygenase.[39] Recently, we have demonstrated that a negatively charged residue (Glu53) in the CD-D region of human Ngb is involved in the interaction with Gα (FIG. 3).[33] Moreover, an Ngb double mutant (C55S, C120S) that is linked by an intermolecular disulfide bond at Cys46-Cys46 cannot function as a GDI, whereas its dithiothreitol-reduced monomeric form has GDI activity,[18] suggesting that the CD-D region in which Cys46 is located is important for protein-protein interactions between ferric Ngb and $G\alpha_{i1}$. Thus, it can be speculated that the structural alterations around the CD-D region of Ngb trigger changes in its affinity for binding Gα.

Moreover, to delineate the region within modules M2–M4 of the human Ngb that is responsible for GDI activity, we pinpointed key differences between the human and zebra fish Ngb sequences, with a particular focus on exposed residues with positive or negative charges. Our site-directed mutagenesis experiments verified that some Ngb residues in modules M3–M4 (Arg97, Glu118, and Glu151) are involved in the regulation of Gα by Ngb (FIG. 3).[33] Further tertiary structural analyses clarified that the residues critical for GDI activity in Ngb correspond to residues that are essential for interactions with Gα in RGS domains: in other words, the relative structural positions of Glu53, Arg97, and Glu118 in Ngb are similar to those of Glu83, Arg134, and Glu161 in RGS4 (205-amino-acid protein), respectively (FIGS. 4A and 4B). It has been reported that a mutant of the RGS domain from G protein–coupled receptor kinase 2 (GRK2) can bind to the GDP-bound form of Gα;[40] thus, Ngb may interact with GDP-bound Gα in a manner similar to the interactions of RGS domains.

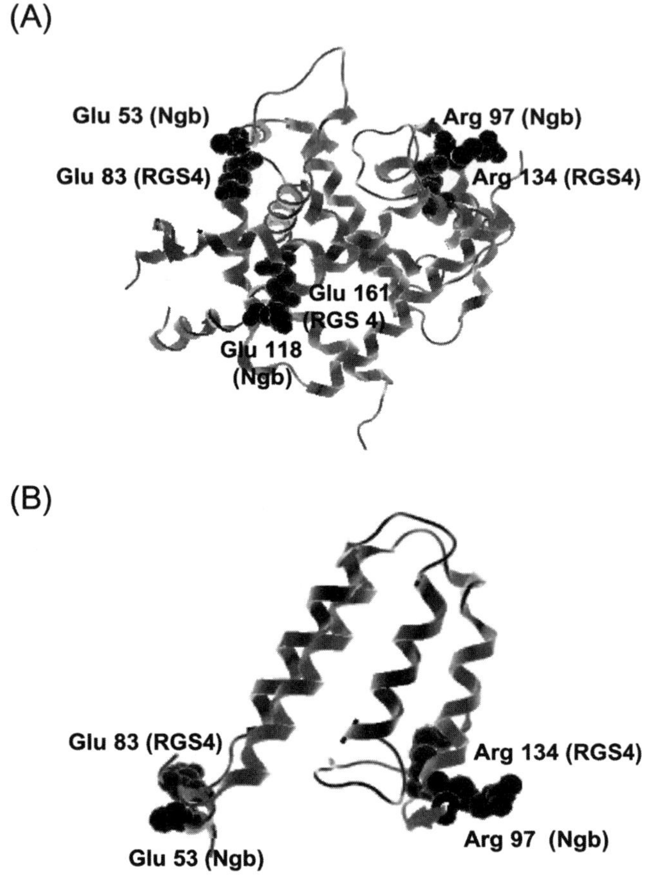

FIGURE 4. **(A)** Comparison of tertiary structure between the residues that are critical for GDI activity in Ngb and the residues that are essential for interacting with Gα in RGS4. **(B)** Partial comparison of the tertiary structure of human Ngb and RGS4.

ASSOCIATION OF NGB WITH FLOTILLIN-1, A LIPID RAFT MICRODOMAIN-ASSOCIATED PROTEIN

To search for proteins that could interact with human Ngb, a yeast two-hybrid analysis was performed in which flotillin-1 was identified as another protein that interacts with Ngb.[41] This interaction was further verified using GST pull-down assays.[41] Flotillin-1, also known as reggie-2,[42] is a component of lipid rafts, which are critical for signal transduction.[43] For example, contained within the lipid rafts of rat brain are heterotrimeric G proteins, Src family protein kinase, and some glycosyl-phosphatidylinositol-anchored proteins.[44] Flotillin-1 has been shown to recruit signaling proteins to lipid rafts, which then mediate the compartmentalization of crucial signal transduction pathways.[45,46] Furthermore, massive intracellular transport of Ngb after its translation has been observed.[7] Because Ngb interacts with Gα, which is also present in lipid rafts,[47,48] flotillin-1 might recruit Ngb to lipid rafts as a means of preventing neuronal death.

NGB INTERACTS WITH CYSTATIN C, A CYSTEINE PROTEINASE INHIBITOR

Cystatin C, a cysteine proteinase inhibitor, has been identified as another human Ngb-binding protein by using a yeast two-hybrid system.[49] SPR experiments verified that human Ngb binds to cystatin C dimers, but not to the monomers.[49] Although cystatin C is known to be a potent endogenous inhibitor of cysteine proteinases such as cathepsin B, H, or L, its precise role in the brain remains unclear. Cystatin C has been reported to be involved in apoptosis induced by oxidative stress in cultured neurons.[50] It has been shown that cathepsin inhibitors can save postischemic CA1 neurons from delayed death and can rescue hippocampal slices from cell death induced by oxygen and/or glucose deprivation.[51,52] Because cystatin C is also an inhibitor of cathepsins, it may be important in preventing neuronal death after severe ischemic damage to the brain through the regulation of cysteine proteinase activity. Further, because oxidative stress rapidly initiates the translocation of cathepsins B and L from lysosomes to the cytosol, owing to injury or rupture of the lysosomal membrane,[53,54] it is possible that cystatin C may be also released from lysosomes into the cytoplasm, where Ngb exists during oxidative stress.

Cystatins are known to function as dimers during intracellular trafficking.[55] Thus, under conditions of oxidative stress, Ngb, by interacting with cystatin C dimers, may modulate intracellular transport or processing through the secretory pathway of cystatin C to protect against neuronal death. Furthermore, an amyloidogenic variant of cystatin C also forms dimers;[56] hence, Ngb may be linked to the development of neurodegenerative diseases.

CONCLUDING REMARKS

In this review, we have highlighted the novel function of Ngb as a regulator of signal transduction. We have demonstrated that human Ngb acts a novel GDI for $G\alpha_{i/o}$ and have identified flotillin-1 and cystatin C as other Ngb-binding proteins. Further studies will be required to elucidate the physiological interactions of Ngb with Gα, flotillin-1, or cystatin C in neurons and to clarify the involvement of Ngb in regulating neuronal death and/or proliferation *in vivo*.

Finally, recent results from Western blot analyses have indicated that the apparent molecular mass of the native Ngb is about 1 kDa larger than that of the recombinant protein,[7,31] implying that Ngb may be posttranslationally modified. Further studies should aim to identify these posttranslational modifications of Ngb and to clarify how they influence the regulation of protein-protein interactions of Ngb. Such research will shed further light on the physiological functions of Ngb and will aid the development of pharmaceutical drugs such as neuroprotective agents.

ACKNOWLEDGMENTS

This work was supported in part by Grants-in-Aid 13780532 and 15770085 for Young Scientists (B) (to K. Wakasugi), Grant-in-Aid 12215077 for Scientific Research on Priority Areas (to K. Wakasugi), and Grant-in-Aid 12002008 for Specially Promoted Research (to I. Morishima) from the Ministry of Education, Culture, Sports, Science, and Technology of Japan, as well as by the Kowa Life Science Foundation (to K. Wakasugi).

REFERENCES

1. Burmester, T., B. Weich, S. Reinhardt & T. Hankeln. 2000. A vertebrate globin expressed in the brain. Nature **407:** 520–523.
2. Awenius, C., T. Hankeln & T. Burmester. 2001. Neuroglobins from the zebrafish *Danio rerio* and the pufferfish *Tetraodon nigroviridis*. Biochem. Biophys. Res. Commun. **287:** 418–421.
3. Dewilde, S., L. Kiger, T. Burmester *et al.* 2001. Biochemical characterization and ligand binding properties of neuroglobin, a novel member of the globin family. J. Biol. Chem. **276:** 38949–38955.
4. Trent, J.T., R.A. Watts & M.S. Hargrove. 2001. Human neuroglobin, a hexacoordinate hemoglobin that reversibly binds oxygen. J. Biol. Chem. **276:** 30106–30110.
5. Erecińska, M. & I.A. Silver. 2001. Tissue oxygen tension and brain sensitivity to hypoxia. Respir. Physiol. **128:** 263–276.
6. Geuens, E., I. Brouns, D. Flamez *et al.* 2003. A globin in the nucleus. J. Biol. Chem. **278:** 30417–30420.
7. Schmidt, M., A. Giel, T. Laufs *et al.* 2003. How does the eye breathe? Evidence for neuroglobin-mediated oxygen supply in the mammalian retina. J. Biol. Chem. **278:** 1932–1935.
8. Laufs, T.L., S. Wystub, S. Reuss *et al.* 2004. Neuron-specific expression of neuroglobin in mammals. Neurosci. Lett. **362:** 83–86.
9. Sun, Y., K. Jin, X.O. Mao *et al.* 2001. Neuroglobin is up-regulated by and protects neurons from hypoxic-ischemic injury. Proc. Natl. Acad. Sci. USA **98:** 15306–15311.
10. Sun, Y., K. Jin, A. Peel *et al.* 2003. Neuroglobin protects the brain from experimental stroke *in vivo*. Proc. Natl. Acad. Sci. USA **100:** 3497–3500.
11. Pitcher, J.A., N.J. Freedman & R.J. Lefkowitz. 1998. G protein–coupled receptor kinases. Annu. Rev. Biochem. **67:** 653–692.
12. Zheng, B., L. De Vries & M.G. Farquhar. 1999. Divergence of RGS proteins: evidence for the existence of six mammalian RGS subfamilies. Trends Biochem. Sci. **24:** 411–414.
13. Gilman, A.G. 1987. G proteins: transducers of receptor-generated signals. Annu. Rev. Biochem. **56:** 615–649.
14. Hepler, J.R. & A.G. Gilman. 1992. G proteins. Trends Biochem. Sci. **17:** 383–387.
15. Sprang, S.R. 1997. G protein mechanisms: insights from structural analysis. Annu. Rev. Biochem. **66:** 639–678.
16. Siderovski, D.P., M.A. Diversé-Pierluissi & L. De Vries. 1999. The GoLoco motif: a $G\alpha_{i/o}$ binding motif and potential guanine-nucleotide-exchange factor. Trends Biochem. Sci. **24:** 340–341.
17. Willard, F.S., R.J. Kimple & D.P. Siderovski. 2004. Return of the GDI: the GoLoco motif in cell division. Annu. Rev. Biochem. **73:** 925–951.
18. Wakasugi, K., T. Nakano & I. Morishima. 2003. Oxidized human neuroglobin as a heterotrimeric $G\alpha$ protein guanine nucleotide dissociation inhibitor. J. Biol. Chem. **278:** 36505–36512.
19. Esplugues, J.V. 2002. NO as a signaling molecule in the nervous system. Br. J. Pharmacol. **135:** 1079–1095.
20. Dröge, W. 2002. Free radicals in the physiological control of cell function. Physiol. Rev. **82:** 47–95.

21. Brunori, M. 2001. Nitric oxide moves myoglobin center stage. Trends Biochem. Sci. **26:** 209–210.
22. Flögel, U., M.W. Merx, A. Gödecke *et al.* 2001. Myoglobin: a scavenger of bioactive NO. Proc. Natl. Acad. Sci. USA **98:** 735–740.
23. Joshi, M.S., T.B. Ferguson, Jr., T.H. Han *et al.* 2002. Nitric oxide is consumed, rather than conserved, by reaction with oxyhemoglobin under physiological conditions. Proc. Natl. Acad. Sci. USA **99:** 10341–10346.
24. Mammen, P.P.A., J.M. Shelton, S.C. Goetsch *et al.* 2002. Neuroglobin, a novel member of the globin family, is expressed in focal regions of the brain. J. Histochem. Cytochem. **50:** 1591–1598.
25. Nishida, M., Y. Maruyama, R. Tanaka *et al.* 2000. $G\alpha_i$ and $G\alpha_o$ are target proteins of reactive oxygen species. Nature **408:** 492–495.
26. Nishida, M., K.L. Schey, S. Takagahara *et al.* 2002. Activation mechanism of G_i and G_o by reactive oxygen species. J. Biol. Chem. **277:** 9036–9042.
27. Lewerenz, J., J. Letz & A. Methner. 2003. Activation of stimulatory heterotrimeric G proteins increases glutathione and protects neuronal cells against oxidative stress. J. Neurochem. **87:** 522–531.
28. Aikawa, R., I. Komuro, T. Yamazaki *et al.* 1997. Oxidative stress activates extracellular signal–regulated kinases through Src and Ras in cultured cardiac myocytes of neonatal rats. J. Clin. Invest. **100:** 1813–1821.
29. Sonoda, Y., S. Watanabe, Y. Matsumoto *et al.* 1999. FAK is the upstream signal protein of the phosphatidylinositol 3-kinase–Akt survival pathway in hydrogen peroxide–induced apoptosis of a human glioblastoma cell line. J. Biol. Chem. **274:** 10566–10570.
30. Schwindinger, W.F. & J.D. Robishaw. 2001. Heterotrimeric G-protein $\beta\gamma$-dimers in growth and differentiation. Oncogene **20:** 1653–1660.
31. Fuchs, C., V. Heib, L. Kiger *et al.* 2004. Zebrafish reveals different and conserved features of vertebrate neuroglobin gene structure, expression pattern, and ligand binding. J. Biol. Chem. **279:** 24116–24122.
32. Go, M. 1981. Correlation of DNA exonic regions with protein structural units in haemoglobin. Nature **291:** 90–92.
33. Wakasugi, K. & I. Morishima. 2005. Identification of residues in human neuroglobin crucial for guanine nucleotide dissociation inhibitor activity. Biochemistry **44:** 2943–2948.
34. Wakasugi, K., K. Ishimori, K. Imai *et al.* 1994. "Module" substitution in hemoglobin subunits: preparation and characterization of a "chimera $\beta\alpha$-subunit". J. Biol. Chem. **269:** 18750–18756.
35. Wakasugi, K., K. Ishimori & I. Morishima. 1997. "Module"-substituted globins: artificial exon shuffling among myoglobin, hemoglobin α- and β-subunits. Biophys. Chem. **68:** 265–273.
36. Wakasugi, K., C. Quinn, N. Tao & P. Schimmel. 1998. Genetic code in evolution: switching species-specific aminoacylation with a peptide transplant. EMBO J. **17:** 297–305.
37. Pesce, A., S. Dewilde, M. Nardini *et al.* 2003. Human brain neuroglobin structure reveals a distinct mode of controlling oxygen affinity. Structure **11:** 1087–1095.
38. Tarricone, C., A. Galizzi, A. Coda *et al.* 1997. Unusual structure of the oxygen-binding site in the dimeric bacterial hemoglobin from *Vitreoscilla* sp. Structure **5:** 497–507.
39. Lee, S.Y., B.C. Stark & D.A. Webster. 2004. Structure-function of the *Vitreoscilla* hemoglobin D-region. Biochem. Biophys. Res. Commun. **316:** 1101–1106.
40. Sterne-Marr, R., J.J.G. Tesmer, P.W. Day *et al.* 2003. G protein–coupled receptor kinase $2/G\alpha_{q/11}$ interaction: a novel surface on a regulator of G protein signaling homology domain for binding $G\alpha$ subunits. J. Biol. Chem. **276:** 6050–6058.
41. Wakasugi, K., T. Nakano, C. Kitatsuji & I. Morishima. 2004. Human neuroglobin interacts with flotillin-1, a lipid raft microdomain-associated protein. Biochem. Biophys. Res. Commun. **318:** 453–460.
42. Schulte, T., K.A. Paschke, U. Laessing *et al.* 1997. Reggie-1 and reggie-2, two cell surface proteins expressed by retinal ganglion cells during axon regeneration. Development **124:** 577–587.

43. BICKEL, P.E., P.E. SCHERER, J.E. SCHNITZER *et al.* 1997. Flotillin and epidermal surface antigen define a new family of caveolae-associated integral membrane proteins. J. Biol. Chem. **272:** 13793–13802.
44. MAEKAWA, S., S. IINO & S. MIYATA. 2003. Molecular characterization of the detergent-insoluble cholesterol-rich membrane microdomain (raft) of the central nervous system. Biochim. Biophys. Acta **1610:** 261–270.
45. BAUMANN, C.A., V. RIBON, M. KANZAKI *et al.* 2000. CAP defines a second signaling pathway required for insulin-stimulated glucose transport. Nature **407:** 202–207.
46. KIMURA, A., C.A. BAUMANN, S.H. CHIANG & A.R. SALTIEL. 2001. The sorbin homology domain: a motif for the targeting of proteins to lipid rafts. Proc. Natl. Acad. Sci. USA **98:** 9098–9103.
47. MOFFETT, S., D.A. BROWN & M.E. LINDER. 2000. Lipid-dependent targeting of G proteins into rafts. J. Biol. Chem. **275:** 2191–2198.
48. OH, P. & J.E. SCHNITZER. 2001. Segregation of heterotrimeric G proteins in cell surface microdomains: G(q) binds caveolin to concentrate in caveolae, whereas G(i) and G(s) target lipid rafts by default. Mol. Biol. Cell **12:** 685–698.
49. WAKASUGI, K., T. NAKANO & I. MORISHIMA. 2004. Association of human neuroglobin with cystatin C, a cysteine proteinase inhibitor. Biochemistry **43:** 5119–5125.
50. NISHIO, C., K. YOSHIDA, K. NISHIYAMA *et al.* 2000. Involvement of cystatin C in oxidative stress–induced apoptosis of cultured rat CNS neurons. Brain Res. **873:** 252–262.
51. TSUCHIYA, K., Y. KOHDA, M. YOSHIDA *et al.* 1999. Postictal blockade of ischemic hippocampal neuronal death in primates using selective cathepsin inhibitors. Exp. Neurol. **155:** 187–194.
52. GRAY, J., M.M. HARAN, K. SCHNEIDER *et al.* 2001. Evidence that inhibition of cathepsin-B contributes to the neuroprotective properties of caspase inhibitor Tyr-Val-Ala-Asp-chloromethyl ketone. J. Biol. Chem. **276:** 32750–32755.
53. KOHDA, Y., T. YAMASHIMA, K. SAKUDA *et al.* 1996. Dynamic changes of cathepsins B and L expression in the monkey hippocampus after transient ischemia. Biochem. Biophys. Res. Commun. **228:** 616–622.
54. KAGEDAL, K., U. JOHANSSON & K. ÖLLINGER. 2001. The lysosomal protease cathepsin D mediates apoptosis induced by oxidative stress. FASEB J. **15:** 1592–1594.
55. MERZ, G.S., E. BENEDIKZ, V. SCHWENK *et al.* 1997. Human cystatin C forms an inactive dimer during intracellular trafficking in transfected CHO cells. J. Cell. Physiol. **173:** 423–432.
56. ABRAHAMSON, M. & A. GRUBB. 1994. Increased body temperature accelerates aggregation of the Leu68→Gln mutant cystatin C, the amyloid-forming protein in hereditary cystatin C amyloid angiopathy. Proc. Natl. Acad. Sci. USA **91:** 1416–1420.

The Impact of Aging, Dietary Restriction, and Glucocorticoids on *ApoE* Gene Expression in Rat Brain

S. RUZDIJIC, M. PEROVIC, A. MLADENOVIC, D. MILANOVIC, L. RAKIC, S. PETANCESKA, AND S. KANAZIR

Department of Neurobiology and Immunology, Institute for Biological Research, 11060 Belgrade, Serbia and Montenegro

KEYWORDS: **Alzheimer's disease (AD); *ApoE*; aging; dietary restriction (DR); glucocorticoids**

The neuroprotective effect of long-term dietary restriction (DR) is widely recognized. Long-term DR is associated with increased production of neurotrophins, enhanced cellular stress response, decreased oxidative stress, increased survival of newly born neuronal cells in the hippocampus, increased glucose utilization, and other neuroprotective and neurorestorative processes. Long-term DR has a positive impact on insulin sensitivity and lipid metabolism. Insulin resistance (type 2 diabetes) and hypercholesterolemia are conditions that are associated with increased risk of Alzheimer's disease (AD).

Glucocorticoids have a profound and complex effect on cognition, particularly on the functioning of the hippocampus, a brain area rich in glucocorticoid receptors and particularly vulnerable in AD. While a transient increase in glucocorticoids can facilitate synaptic efficacy, long-term elevations in circulating glucocorticoids due to exogenous administration are associated with decreased synaptic efficacy, decreased adult neurogenesis, and neuronal atrophy in the hippocampus. Although DR results in increased levels of circulating glucocorticoids, it confers neuroprotection against different acute injuries such as excitotoxic insult and ischemia, a phenomenon known as "the glucocorticoid paradox". The ability of long-term DR to protect the brain against the negative impact of chronic stress (chronic elevations of glucocorticoids) has not been investigated.

The aim of the present study was to examine the effects of aging, DR, and acute glucocorticoid treatment on the expression of *ApoE* in rat cortex and hippocampus. In the course of the experiment, the animals' body weight, body temperature, and general well-being were carefully monitored. As expected, DR prevented the age-associated increase in body weight and was associated with a decrease in basal body temperature [i.e., 34.06 ± 0.43°C for 18-month-old rats on DR compared to 36.0 ± 0.77°C for 18-month-old rats fed *ad libitum* (AL); $P < 0.05$]. We measured the levels of free plasma corticosterone in DR rats and AL rats at 6 and 12 months of

Address for correspondence: S. Ruzdijic, Department of Neurobiology and Immunology, Institute for Biological Research, 11060 Belgrade, Serbia and Montenegro.

Ann. N.Y. Acad. Sci. 1053: 231–232 (2005). © 2005 New York Academy of Sciences. doi: 10.1196/annals.1344.055

age. In the AL rats, we observed a significant increase in free plasma corticosterone at 12 months compared to 6 months ($P < 0.01$). Rats on DR had significantly higher levels of free corticosterone in the plasma compared to rats fed AL, and this increase was exacerbated by age. To evaluate possible effects of DR, aging, and glucocorticoids, we assessed the expression of *ApoE*, a molecule involved in the metabolism of the AD amyloid precursor protein using Q-RT-PCR analyses. *ApoE* mRNA levels were significantly higher in the cortex and in the hippocampus of 12-month-old rats fed AL compared to 6-month-old AL rats. DR reversed the effect of age on *ApoE* mRNA levels in the cortex, but had no effect on *ApoE* expression in the hippocampus. Acute dexamethasone treatment of 6-month-old rats fed AL resulted in ~50% increase in *ApoE* mRNA in the hippocampus compared to vehicle-treated rats.

In summary, these findings suggest that aging, dietary restriction, and glucocorticoids can modulate the metabolism of the AD amyloid precursor protein by altering the expression of protein involved in APP processing and Aβ peptide clearance/deposition.

Questions and Answers

Session V: Neuroprotective Approaches and Models

QUESTION FOR LARS WIKLUND

From Gary Fiskum

As early oxidative stress contributes to reperfusion injury after global cerebral ischemia, is it necessarily beneficial to increase brain blood flow with, for example, vasopressin, during resuscitation?

ANSWER: As far as is known today, flow support seems to be beneficial. However, this has never been totally proven. In one of our studies, gentle vasodilation during the time after restoration of spontaneous circulation resulted in slightly greater signs of peroxidation (8-iso-PGF2α) of cerebral lipids. In another group given *S*-PBN as a scavenger, the signs of peroxidation were slightly less and autoregulation of cerebral blood flow functioned slightly better. This was interpreted as a vasodilation possibly resulting in hyperperfusion in some cerebral regions and less perfusion in others, resulting in somewhat greater total peroxidation of cerebral lipids. Thus, probably a well-functioning autoregulation of blood flow is the optimal condition and not necessarily uneven hyper/hypoperfusion in other areas.

QUESTIONS FOR DE-MAW CHUANG

From William Slikker, Jr.

Are there any epidemiological or clinical studies that demonstrate Li protection against PD or AD?

ANSWER: Neuroprotective effects of lithium have been demonstrated in several cellular and animal models of PD and AD. To my knowledge, clinical studies using lithium for both diseases are being planned. One epidemiological study conducted by Paula Nunes and colleagues from the University of São Paulo, Brazil, employed 74 elderly people with bipolar disorder. Four percent of those taking lithium had AD, compared with 21% of patients who were not taking the drug. These results were presented at the Ninth International Conference on AD and Related Disorders in Philadelphia, PA, in July 2004. Although the number of AD patients involved is relatively small, the study outcome does look very encouraging.

From Xiaoyang Xi

What is the metabolic rate of lithium in brain? What is the toxic dose in animals?

ANSWER: Lithium is rapidly absorbed by the gastrointestinal system when taken orally. Usually, the plasma lithium level reaches its peak within 1–2 h following

Ann. N.Y. Acad. Sci. 1053: 233–236 (2005). © 2005 New York Academy of Sciences.
doi: 10.1196/annals.1344.064

administration of a lithium carbonate tablet or some other soluble lithium salt. The concentration of lithium in the whole brain is approximately the same as that found in the serum as this ion readily passes through the blood-brain barrier. Although there are some regional differences in lithium concentration, no brain area accumulates this drug to a high level. During lithium treatment for bipolar disorder, the steady-state drug concentration in the serum is maintained in the range of 0.3 to 1.0 mM. This is routinely determined from a blood sample taken 12 h after the last intake of lithium and is thus considered to be the mean serum level for that 24-h period. When the plasma lithium concentration reaches the range of 2 to 10 mM, toxic effects including nausea, vomiting, diarrhea, and tremors can develop in humans and animals. Lithium is eliminated almost exclusively through the kidney. After filtration through the glomerular membrane, lithium can be reabsorbed. The elimination half-time of lithium from the body is about 24 h. For details, see *Lithium and the Cell: Pharmacology and Biochemistry* (1991. Academic Press. New York/London).

From Naren Banik

Does lithium have any effects on calcium channels other than NMDA-receptor-mediated calcium influx? Have you looked at calpain activity in your system since Ca^{2+} is upregulated?

ANSWER: Besides inhibiting the NMDA-receptor-mediated calcium influx that we reported, long-term lithium was shown to suppress the intracellular calcium increase induced by β-bungarotoxin in cultured cerebellar granule neurons and to protect against neuronal death induced by this toxin (TSENG & LIN-SHIAU. 2002. Neurosci. Res. **69:** 633–641). Lithium also inhibits calcium release from the endoplasmic reticulum (ER) induced by thapsigargin and rescues cells from the ER stress (HIROI *et al.* 2005. Pharmacogenomics J. **5:** 102–111). Indeed, NMDA receptor stimulation results in rapid activation of the calcium-dependent protease, calpain. A recent study showed that NMDA receptor activation leads to rapid calpain-specific proteolysis of the spectrum and decreased levels of NR2A/2B subunits, giving rise to active NMDA receptor forms present on the cell surface (SIMPKINS *et al.* 2003. J. Neurosci. **23:** 11322–11331). We have not yet studied the effects of lithium on NMDA-receptor-mediated calpain activation. However, since lithium inactivates NMDA receptors, we would expect receptor-mediated calpain activation to be inhibited as well. Recently, our preliminary results showed that lithium inhibits glutamate-induced, NMDA-receptor-mediated β-tubulin degradation. We have yet to study whether the β-tubulin degradation is mediated by calpain.

From Philip Lazarovici

Lithium at therapeutic concentrations inhibits lipid phosphatases. Have you looked at your models of neuroprotection for lipid phosphatase activity or level?

ANSWER: Indeed, it has been shown that chronic treatment of rodents with therapeutic doses of lithium downregulates brain phospholipase A_2 (PLA_2) and its downstream arachidonic acid cascade (RAPOPORT & BOSETTI. 2002. Arch. Gen. Psychiatry **59:** 592–596), and blocks 5-$HT_{2A/2C}$ receptor–mediated PLA_2/arachidonate signaling in the brain (BASSELIN *et al.* 2005. Neuropsychopharmacology **30:** 461–472). We have not yet studied whether PLA_2 activation is involved in glutamate excitotoxicity and lithium neuroprotection in cellular or animal models.

QUESTIONS FOR ANTHONY SCHAPIRA

From William Slikker, Jr.

Is there evidence that coenzyme Q10 reaches its CNS target?

ANSWER: There is direct evidence in rats that oral coenzyme Q10 penetrates the CNS, but there is no direct evidence in humans.

From Russell J. Andrews

In keeping with the interdisciplinary aspect of the conference, would you comment on the neuroprotective effects of deep brain stimulation (specifically, subthalamic nucleus) in Parkinson's disease? In particular, I am thinking of the recent 5-year follow-up report from the Grenoble Group (BENABID *et al.*) showing quite impressive maintenance of UPORS scores, etc., over a 5-year period. Also, what are your thoughts on the interaction between DBS and pharmacological agents for PD?

ANSWER: The hypothetical basis to STN stimulation is the identification of excitotoxic innervation of the substantia nigra pars compacta by the STN. The long-term clinical study certainly demonstrates the continuing efficacy of STN stimulation, but does not of course demonstrate neuroprotection. This would require a study with a different design. At present, STN stimulation is confined to those patients who have, in the most part, motor complications not controlled by medical therapy, and it is unlikely that STN stimulation will be widely used beyond this.

From Philip Lazarovici

Can you comment on the criteria to measure neuroprotection in *in vivo* animal models?

ANSWER: To date, *in vivo* animal models have not provided a good indication for translation of neuroprotective effects to humans. The MPTP, rotenone, and 6-hydroxydopamine models, while effective for certain aspects of PD modeling and used in identifying drugs for neuroprotection, do have their limitations. It might be that such models are useful for screening potential compounds, but we need improved models that provide more reliable indications of efficacy in humans.

QUESTIONS FOR MOUSSA YOUDIM

From Ziaoyang Qi

Cancer cells have genetic deficits to escape apoptosis. Have you seen any interference of the gene defects in your drug development?

ANSWER: I really do not understand what you mean by this. As far as what we have observed in the type of apoptosis that we induce, M30 causes neuroprotection *in vivo* with the MPTP model of PD and kainite-induced hippocampal degeneration in mice.

From Winston Ko

I agree with your hypothesis and appreciate your evidence that drugs developed to act on a single molecular target involve a "domino" cascade of events. By extension of your hypothesis, would you agree that there are compounds on a higher level that can trigger multiple pathways and autophosphorylation, and that these compounds are highly specific and should be found at the developmental stage of the human fetus?

ANSWER: In fact, we have recently shown with gene expression and proteomic analysis that our anti-Parkinson drug, rasagiline, a selective irreversible monoamine oxidase B inhibitor, activates several cell survival gene pathways, while down-regulating proapoptotic ones.

From Philip Lazarovici

What is the cation selectivity of the M30 compound?

ANSWER: There is some evidence that M30 is an iron chelator with a potency very similar to desferrioxamine (Desferal). It also has affinity for zinc, but this is not as strong.

From William Slikker, Jr.

Is there evidence of functional rescue associated with postinsult administration of M30?

ANSWER: We have recently submitted a paper for publication on this very subject, namely neurorescue. In a well-known model of serum deprivation, neuroblastoma cells were incubated for 24 h with full serum and then incubated for 3 days in serum-free medium and incubated for 24 h with fresh serum-free medium to which M30 was added (1–10 μM). The cells in serum-free medium underwent apoptosis as determined by Dappi, while cells that were treated with M30 recovered and showed increased GAP43 and neurite formation. Western analysis revealed increased Bcl-2, with decreases in Bad and caspase-3, opposite to that seen with the cells in serum-free medium.

Saposin C: Neuronal Effect and CNS Delivery by Liposomes

ZHENGTAO CHU,[a] YING SUN,[a] CHIA YI KUAN,[b] GREGORY A. GRABOWSKI,[a] AND XIAOYANG QI[a]

[a]*Division and Program in Human Genetics,* [b]*Division of Developmental Biology, Children's Hospital Research Foundation, University of Cincinnati, Cincinnati, Ohio 45229-3039, USA*

Abstract: Saposin C is one of four small lipid-binding proteins that derive from a single precursor protein, named prosaposin (PSAP). PSAP has several neuronal effects, including neurite outgrowth stimulation, neuron preservation, and nerve regeneration enhancement. A minimal domain required for PSAP's neurotrophic function is located in the amino-terminal half of saposin C. Genetic defects of the PSAP gene in humans and mice lead to a complex lysosomal storage disease. The skin fibroblasts from PSAP- and saposin C–deficient patients have a massive accumulation of multivesicular bodies (MVBs). Incorporation of exogenous saposin C–containing liposomes into the cultured PSAP–/– cells reduced the accumulated MVBs to normal levels. Internalized saposin C was localized to late endosomes and lysosomes. MVBs are crucial for maintaining the cellular homeostasis required for neuronal development and growth. PSAP–/– mice have a short life span (30 days) and central nervous system (CNS) neuronal degeneration. Similar to PSAP–/– fibroblasts, excessive MVBs accumulated in CNS neurons and brain tissues of PSAP-null mice. Cultured cortical and hippocampal neurons from PSAP–/– mice had poor survival and displayed a neurite degenerative pattern. Delivery of saposin C *ex vivo* into cultured neurons and *in vivo* into brain neuronal cells in mice across the blood-brain barrier was accomplished with intravenously administered dioleoylphosphatidylserine (DOPS) liposomes. These studies may yield a new therapeutic approach for neuron protection, preservation, and regeneration.

Keywords: prosaposin; phosphatidylserine; liposome; blood-brain barrier; multivesicular body

INTRODUCTION

Saposin C is a small (80-amino-acid), multifunctional glycoprotein that is present in all normal tissues and cells. This protein along with saposins A, B, and D are proteolytically processed from a precursor protein, named prosaposin (PSAP).[1–5] Saposin C has been localized on the endosomal/lysosomal membrane using immunoelectron microscopy.[6] A saposin-fold structure, a helical-bundle conformation with

Address for correspondence: Xiaoyang Qi, Ph.D., Assistant Professor, Division and Program in Human Genetics, 3333 Burnet Avenue, Cincinnati, OH 45229-3039. Voice: 513-636-5964; fax: 513-636-3486.
qix0@chmcc.org

Ann. N.Y. Acad. Sci. 1053: 237–246 (2005).
doi: 10.1196/annals.1344.021

three intradisulfide bridges, leads to the heat-stable and protease-resistance properties of saposin C.[7–9] Glycosylation is not required for its biological activities.[10,11] The primary physiological function of saposin C has been defined by a glycosphingolipid (GSL) storage disease similar to neuronopathic "Gaucher's disease" in patients with a deficiency of the protein.[12,13] Thus, saposin C is a critical physiologic activator for the lysosomal enzyme, acid β-glucosidase. The enzymatic activation domain was localized to the carboxyl-terminal-half region *in vitro* and *ex vivo*.[14,15]

In addition to stimulating the glucosylceramide degradation by acid β-glucosidase, saposin C has several other potential roles. These include inter-membrane transport of gangliosides and GSLs,[16] reorganization and destabilization of phospholipid-containing membranes,[17–19] and fusion of acidic phospholipid vesicles.[20,21] Saposin C associates with phosphatidylserine (PS) membranes by embedding its amino- and carboxyl-end helices into the outer leaflet of membranes.[22] Increasing evidence indicates that interactions of saposins with appropriate membranes are crucial for their specificity and activity. Moreover, PSAP, the precursor of saposins, is a neurotrophic factor with *in vitro* neuritogenic,[14,23,24] *in vivo* nerve growth promoting, and apoptosis protection properties.[25–27] Such neuritogenic functions are mediated through sequences in the NH_2-terminal half of saposin C.[14,28] The minimum sequence required for *in vitro* neuritogenic activity spans amino acid residues 22–31 of saposin C in humans and mice. Neurological functions of PSAP and saposin C are mediated by activation of the enzymes in the MAPK pathway through a G-protein-associated cell membrane receptor in a number of neuroglia-derived cells.[29,30]

Human and mouse PSAP genetic defects result in total saposin deficiency.[31–33] Aberrant accumulation of multivesicular bodies (MVBs) was present in the skin fibroblasts from PSAP-deficient patients.[31,34] The sinusoidal cells in liver from a PSAP-deficient patient were crowded with multivesicular inclusions.[12,31] Similar MVB structures also were found in fibroblasts from a saposin C–deficient patient.[13] In PSAP–/– mice, inclusions consisting of numerous concentric lamellar bodies and dense granular structures were noted in a variety of tissues and cells.[35] Thin sections of mouse PSAP–/– cells revealed a selective accumulation of MVBs by electron microscopy.[36] In this report, we observed the altered MVB structures in neuronal cells and brain tissues from PSAP–/– mice.

MVBs, a subset of the late endosomes, have a crucial role in communications by vesicular transport between the *trans*–Golgi network, the plasma membrane, and lysosomal/vacuolar organelles.[37] One of their functions is to maintain the cellular homeostasis required for neuronal development and growth. The hypothetic "signaling endosome" model explains that the ligand-receptor complex on an endosomal signaling platform is transported retrogradely from the distal axon to the cell body to promote gene expression and neuron survival.[38] The altered MVB structures in neurons of PSAP–/– mice may disrupt the retrograde movement of neurotrophins via vesicular signaling transports and may impair the development of neuronal cells in the CNS. The present and previous observations[35,39] showed the neuronal degeneration and defect in CNS of PSAP–/– mice. Thus, PSAP–/– mice provide a model to investigate the causes of massive MVB structures in neuronal defects.

Introducing exogenous PSAP or saposin C into the medium of cultured fibroblasts from the PSAP-deficient patient reversed the aberrant accumulation of MVBs.[34,40] This result suggests that saposin C is a key regulatory molecule in MVB formation. To date, little is known *in vivo* regarding specificity and mechanisms of action of saposin C in the MVB pathway. Thus, elucidation of the effects of saposin C in biogenesis and function of MVBs is needed to understand its physiological roles in CNS. Our approach is to correct MVB structures and neuron defects in CNS by transport of exogenous saposin C into the brain of PSAP–/– mice. Delivery of macromolecular therapeutic agents into the brain, for example, glycoproteins, remains an obstacle to effective treatments for patients with neurological diseases. The blood-brain barrier (BBB) is exclusive for such macromolecules.[41,42] Liposomes hold promise for delivery of genes, proteins, and other biological molecules across the BBB into brain.[41,42] Liposomes are colloid, spherical, self-closed vesicles with well-defined lipid layers. Such liposome delivery systems can be used to improve the therapeutic and pharmacological properties of drugs through parenteral administration. Saposin C has strong binding activity with liposomal membranes containing the negatively charged lipid, dioleoylphosphatidylserine (DOPS).[22] This protein-lipid complex was used to successfully transport saposin C into CNS neurons via intravenous administration.

EXPERIMENTAL PROCEDURES

Materials

The following materials were from commercial sources: mouse laminin, penicillin, streptomycin, fetal bovine serum, DMEM, and Neurobasal medium with B27 supplement (Gibco BRL, Gaithersburg, MD); restriction endonucleases (New England Biolabs, Beverly, MA); pET21a(+) DNA vector, *E. coli* host strain [BL21(DE3)], and His·Bind resin (Novagen, Madison, WI); monoclonal anti-His antibody conjugated with Alexa Fluor488 (QIAGEN, Valencia, CA); fluorescein-conjugated goat anti-rabbit and rhodamine-conjugated sheep anti-mouse antibodies (ICN/CAPPEL, Aurora, OH); antifade reagent (Ventana Medical Systems, Tucson, AZ); C4 reverse-phase HPLC column (Alltech Association, Deerfield, IL); DOPS and 1,2-dioleoyl-*sn*-glycero-3-phospho-L-serine-*N*-(7-nitro-2-1,3-benzoxadiazol-4-yl) (NBD-DOPS) as stock solutions in chloroform (Avanti Polar Lipids, Alabaster, AL); and polyethylenimine (PEI) and papain (Sigma, St. Louis, MO). Anionic lipids were sodium salts. All other chemicals were reagent grade or better.

Fibroblast Cell Cultures

Human and mouse primary fibroblasts were used for all experiments and established with standard procedures in this laboratory.[15] Mouse PSAP-deficient fibroblasts were cultured from PSAP–/– mice as previously described.[15] All the cells were cultured in DMEM/fetal bovine serum (10%) medium at 37°C in monolayer for future use.

Primary Cortical Neuron Cultures

Cortical neurons were cultured in serum-free Neurobasal medium with B27 supplements as described by Whitmarsh *et al.*[43] E16 mouse embryos were dissected in ice-cold Ca/Mg-free Hanks' balanced salt solution (HBSS) to remove the head.

The cerebral cortex was dissected with a curved fine surgical scissors and collected into ice-cold HBSS. The cortical tissue was placed into papain HBSS for 15–20 min at room temperature and dissociated by mechanical trituration. Fisherbran 12-546 (18CIR-2) cover glasses in 12-well plates were coated with PEI containing laminin overnight. The isolated cortical tissues were cultured on the PEI-coated cover glass in the plate with Neurobasal/B27 medium.

Saposin C and Liposome Preparation

Recombinant saposin C was produced using the IPTG-inducing pET system in *E. coli* cells.[11] All expressed proteins contained a His-tag and were purified on a nickel column and with C4 reverse-phase HPLC chromatography using a linear (0–100%) gradient of acetonitrile in 0.1% trifluoroacetic acid. The major protein peak was collected and lyophilized. The protein concentrations were determined as previously described.[11]

DOPS (16.2 μg) in chloroform was dried under N_2 and vacuum to form a lipid film. Saposin C (79 μg) was added into the lipid film and suspended in 50 μL of 0.1 M citric acid/0.2 M phosphate (pH 4.7). Additional medium or PBS was added to a final volume to 1 mL. Large unilamellar vesicles (LUVs) were prepared by bath sonications.[14] Liposome size was assessed by photon correlation spectroscopy with an N4+ submicron particle size analyzer (Coulter, Miami, FL). The populations of LUVs had an average diameter of 250 ± 100 nm.

Delivery of Saposin C–DOPS Proteoliposomes **In Vitro** *and* **In Vivo**

Cells (10^5) were grown in DMEM for 48 h in an 8-well chamber slide with cover glass (Lab-Tek II, Nalge Nunc International). Saposin C–DOPS complexes in DMEM were added into cell cultures. After incubation (37°C, 48 h), the cells were washed with PBS twice and fixed with 2% paraformaldehyde for immunofluorescence studies. The proteoliposomes in PBS were injected into tail veins for *in vivo* evaluations. Mouse brain tissues were collected at 48 h after administration of the protein-lipid complex.

Immunofluorescence and Electron Microscopy (EM)

Immunofluorescence staining was as described with minor modification.[15] Cultured cells (1×10^5) in a dish with coverslips were washed with PBS and fixed with 2% paraformaldehyde for 10 min at room temperature. After treatment with 0.1% Triton X-100 in PBS, the samples were incubated with each respective primary antiserum (for 2 h) and fluorescence-conjugated secondary antibody (for 1 h) at 37°C. The dilutions of primary and secondary antibodies were 1:30 and 1:60, respectively. Mouse brain tissue sections fixed in 4% paraformaldehyde were incubated with a blocking solution containing 5% mouse serum prior to addition of primary anti-His antibody. Rhodamine-conjugated anti-mouse antibody was used as secondary antibody for detection. Antifade was added on the section to decrease fluorescence quenching. Fluorescence signals were detected by a confocal microscope (LSM510, Zeiss) or by a fluorescence microscope (Zeiss Axioskop).

EM analysis was as previously described.[40] Briefly, neuronal cells were fixed in 3% glutaraldehyde in 0.175 M cacodylate buffer and postfixed in 1% osmic acid before embedding in Epon 812. Uranyl acetate–stained thin sections were examined with a Phillips 400 transmission electron microscope.

RESULTS AND DISCUSSION

Neuronal Degeneration in PSAP–/– Mice

Onset of the neurologic phenotype in the PSAP–/– mice is about 18 days. At this age, they develop tremors and over the next 10 days deteriorate neurologically. The mice develop severe weakness of all limbs, gait ataxia, and terminally a tonic status epilepticus at 30–35 days. Their body weights were one-quarter to one-half of those for their normal littermates. In brain sections of 30-day PSAP–/– mice, degenerated neurons and axonal globoid bodies were present in the thalamus, striatum, brain stem, and cerebral cortex.[35,39]

Cortical neurons were collected from E16 embryos of wild-type and PSAP–/– mice.[44] Initially, neurons from the PSAP–/– mice and wild-type littermates showed similar morphology, neurite growth pattern, and density. After culturing for about 5 days, the PSAP–/– neurons changed their morphology to a larger and flatter cell body (see *arrows* in FIG. 1B). At day 7, decreased neuronal density and increased neuron death were observed when compared to wild-type neurons (FIG. 1A). Also, neurites, stained with anti-β-tubulin III, from the surviving PSAP–/– neurons were degenerating and had a far-shortened appearance (data not shown). These changes were not observed in wild-type cells. These data suggest that PSAP is crucial for neuron survival and growth.

MVB Accumulation in Neurons of PSAP–/– Mice

Excessive accumulation of MVBs is a major pathological defect in human PSAP–/– fibroblasts. These MVBs were large in size (>0.5 μm) and contained vesicular structures.[40] Massive MVB structures also were observed in cultured cortical neurons from

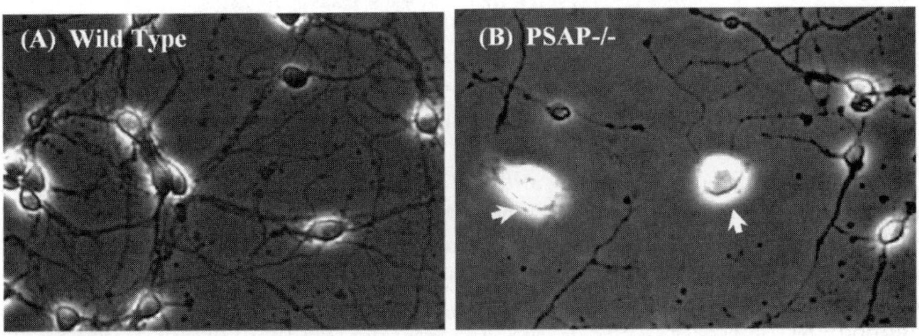

FIGURE 1. Cortical neuron cultures from wild-type (**A**) and PSAP–/– (**B**) mouse brains: phase-contrast images (×400). Cells were cultured for 8 days. Photos of cultured neuronal cells were taken under a microscope (Leica DM IRE2, Leica, GMBH, Germany). The dying cells were marked with *arrows*. [Images reduced to 90%.]

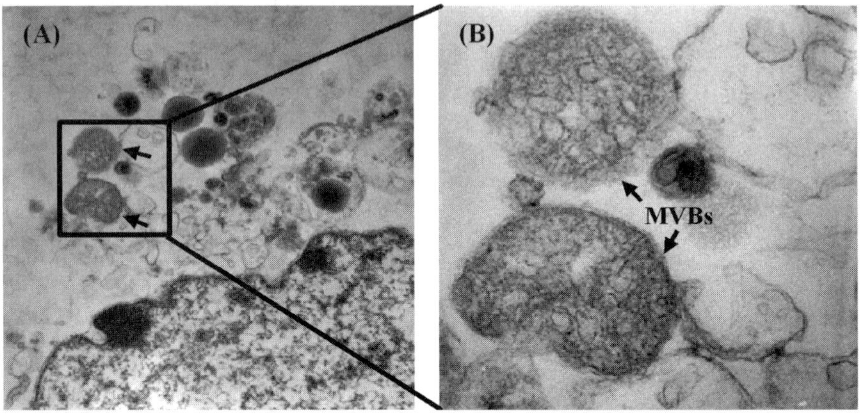

FIGURE 2. Electron micrographs of the cortical neurons from PSAP–/– mouse brains. Cells were cultured for 8 days. MVBs with intravesicular structures are indicated with *arrows*. Magnification: **(A)** ×12,500; **(B)** ×50,000. [Images reduced to 94%.]

PSAP–/– mice (FIGS. 2A and 2B; see *arrows*). Similar MVB structures were found in neurons of brain tissues from PSAP–/– mice (data not shown). MVBs did not accumulate in the neurons and brain tissues from wild-type littermates. These results indicate that saposins are important in regulation of MVB formation. The altered MVB structure correlates with neuronal defects in PSAP–/– mice.

Internalization of Saposin C into Neuronal Cells

Preliminary studies showed that saposin C was transported into the cultured mouse cortical and hippocampal neurons, and was facilitated by complexes with DOPS liposomes. Since exogenous saposin C has a hexahistidine tag, internalization of saposin C was demonstrated using monoclonal anti-His antibody conjugated with Alexa Fluor488 (QIAGEN) by immunohistochemical analysis (FIG. 3). The fluorescence signal (see white granular signals indicated by *arrows* in FIG. 3A) had a punctate pattern in these neuronal cells. The internalization of the saposin C–DOPS proteoliposomes did not affect the neuronal cell growth. No signal was detected in the neurons without the treatment of saposin C–DOPS.

Subcellular localization of internalized saposin C was evaluated by immunofluorescence with antisera for endosomal/lysosomal compartments. Antiserum against lysobisphosphatidic acid (LBPA) was used as a marker for late endosomes, and anti-LAMP-1 was the lysosomal marker.[15,40] LBPA is an abundant phospholipid in the complex system of membranes in the lumen of late endosomes.[45] Colocalization patterns of exogenous saposin C and LBPA/LAMP-1 were found in cultured fibroblasts (Qi *et al.*, unpublished data). These results indicated that exogenous saposin C was transported to the endosomal and lysosomal compartments. Exogenous saposin C also has biological activity in PSAP-deficient fibroblasts since it was a reduction of the accumulated MVBs.[40] These results support the feasibility for *in vivo* correction of neuron defects caused by MVB accumulation if saposin C could be delivered into the brain.

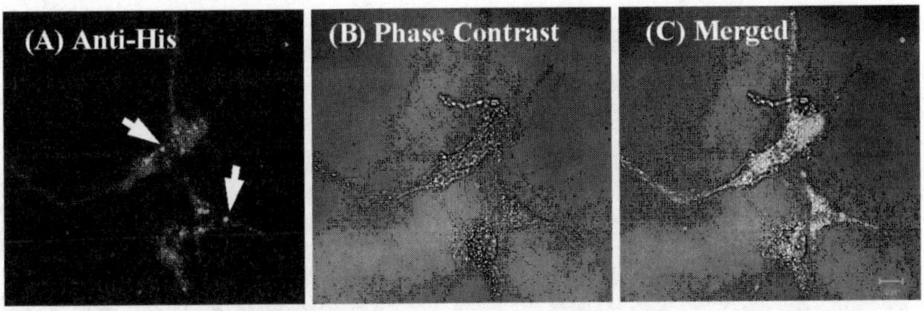

FIGURE 3. Internalization of saposin C into cortical neurons from brains of wild-type mouse embryos (E16): **(A)** exogenous saposin C (see *arrows*) stained with anti-His antibody conjugated with Alexa Fluor488; **(B)** phase-contrast imaging; **(C)** merged with (A) and (B). Bar: 20 μm (C). Photos were taken using a confocal microscope (LSM510, Zeiss).

Saposin C Transport into Mouse Brain by Liposomes

Exogenous saposin C and DOPS proteoliposome was injected into adult mice via tail vein. NBD-DOPS was detected in brain sections at 4 h after intravenous injection. No fluorescence was detected in brain sections from the phosphate-buffered saline (PBS)–treated mice under the same experimental conditions. At 48 h after injection, saposin C and NBD-DOPS were detected in brain tissue sections (FIG. 4). NBD is a green fluorophore with an emission wavelength at 534 nm. NBD-DOPS lipids were detected as punctate patterns in Purkinje cells (p) and granular cells (g) of the cerebellum (FIG. 4A). Similar staining patterns were observed in neuronal cells in cornu Ammonis (CA, hippocampus), dentate gyrus (DG), and cortex regions (data not shown). The majority of exogenous saposin C stained with anti-His antibody (FIG. 4D) colocalized with NBD-DOPS with green fluorescence in Purkinje cells (FIG. 4C) and cells in the hippocampus and dentate gyrus (data not shown). No signals were detected in the control experiments with PBS administration (FIGS. 4B, 4E, and 4F). These experiments demonstrate the feasibility of delivery of saposin C across the BBB into the brain by DOPS liposomes.

Our previous results indicated that exogenous saposin C reversed MVB structures in human PSAP–/– and saposin C-deficient fibroblasts.[40] A similar approach can be used to reduce the accumulation of MVBs in mouse neuron cultures since saposin C can internalize into these neurons. *In vivo* rescue of neurological symptoms in PSAP–/– mice is our ultimate goal. The present studies of saposin C transport into CNS neurons *in vitro* and *in vivo* by DOPS liposomes provide supportive information for our proposed rescue experiments with saposin C. Based on the above findings, we propose that delivery of saposin C–DOPS liposome complexes could rescue the defects of PSAP-null neurons *in vivo* as a novel therapeutic approach for treatment of lysosomal storage diseases with abnormalities in the CNS.

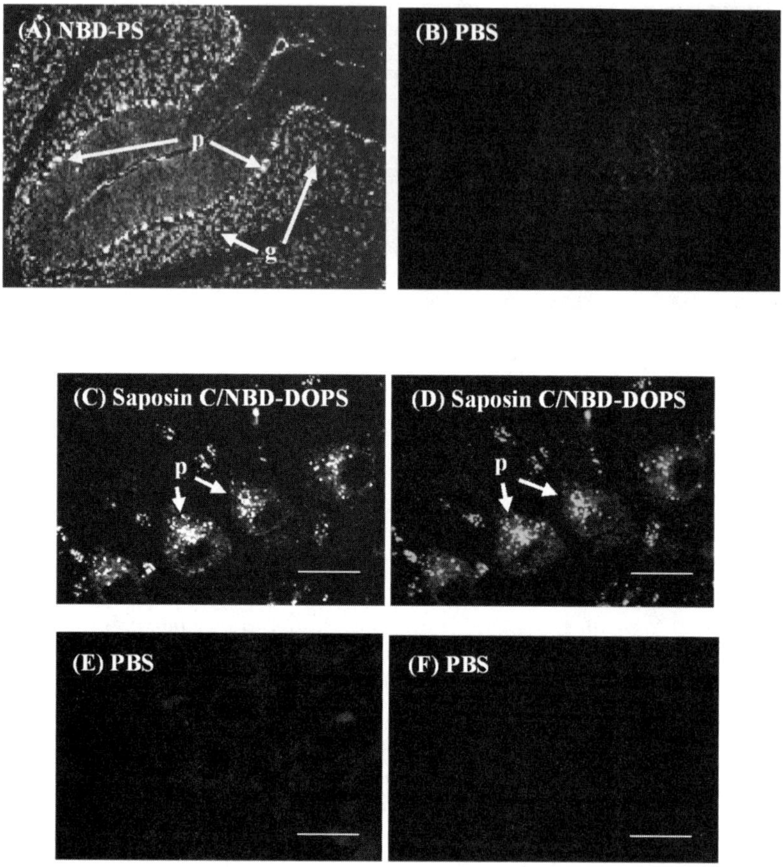

FIGURE 4. Transport of NBD-DOPS and saposin C into cerebellum of mouse brains. NBD-DOPS–saposin C proteoliposomes **(A, C, D)** and PBS **(B, E, F)** were administrated through tail veins of FVB/N adult mice. Frozen cerebellum sections were prepared at 48 h after injection. NBD green fluorescence for detecting DOPS in (A) and (B) was visualized using a microscope (Zeiss Axioskop, ×100). NBD green fluorescence (C and E) and anti-His antibody (a rhodamine-conjugated secondary antibody, red fluorescence) for detecting saposin C (D and F) in Purkinje cells were imaged under a confocal microscope (LSM510, Zeiss). Bar: 20 μm (C–F). Terms: p = Purkinje cells; g = granular cells.

ACKNOWLEDGMENTS

We thank Jean Snyder for assistance with the EM analysis. This work was supported by NIH Grant No. DK 57690 (to X. Qi) through the Cincinnati Children's Hospital Research Foundation.

REFERENCES

1. NAKANO, T., K. SANDHOFF *et al.* 1989. Structure of full-length cDNA coding for sulfatide activator, a co-beta-glucosidase and two other homologous proteins: two alternate forms of the sulfatide activator. J. Biochem. (Tokyo) **105:** 152–154.
2. RORMAN, E.G. & G.A. GRABOWSKI. 1989. Molecular cloning of a human co-beta-glucosidase cDNA: evidence that four sphingolipid hydrolase activator proteins are encoded by single genes in humans and rats. Genomics **5:** 486–492.
3. FUJIBAYASHI, S. & D.A. WENGER. 1986. Synthesis and processing of sphingolipid activator protein-2 (SAP-2) in cultured human fibroblasts. J. Biol. Chem. **261:** 15339–15343.
4. FUJIBAYASHI, S. & D.A. WENGER. 1986. Biosynthesis of the sulfatide/GM1 activator protein (SAP-1) in control and mutant cultured skin fibroblasts. Biochim. Biophys. Acta **875:** 554–562.
5. LEONOVA, T., X. QI *et al.* 1996. Proteolytic processing patterns of prosaposin in insect and mammalian cells. J. Biol. Chem. **271:** 17312–17320.
6. PATON, B.C., J.L. HUGHES *et al.* 1990. Immunocytochemical localization of sphingolipid activator protein 2 (SAP-2) in normal and SAP-deficient fibroblasts. Eur. J. Cell Biol. **51:** 157–164.
7. KISHIMOTO, Y., M. HIRAIWA *et al.* 1992. Saposins: structure, function, distribution, and molecular genetics. J. Lipid Res. **33:** 1255–1267.
8. VACCARO, A.M., R. SALVIOLI *et al.* 1995. Structural analysis of saposin C and B: complete localization of disulfide bridges. J. Biol. Chem. **270:** 9953–9960.
9. HIRAIWA, M., B.M. MARTIN *et al.* 1997. Lysosomal proteolysis of prosaposin, the precursor of saposins (sphingolipid activator proteins): its mechanism and inhibition by ganglioside. Arch. Biochem. Biophys. **341:** 17–24.
10. HIRAIWA, M., S. SOEDA *et al.* 1993. The effect of carbohydrate removal on stability and activity of saposin B. Arch. Biochem. Biophys. **303:** 326–331.
11. QI, X., T. LEONOVA *et al.* 1994. Functional human saposins expressed in *Escherichia coli*: evidence for binding and activation properties of saposins C with acid beta-glucosidase. J. Biol. Chem. **269:** 16746–16753.
12. SANDHOFF, K., T. KOLTER *et al.* 2000. Sphingolipid activator proteins. *In* The Metabolic and Molecular Bases of Inherited Disease, pp. 3371–3388. McGraw–Hill. New York.
13. PAMPOLS, T., M. PINEDA *et al.* 1999. Neuronopathic juvenile glucosylceramidosis due to sap-C deficiency: clinical course, neuropathology, and brain lipid composition in this Gaucher disease variant. Acta Neuropathol. (Berlin) **97:** 91–97.
14. QI, X., W. QIN *et al.* 1996. Functional organization of saposin C: definition of the neurotrophic and acid beta-glucosidase activation regions. J. Biol. Chem. **271:** 6874–6880.
15. QI, X., K. KONDOH *et al.* 2002. *Ex vivo* localization of the mouse saposin C activation region for acid beta-glucosidase. Mol. Genet. Metab. **76:** 189–200.
16. HIRAIWA, M., S. SOEDA *et al.* 1992. Binding and transport of gangliosides by prosaposin. Proc. Natl. Acad. Sci. USA **89:** 11254–11258.
17. YOU, H.X., L. YU *et al.* 2001. Phospholipid membrane restructuring induced by saposin C: a topographic study using atomic force microscopy. FEBS Lett. **503:** 97–102.
18. YOU, H.X., X. QI *et al.* 2003. Phospholipid membrane interactions of saposin C: *in situ* atomic force microscopic study. Biophys. J. **84:** 2043–2057.
19. VACCARO, A.M., M. TATTI *et al.* 1994. Saposin C induces pH-dependent destabilization and fusion of phosphatidylserine-containing vesicles. FEBS Lett. **349:** 181–186.
20. WANG, Y., G.A. GRABOWSKI *et al.* 2003. Phospholipid vesicle fusion induced by saposin C. Arch. Biochem. Biophys. **415:** 43–53.
21. QI, X. & Z. CHU. 2004. Fusogenic domain and lysines in saposin C. Arch. Biochem. Biophys. **424:** 210–218.
22. QI, X. & G.A. GRABOWSKI. 2001. Differential membrane interactions of saposin A and C: implications for the functional specificity. J. Biol. Chem. **276:** 27010–27017.
23. O'BRIEN, J.S., G.S. CARSON *et al.* 1994. Identification of prosaposin as a neurotrophic factor. Proc. Natl. Acad. Sci. USA **91:** 9593–9596.
24. QI, X., K. KONDOH *et al.* 1999. Conformational and amino acid residue requirements for the saposin C neuritogenic effect. Biochemistry **38:** 6284–6291.

25. Kotani, Y., S. Matsuda *et al.* 1996. Prosaposin facilitates sciatic nerve regeneration *in vivo*. J. Neurochem. **66:** 2019–2025.
26. Kotani, Y., S. Matsuda *et al.* 1996. A hydrophilic peptide comprising 18 amino acid residues of the prosaposin sequence has neurotrophic activity *in vitro* and *in vivo*. J. Neurochem. **66:** 2197–2200.
27. Tsuboi, K., M. Hiraiwa *et al.* 1998. Prosaposin prevents programmed cell death of rat cerebellar granule neurons in culture. Brain Res. Dev. Brain Res. **110:** 249–255.
28. O'Brien, J.S., G.S. Carson *et al.* 1995. Identification of the neurotrophic factor sequence of prosaposin. FASEB J. **9:** 681–685.
29. Campana, W.M., M. Hiraiwa *et al.* 1996. Induction of MAPK phosphorylation by prosaposin and prosaptide in PC12 cells. Biochem. Biophys. Res. Commun. **229:** 706–712.
30. Hiraiwa, M., W.M. Campana *et al.* 1997. Prosaposin receptor: evidence for a G-protein-associated receptor. Biochem. Biophys. Res. Commun. **240:** 415–418.
31. Harzer, K., B.C. Paton *et al.* 1989. Sphingolipid activator protein deficiency in a 16-week-old atypical Gaucher disease patient and his fetal sibling: biochemical signs of combined sphingolipidoses. Eur. J. Pediatr. **149:** 31–39.
32. Hulkova, H., M. Cervenkova *et al.* 2001. A novel mutation in the coding region of the prosaposin gene leads to a complete deficiency of prosaposin and saposins, and is associated with a complex sphingolipidosis dominated by lactosylceramide accumulation. Hum. Mol. Genet. **10:** 927–940.
33. Fujita, N., K. Suzuki *et al.* 1996. Targeted disruption of the mouse sphingolipid activator protein gene: a complex phenotype, including severe leukodystrophy and wide-spread storage of multiple sphingolipids. Hum. Mol. Genet. **5:** 711–725.
34. Burkhardt, J.K., S. Huttler *et al.* 1997. Accumulation of sphingolipids in SAP-precursor (prosaposin)–deficient fibroblasts occurs as intralysosomal membrane structures and can be completely reversed by treatment with human SAP-precursor. Eur. J. Cell Biol. **73:** 10–18.
35. Oya, Y., H. Nakayasu *et al.* 1998. Pathological study of mice with total deficiency of sphingolipid activator proteins (SAP knockout mice). Acta Neuropathol. (Berlin) **96:** 29–40.
36. Morales, C.R., Q. Zhao *et al.* 1999. Biogenesis of lysosomes by endocytic flow of plasma membrane. Biocell **23:** 149–160.
37. Katzmann, D.J., G. Odorizzi *et al.* 2002. Receptor downregulation and multivesicular-body sorting. Nat. Rev. Mol. Cell Biol. **3:** 893–905.
38. Ginty, D.D. & R.A. Segal. 2002. Retrograde neurotrophin signaling: Trk-ing along the axon. Curr. Opin. Neurobiol. **12:** 268–274.
39. Sun, Y., X. Qi *et al.* 2002. Prosaposin: threshold rescue and analysis of the "neuritogenic" region in transgenic mice. Mol. Genet. Metab. **76:** 271–286.
40. Chu, Z., D.P. Witte *et al.* 2005. Saposin C–LBPA interaction in late-endosomes/ lysosomes. Exp. Cell Res. **303:** 300–307.
41. Cornford, E.M. & M.E. Cornford. 2002. New systems for delivery of drugs to the brain in neurological disease. Lancet Neurol. **1:** 306–315.
42. Pardridge, W.M. 2002. Drug and gene delivery to the brain: the vascular route. Neuron **36:** 555–558.
43. Whitmarsh, A.J., C.Y. Kuan *et al.* 2001. Requirement of the JIP1 scaffold protein for stress-induced JNK activation. Genes Dev. **15:** 2421–2432.
44. Kuan, C.Y., A.J. Whitmarsh *et al.* 2003. A critical role of neural-specific JNK3 for ischemic apoptosis. Proc. Natl. Acad. Sci. USA **100:** 15184–15189.
45. Kobayashi, T., E. Stang *et al.* 1998. A lipid associated with the antiphospholipid syndrome regulates endosome structure and function. Nature **392:** 193–197.

Brain-Derived Neurotrophic Factor Is Neuroprotective against Human Immunodeficiency Virus-1 Envelope Proteins

ALESSIA BACHIS AND ITALO MOCCHETTI

Department of Neuroscience, Georgetown University Medical Center, Washington, District of Columbia 20057, USA

ABSTRACT: Human immunodeficiency virus type 1 (HIV-1)–positive patients in the late phase of infection develop AIDS dementia complex, an array of neurological complications that include extrapyramidal symptoms, cognitive impairments, and psychiatric disturbances. Brains of these patients exhibit brain injury. The HIV-1 envelope glycoprotein 120 (gp120) has been suggested to be a causal agent of neuronal loss; however, several strains of gp120 exist during the infection and the relative neurotoxic potential of each strain is presently unknown. Using cultured cerebellar granule neurons, we determined whether two strains of gp120, gp120IIIB and gp120BaL, which bind to CXCR4 and CCR5 chemokine receptors, respectively, induce cell death. Apoptotic cell death and activated caspase-3 were evident within a few hours in neurons exposed to low nanomolar concentrations of either gp120IIIB or gp120BaL. However, the neurotoxic effect of gp120IIIB was more rapid and occurred at lower concentrations than that of gp120BaL, suggesting that cerebellar granule cells may be more sensitive to apoptotic signals activated by the CXCR4 receptor. The neurotrophin brain-derived neurotrophic factor (BDNF) has been shown to block neuronal apoptosis. Therefore, we examined whether BDNF protects against both strains of gp120. Preexposure of cerebellar granule cells to BDNF prior to both gp120s decreased apoptosis and consequently enhanced their survival. These findings underlie the rationale for exploring the ability of BDNF to reduce HIV-1-mediated neuronal cell death *in vivo*.

KEYWORDS: AIDS; apoptosis; BDNF; caspase-3; gp120BaL; gp120IIIB; neuroprotection; RANTES

INTRODUCTION

Acquired immune deficiency syndrome–associated dementia complex (ADC) is frequent in human immunodeficiency virus type 1 (HIV-1)–positive patients in the late phase of infection, resulting in dysfunction of the central nervous system (CNS) and ultimately neuronal cell death. These patients usually have a rapid progression of their symptoms, with a survival rate of a few months. Neurological complications

Address for correspondence: Italo Mocchetti, Georgetown University Medical Center, Research Building, Room EP04, Box 571464, Washington, D.C. 20057. Voice: 202-687-1197; fax: 202-687-0617.

moccheti@georgetown.edu

Ann. N.Y. Acad. Sci. 1053: 247–257 (2005).
doi: 10.1196/annals.1344.022

associated with this disease include extrapyramidal symptoms, cognitive impairments, and psychiatric disturbances.[1,2] *Ex vivo* examinations of autoptic brains of HIV-positive individuals[3–5] as well as quantitative MRI[6–9] have revealed several pathological features, including ventricular enlargement and cortical and subcortical atrophy. The pathology of HIV-1 infection in the CNS is also characterized by widespread reactive astrocytosis, myelin pallor, and infiltration by monocytoid cells, including blood-derived macrophages, microglia, and multinucleated giant cells.[10] Moreover, neurons in HIV-infected brains show dendritic and synaptic damage.[11] These abnormalities may explain the onset of cognitive and motor deficits observed in these patients.

A better understanding of the pathogenic mechanisms mediating HIV-1 neurotoxicity is crucial for developing effective neuroprotective therapies against ADC. HIV-associated neuronal loss is generally thought to result from neurotoxic factors released from infected macrophages or microglia. Considerable experimental data indicate that the HIV-1 exterior envelope glycoprotein gp120, which is shed from the virus, may be one of the agents causing neuronal cell death and other debilitating neuropathological consequences of HIV infection observed in ADC. Indeed, brains of mice overexpressing gp120 are characterized by loss of neurons,[12] and exposure of neuronal cultures to gp120 causes apoptotic cell death.[13–16] Infusion of recombinant gp120 into rat brain[17–20] causes widespread neuronal cell death. Thus, therapeutic intervention aimed at reducing gp120 toxicity may be important for ADC.

GP120 CAUSES CELL DEATH IN CEREBELLAR GRANULE NEURONS

Macrophages are major reservoirs of HIV-1. The viral entry into macrophages is initiated by binding of gp120 to CD4 followed by interaction with chemokine receptors, CXCR4 or CCR5.[21] Indeed, M-tropic viruses can infect macrophages and $CD4^+$ cells using CCR5, while T-tropic viruses infect primarily $CD4^+$ T cells expressing CXCR4. Engagement of CD4 and chemokine receptors by gp120 is the initial step required for HIV-1 entry and infection. However, this interaction can also occur apart from infection as a result of soluble gp120 shed from virus particles or infected cells. Moreover, recent studies have demonstrated that gp120 has neurotoxic properties in CD4-negative neurons,[16] implying that gp120 may be neurotoxic in the absence of HIV-1 by binding directly to chemokine receptors. In the brain, both glia cells and CD4-negative neurons express CXCR4 or CCR5. Therefore, it has been proposed that gp120 neurotoxicity may occur through inflammatory events associated with activated glia.[22]

To examine the relative sensitivity of neurons to gp120-mediated cell death in the absence of glia and CD4, we used rat cerebellar granule cells prepared according to an established method from 8-day-old pups.[16,23] Cultures were grown for 7 days in the presence of cytosine arabinoside to prevent glia proliferation. At 8 days *in vitro*, a minimal number of glial cells are present (~5% of the entire cell population) and neurons express both CXCR4 and CCR5 receptors.[16] Cultures were exposed to inactivated (boiled) gp120 as a control or low nanomolar concentrations (5 nM) of two strains of gp120, IIIB and BaL, for various times. These two strains of gp120 recognize only CXCR4 or CCR5, respectively.[21] We then measured mitochondrial dehydrogenase [3(4,5-dimethylthiazol-2-yl)-2,5-diphenyltetrazolium bromide] (MTT) activity, a marker of cell death, as previously described.[16,24] In control neurons (exposed to inactivated gp120), a very modest (5%) induction of MTT was observed. Instead, both strains of gp120 induced a time-dependent neurotoxicity. Activation of MTT by gp120IIIB was observed as early as 12 h and remained activated even 24 h later (FIG. 1A). Instead, gp120BaL caused a significant increase in MTT activity only at 24 h (FIG. 1A). Thus, these strains of gp120 may exhibit a similar neurotoxic effect, but different kinetics of cell death activation.

CELL DEATH BY GP120s IS MAINLY APOPTOTIC

Neuronal apoptosis is a hallmark of ADC. To establish whether gp120 induces apoptosis, cerebellar granule cells were exposed to either strain of gp120 for various times. Apoptosis was then examined by determining *in situ* terminal deoxynucleotidyl transferase–mediated biotinylated UTP nick end labeling (TUNEL) as previously described.[16,24] To distinguish neuronal versus glial apoptosis, cells were counterstained with a microtubule activating protein-2 (MAP-2) antibody or Nissl, two neuronal specific markers. By 12 h, ~30% of cells exposed to gp120IIIB were TUNEL-positive (FIG. 1B). A significant greater number of cells (~55%) were TUNEL-positive at 24 h (FIG. 1B). Instead, in cultures exposed to gp120BaL, a significant increase in the number of TUNEL-positive cells was observed only at 24 h (FIG. 1B). All TUNEL-positive cells were MAP-2- or Nissl-positive (data not shown),

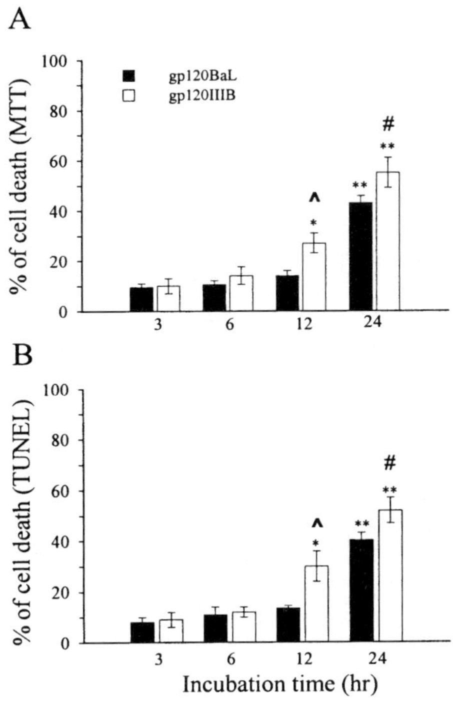

FIGURE 1. Gp120IIIB and gp120BaL induce cell death in cerebellar granule cells. Cerebellar granule cells were obtained from P8 rats, cultured, and used at day 8 *in vitro* as previously described.[16,24] Neurons were exposed for the indicated times to both gp120s (5 nM, each) in 0.1% BSA. Control cells received inactivated (boiled) gp120 in 0.1% BSA. Cell death was analyzed by MTT assay **(A)** or by counting the number of TUNEL-positive cells **(B)** as previously described.[16,24] Neurons exposed to medium alone or to inactivated gp120 showed a similar percent of cell death (~5%). Data are the mean ± SEM of 3 separate experiments ($n = 4$, each experiment, each group). $^{*}P < 0.05$, $^{**}P < 0.001$ vs. control; $^{\#}P < 0.05$, $^{\wedge}P < 0.01$ vs. gp120BaL (ANOVA and Tukey's test).

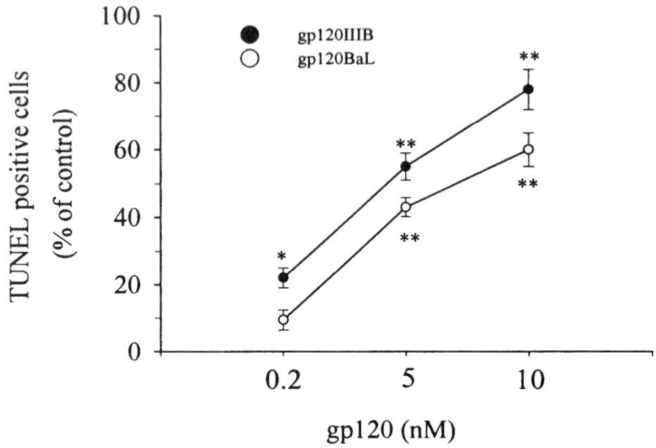

FIGURE 2. Concentration-dependent cell death. Cerebellar granule cells were exposed for 24 h to either gp120 strain at the indicated concentrations. Control cells were exposed to heat-inactivated gp120. Apoptosis was analyzed by counting the number of TUNEL-positive cells. Data are the mean ± SEM ($n = 12$, each data point). *$P < 0.05$, **$P < 0.001$ vs. control (ANOVA and Tukey's test).

indicating neuronal apoptosis. Cerebellar granule cells were then exposed to different concentrations of gp120s to examine their relative neurotoxic potency. TUNEL-positive neurons were seen following concentrations of gp120IIIB as low as 0.2 nM (FIG. 2). Gp120BaL was effective in causing apoptosis starting at 5 nM (FIG. 2). Thus, it appears that cerebellar granule cells are more sensitive to gp120IIIB than gp120BaL.

The concordance of cell death measured by both MTT and TUNEL assays is remarkable, suggesting that the main form of cell death evoked by gp120 is apoptosis. However, TUNEL alone may not distinguish between necrosis and apoptosis. Thus, to confirm apoptosis, we examined whether gp120 activates caspase-3, a protease essential in neuronal apoptosis.[25] Both strains of gp120 elicited a time-dependent activation of caspase-3, an effect that peaked between 6 and 12 h (FIG. 3). These data, taken together, suggest that neurons are sensitive to M-tropic and T-tropic viral proteins even if they are cultured in the absence of glia, and that neuronal cell death can occur independently from the presence of CD4.[26]

CHEMOKINE RECEPTOR–MEDIATED NEUROTOXICITY

The neurotoxic profiles of gp120IIIB and gp120BaL show relevant differences. In fact, apoptosis seen after gp120BaL occurs with a time delay of several hours when compared to gp120IIIB (FIG. 3). These results parallel those shown in FIGURE 2 in which gp120IIIB induces neuronal cell death at lower concentrations than gp120BaL. Thus, it appears that gp120IIIB might be more neurotoxic than gp120BaL. This consideration poses the question as to what role chemokine receptors play in the neurotoxic effect of gp120. As noted above, different HIV-1 envelope

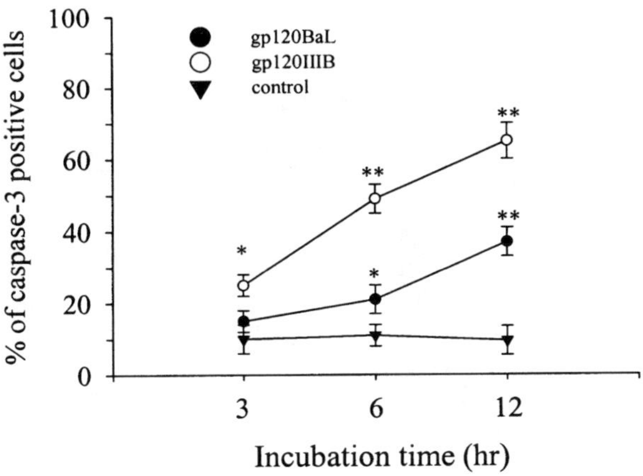

FIGURE 3. Gp120s activate caspase-3. Neurons were exposed to control medium containing boiled gp120 or to gp120s (5 nM each) for the indicated times. Cells were fixed with 4% paraformaldehyde and incubated with an antibody against cleaved caspase-3 (1:150 dilution; Cell Signaling, Beverly, MA) for 48 h at 4°C. Cells were washed and then incubated with fluorescein secondary antibodies as described previously.[16] Immunofluorescence was analyzed with Nikon inverted fluorescent microscope ECLIPSE TE300. Optronics Magnafire software (Optronics, Goleta, CA) was used to analyze immunoreactive cells. Data are the mean ± SEM of 9 samples for each point. $*P < 0.05$, $**P < 0.001$ vs. control (ANOVA and Tukey's test).

proteins bind to different chemokine receptors. CXCR4 and CCR5 belong to the rhodopsin-like receptor family and they signal through G_i proteins.[21] To examine whether receptor specificity underlies the ability of gp120s to induce neurotoxicity, cerebellar granule cells were exposed for 24 h to RANTES, a CCR5-preferred ligand, or stromal derived factor-1α (SDF), the endogenous ligand for CXCR4. RANTES did not affect neuronal viability per se, while SDF elicited a 60% decrease in neuronal survival (FIG. 4A). While these findings support previous data demonstrating that activation of neuronal CXCR4 (but not CCR5) is sufficient to evoke apoptosis,[16,27] they also pose the question as to whether gp120BaL may indirectly bind to CXCR4. Neurons were then incubated with RANTES or AMD3100 (AMD), a selective CXCR4 antagonist,[28] at 15 min prior to gp120s. RANTES completely blocked the neurotoxic effect of gp120BaL, but was ineffective in reducing the neurotoxic activity of gp120IIIB (FIG. 4A). AMD instead inhibited the effect of gp120IIIB, but failed to diminish gp120BaL-mediated cell death (FIG. 4A). Therefore, the neurotoxic effect of gp120BaL stems from its ability to bind CCR5. These data support the current view that CCR5 and CXCR4, two receptors most involved in HIV-1 infection, also play a substantial role in neurotoxicity of viral proteins by activating an intracellular mechanism crucial for apoptosis. Thus, compounds that block chemokine receptor activation may interfere with viral infection as well as with the cascade of neurotoxic events responsible for ADC.

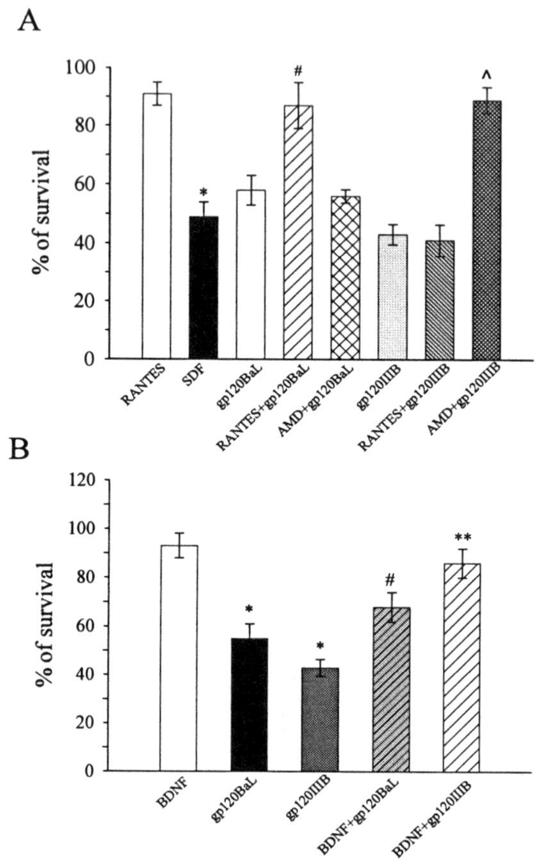

FIGURE 4. Gp120-induced cell death is mediated by chemokine receptors and attenuated by BDNF. **(A)** Cerebellar granule cells were exposed to RANTES or SDF (20 nM, each) for 24 h. Cell death was then determined by counting TUNEL-positive cells. Neurons were also exposed to RANTES (20 nM) or AMD (5 nM) at 15 min prior to gp120s (5 nM, each), and TUNEL determined 24 h later. **(B)** Neurons were exposed to BDNF (50 ng/mL) alone or at 12 h prior to gp120s (5 nM, each). TUNEL-positive cells were determined 24 h later. Data are the mean ± SEM of 8 independent samples for each treatment. **(A)** $^{*}P < 0.001$ vs. control; $^{\#}P < 0.01$ vs. gp120BaL; $^{\wedge}P < 0.01$ vs. gp120IIIB. **(B)** $^{*}P < 0.001$ vs. control; $^{\#}P < 0.05$ vs. gp120BaL; $^{**}P < 0.005$ vs. gp120IIIB (ANOVA and Tukey's test).

BRAIN-DERIVED NEUROTROPHIC FACTOR AND NEUROPROTECTION

Brain-derived neurotrophic factor (BDNF) belongs to the neurotrophin family of growth factors, which includes nerve growth factor, neurotrophin-3 (NT-3), and NT4/5.[29] During CNS development, BDNF affects a variety of events associated with neuronal plasticity.[30] In the adult CNS, BDNF exhibits neuroprotective properties. For instance, this neurotrophin is a survival factor for dopaminergic neurons as it protects against neurotoxins such as *N*-methyl-4-phenyl-1,2,3,6-tetrahydropyridine and 6-OH-dopamine,[31,32] and for glutamatergic neurons as it prevents excitatory amino acid–mediated neuronal injury.[23,33] BDNF also rescues neurons from stroke-mediated secondary injury.[34]

Recently, several lines of independent investigation have suggested that BDNF may prevent the neurotoxic effect of HIV proteins. In fact, BDNF enhances survival of cerebellar granule cells exposed to gp120IIIB[16] or the HIV-1 transcriptional transactivator Tat.[35] However, the relative potency of BDNF in preventing the neurotoxic effect of gp120BaL has never been tested. Cerebellar granule cells were incubated with BDNF (50 ng/mL) for 12 and 24 h prior to gp120IIIB or gp120BaL. TUNEL-positive cells were then examined. BDNF prevented the increase in TUNEL-positive cells by gp120IIIB and gp120BaL (FIG. 4B), suggesting that BDNF is neuroprotective against different strains of gp120. However, the neuroprotection of BDNF against gp120IIIB was significantly stronger than that against gp120BaL. In fact, in the presence of BDNF, 90% and 70% of neurons survived against gp120IIIB and gp120BaL, respectively. It will be interesting in the future to explore in more detail the molecular mechanisms by which BDNF is neuroprotective against multiple strains of gp120.

SUMMARY AND BRIEF DISCUSSION

Productive HIV-1 infection is confined to macrophages and related microglial cells, whereas neurons are not infected. Yet, neuronal degeneration is commonly seen in ADC.[1–3] Several lines of prior research support the hypothesis that gp120 may be an etiological agent causing neuronal atrophy in the HIV-1-infected brain. Gp120 is shed into the extracellular environment by HIV-infected cells and soluble gp120 has been shown to cause neuronal apoptosis and neuronal atrophy *in vivo*[17–20,36] and *in vitro*.[13,16,24] Transgenic mice expressing and secreting gp120 in the CNS develop apoptosis-mediated dendrite degeneration.[12] In conjunction with reports that other HIV proteins, such as tat, nef, and vpr, can all induce cell death,[37] the data presented here support the hypothesis that widespread apoptosis seen in the majority of ADC cases may not be caused by the direct viral infection of neurons, but rather due to release of neurotoxic HIV proteins. In the present study, we sought to determine whether cerebellar granule cells are equally sensitive to different strains of gp120 and whether they can be rescued by BDNF from the toxic effect of gp120. We report that BDNF prevents neuronal cell death induced by gp120IIIB and gp120BaL, the envelope proteins of the T- and M-tropic strains of HIV, respectively. Thus, it is plausible that BDNF attenuates neurotoxic processes that are activated by multiple strains of HIV protein. Future studies will investigate whether BDNF is neuroprotective *in vivo* in animal models of HIV-1. These studies are crucial because no alternative strategies are currently available to limit neuronal loss in ADC.

CXCR4 and CCR5 are chemokine receptors abundant in mammalian brain.[38–40] They belong to a family of G protein–coupled receptors that share common structural features, including an extracellular N-terminus, three extracellular and intracellular loops, and an intracellular C-terminal tail.[41] In addition to important biological processes, these receptors act as coreceptors along with CD4 to regulate viral entry and, consequently, the lethal infection of cells.[42–44] Indeed, transmission of HIV-1 is almost always associated with viruses that utilize CCR5 during the acute phase of infection, and CXCR4 or both in the late progression of the disease. The importance of CCR5 receptor in HIV-1 pathogenesis is underscored by the observation that individuals deficient in CCR5 are resistant to infection by HIV-1.[42,45] Moreover, CCR5 and CXCR4 perform essentially the same function in HIV entry and promote infection with similar efficiency. Therefore, we were expecting a robust neurotoxic effect from gp120BaL. Instead, we were surprised to discover that gp120IIIB is more neurotoxic than gp120BaL, at least in cerebellar granule cells. Paradoxically, in our study, the CCR5 agonist RANTES prevented gp120BaL neurotoxicity, while the CXCR4 endogenous ligand SDF was neurotoxic, supporting previous results from other investigators indicating that RANTES may be neuroprotective.[27,46] The reason for this discrepancy is unclear at present. The affinity of different strains of the envelope protein for CCR5 may be significantly higher than that for CXCR4.[47] These two receptors, although coupled to the same G protein, may use different intracellular signals, which in turn may have different efficacy in activating the apoptotic pathway. RANTES may also block gp120 interactions with CCR5 or cause internalization and breakdown of this receptor.[48] On the other hand, while we speculate that CXCR4-binding envelope protein may be more lethal, we also need to consider the experimental model used to obtain these data. CXCR4 plays a key role in cerebellar development and migration of neurons.[49] Thus, cerebellar granule cells may be more sensitive to CXCR4 activation and apoptosis, a process that is physiologically important during development. Cerebellar granule neurons may also express more CXCR4 receptors than CCR5 receptors. Clearly, more experiments are needed before reaching any conclusion.

In this study, we have examined the ability of BDNF to reduce the neurotoxic effect of two strains of gp120 and found that the neuroprotective effect of this neurotrophin is more dramatic against gp120IIIB. Although preliminary, these data are of paramount interest because they suggest that BDNF may not be suitable to completely block the neurotoxic effect of CCR5 ligands, such as gp120BaL. To this end, it is crucial to define the molecular mechanisms of neuroprotection. While we cannot rule out that a different intracellular mechanism may contribute to CCR5- and CXCR4-mediated neurotoxicity, the weaker effect of BDNF against gp120BaL might be explained by considering the ability of BDNF to alter CXCR4 levels, but not those of CCR5. In fact, we have previously demonstrated that BDNF promotes a time-dependent downregulation of CXCR4 receptors without affecting CCR5 expression.[16] Reduced CXCR4 levels correlated with neuroprotection.[16] Moreover, BDNF has been shown to block the neurotoxic and apoptotic effect of SDF[24] and to share a pharmacological profile similar to AMD, a specific antagonist of CXCR4.[28] These considerations indicate that BDNF may act through a different molecular and cellular mechanism to prevent the neurotoxic effect of gp120BaL. Nonetheless, it will be important to determine the effect of BDNF on CXCR4 and CCR5 expression *in vivo* both in normal brain and under gp120-related conditions.

BDNF is a neuroprotective agent against a variety of neurotoxins. Through the use of an *in vitro* model of HIV-induced neuronal injury, this and previous studies have established fundamental observations regarding the neuroprotective activity of BDNF against gp120. First, BDNF prevents gp120-mediated cell death by inhibiting caspase-3 activation seen after exposure of neurons to low concentrations of gp120. Second, the effect of BDNF occurs through the TrkB receptor.[50] These results may have clinical implications. In fact, in rodent brains, gp120 activates a caspase-3 apoptotic pathway,[20] and caspase-3 activation has been described in postmortem brain tissues of HIV-positive patients.[51] Thus, BDNF, which inhibits stroke-evoked caspase-3 activation in rat brain,[34] may block the neurotoxic effect of gp120 in animals as well. These studies are crucial because they may ultimately promote neuronal survival in ADC patients. It remains to be established whether a protein such as BDNF can be administered to animals or clinically in patients without disrupting the blood-brain barrier. Alternatively, lipophilic agents that mimic BDNF[52] should be tested to establish if they exhibit protective effects similar to those of BDNF. A search for such agents seems warranted to attempt to develop therapies against HIV-1-mediated neuronal loss.

ACKNOWLEDGMENTS

This work was financially supported by National Institutes of Health Grant Nos. NS040670 and NS047977.

REFERENCES

1. McArthur, J.C. *et al.* 2003. Human immunodeficiency virus–associated dementia: an evolving disease. J. Neurovirol. **9:** 205–221.
2. Neuenburg, J.K. *et al.* 2002. HIV-related neuropathology, 1985 to 1999: rising prevalence of HIV encephalopathy in the era of highly active antiretroviral therapy. J. Acquired Immune Defic. Syndr. **31:** 171–177.
3. Wiley, C.A. *et al.* 1991. Neocortical damage during HIV infection. Ann. Neurol. **29:** 651–657.
4. Everall, I.P. *et al.* 1995. Decreased expression of AMPA receptor messenger RNA and protein in AIDS: a model for HIV-associated neurotoxicity. Nat. Med. **1:** 1174–1178.
5. Gelbard, H.A. & L.G. Epstein. 1995. HIV-1 encephalopathy in children. Curr. Opin. Pediatr. **7:** 655–662.
6. Aylward, E.H. *et al.* 1995. Magnetic resonance imaging measurement of gray matter volume reductions in HIV dementia. Am. J. Psychiatry **152:** 987–994.
7. Dal Pan, G.J. *et al.* 1992. Patterns of cerebral atrophy in HIV-1-infected individuals: results of a quantitative MRI analysis. Neurology **42:** 2125–2130.
8. Stout, J.C. *et al.* 1998. Progressive cerebral volume loss in human immunodeficiency virus infection: a longitudinal volumetric magnetic resonance imaging study—HIV Neurobehavioral Research Center Group. Arch. Neurol. **55:** 161–168.
9. Lopez-Villegas, D., R.E. Lenkinski & I. Frank. 1997. Biochemical changes in the frontal lobe of HIV-infected individuals detected by magnetic resonance spectroscopy. Proc. Natl. Acad. Sci. USA **94:** 9854–9859.
10. Kolson, D.L. 2002. Neuropathogenesis of central nervous system HIV-1 infection. Clin. Lab. Med. **22:** 703–717.
11. Masliah, E. *et al.* 1997. Dendritic injury is a pathological substrate for human immunodeficiency virus–related cognitive disorders: HNRC Group—The HIV Neurobehavioral Research Center. Ann. Neurol. **42:** 963–972.
12. Toggas, S.M. & L. Mucke. 1996. Transgenic models in the study of AIDS dementia complex. Curr. Top. Microbiol. Immunol. **206:** 223–241.
13. Meucci, O. & R.J. Miller. 1996. Gp120-induced neurotoxicity in hippocampal pyramidal neuron cultures: protective action of TGF-β1. J. Neurosci. **16:** 4080–4088.
14. Hesselgesser, J. *et al.* 1998. Neuronal apoptosis induced by HIV-1 gp120 and the chemokine SDF-1α is mediated by the chemokine receptor CXCR4. Curr. Biol. **8:** 595–598.

15. DREYER, E.B. & S.A. LIPTON. 1995. The coat protein gp120 of HIV-1 inhibits astrocyte uptake of excitatory amino acids via macrophage arachidonic acid. Eur. J. Neurosci. **7:** 2502–2507.
16. BACHIS, A., E.O. MAJOR & I. MOCCHETTI. 2003. Brain-derived neurotrophic factor inhibits human immunodeficiency virus-1/gp120–mediated cerebellar granule cell death by preventing gp120 internalization. J. Neurosci. **23:** 5715–5722.
17. BAGETTA, G. *et al.* 1995. HIV-1 gp120 produces DNA fragmentation in the cerebral cortex of rat. Biochem. Biophys. Res. Commun. **211:** 130–136.
18. BANSAL, A.K. *et al.* 2000. Neurotoxicity of HIV-1 proteins gp120 and Tat in the rat striatum. Brain Res. **879:** 42–49.
19. CORASANITI, M.T. *et al.* 1998. The HIV envelope protein gp120 in the nervous system: interactions with nitric oxide, interleukin-1beta, and nerve growth factor signalling, with pathological implications *in vivo* and *in vitro*. Biochem. Pharmacol. **56:** 153–156.
20. ACQUAS, E. *et al.* 2004. Human immunodeficiency virus type 1 protein gp120 causes neuronal cell death in the rat brain by activating caspases. Neurotox. Res. **5:** 605–615.
21. BERGER, E.A., P.M. MURPHY & J.M. FARBER. 1999. Chemokine receptors as HIV-1 co-receptors: roles in viral entry, tropism, and disease. Annu. Rev. Immunol. **17:** 657–700.
22. BEZZI, P. *et al.* 2001. CXCR4-activated astrocyte glutamate release via TNFα: amplification by microglia triggers neurotoxicity. Nat. Neurosci. **4:** 702–710.
23. MARINI, A.M. *et al.* 1998. Activity-dependent release of brain-derived neurotrophic factor underlies the neuroprotective effect of *N*-methyl-D-aspartate. J. Biol. Chem. **273:** 29394–29399.
24. BACHIS, A. & I. MOCCHETTI. 2004. The chemokine receptor CXCR4 and not the *N*-methyl-D-aspartate receptor mediates gp120 neurotoxicity in cerebellar granule cells. J. Neurosci. Res. **75:** 75–82.
25. BOATRIGHT, K.M. & G.S. SALVESEN. 2003. Mechanisms of caspase activation. Curr. Opin. Cell Biol. **15:** 725–731.
26. ENDRES, M. *et al.* 1996. CD4-independent infection by HIV-2 is mediated by fusin/CXCR4. Cell **87:** 745–756.
27. MEUCCI, O. *et al.* 1998. Chemokines regulate hippocampal neuronal signaling and gp120 neurotoxicity. Proc. Natl. Acad. Sci. USA **95:** 14500–14505.
28. DONZELLA, G.A. *et al.* 1998. AMD3100, a small molecule inhibitor of HIV-1 entry via the CXCR4 co-receptor. Nat. Med. **4:** 72–77.
29. REICHARDT, L.F. 2001. Neurotrophic Factors: A Window into the Nervous System. F. P. Graham Pub. Johnson City, TN.
30. THOENEN, H. 1995. Neurotrophins and neuronal plasticity. Science **270:** 593–598.
31. ALTAR, C.A. *et al.* 1992. Brain-derived neurotrophic factor augments rotational behavior and nigrostriatal dopamine turnover *in vivo*. Proc. Natl. Acad. Sci. USA **89:** 11347–11351.
32. HYMAN, C. *et al.* 1991. BDNF is a neurotrophic factor for dopaminergic neurons of the substantia nigra. Nature **350:** 230–232.
33. LINDHOLM, D. *et al.* 1993. Brain-derived neurotrophic factor is a survival factor for cultured rat cerebellar granule neurons and protects them against glutamate-induced neurotoxicity. Eur. J. Neurosci. **5:** 1455–1464.
34. HAN, B.H. *et al.* 2000. BDNF blocks caspase-3 activation in neonatal hypoxia-ischemia. Neurobiol. Dis. **7:** 38–53.
35. RAMIREZ, S.H. *et al.* 2001. Neurotrophins prevent HIV Tat-induced neuronal apoptosis via a nuclear factor-kappaB (NF-kappaB)–dependent mechanism. J. Neurochem. **78:** 874–889.
36. CORASANITI, T. *et al.* 2001. Exploitation of the HIV-1 coat glycoprotein, gp120, in neurodegenerative studies *in vivo*. J. Neurochem. **79:** 1–8.
37. MARAGOS, W.F. *et al.* 2003. Neuronal injury in hippocampus with human immunodeficiency virus transactivating protein, Tat. Neuroscience **117:** 43–53.
38. BANISADR, G. *et al.* 2002. Neuroanatomical distribution of CXCR4 in adult rat brain and its localization in cholinergic and dopaminergic neurons. Eur. J. Neurosci. **16:** 1661–1671.
39. VAN DER MEER, P. *et al.* 2000. Immunohistochemical analysis of CCR2, CCR3, CCR5, and CXCR4 in the human brain: potential mechanisms for HIV dementia. Exp. Mol. Pathol. **69:** 192.

40. KLEIN, R.S. *et al.* 1999. Chemokine receptor expression and signaling in macaque and human fetal neurons and astrocytes: implications for the neuropathogenesis of AIDS. J. Immunol. **163:** 1636–1646.
41. ROSSI, D. & A. ZLOTNIK. 2000. The biology of chemokines and their receptors. Annu. Rev. Immunol. **18:** 217–242.
42. SAMSON, M. *et al.* 1996. Resistance to HIV-1 infection in caucasian individuals bearing mutant alleles of the CCR-5 chemokine receptor gene. Nature **382:** 722–725.
43. ZHENG, J. *et al.* 1999. Intracellular CXCR4 signaling, neuronal apoptosis, and neuropathogenic mechanisms of HIV-1-associated dementia. J. Neuroimmunol. **98:** 185–200.
44. HE, J. *et al.* 1997. CCR3 and CCR5 are co-receptors for HIV-1 infection of microglia. Nature **385:** 645–649.
45. DEAN, M. *et al.* 1996. Genetic restriction of HIV-1 infection and progression to AIDS by a deletion allele of the CKR5 structural gene: Hemophilia Growth and Development Study, Multicenter AIDS Cohort Study, Multicenter Hemophilia Cohort Study, San Francisco City Cohort, ALIVE Study. Science **273:** 1856–1862.
46. KAUL, M. & S.A. LIPTON. 1999. Chemokines and activated macrophages in HIV gp120-induced neuronal apoptosis. Proc. Natl. Acad. Sci. USA **96:** 8212–8216.
47. HOFFMAN, T.L. *et al.* 2000. A biosensor assay for studying ligand-membrane receptor interactions: binding of antibodies and HIV-1 Env to chemokine receptors. Proc. Natl. Acad. Sci. USA **97:** 11215–11220.
48. ARAMORI, I. *et al.* 1997. Molecular mechanism of desensitization of the chemokine receptor CCR-5: receptor signaling and internalization are dissociable from its role as an HIV-1 co-receptor. EMBO J. **16:** 4606–4616.
49. MA, Q. *et al.* 1998. Impaired B-lymphopoiesis, myelopoiesis, and derailed cerebellar neuron migration in CXCR4- and SDF-1-deficient mice. Proc. Natl. Acad. Sci. USA **95:** 9448–9453.
50. MOCCHETTI, I. & A. BACHIS. 2004. Brain-derived neurotrophic factor activation of TrkB protects neurons from HIV-1/gp120-induced cell death. Crit. Rev. Neurobiol. **16:** 51–57.
51. JAMES, H.J. *et al.* 1999. Expression of caspase-3 in brains from paediatric patients with HIV-1 encephalitis. Neuropathol. Appl. Neurobiol. **25:** 380–386.
52. BACHIS, A. *et al.* 2002. Gangliosides prevent excitotoxicity through activation of TrkB receptor. Neurotox. Res. **4:** 225–234.

Nicotinamide Modulates Energy Utilization and Improves Functional Recovery from Ischemia in the *In Vitro* Rabbit Retina

DIAMOND TAM,[a] MAJESTIC TAM,[b] AND KENNETH I. MAYNARD[c]

[a]*Department of Ophthalmology, Beckman Vision Center, University of California, San Francisco, California, USA*

[b]*Royal College of Surgeons, Dublin, Ireland*

[c]*Neurosurgical Service, Massachusetts General Hospital and Harvard Medical School, Boston, Massachusetts, USA*

ABSTRACT: The central nervous system depends critically on a regular supply of oxygen and glucose for the formation of adenosine triphosphate (ATP) and the sustenance of its energy metabolism. Consequently, a significant reduction in the supply of oxygen and glucose to neuronal tissue causes an imbalance between the energy supply and demand, inducing the onset of neuronal ischemia and triggering many metabolic cascades leading to irreversible injury and cell death. Nicotinamide (NAm), an essential precursor to nicotinamide adenine dinucleotide (NAD^+), which raises brain ATP levels, may improve cerebral blood flow and is neuroprotective against ischemia-induced injury. We therefore chose to examine the metabolic and electrophysiologic/functional effects of NAm (0.1 mM, 1.0 mM, 10.0 mM) under normal, control, and ischemic conditions, as well as following the early stages of reperfusion ("return-to-control" conditions) using an *in vitro* rabbit retina model where blood flow effects are excluded. Under nonischemic, control conditions, the protective concentration of NAm (10.0 mM) increased glucose utilization (34%, $P < 0.01$) and decreased lactate production (44%, $P < 0.01$), but had no significant effect on electrophysiologic function. After 2 h of ischemia, glucose utilization was significantly decreased (41%, $P < 0.01$) and lactate production was unaffected by NAm (10 mM). Following 3 h of "reperfusion", NAm (10 mM) significantly improved glucose utilization (217%, $P < 0.01$), lactate production (40%, $P < 0.01$), and electrophysiologic function (264%, $P < 0.01$) relative to controls. Thus, the functional neuroprotective effects of NAm may be independent of blood flow effects, but related, at least in part, to its improvement of tissue glucose utilization and lactate production.

KEYWORDS: nicotinamide (NAm); neuroprotection; stroke; hypoxia; niacin; neuronal energy metabolism

Address for correspondence: Dr. Kenneth I. Maynard, Sanofi-Aventis, Inc., 200 Crossing Boulevard, BX2-306A, Bridgewater, NJ 08807-0800. Voice: 908-304-6352; fax: 908-304-6730. kenneth.maynard@sanofi-aventis.com

Ann. N.Y. Acad. Sci. 1053: 258–268 (2005). © 2005 New York Academy of Sciences. doi: 10.1196/annals.1344.023

INTRODUCTION

A reduction in the supply of oxygen and glucose to neuronal tissue causes an imbalance between the energy supply and demand, signaling the onset of neuronal ischemia. Consequently, the resulting lack of adenosine triphosphate (ATP) leads to the reversal of the Na^+/K^+/ATPase pump, causing an influx of Na^+ intracellularly. Spontaneous depolarization of neurons occurs, intracellular Ca^{2+} levels increase, and various cascades are triggered, all potentially leading to irreversible cell injury or cell death.[1,2] Previously, we showed that protection against neuronal ischemia was attainable using a pharmacologic cocktail aimed at the temporary blockade of non-essential, function-related processes.[3] Many of the drugs with which the cocktail was composed, however, were unfit for clinical use in the treatment of retinal ischemia or stroke. In subsequent studies, we showed that Mg^{2+} [a blocker of various subtypes of Ca^{2+} channels and *N*-methyl-D-aspartate (NMDA) channels that have been implicated in excitotoxicity] and mexiletine (a voltage-dependent Na^+-channel blocker), when used individually or combined, exhibited various degrees of neuro-protection in both metabolic as well as electrophysiologic studies in the *in vitro* rabbit retina preparation.[4] We subsequently provided evidence to support a mechanism of action, which we proposed was the reduction of the energy requirements of neurons at risk of cell death via the temporary blockade of nonvital cellular functions.[5]

While the above studies achieved neuroprotection via reducing neuronal energy demands, in theory, the ischemia-induced energy imbalance between reduced supply and normal neuronal energy demand may also be corrected by increasing neuronal energy reserves. Thus, we chose to examine the effects of nicotinamide (NAm) in the *in vitro* rabbit retina as a model of the central nervous system (CNS) to determine its effects on CNS energy metabolism and functional outcome prior to, during, and following ischemia. NAm (vitamin B_3) is a soluble B-group vitamin, which is an essential precursor of nicotinamide adenine dinucleotide (NAD^+). It is reported to prevent the depletion of neuronal ATP in the presence of chemical toxins as well as boost the amount of ATP in the brain following ischemia.[6–8] By enhancing the neuronal energy supply of the tissue at risk, NAm should therefore be capable of protecting the CNS against the initial energy imbalance induced by ischemia. We examined a range of concentrations of NAm (0.1 mM, 1.0 mM, and 10.0 mM) on isolated rabbit retinas using a model that was developed and established in our laboratory specifically for testing the effect of agents on glucose utilization, lactate production, and light-evoked compound action potentials (CAPs) of retinas under normal conditions and before, during, and following ischemia.[3,4,9–11]

MATERIALS AND METHODS

All procedures performed on the animals in this study were approved by the Subcommittee on Research Animal Care of the Massachusetts General Hospital, whose standards concur with those of the Federal (NIH) and State (Massachusetts) reviewing organizations. As previously described,[3,11] retinas with 4–5 mm of optic nerve were isolated from dark-adapted, anesthetized (70 mg/kg ketamine and 25 mg/kg xylazine, im) New Zealand White male rabbits (2.5–4 kg).

Biochemical Studies

The isolated rabbit retinas were placed in glass boats containing a liquid medium of artificial cerebrospinal fluid containing 6 mM glucose (Ames' medium, Sigma Chemical) and a continuous supply of gas (95% O_2 and 5% CO_2) passing over the Ames' medium into the boat. The boats were maintained at 36.5 ± 0.5°C and rocked at ~1 Hz along the longitudinal axis to facilitate exchange between the medium, the gas, and the retina. The retina was allowed to equilibrate in these conditions for 1 h. Following equilibration, the medium was sampled before and after each subsequent incubation period. Retinas were incubated for 1 h in 5 mL of Ames' medium alone (control), and then for 35 min in 5 mL of Ames' medium containing 0.1, 1.0, or 10.0 mM NAm (Sigma Chemical) or Ames' medium without NAm. The retinas then underwent 2 h of ischemia with or without (control) the same concentration of NAm from the preischemia incubation period. They were then returned to control (i.e., normal, nonischemic) conditions for 3 h with fresh Ames' medium without NAm. At the end of the experiments, the retinas were removed from the medium, frozen in liquid nitrogen, weighed (wet weight), and stored in –80°C conditions. The incubation samples of medium obtained were analyzed for glucose (Boehringer Mannheim) and lactate (Sigma Chemical) levels using standard enzymatic determination reaction kits.

Electrophysiological Studies

The isolated rabbit retina was placed in an incubation chamber containing Ames' medium that was gassed with 95% O_2 and 5% CO_2 and maintained at 36–37°C. A dim 1-s light flash was used to evoke CAPs, which were recorded using a Grass pen amplifier/recorder (Grass-Astromed Model CP511). In response to the dim light stimulus, the light-evoked CAPs measured from the optic nerve consisted of "on" and "off" responses. Light-evoked CAPs were recorded every 10–15 min for 60 min. Recordings were continued while the retinas underwent incubation with 0.1, 1.0, or 10.0 mM NAm or Ames' medium without NAm (control) for 35 min. The retinas then underwent 1 h of ischemia (15% O_2, 5% CO_2, and 80% N_2 in 1 mM glucose containing Ames' solution) with the same corresponding concentrations of NAm from the preischemia period. During recovery ("return-to-control") conditions, the Ames' medium with or without (control) NAm was maintained for 15 min and subsequently replaced with fresh Ames' medium without NAm for the final 2 h and 45 min while light-evoked CAPs were recorded.

Data Calculation and Analysis

Analysis of glucose utilization and lactate production under nonischemic conditions was carried out using a Tukey/Kramer statistical analysis. For the electrophysiological studies, data were calculated as a percentage of the control light-evoked CAPs (100%) for each individual retina. Prior to the introduction of ischemic conditions to the retina preparation, four light-evoked CAP recordings, both "on" and "off", were taken and averaged to determine the control response. Analyses for ischemic and "return-to-control" data were performed using repeated measure analysis of variance (ANOVA) followed by Fisher's LSD (protected *t*) post-hoc test for both biochemical and electrophysiological studies. These tests were justified since data were collected from one retina over various time points throughout the entire procedure. All data are presented as mean ± SEM.

RESULTS

Biochemical Data

Glucose utilization and lactate production were both measured prior to, during, and after ischemia for control retinas as well as for retinas exposed to 0.1, 1.0, and 10.0 mM NAm. During preischemia (preincubation), retinal glucose utilization was significantly increased at all concentrations of NAm ($P < 0.05$, $n = 6$, FIG. 1) compared to control retinas (0.81 ± 0.11 μmol/min/g wet weight of tissue). In addition, retinas treated with 10.0 mM NAm exhibited significantly increased glucose utilization compared to 0.1 and 1.0 mM NAm-treated retinas (FIG. 1). In contrast, lactate production was decreased significantly in retinas preincubated with 10.0 mM NAm ($P < 0.005$, $n = 6$, FIG. 1) when compared to untreated (control) retinas (3.75 ± 0.32 μmol/min/g wet weight of tissue for control retinas), or those treated with 0.1 or 1.0 mM NAm prior to ischemia, which were no different from control retinas.

During the 2-h ischemic period, glucose utilization was significantly decreased in retinas treated with 10.0 mM NAm ($P < 0.005$, $n = 6$, FIG. 2) compared to untreated (control) retinas for the entire 2-h duration of ischemia. Lactate production during the first hour of ischemia was not significantly different between NAm-treated retinas and untreated (control) retinas. However, 0.1 mM and 1.0 mM NAm–exposed retinas, but not 10.0 NAm–treated retinas, showed increased lactate production during the second hour of ischemia ($P < 0.05$, $n = 6$, FIG. 2).

During return-to-control conditions, following 2 h of ischemia, glucose utilization was significantly improved in all of the experimental groups as compared to the control retinas when measured 3 h postischemia ($P < 0.005$, $n = 6$, FIG. 3). Furthermore, glucose utilization in 10.0 mM NAm–treated retinas was found to be signifi-

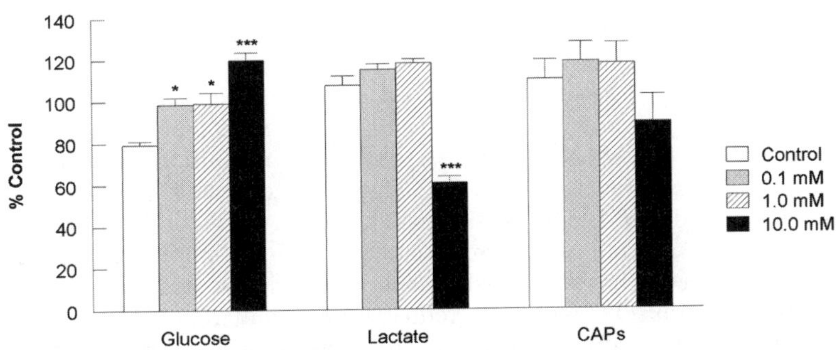

FIGURE 1. Histograms showing the relative rate (compared to a group of control retinas) of glucose utilization, lactate production, and light-evoked compound action potentials (CAPs) following 35-min preincubation with nicotinamide (NAm: 0.1, 1.0, 10.0 mM) under control (6 mM glucose and 95% O_2/5% CO_2) conditions in Ames' medium. Data are represented as mean ± SEM; *$P < 0.05$; ***$P < 0.005$.

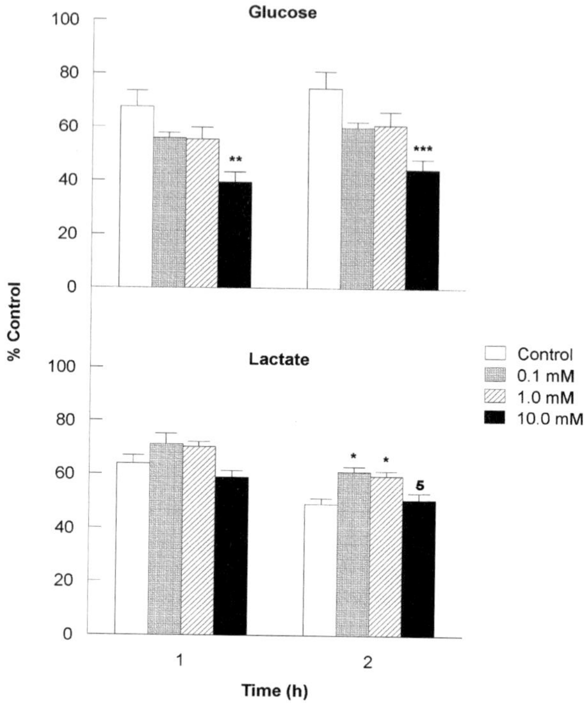

FIGURE 2. Histograms showing the relative rate (compared to a group of control retinas) of glucose utilization and lactate production during and up to 2 h of ischemia (i.e., from 6 mM to 1 mM glucose and from 95% O_2/5% CO_2 to 15% O_2/5% CO_2/80% nitrogen) in the presence of nicotinamide (NAm: 0.1, 1.0, 10.0 mM) in Ames' medium. Data are represented as mean ± SEM; *$P < 0.05$; **$P < 0.01$; ***$P < 0.005$.

cantly improved compared to retinas treated with 0.1 and 1.0 mM NAm (FIG. 3). Although glucose utilization recovery was noted in retinas exposed to 0.1 mM NAm during the first and third hours of "return-to-control" conditions, there was a marked decline and failure in glucose utilization over the course of 3 h of postischemia with retinas treated with 0.1 mM NAm (FIG. 3). Interestingly, retinas treated with 1.0 mM NAm exhibited a mild reversal of the declining trend in glucose utilization seen in retinas exposed to 0.1 mM NAm. With regard to lactate production, following 1 h of "return-to-control" conditions, only retinas treated with 10.0 mM NAm showed significant improvement when compared to control retinas ($P < 0.05$, $n = 6$, FIG. 3). At 2 h of "return-to-control" conditions, retinas treated with 10.0 mM NAm showed additional improvement when compared to all other groups ($P < 0.005$, $n = 6$, FIG. 3). At the 3-h time point postischemia, the recovery of lactate production was further increased in retinas treated with 1.0 and 10.0 mM NAm when compared with untreated (control) retinas (FIG. 3). Retinas treated with 10.0 mM NAm exhibited improved recovery of lactate production over both 0.1 and 1.0 mM NAm–treated groups (FIG. 3).

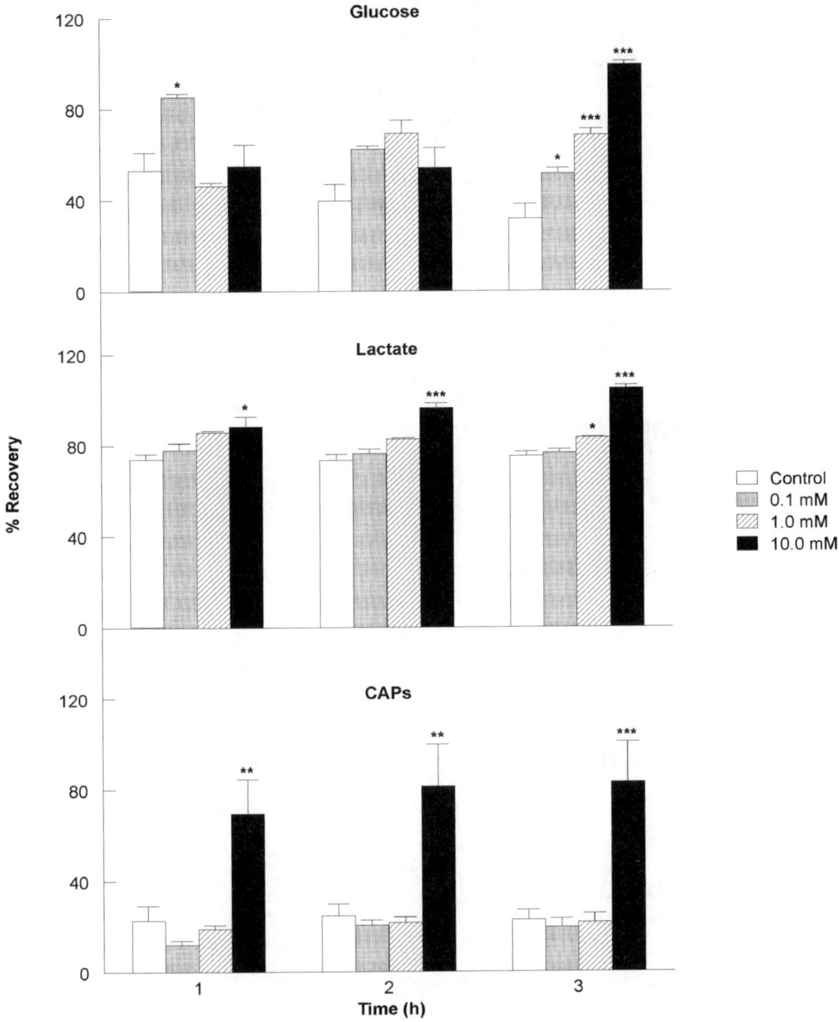

FIGURE 3. Histograms showing the relative rate (compared to a group of control retinas) of glucose utilization, lactate production, and light-evoked compound action potentials (CAPs) up to 3 h following "return-to-control" conditions (6 mM glucose and 95% O_2/5% CO_2) after exposure to nicotinamide (NAm: 0.1, 1.0, 10.0 mM) in Ames' medium. Data are represented as mean ± SEM; $*P < 0.05$; $**P < 0.01$; $***P < 0.005$.

Electrophysiological Data

Prior to preincubation and ischemia, the average sizes of "on" and "off" light-evoked CAPs were 894 ± 67 μV and 343 ± 30 μV, respectively (FIG. 4). No significant differences in the amplitudes of the light-evoked "on" and "off" CAPs between all groups were found prior to preincubation with NAm and ischemia. Following preincubation with NAm (0.1, 1.0, and 10.0 mM), no significant differences were found in all groups with respect to the amplitude of the "on" and "off" light-evoked CAPs (data not shown). Within 5 min of inducing ischemia, light-evoked CAPs were suppressed in all retinas across all groups.

Upon "return-to-control" (postischemic/recovery) conditions following ischemia, light-evoked CAPs recovered partially in all groups (FIG. 3), but robust recovery was only found in retinas exposed to 10.0 mM NAm. Recovery of the light-evoked CAPs from ischemia in untreated (control) retinas was 22.6% ($n = 7$), while retinas treated with 10 mM NAm recovered 83.0% ($P < 0.005$, $n = 6$, FIGS. 3 and 4) at 3-h postischemia. Retinas treated with 0.1 mM NAm (19.4%, $n = 6$) or 1 mM NAm (21.5%, $n = 6$) recovered similarly to the control (untreated) retinas throughout the 3-h postischemic course of the protocol (FIG. 3).

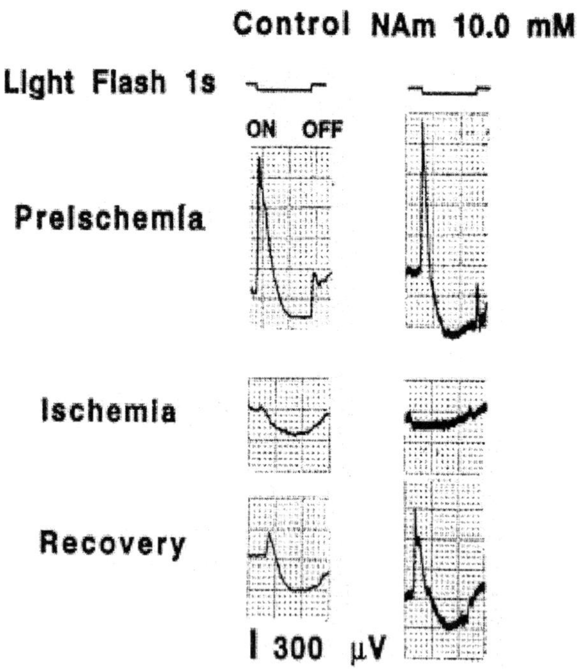

FIGURE 4. Representative original traces showing the effect of nicotinamide (NAm, 10 mM) on the "on" and "off" light-evoked compound action potentials (CAPs) under control ("preischemia"), "ischemia", and return-to-control ("recovery") conditions recorded from *in vitro* rabbit retinas. "Ischemia" consisted of oxygen-glucose deprivation (reduction of glucose from 6 mM to 1 mM and of O_2 from 95% to 15%). "On" and "off" CAPs were evoked in response to a 1-s, dim light flash and recorded from the rabbit optic nerve attached to the *in vitro* retina.

DISCUSSION

This isolated *in vitro* rabbit retina preparation is an established model of the CNS developed and modified in our laboratory to examine the effect of agents acting directly on neural (i.e., neurons and glial) cells.[3,9–12] In these experiments, we have used it to begin to examine the mechanism(s) of action of the protective effects of NAm reported in the CNS. The concentration range of NAm used in our studies was based upon previous reports of neuroprotection observed by exogenous NAm *in vitro*.[13–16] One of these reports showed that up to 25 mM NAm was not toxic to neurons.[14] Further, it was observed that NAm exhibited a concentration-dependent protective effect against NO-induced toxicity in *in vitro* rat hippocampal neurons, with optimal protection observed between 7.5 and 15 mM NAm and declining neuronal survival at higher or lower exogenous concentrations.[14] Thus, we selected 10 mM NAm as our maximal and potentially optimal concentration. Our study showed a robust protective effect, demonstrated by marked biochemical and electrophysiologic/functional improvement of retinas against ischemic conditions when treated with 10 mM exogenous NAm, and this corresponds well with previously documented neuroprotective concentrations of NAm.[13,14] In addition, since the rabbit retina preparation used in these experiments is avascular, it is clear that the acute retinal or neural protective effects of NAm noted in these studies are independent of any potential beneficial vascular effects of the agent.

Under normal, control conditions and prior to the onset of ischemia, NAm increased glucose utilization significantly and only at 10 mM NAm did it inhibit lactate production. These changes suggest that, as is seen *in vivo*,[6,7,17] treatment with NAm boosts neural tissue energy levels, perhaps at least partially, via glycolysis under control, nonischemic conditions. The marked reduction in lactate production at 10.0 mM NAm not only shows that NAm boosts tissue energy levels by increasing glucose utilization, but it also eliminates the accumulation of lactic acid that may also be protective as has been reported *in vitro*[16] and in humans by attenuating stroke-induced lactacidemia.[18] Thus, we propose that under normal, nonischemic conditions, since glycolysis and especially the citric acid cycle are highly dependent upon the availability of NAD^+, the precursor of which is NAm, administration of a high concentration of NAm (e.g., 10.0 mM) may enable the citric acid cycle to operate optimally, hence diverting pyruvate away from being converted to lactate and resulting in the reduction of lactate production. As a result of this diversion, aerobic respiration may boost ATP production and hence neuronal energy reserves. Under control, nonischemic conditions, there was a nonsignificant tendency towards reduced light-evoked CAPs at 10 mM NAm exposure. Since an increase in neuronal energy reserve is not required for normal function, an excess of energy supply to these retinas would not be expected to affect their functional capacity. Thus, since neuronal energy demands are not expected to increase with improved neuronal energy supply or reserve, it is reasonable to expect that treatment with NAm would have no significant effect on neuronal function.

During ischemia, although all concentrations of NAm caused a reduction in glucose utilization when compared to control retinas, only 10.0 mM NAm treatment resulted in a significant reduction. Lactate production increased at low concentrations (0.1 mM, 1.0 mM) of NAm, although significance was not observed until the second hour of ischemia. Nevertheless, at the protective concentration of 10.0 mM

NAm, lactate production was not significantly different from control retinas. The increase in NAm, and hence NAD^+, which feeds the electron transport chain means that energy obtained by glycolysis may not have been needed since energy may have been supplied via oxidative metabolism in the presence of excess NAD^+ supplied by NAm. In addition, since NAm pretreatment enhanced neuronal energy reserves compared to untreated retinas, survival of neural cells of the retina was likely maintained, at least initially, during the period of ischemia via these excess energy stores. Paradoxically, although the glucose utilization was reduced, the lactate production increased significantly at the lower concentrations of NAm. This may be explained if it is realized that the increase in energy reserves, once used, will produce increased lactate levels (following conversion from pyruvate via glycolysis), although the protective concentration of NAm may also protect against the effects of accumulated lactic acid,[18] perhaps by decreasing the release of lactate dehydrogenase.[16] With 10 mM NAm exposure during ischemia, rapid accumulation of acidic metabolic intermediates may ensue, causing inhibition of glycolysis and the citric acid cycle as evidenced by the drastic drop in glucose utilization. However, at the lower concentrations of exogenous NAm, insufficient energy reserves may have accumulated during pretreatment and, in addition, the loss of the electron transport chain efficacy during ischemia may have resulted in decreased neuronal survival. These various metabolic effects may underlie the robust biochemical, bioenergetic, and electrophysiologic/functional protection (or lack thereof at the lower concentrations of NAm) observed in retinas, as revealed by the measurements of glucose utilization, lactate production, and light-evoked CAPs exhibited only in retinas treated with 10 mM NAm.

It is well known that moderate to severe transient neuronal ischemia causes secondary energy failure from 1 to 48 h postischemia, which results in cell death.[19–21] This phenomenon was observed in our investigations since glucose utilization was decreased relative to preischemic, control metabolism in both NAm-treated and untreated retinas for the entire "return-to-control", postischemic period. In general, following "return-to-control", postischemic conditions, there was a reversal of the secondary energy failure indicated by improved glucose utilization in retinas treated with 10 mM NAm compared to untreated retinas. Milder, but similar effects were seen on the recovery of lactate production, but with a robust and significant effect seen at 10 mM NAm. Specifically, at 3 h following "return-to-control" conditions, all groups treated with NAm exhibited significantly improved glucose utilization relative to untreated retinas. More interestingly, the trend towards bioenergetic recovery was seen by realizing that, at 0.1 mM NAm exposure, glucose utilization continued to show a downward trend following "return-to-control" conditions over the 1- to 3-h period. In contrast, retinas treated with 1.0 mM NAm showed a continual improvement in their glucose utilization throughout the 3-h return-to-control period, with the most robust improvement seen with retinas treated with 10 mM NAm. These data are signs of a concentration-dependent, acute recovery from secondary energy failure induced by the ischemic insult and they strongly indicate that exogenous NAm (1.0 and 10.0 mM) acutely reversed the secondary energy failure and likely contributed to the subsequent electrophysiologic/functional protection observed throughout the "return-to-control", postischemic period. Interestingly, although lactate production remained more or less constant following "return-to-control" conditions, 1.0 and 10.0 mM NAm–treated retinas showed enhanced and normalized lactate production relative to controls by 3 h following "return-to-control", postischemic conditions.

Although we showed that NAm has extensive effects on glucose utilization and lactate production (i.e., glycolysis), and hence the citric acid cycle, it is also well known that NAm inhibits the activity of poly-ADP ribose polymerase (PARP), an ATP-dependent enzyme that plays a significant role in repair of damaged DNA incurred from events such as ischemia.[22,23] Neuronal energy reserve depletion brought about by PARP activity during ischemia would add further insult to injury caused by the already ensuing deleterious intracellular cascades, resulting in irreversible cell injury/death. Hence, inhibition of PARP by NAm could also act to preserve neuronal energy reserves in order to maintain vital cell functions for neuronal survival.

The protective effects of NAm in animal models of stroke are well established.[24,25] Nevertheless, further studies are required to elucidate the mechanism(s) of action by which NAm protects against stroke. It has been proposed that NAm is profoundly protective in the brain due to its various advantageous mechanisms of action.[8,24,26] Although the current studies begin to examine some of the mechanisms that may contribute to acute biochemical and functional protection of neurons and glia of the CNS, using the retina as a model, further mechanistic studies are needed to clarify how NAm protects against stroke-induced necrosis and apoptosis in the brain, particularly following delayed administration.

REFERENCES

1. SIESJO, B.K. 1992. Pathophysiology and treatment of focal cerebral ischemia. Part I: pathophysiology. J. Neurosurg. **77:** 169–184.
2. MERGENTHALER, P., U. DIRNAGL & A. MEISEL. 2004. Pathophysiology of stroke: lessons from animal models. Metab. Brain Dis. **19:** 151–167.
3. AMES, A., III, K.I. MAYNARD & S. KAPLAN. 1995. Protection against CNS ischemia by temporary interruption of function-related processes of neurons. J. Cereb. Blood Flow Metab. **15:** 433–439.
4. MAYNARD, K.I., A. QUIÑONES & C.S. OGILVY. 1998. Magnesium plus mexiletine inhibit energy usage and protect retinas against ischemia. NeuroReport **9:** 4141–4144.
5. MAYNARD, K.I., A. QUIÑONES-HINOJOSA & J. MALEK. 1999. Neuroprotection against ischemia by metabolic inhibition revisited: a comparison of hypothermia, a pharmacologic cocktail, and magnesium plus mexiletine. Ann. N.Y. Acad. Sci. **890:** 240–254.
6. BEAL, M.F., D.R. HENSHAW, B.G. JENKINS *et al.* 1994. Co-enzyme Q10 and nicotinamide block striatal lesions produced by the mitochondrial toxin malonate. Ann. Neurol. **36:** 882–888.
7. YANG, J., L.K. KLAIDMAN, A. NALBANDIAN *et al.* 2002. The effects of nicotinamide on energy metabolism following transient focal cerebral ischemia in Wistar rats. Neurosci. Lett. **333:** 91–94.
8. KLAIDMAN, L., M. MORALES, S. KEM *et al.* 2003. Nicotinamide offers multiple protective mechanisms in stroke as a precursor for NAD^+, as a PARP inhibitor, and by partial restoration of mitochondrial function. Pharmacology **69:** 150–157.
9. MAYNARD, K.I., D. CHEN, P.M. ARANGO *et al.* 1996. Nitro-*l*-arginine worsens and *l*-arginine improves functional recovery when added during ischemia in the *in vitro* rabbit retina. NeuroReport **8:** 81–85.
10. MAYNARD, K.I., P.M. ARANGO, D. CHEN *et al.* 1998. Acetylsalicylate administered during simulated ischemia impairs the recovery of neuronal function in the *in vitro* rabbit retina. Neurosci. Lett. **249:** 159–162.
11. QUIÑONES-HINOJOSA, A., A. AMES III, J.Y. MALEK *et al.* 1999. An *in vitro* rabbit retina model to study electrophysiologic and metabolic function during and following ischemia. J. Neurosci. Methods **90:** 107–115.
12. ZAGER, E.L. & A. AMES III. 1988. Reduction of cellular energy requirements: screening for agents that may protect against CNS ischemia. J. Neurosurg. **69:** 568–579.

13. WALLIS, R.A., K.L. PANIZZON, D. HENRY *et al.* 1993. Neuroprotection against nitric oxide injury with inhibitors of ADP-ribosylation. NeuroReport **5:** 245–248.
14. LIN, S.H., A. VINCENT, T. SHAW *et al.* 2000. Prevention of nitric oxide–induced neuronal injury through the modulation of independent pathways of programmed cell death. J. Cereb. Blood Flow Metab. **20:** 1380–1391.
15. SONEE, M., J.R. MARTENS, M.R. EVERS *et al.* 2003. The effects of tertiary butylhydroperoxide and nicotinamide on human cortical neurons. Neurotoxicology **24:** 443–448.
16. SHEN, C-C., H-M. HUANG, H-C. OU *et al.* 2004. Protective effect of nicotinamide on neuronal cells under oxygen and glucose deprivation and hypoxia/reoxygenation. J. Biomed. Sci. **11:** 472–481.
17. SADANAGA-AKIYOSHI, F., H. YAO, S. TANUMA *et al.* 2003. Nicotinamide attenuates focal cerebral ischemic brain injury in rats: with special reference to changes in nicotinamide and NAD^+ levels in ischemic core and penumbra. Neurochem. Res. **28:** 1227–1234.
18. MAJAMAA, K., H. RUSANEN, A.M. RENNES *et al.* 1996. Increase of blood NAD^+ and attenuation of lactacidemia during nicotinamide treatment of a patient with MELAS syndrome. Life Sci. **58:** 691–699.
19. KURODA, S., K.I. KATSURA, R. TSUCHIDATE *et al.* 1996. Secondary bioenergetic failure after transient focal ischaemia is due to mitochondrial injury. Acta Physiol. Scand. **156:** 149–150.
20. SIESJO, B.K., E. ELMER, S. JANELIDZE *et al.* 1999. Role and mechanisms of secondary mitochondrial failure. Acta Neurochir. Suppl. (Wien) **73:** 7–13.
21. LUST, W.D., C. TAYLOR, S. PUNDIK *et al.* 2002. Ischemic cell death: dynamics of delayed secondary energy failure during reperfusion following focal ischemia. Metab. Brain Dis. **17:** 113–121.
22. KLAIDMAN, L.K., S.K. MUKHERJEE & J.D. ADAMS, JR. 2001. Oxidative changes in brain pyridine nucleotides and neuroprotection using nicotinamide. Biochim. Biophys. Acta **1525:** 136–148.
23. VIRAG, L. & C. SZABO. 2001. Purines inhibit poly(ADP-ribose) polymerase activation and modulate oxidant-induced cell death. FASEB J. **15:** 99–107.
24. MAYNARD, K.I. 2002. Natural neuroprotectants after stroke. Sci. Med. **Sept/Oct:** 258–267.
25. MACLEOD, M.R., T. O'COLLINS, D.W. HOWELLS *et al.* 2004. Pooling of animal experimental data reveals influence of study design and publication bias. Stroke **35:** 1203–1208.
26. LI, F., Z.Z. CHONG & K. MAIESE. 2004. Navigating novel mechanisms of cellular plasticity with the NAD^+ precursor and nutrient nicotinamide. Front. Biosci. **9:** 2500–2520.

Mechanisms of Disease: Motoneuron Disease Aggravated by Transgenic Expression of a Functionally Modified AMPA Receptor Subunit

ROHINI KUNER,[a] ANTHONY J. GROOM,[b] GERALD MÜLLER,[c] HANS-CHRISTIAN KORNAU,[d] VANYA STEFOVSKA,[e] IRIS BRESINK,[f] BETTINA HARTMANN,[a] KARSTEN TSCHAUNER,[g] STEFAN WAIBEL,[g] ALBERT C. LUDOLPH,[g] CHRYSANTHY IKONOMIDOU,[e] PETER H. SEEBURG,[h] AND LECHOSLAW TURSKI[i]

[a]*Institute of Pharmacology, University of Heidelberg, D-69120 Heidelberg, Germany*

[b]*Eisai London Research Laboratories, University College London, London WC1E 6BT, United Kingdom*

[c]*Hönower Strasse 152, D-12623 Berlin, Germany*

[d]*Center for Molecular Neurobiology (ZMNH), University of Hamburg, D-20251 Hamburg, Germany*

[e]*Department of Pediatric Neurology, Children's Hospital, Technical University, D-01307 Dresden, Germany*

[f]*Research and Development, Asche AG, D-22763 Hamburg, Germany*

[g]*Department of Neurology, University of Ulm, D-89081 Ulm, Germany*

[h]*Department of Molecular Neurobiology, Max-Planck-Institute for Medical Research, D-69120 Heidelberg, Germany*

[i]*Solvay Pharmaceuticals Research Laboratories, 1381 CP Weesp, the Netherlands*

ABSTRACT: To reveal whether increased Ca^{2+} permeability of glutamate AMPA channels triggered by the transgene for GluR-B(N) induces decline in motor functions and neurodegeneration in the spinal cord, we evaluated growth, motor coordination, and spinal reflexes in transgenic GluR-B(N) and wild-type (wt) mice. To reveal whether the transgenic GluR-B(N) expression aggravates the course of motoneuron disease in SOD1 mice, we mated heterozygous GluR-B(N) and SOD1 [C57BL6Ico-TgN(hSOD1-G93A)1Gur] mice to generate double-transgenic progeny. The phenotypic sequelae in mice carrying mutations were evaluated by monitoring growth, motor coordination, and survival. Neuronal degeneration was assessed by morphological and stereological analysis of spinal cord and brain. We found that transgenic expression in mice of GluR-B(N)-containing glutamate AMPA receptors with increased Ca^{2+} per-

Address for correspondence: Prof. Dr. med. L. Turski, Solvay Pharmaceuticals Research Laboratories, C. J. van Houtenlaan 36, 1381 CP Weesp, the Netherlands. Voice: +31-294-479498; fax: +31-294-477109.
les.turski@solvay.com

Ann. N.Y. Acad. Sci. 1053: 269–286 (2005).
doi: 10.1196/annals.1344.024

meability leads to a late-onset degeneration of neurons in the spinal cord and decline of motor functions. Neuronal death progressed over the entire life span, but manifested clinically in late adulthood, resembling the course of a slow neurodegenerative disorder. Additional transgenic expression of mutated human SOD1 accelerated disease progression, aggravated severity of motor decline, and decreased survival. These observations reveal that moderate, but persistently elevated Ca^{2+} influx via glutamate AMPA channels causes degeneration of spinal motoneurons and motor decline over the span of life. These features resemble the course of sporadic amyotrophic lateral sclerosis (ALS) in humans and suggest that modified function of glutamate AMPA channels may be causally linked to pathogenesis of ALS.

KEYWORDS: amyotrophic lateral sclerosis; AMPA channels; GluR-B subunits; glutamate; spinal reflexes; neurodegeneration

INTRODUCTION

Amyotrophic lateral sclerosis (ALS) is a devastating disorder of the central nervous system in middle and old age, leading to grave disability and early death in humans.[1] Progressive loss of spinal motoneurons is a pathological hallmark of ALS.[2] The dominant early clinical symptoms are progressive asymmetric muscle weakness and atrophy.[2] Transgenic mice overexpressing mutated human Cu^{2+}/Zn^{2+} superoxide dismutase 1 (SOD1) reproduce clinical features of the familial form of ALS.[3] However, changes in SOD1 activity do not correlate with severity of motor decline in sporadic cases,[4] indicating that targets unrelated to superoxide metabolism contribute to pathogenesis of the disease.

Glutamate is suspected to contribute to the etiology of ALS.[5,6] Cerebrospinal fluid (CSF) from ALS patients is toxic to rat cortical neurons in culture,[7] and glutamate antagonists are effective in preventing death of cortical neurons exposed to CSF from ALS patients or of motoneurons in spinal cord explants subjected to glutamate uptake inhibition.[8,9] Agonists at glutamate AMPA/kainate (but not NMDA) receptors injure spinal motoneurons and induce in rodents pathology resembling that seen in patients suffering from ALS.[10,11] Furthermore, SOD1 mutants inactivate the high-affinity glutamate transporter GLT1, which is the predominant isoform involved in keeping extracellular glutamate at nontoxic concentrations.[12]

AMPA receptors assemble from subsets of four subunits, GluR-A to -D (GluR1 to 4). The GluR-B subunit imparts on heteromeric AMPA channels low Ca^{2+} permeability and insensitivity to polyamines by virtue of an arginine (R607) in its pore-forming M2 region, which results from RNA editing of primary GluR-B transcripts at the codon for the Q/R site.[13,14] A reduction in the extent of RNA editing of primary GluR-B transcripts generates a seizure-prone phenotype in mice.[15,16] In contrast, transgenic mice expressing a minigene for GluR-B(N) with an R to N mutation at the Q/R site are viable and fertile.[17] GluR-B(N) subunits confer on recombinant AMPA channels increased Ca^{2+} permeability, but without the current rectification that characterizes Ca^{2+}-permeable AMPA channels configured of subunits with Q at their Q/R site.[14] The combined expression of the GluR-B(N) transgene and the endogenous GluR-B alleles leads in neurons of the transgenic mice to a moderately (twofold) increased Ca^{2+} permeability of the AMPA channel population without significantly affecting macroscopic AMPA conductance.[17]

To reveal whether the increased Ca^{2+} permeability of AMPA channels triggered by the transgene for GluR-B(N) induces decline in motor functions and neurodegeneration in the spinal cord, we evaluated growth (body weight, skeleton), motor coordination (exploratory activity, gait patterns, righting reflex, tremor), and spinal reflexes in transgenic GluR-B(N) and wild-type (wt) mice. Moreover, neuronal degeneration was assessed by morphological and stereological analysis of spinal cord and brain.

SOD1 transgenic mice are known to develop motoneuron disease with a course characterized by early-onset motor dysfunction, tremor and paralysis of the extremities in terminal stages (within 27–32 weeks), and death (within 30–35 weeks).[3] To reveal whether the transgenic GluR-B(N) expression aggravates the course of motoneuron disease in SOD1 mice, we mated heterozygous GluR-B(N) and SOD1 [C57BL6Ico-TgN(hSOD1-G93A)1Gur][3] mice to generate double-transgenic progeny. The phenotypic sequelae in mice carrying both mutations were evaluated by monitoring growth (body weight), motor coordination (righting reflex, tremor), and survival.

MATERIALS AND METHODS

Growth and Skeletal Anomalies

GluR-B(N), SOD1, GluR-B(N)/SOD1, and wt mice were housed under environmentally controlled conditions (6:00 A.M. to 6:00 P.M.; 12-h light/dark cycle; 22–24°C; 40–60% humidity) and permitted free access to food and water. Body weight was monitored by means of a Sartorius model U6100 balance. The measurements were performed weekly between 8:00 and 9:00 A.M. Assessment of skeleton was performed by means of X-ray radiographs taken during ketamine/xylazine anesthesia at the age of 37 and 100 weeks.

Locomotor Activity Patterns

To estimate changes in exploratory activity, groups of nonhabituated GluR-B(N) and wt mice were monitored by means of a Digiscan-16 Animal Activity System (Omnitech, Columbus, OH) for up to 83 weeks starting at the age of 19 weeks. The number of interruptions of the horizontal sensors was taken as a measure of horizontal activity, while that of vertical sensors was taken as a measure of vertical activity. The distance travelled was measured in cm, while average speed of movements was measured in cm/s. Furthermore, the time spent by mice moving in close proximity to the walls (closer than 1 cm) or in the center (>1 cm), indicating fear, was monitored,[18] and the center time/margin time ratio was used as a measure of anxiety.[19] Monitoring of locomotor activity and movement tracking were performed every 4 weeks in independent groups of mice for 2 min between 9:00 and 10:00 A.M.

Elevated Plus-Maze

The elevated plus-maze consisted of two open arms, 50 × 10 cm, and two closed arms, 50 × 10 × 40 cm, with an open roof, arranged such that the open arms were opposite to each other.[20] The maze was elevated to a height of 50 cm and illuminated with 550 Lux. Mice were placed individually in the center of the maze, facing one of the open arms. The number of entries into either the open or closed arms and the time spent in the open arms were recorded. Monitoring of performance in elevated plus-maze was done in groups of GluR-B(N) and wt mice aged 19, 35, 55, and 75 weeks for 5 min between 9:00 and 10:00 A.M. Each mouse was tested only once.

Four-Plate Test

Mice were placed individually in the center of a rectangular chamber (23 × 18 × 30 cm), the floor of which consisted of four metal plates, and were allowed to freely explore for 20 s. During the subsequent 60 s, the mouse received mild shock (1 mA, 60 ms) each time it crossed from one plate to another. The number of crossings was recorded over 60 s.[21] Monitoring of performance in the four-plate test was done in groups of GluR-B(N) and wt mice aged 19, 35, 55, and 75 weeks between 9:00 and 10:00 A.M.

Motor Disturbances

Righting reflex, plantar flexion, and tremor were assessed in an open field (60 × 45 cm) for at least 3 min. Inability of mice to regain upright position within 30 s was scored as a loss of righting reflex. Tremor was defined as rhythmic whole body trembling for longer than 30 s. Plantar flexion was determined in mice at the time of maximal stretching of the body. Measurements were performed weekly.

Assessment of Gait Patterns

Stride length, width, 1–5 toe spreading, and outward rotation angle were assessed monthly starting at the age of 19 weeks. The gait analysis was performed according to the methods of Parker and Clarke.[22] The mouse had to walk through an 80-cm-long and 5-cm-broad tunnel, which had 30-cm-high black walls and was equipped with a Perspex bottom for videotaping. The tunnel was placed in a soundproof room. The legs of each mouse were stained with washable ink. Up to 20 steps were made by the freely moving mouse, which were videotaped, digitized, and subsequently analyzed (Image 1.51, NIH, Bethesda, MD).

Electromyography and Spinal Reflexes

The spinal reflexes in mice were recorded under α-chloralose (Merck; 80 mg/kg ip)/urethane (Sigma; 400 mg/kg ip) anesthesia. To record muscle (M) wave and Hoffmann (H) reflex, the tibial nerve was stimulated by single square-wave shocks of 0.2-ms duration until the respective maximal response (M_{max} or H_{max}) was reached. Electromyogram (EMG) was recorded with a pair of skin-clip surface electrodes from the plantar foot muscle. For every measurement, 20 consecutive EMG responses were averaged; the magnitude of EMG responses was evaluated by measuring the peak-to-peak amplitude. For recording flexor reflexes and determining the reflex stimulation-response relationship, the tibial nerve was stimulated electrically (5 square-wave shocks at 500 Hz, 0.2-ms duration) at 1.5, 1.8, 2.0, 2.5, and 3.0 times the nerve threshold (T_n). EMG was recorded with a pair of wire electrodes inserted percutaneously into the ipsilateral tibial muscle. For every stimulation level, 20 consecutive EMG responses were averaged; the magnitude of flexor reflexes was evaluated by measuring the area bounded by the averaged response and the baseline.[18]

Morphology

For morphological examination, mice were deeply anesthetized with pentobarbital and perfused with a fixative containing 4% paraformaldehyde and 0.5% glutaraldehyde in phosphate-buffered saline (for combined light and electron microscopy) or containing 10% formaldehyde, 10% glacial acetic acid, and 80% methanol (for light microscopy). Sections of the brain and lumbar spinal cord were cut, 10–15 µm thick, were mounted on a glass slide, and stained with cresyl violet or hematoxylin and eosin. For electron microscopy, the tissue was processed in osmium tetroxide and uranyl acetate, dehydrated in graded ethanols, cleared in propylene oxide, embedded in araldite, and examined by transmission electron microscope. For light microscopy, semithin sections, 1-µm-thick, were cut and stained with toluidine blue. For glial fibrillary acidic protein (GFAP) staining of astrocytes in the brain and spinal cord, murine monoclonal antibody (Dako) was used. A rabbit polyclonal anti-GluR-B antiserum (Chemicon, Hofheim, Germany) was used to detect GluR-B expression. Freshly frozen tissue was cut into 20-µm-thick sections, fixed in ethanol, incubated with primary antibody, and washed before a biotinylated antibody against mouse IgG (Vector Laboratories) was added. Peroxidase-labeled avidin-biotin complex (ABC; Vector Laboratories) was added to the sections, and peroxidase activity was detected in a 3,3′-diaminobenzidine (Sigma) solution in phosphate-buffered saline containing 0.01% hydrogen peroxide. Rinsed sections were counterstained in cresyl violet, dehydrated in a series of increasing alcohol concentrations, cleared in xylene, and mounted on glass slides. Sections with no primary antibody were included as controls. The density of immunostaining was semiquantitatively assessed in digitized microscopic images (Leica, Bensheim, Germany) of sections from the brain or spinal cord of mice (n = 4–6/group) using NIH Image (NIH, Bethesda, MD) software. To provide an estimate for possible neuronal loss in the brain and spinal cord, an unbiased stereologic dissector technique[23] was used to estimate the mean numerical density (N_v). The N_v for each brain or spinal cord region was determined with 8–10 dissectors. An unbiased counting frame (0.1 mm × 0.1 mm; dissector height = 0.015 mm) and a high-aperture objective (×100) were used for the sampling. Normal neurons were identified by the presence of the typical nuclei with clear nucleoplasm and distinct nucleolus surrounded by cytoplasm. In the spinal cord, an arbitrary horizontal line connecting the lateral ends of the spinal cord and crossing the ventral edge of the central commissure was considered a junction between intermediate zone and ventral horns. An arbitrary parallel horizontal line crossing the dorsal edge of the central commissure was considered a junction between intermediate zone and dorsal horns. The gray matter of the ventral horns contains motoneurons controlling function of the limbs and trunk, and interneurons. The intermediate zone contains sensory neurons projecting towards the cerebellum, preganglionic autonomic neurons, and interneurons. The dorsal horns contain sensory projection neurons connecting supraspinal centers. Data were analyzed statistically by means of analysis of variance and Student's t test.

mRNA In Situ *Hybridization*

Specific detection of mRNAs for total GluR-B or the GluR-B(N) transgene was performed using ^{35}S-labeled, GluR-B-pan or transgenic oligonucleotide probes on 16-µm frozen spinal sections from GluR-B(N) or wt mice.[17] Competition of hybridization with an excess of the respective cold (unlabeled) oligoprobes was done to verify specificity of *in situ* staining. Sections were subsequently developed for 6 weeks in photographic emulsion and analyzed using dark-field microscopy to permit quantification of cellular distribution of mRNAs, which was performed by counting photographic grains representing mRNA signals on individual neurons (at least 15–20 neurons per section, at least 5–6 sections per mouse).

Cobalt Uptake in Mouse Spinal Cord Slices

We used kainate-induced cobalt uptake as a functional marker for cells expressing Ca^{2+}-permeable AMPA receptors.[24] Lumbar spinal cord was rapidly removed from 4-month-old GluR-B(N) and wt mice under ether anesthesia and sliced at 400 μm on a vibratome in 95% CO_2/5% O_2–bubbled Krebs buffer; treated with 250 μM kainic acid (Sigma) and 1.5 mM cobalt chloride in Krebs buffer containing 0.5 μM tetrodotoxin (Sigma) and the NMDA receptor antagonist, D-aminophosphonopentanoic acid (AP5, Tocris), for 20 min; and processed for cobalt histochemistry with ammonium sulfide. Slices were fixed overnight with 4% PFA in PBS, immersed overnight in sucrose, cryosectioned at 20 μm, and subjected to silver intensification. The numbers of cobalt-positive cells were counted in specified spinal laminae, which were judged by cresyl violet staining on adjacent sections [15 sections/slice, at least 2 slices/mouse, $n = 3$ for GluR-B(N) and wt mice].

RESULTS

Growth of GluR-B(N) and wt mice was monitored for up to 83 weeks starting at the age of 19 weeks. FIGURE 1a shows that body weight in GluR-B(N) mice increased less than in age-matched wt mice [$F_{19–83}(1,222) = 355.73$, $P < 0.001$]. The body weight in GluR-B(N) mice increased from 26.0 ± 0.71 g at the age of 19 weeks to 29.53 ± 1.11 g at the age of 87 weeks (13.5%), while wt mice grew from 30.21 ± 0.49 g to 37.67 ± 1.23 g during this period (25%) (FIG. 1a). No skeletal anomalies were detected on X-ray radiographs of GluR-B(N) and wt mice aged 37 and 100 weeks. The analysis of growth and skeleton showed that weight gain in GluR-B(N) mice was slower than in wt mice, whereas gross skeletal anomalies were not detected.

Assessment of motor coordination revealed that horizontal exploratory activity[18] in wt mice increased from 2000 to 3500 counts/2 min, while in GluR-B(N) mice it increased from 1500 to 2500 counts/2 min between 19 and 47 weeks of age (FIG. 1b). Between 47 and 83 weeks of age, horizontal activity progressively decreased in wt and GluR-B(N) mice, but remained lower in GluR-B(N) mice (FIG. 1b). Analysis of total distance revealed that GluR-B(N) mice moved less than wt mice between 35 and 83 weeks of age (FIG. 1c), while average speed of movements did not differ in wt and GluR-B(N) mice over the initial 59 weeks (FIG. 1d). Average speed of movements was lower in GluR-B(N) than in wt mice between 63 and 83 weeks of age (FIG. 1d). Vertical activity increased in wt mice between 19 and 55 weeks of age and rapidly waned thereafter (FIG. 1e). GluR-B(N) mice demonstrated no vertical activity up to the age of 83 weeks (FIG. 1e). Thus, GluR-B(N) mice were less mobile than wt mice.

The center/margin time ratio[18,19] was lower in GluR-B(N) than in wt mice, indicating that GluR-B(N) mice avoided the center of the open field (FIG. 1f). Since low

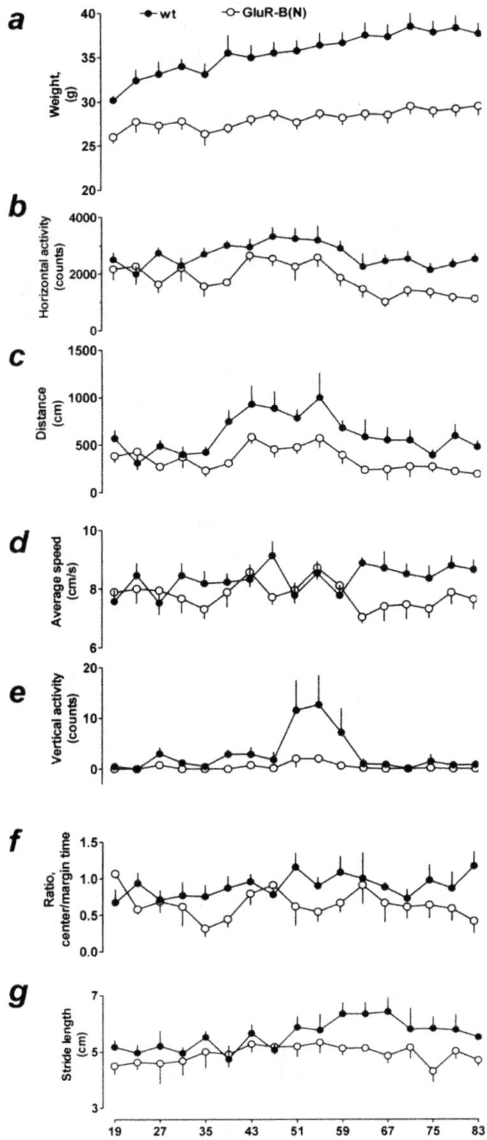

FIGURE 1. Growth **(a)**, locomotor activity **(b–f)**, and gait patterns **(g)** in GluR-B(N) and wt mice between 19 and 83 weeks of age. Growth (a) was monitored by measurements of body weight in GluR-B(N) ($n = 9$) and wt ($n = 15$) mice and is expressed in grams. Analysis of variance showed that, although growth in GluR-B(N) and wt mice was dependent on age [$F_{19–83}(16,222) = 3.35$, $P < 0.001$], it was significantly lower in GluR-B(N) than in wt mice [$F_{19–83}(1,222) = 355.73$, $P < 0.001$]. Locomotor activity was monitored by means of horizontal activity (b), total distance (c), average speed (d), and vertical activity (e) in independent groups of 5–11 GluR-B(N) and 4–7 wt mice. Analysis of variance revealed that changes in

center/margin time ratio and avoidance of rearing (vertical activity) may suggest fear,[18] we subjected mice to trials in an elevated plus-maze[20] and four-plate test,[21] which measure anxiety, at the age of 19, 35, 55, and 75 weeks. GluR-B(N) mice consistently avoided open arms of the maze, entering them less frequently [$F_{19–75}(1,97) = 6.62$, $P < 0.02$] and spending less time in open arms [$F_{19–75}(1,90) = 4.05$, $P < 0.05$] than wt mice in all trials. Similarly, GluR-B(N) mice consistently avoided punished crossings in the four-plate test [$F_{19–75}(1,49) = 31.68$, $P < 0.001$]. These data indicate that GluR-B(N) mice showed anxiety between 19 and 75 weeks of age.

Motor disturbances such as plantar flexion, tremor, and righting reflex were assessed in an open field beginning at the age of 19 weeks. Plantar flexion, which suggests dysfunction of supraspinal control of anterior horn neurons, was first seen in 33% of GluR-B(N) mice aged 35 weeks, became progressively evident in 83% of GluR-B(N) mice beginning with 47 weeks, and persisted up to the age of 83 weeks. Of wt mice, 15–25% showed plantar flexion at more advanced ages only. Righting reflex in GluR-B(N) mice was preserved over 83 weeks, and no tremor occurred up to the age of 83 weeks.

Analysis of gait patterns[22] showed that stride length in GluR-B(N) and wt mice remained similar between 19 and 47 weeks (FIG. 1g). It increased from 5.17 ± 0.24 cm at the age of 19 weeks to 6.42 ± 0.43 cm in 67-week-old wt mice (FIG. 1g). In GluR-B(N) mice, stride length increased from 4.51 ± 0.29 cm at the age of 19 weeks to 5.33 ± 0.38 cm at 55 weeks (FIG. 1g). The stride length decreased in wt mice after 67 weeks to reach 5.52 ± 0.1 cm at 83 weeks, while stride length in GluR-B(N) mice decreased after 55 weeks to reach 4.71 ± 0.22 cm at the age of 83 weeks (FIG. 1g). No changes in stride width, spreading between toes 1 and 5, and outward rotation angle were detected between GluR-B(N) and wt mice over 83 weeks. Analysis of gait patterns demonstrated that GluR-B(N) mice kept their strides shorter than the age-matched wt mice between 19 and 83 weeks of age.

---

horizontal activity (b) in GluR-B(N) and wt mice were age-dependent [$F_{19–83}(16,191) = 4.19$, $P < 0.001$]. The horizontal activity increased in GluR-B(N) and wt mice up to the age of 43–47 weeks and then gradually decreased, remaining significantly lower in GluR-B(N) than in wt mice over the entire observation period [$F_{19–83}(1,16) = 59.89$, $P < 0.001$]. Analysis of the distance traveled (c) showed age-dependent changes in GluR-B(N) and wt mice [$F_{19–83}(16,189) = 3.90$, $P < 0.001$], confirming initial increase of activity lasting up to the age of 43–47 weeks followed by gradual decrease of activity up to the age of 83 weeks. GluR-B(N) mice moved significantly less than wt mice between 35 and 83 weeks of age [$F_{19–83}(1,189) = 46.58$, $P < 0.001$]. Average speed of movements (d) in GluR-B(N) and wt mice did not show age-dependent changes [$F_{19–83}(16,189) = 0.67$, $P > 0.05$]. However, GluR-B(N) mice moved with lower speed between 59 and 83 weeks of age [$F_{19–83}(1,189) = 10.91$, $P < 0.05$]. Analysis of changes in vertical activity (e) revealed age-dependent [$F_{19–83}(16,192) = 4.25$, $P < 0.001$] increase between 27 and 55 weeks of age in wt mice, while GluR-B(N) mice displayed little or no vertical activity [$F_{19–83}(1,192) = 22.18$, $P < 0.001$]. The center/margin time ratio (f) did not show age-dependent changes [$F_{19–83}(16,135) = 0.70$, $P > 0.05$] in GluR-B(N) and wt mice, but it was significantly lower in GluR-B(N) than in wt mice [$F_{19–83}(1,135) = 21.52$, $P < 0.001$], indicating that GluR-B(N) mice avoided the center of the open field. Analysis of variance revealed also that stride length (g) in GluR-B(N) mice was significantly shorter than that in wt mice [$F_{19–83}(1,133) = 22.20$, $P < 0.001$]. Reprinted (a–d, f, g) from KUNER, R. *et al.* 2005. Proc. Natl. Acad. Sci. USA **102:** 5826–5831 (copyright: 2005, National Academy of Sciences of the USA).

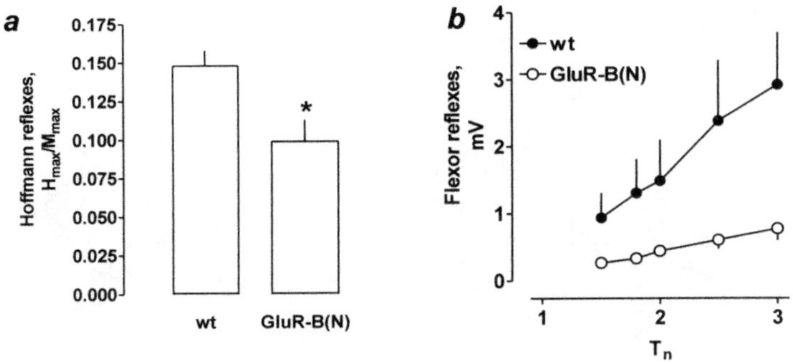

FIGURE 2. Hoffmann (monosynaptic) and flexor reflexes (polysynaptic) in 24-month-old GluR-B(N) and wt mice. Magnitude of Hoffmann reflexes **(a)** is expressed as a ratio between H_{max} and M_{max}.[11] $*P < 0.02$ vs. wt mice (Student's t test; $n = 6–10$). Differences between flexor reflexes **(b)** are shown as a shift of the reflex stimulation-response curve established at different nerve thresholds (T_n; 1.5, 1.8, 2.0, 2.5, and 3.0). Analysis of variance showed that the magnitude of flexor reflexes was significantly lower in GluR-B(N) vs. wt mice [$F(1,70) = 32.21$, $P < 0.001$; $n = 6–10$]. Reprinted from KUNER, R. *et al.* 2005. Proc. Natl. Acad. Sci. USA **102:** 5826–5831 (copyright: 2005, National Academy of Sciences of the USA).

Recording of spinal reflexes[18] in 24-month-old mice showed that both the H-reflexes (monosynaptic) (FIG. 2a) and flexor reflexes (polysynaptic) (FIG. 2b) were decreased in GluR-B(N) mice, suggesting dysfunction of spinal cord. To determine the reasons for disturbances in motor control, we subjected lumbar spinal cords and brains from 1-, 4-, 12-, and 24-month-old GluR-B(N) and wt mice to morphological examination by light and electron microscopy, and stereology.[23]

Expression analysis revealed that the transgene was abundant in the spinal cord of GluR-B(N) mice (FIG. 3). *In situ* hybridization on sections of the lumbar spinal cord with a pan-GluR-B oligoprobe recognizing both endogenous and transgenic GluR-B mRNA revealed a significantly higher content of GluR-B mRNA in ventral horn neurons in GluR-B(N) than in wt mice (FIG. 3a). A high level of expression of the GluR-B(N) transgene in spinal motoneurons was further indicated by an oligoprobe specifically recognizing the GluR-B(N) mRNA sequence, which is largely of rat origin (FIG. 3a). In addition, prominent expression of the GluR-B(N) minigene was manifest in young adult GluR-B(N) mice as an approximately threefold increase in the level of GluR-B immunoreactivity on neurons in spinal motor laminae (FIG. 3b). To assess whether the protein encoded by the GluR-B(N) minigene was incorporated into functional AMPA receptors in spinal motoneurons, we measured AMPA receptor agonist–induced cobalt uptake, which identifies cells expressing Ca^{2+}-permeable AMPA receptors,[24] in living neurons in spinal slices of 4-month-old GluR-B(N) and wt mice. In the presence of saturating concentration of the NMDA receptor antagonist, D-aminophosphonopentanoic acid (AP5), kainate-induced cobalt uptake was observed in significantly higher cell numbers in the spinal interneuron lamina VII and the spinal motor lamina IX of GluR-B(N) than age-matched wt mice (FIG. 3c), indicating that the GluR-B(N) protein is indeed part of functional AMPA receptors in spinal ventral horn neurons and renders them more permeable to Ca^{2+}.

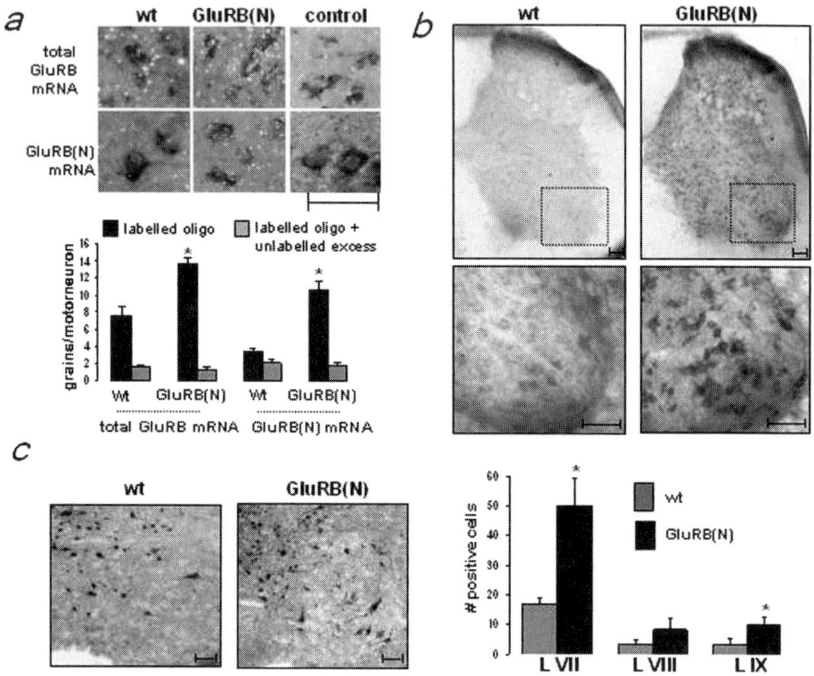

FIGURE 3. **(a)** Representative images of mRNA *in situ* hybridization of lumbar spinal cord sections of GluR-B(N) and wt mice processed in parallel with a pan-probe recognizing native as well as transgenic GluR-B mRNA (total GluR-B mRNA) and with a probe specifically recognizing the GluR-B(N) transgene [GluR-B(N) mRNA]. Sections of spinal cord from GluR-B(N) mice processed in parallel and treated with the labeled probes and an excess of the respective unlabeled probes served as specificity controls. Scale bar: 100 μm. Quantification of positive grains from several sections is represented in the bar graphs below. Ventral horn neurons of GluR-B(N) mice show an increase in GluR-B mRNA-positive grains over wt mice. Furthermore, transgenic GluR-B(N) mice, but not wt mice, show specific expression of the GluR-B(N) transgene. **(b)** Immunostaining of the lumbar spinal cords of 4-month-old wt mice and age-matched GluR-B(N) transgenics with an anti-GluR-B antibody that recognizes the native GluR-B protein as well as the GluR-B(N) transgene. Boxed areas of ventral horns are shown at a higher magnification in the lower panels. GluR-B(N) mice show a significant increase in GluR-B immunoreactivity. Scale bar: 100 μm. **(c)** Labeling of functional AMPA receptors in lumbar spinal cord sections of GluR-B(N) transgenics and wt mice via ligand-induced cobalt uptake. Scale bar: 100 μm. Quantification of cobalt-positive cells in several sections derived from 3 mice/group is demonstrated in the bar graph. The numbers of neurons demonstrating functional AMPA receptors are significantly higher in the spinal ventral laminae VII and IX of GluR-B(N) transgenic mice as compared to wt mice. Reprinted (in modified form) from KUNER, R. *et al.* 2005. Proc. Natl. Acad. Sci. USA **102:** 5826–5831 (copyright: 2005, National Academy of Sciences of the USA).

TABLE 1. Density of cells in the lumbar spinal cord of GluR-B(N) and wt mice

	Density of neurons in the lumbar spinal cord						
Age (months)	Ventral horns, N_v	%	Intermediate zone, N_v	%	Dorsal horns, N_v	%	*n*
wt							
1	21,813 ± 245	100	152,248 ± 5427	100	479,262 ± 9523	100	3
4	20,996 ± 506	96	139,565 ± 518	92	478,156 ± 8775	100	3
12	20,825 ± 682	95	135,869 ± 4854	89	474,553 ± 11,760	99	8
24	20,636 ± 719	95	133,606 ± 8327	88	457,315 ± 16,628	95	7
GluR-B(N)							
1	21,802 ± 539	100	154,755 ± 2392	100	478,298 ± 1995	100	3
4	20,061 ± 651	92	138,773 ± 3896	90	474,038 ± 5874	99	6
12	18,064 ± 789*	83	135,352 ± 4726	87	471,674 ± 17,752	99	8
24	14,023 ± 724***	64	128,796 ± 3921	83	458,782 ± 11,799	96	13

NOTE: Numerical cell densities (N_v) were determined by means of a stereological dissector. Analysis of variance revealed that cell densities in the ventral horns in GluR-B(N) and wt mice decreased with age [$F_{vhage}(3,43) = 9.46$, $P < 0.001$]. Loss of cells in the ventral horns in GluR-B(N) mice was faster than in wt mice [$F_{vh}(1,43) = 15.49$, $P < 0.001$]. Cell densities in the intermediate zone in GluR-B(N) and wt mice decreased with age [$F_{intage}(3,43) = 3.88$, $P < 0.05$] as well, but the rate of cell loss did not significantly differ [$F_{int}(1,43) = 0.04$, $P > 0.05$]. Cell densities [$F_{dhage}(3,43) = 0.81$, $P > 0.05$] and the rates of cell loss [$F_{age}(1,43) = 0.02$, $P > 0.05$] did not significantly change in the dorsal horns in GluR-B(N) and wt mice with increasing age. *$P < 0.05$, ***$P < 0.001$ vs. age-matched wt mice. N_v values given as mean/mm^3 ± SEM. Reprinted from KUNER, R. *et al.* 2005. Proc. Natl. Acad. Sci. USA **102:** 5826–5831 (copyright: 2005, National Academy of Sciences of the USA).

Morphological analysis showed neurons in different stages of degeneration and reactive gliosis in the ventral horns of lumbar spinal cord, basolateral amygdaloid nucleus, and ventromedial hypothalamic nucleus (FIG. 4). Formation of vacuolar structures in the cytoplasm and darkening of the nucleoplasm and cytoplasm prevailed in degenerating neurons (FIG. 5). Cytoplasmic vacuoles appeared to derive either from dilated cisternae of the endoplasmic reticulum or from the swollen mitochondria (FIG. 5). Preservation of synaptic contacts onto degenerating neurons was a characteristic feature of neuronal degeneration in GluR-B(N) mice (FIG. 5). Preservation of presynaptic elements and degeneration of postsynaptic structures constitute hallmark neuropathological features of excitotoxic neurodegeneration.[25] Stereology revealed that in 24-month-old GluR-B(N) mice the density of cells in the ventral horns of lumbar spinal cord decreased by 32% compared to age-matched wt mice (TABLE 1; FIG. 4). Stereological analysis of the brains from 12- and 24-month-old mice revealed that the density of cells in the basolateral amygdaloid nucleus decreased by 31–37% and in the ventromedial hypothalamic nucleus by 34–37% compared to age-matched wt mice (TABLE 2; FIG. 4). In addition, dark cellular profiles were detected, scattered over layer V of the sensorimotor cortex (pyramidal cells), trigeminal motor nucleus, paraventricular and midline thalamic nuclei, gyrus dentatus and CA3/CA4 subfields in the hippocampus, dorsolateral septum, olfactory

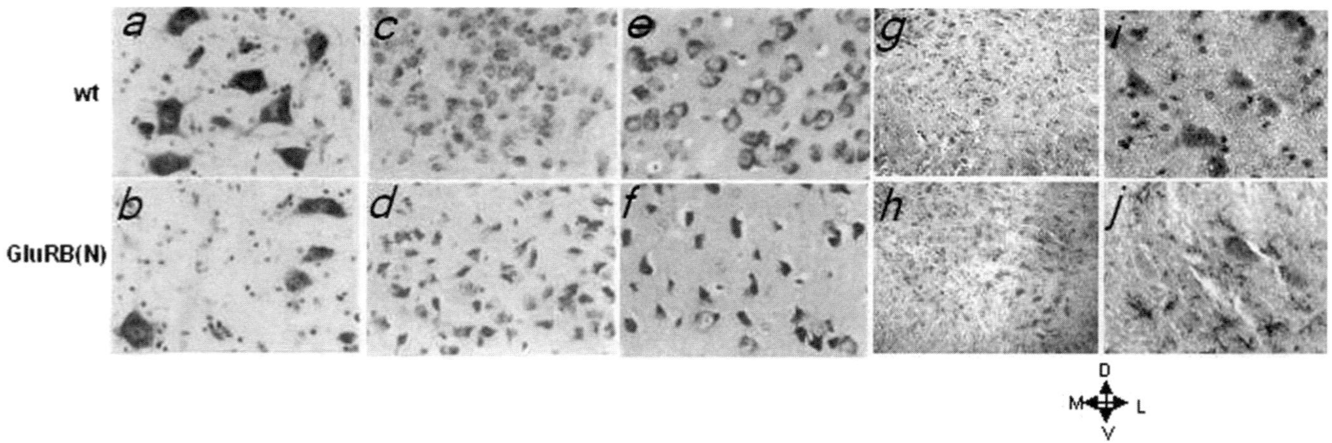

FIGURE 4. **(a)** Ventral horn of the lumbar spinal cord in a 12-month-old wt mouse. **(b)** Extensive neuronal depletion and glial infiltration are prominent within the ventral horn of the lumbar spinal cord of a GluR-B(N) mouse. Shrunken and darkened pyknotic cells displaying narrowings are present throughout the ventral horn. **(c)** No morphological alterations are discernible throughout the basolateral amygdaloid nucleus in the 12-month-old wt mouse. **(d)** Neuronal depletion is remarkable in the basolateral amygdaloid nucleus of an age-matched GluR-B(N) mouse. The cells stain dark and become severely shrunken. **(e)** High-power photomicrograph showing cytoarchitecture of the ventromedial hypothalamic nucleus in the 12-month-old wt mouse. **(f)** Loss of neurons is visible in the ventromedial hypothalamic nucleus in the 12-month-old GluR-B(N) mouse. Shrunken and darkened neuronal somata are interspersed among normal-appearing cells. Cresyl violet stain was used. Magnification: ×40 in a-f. **(g, i)** Immunomicrograph showing ventral horn of the lumbar spinal cord in the 12-month-old wt mouse. **(h, j)** In the GluR-B(N) mouse, cells positive for GFAP (astrocytes) are present in the ventral horn in close proximity to motoneurons. Magnification: ×10 in g and h; ×40 in i and j, counterstained with cresyl violet. [Figure reduced to 66%.]

TABLE 2. Density of neurons in the brain of GluR-B(N) and wt mice aged 12 and 24 months

Mouse type	Age (months)	Brain region	Ventral horns, N_v	n
wt	12	Basolateral amygdaloid nucleus (BLA)	152,677 ± 1570	5
	24		144,000 ± 8901	5
GluR-B(N)	12		105,299 ± 3183***	6
	24		90,330 ± 5938***	11
wt	12	Ventromedial hypothalamic nucleus (VMH)	302,496 ± 10,601	5
	24		282,400 ± 16,118	5
GluR-B(N)	12		192,512 ± 3791***	5
	24		177,192 ± 13,784***	10
wt	12	Purkinje cells, cerebellum	205,924 ± 3052	9
	24		199,930 ± 3528	6
GluR-B(N)	12		202,491 ± 5376	10
	24		199,052 ± 3257	13
wt	12	CA3, hippocampus	298,394 ± 5625	9
	24		307,307 ± 8801	7
GluR-B(N)	12		299,081 ± 5588	10
	24		283,623 ± 10,603	12
wt	12	Pyramidal cells, motor cortex layer V	120,120 ± 6858	4
	24		117,244 ± 3076	8
GluR-B(N)	12		116,840 ± 6901	4
	24		107,711 ± 3175	6
wt	12	Motor trigeminal nucleus	24,120 ± 3031	4
	24		28,667 ± 1022	5
GluR-B(N)	12		25,200 ± 1007	4
	24		28,053 ± 1852	4
wt	12	Lateral septum, dorsal nucleus	123,793 ± 6228	4
	24		121,685 ± 2761	4
GluR-B(N)	12		106,371 ± 12,988	4
	24		109,862 ± 4887	5

NOTE: Numerical densities (N_v) were determined by means of a stereological dissector. Analysis of variance revealed that densities of neurons in the basolateral amygdaloid nucleus and ventromedial hypothalamic nucleus, and not in cerebellum (Purkinje cells), hippocampus (CA3, pyramidal cells), lateral septum (dorsal nucleus), motor cortex (layer V), or motor trigeminal nucleus, were lower in 12- and 24-month-old GluR-B(N) vs. age-matched wt mice [$F_{BLA}(1,23) = 61.40$, $P < 0.001$; $F_{VMH}(1,21) = 55.95$, $P < 0.001$]. ***$P < 0.001$ vs. age-matched wt mice. N_v values given as mean/mm^3 ± SEM. Reprinted from KUNER, R. *et al.* 2005. Proc. Natl. Acad. Sci. USA **102:** 5826–5831 (copyright: 2005, National Academy of Sciences of the USA).

tubercle, and ventral cochlear nucleus. Stereological analysis of these regions did not reveal significant changes in cell densities (TABLE 2).

Morphological analysis indicated that neurodegeneration occurring in the brain and spinal cord of GluR-B(N) mice follows the GluR-B expression pattern[26,27] and is preferentially accelerated in the ventral horns of the spinal cord, basolateral amygdaloid nucleus, and ventromedial hypothalamic nucleus. The ventral horns in

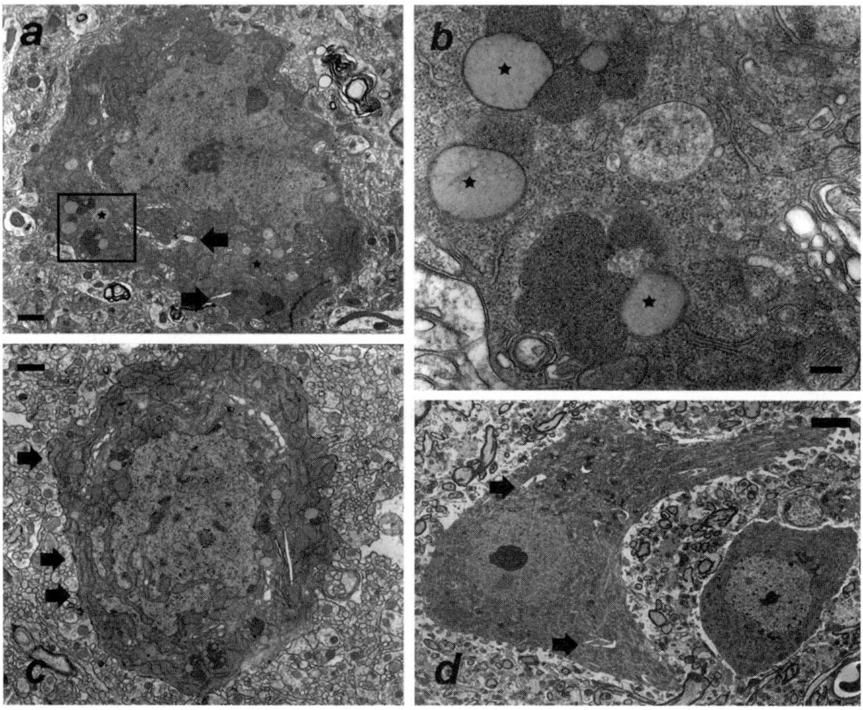

FIGURE 5. Electron micrographs illustrating morphological alterations in the basolateral amygdaloid nucleus **(a–c)** and in the ventral horns of the lumbar spinal cord **(d)** in 12-month-old GluR-B(N) mice. The neuron in **a** appears shrunken, and its cytoplasm has darkened and is filled with vacuolar structures. The *arrows* mark dilated cisternae of the endoplasmic reticulum and the *stars* indicate swollen mitochondria. In **b**, a magnified view of the boxed area in **a** is shown. The dark pigment is lipofuscin and the vacuoles can be identified as swollen mitochondria containing remnants of the mitochondrial cristae. A neuron from basolateral amygdaloid nucleus in **c** displays advanced morphological changes, although synaptic densities at its cytoplasmic membrane remain intact. Preservation of synaptic contacts and degeneration of postsynaptic structures are hallmark neuropathological features of excitotoxic neurodegeneration. A spinal motoneuron depicted in **d** displays pathological alterations consisting of darkening of the cytoplasm, formation of cytoplasmic vacuoles [which partly derive from the endoplasmic reticulum (*arrows*) and partly from the mitochondria], and shrinkage. Morphological changes in spinal motoneurons resemble those seen in neurons of the basolateral amygdaloid nucleus (a–c). Scale bar: 1 μm in a and c; 200 nm in b; 5 μm in d. Reprinted (in modified form) from KUNER, R. *et al.* 2005. Proc. Natl. Acad. Sci. USA **102:** 5826–5831 (copyright: 2005, National Academy of Sciences of the USA).

the spinal cord are essential in the regulation of muscle tone and the execution of movements,[28] the basolateral amygdaloid nucleus has a key role in the perception of fear,[29,30] while the ventromedial hypothalamic nucleus is involved in the regulation of food intake (satiety center).[31] Thus, the clinical effects of the GluR-B(N) mutation, such as motor disturbances, anxiety, and low weight, likely arise from altered AMPA receptor function in the ventral horns of the spinal cord, in the basolateral amygdaloid nucleus, and in the ventromedial hypothalamic nucleus.

Growth of GluR-B(N)/SOD1 and SOD1 mice was monitored for up to 30 weeks after birth. Body weight in GluR-B(N)/SOD1 and SOD1 mice increased over the initial 20 weeks and reached 23.77 ± 0.68 g and 25.82 ± 0.70 g, respectively. The body weight in GluR-B(N)/SOD1 mice subsequently declined to 20.38 ± 0.69 g (14.3%) over 51 ± 3.48 (n = 12) days, while that in the age-matched SOD1 mice fell to 22.73 ± 0.66 g (12%) over 64 ± 6.37 (n = 26) days ($P < 0.05$, Student's t test). Motor disturbances such as tremor and righting reflex were assessed in an open field beginning at the age of 11 weeks. Righting reflex in SOD1 mice was preserved over 20 weeks, while it was lost in GluR-B(N)/SOD1 mice between 12 and 18 weeks of age. Tremor occurred in all 13 double-transgenic mice investigated, but in only 3 of 11 SOD1 mice (27%) ($P < 0.001$, χ^2 test). The onset of tremor in GluR-B(N)/SOD1 double-transgenic mice was accelerated compared to SOD1 mice [87.20 ± 5.50 days vs. 185.0 ± 6.30 days; $P < 0.01$, Student's t test]. GluR-B(N)/SOD1 double-transgenic mice survived 193 ± 2.93 (n = 12) days, whereas SOD1 mice reached 208.4 ± 5.06 (n = 26) days ($P < 0.01$, Student's t test). GluR-B(N) (n = 15) and wt (n = 12) mice survived >350 days ($P < 0.001$, Student's t test). These observations reveal that body weight decline in GluR-B(N)/SOD1 mice was more rapid, motor coordination deteriorated earlier, and tremor was more severe than in age-matched SOD1 mice, indicating that the course of motoneuron disease was aggravated in the GluR-B(N)/SOD1 genotype.

DISCUSSION

Our observations have implications for understanding how moderate, but persistent functional changes in glutamatergic neurotransmission contribute over time to the pathogenesis of brain disorders. We reveal that the transgenic expression of a functionally altered glutamate AMPA receptor subunit can result in a phenotype in mice characterized by a delayed pattern of neurodegeneration and progressive motor decline resembling motoneuron disease in humans. Chronic moderate AMPA channel-mediated Ca^{2+} influx into central principal neurons, as seen in our GluR-B(N)-expressing transgenics, appears not to affect development, but over time consistently leads in adult mice to a selective loss of neurons in the spinal cord, amygdala, and hypothalamus, although the deleterious GluR-B(N) subunit should be operant throughout the entire nervous system.

The selective vulnerability of motoneurons to GluR-B(N) deserves consideration. In humans, spinal motoneurons selectively die from the suspected AMPA agonist, β-*N*-oxalylamino-L-alanine, leading to the symptoms of motoneuron disease (lathyrism).[32] Remarkably, the expression of functionally altered AMPA channels by impaired Q/R site editing of GluR-B leads in mice to severe seizures and premature death during the first postnatal month,[15] which precludes the likely development of motoneuron disease in later life. Intriguingly, the Q/R site–edited GluR-B subunit, which confers low Ca^{2+} permeability on AMPA channels, is at lesser abundance in spinal motoneurons than in dorsal horn neurons,[33] and most other principal neurons of the brain,[33] and hence the AMPA channel population in spinal motoneurons is in part Ca^{2+}-permeable. The deleterious effect of GluR-B(N) on motoneurons therefore strongly indicates that further increases in the population of Ca^{2+}-permeable AMPA channels become harmful for these cells. Our work thus provides a causal link for the intriguing observation that Q/R site editing of GluR-B is incomplete in a large proportion of spinal motoneurons from individuals with sporadic ALS.[34]

The genetic mechanisms controlling GluR-B subunit expression and the extent of Q/R site editing in motoneurons may, if faulty, trigger the phenotype of motoneuron disease by itself, on the background of facilitating environmental factors (lathyrism),[32] excessive exercise (high performance professional athletes),[35–37] or combinations of both. Similar molecular mechanisms may apply to the loss of neurons in the amygdala and hypothalamus in GluR-B(N) mice and ALS,[38,39] resulting in the phenotype of affective lability or low weight, frequently also noted in humans suffering from ALS.[37,40]

Insights into the mechanisms affecting survival of motoneurons in GluR-B(N) and GluR-B(N)/SOD1 mice may provide important guidance for the development of preventive strategies and future remedies to halt progression of ALS and, perhaps, other chronic neurodegenerative disorders.

COMPETING INTEREST: The authors declare that they have no competing financial interests.

REFERENCES

1. ROWLAND, L.P. 1994. *In* Neurodegenerative Diseases, pp. 507–521. Saunders. Philadelphia.
2. LOWE, J., G. LENNOX & P.N. LEIGH. 1997. *In* Greenfield's Neuropathology, pp. 281–366. Arnold. London.
3. GURNEY, M.E., H. PU, A.Y. CHIU *et al.* 1994. Motor neuron degeneration in mice that express a human Cu,Zn superoxide dismutase mutation. Science **264:** 1772–1775.
4. ROSEN, D.R., T. SIDDIQUE, D. PATTERSON *et al.* 1993. Mutations in Cu/Zn superoxide dismutase gene are associated with familial amyotrophic lateral sclerosis. Nature **362:** 59–62.
5. SHAW, P.J. & P.G. INCE. 1997. Glutamate, excitotoxicity, and amyotrophic lateral sclerosis. J. Neurol. **244:** S3–S14.
6. CLEVELAND, D.W. & J.D. ROTHSTEIN. 2001. From Charcot to Lou Gehrig: deciphering selective motor neuron death in ALS. Nat. Rev. Neurosci. **2:** 806–819.
7. COURATIER, P., J. HUGON, P. SINDOU *et al.* 1993. Cell culture evidence for neuronal degeneration in amyotrophic lateral sclerosis being linked to glutamate AMPA/kainate receptors. Lancet **341:** 265–268.
8. ROTHSTEIN, J.D., L. JIN, M. DYKES-HOBERG *et al.* 1993. Chronic inhibition of glutamate uptake produces a model of slow neurotoxicity. Proc. Natl. Acad. Sci. USA **90:** 6591–6595.
9. COURATIER, P., P. SINDOU, F. ESCLAIRE *et al.* 1994. Neuroprotective effects of riluzole in ALS CSF toxicity. Neuroreport **5:** 1012–1014.
10. HUGON, J. & J.M. VALLAT. 1990. Abnormal distribution of phosphorylated neurofilaments in neuronal degeneration induced by kainic acid. Neurosci. Lett. **119:** 45–48.
11. IKONOMIDOU, C., Y. QIN, J. LABRUYERE *et al.* 1996. Motor neuron degeneration induced by excitotoxin agonists has features in common with those seen in the SOD-1 trans-

genic mouse model of amyotrophic lateral sclerosis. J. Neuropathol. Exp. Neurol. **55:** 211–224.
12. Trotti, D., A. Rolfs, N.C. Danbolt *et al.* 1999. SOD1 mutants linked to amyotrophic lateral sclerosis selectively inactivate a glial glutamate transporter. Nat. Neurosci. **2:** 427–433.
13. Burnashev, N., H. Monyer, P.H. Seeburg *et al.* 1992. Divalent ion permeability of AMPA receptor channels is dominated by the edited form of a single subunit. Neuron **8:** 189–198.
14. Seeburg, P.H., M. Higuchi & R. Sprengel. 1998. RNA editing of brain glutamate receptor channels: mechanism and physiology. Brain Res. Rev. **26:** 217–229.
15. Brusa, R., F. Zimmermann, D.S. Koh *et al.* 1995. Early-onset epilepsy and postnatal lethality associated with an editing-deficient GluR-B allele in mice. Science **270:** 1677–1680.
16. Higuchi, M., S. Maas, F.N. Single *et al.* 2000. Point mutation in an AMPA receptor gene rescues lethality in mice deficient in the RNA-editing enzyme ADAR2. Nature **406:** 78–81.
17. Feldmeyer, D., K. Kask, R. Brusa *et al.* 1999. Neurological dysfunctions in mice expressing different levels of the Q/R site–unedited AMPAR subunit GluR-B. Nature Neurosci. **2:** 57–64.
18. Steppuhn, K.G. & L. Turski. 1993. Diazepam dependence prevented by glutamate antagonists. Proc. Natl. Acad. Sci. USA **90:** 6889–6893.
19. Pinna, G., R. Galici, H.H. Schneider *et al.* 1997. Alprazolam dependence prevented by substituting with the β-carboline abecarnil. Proc. Natl. Acad. Sci. USA **94:** 2719–2723.
20. Lister, R.G. 1987. The use of a plus-maze to measure anxiety in the mouse. Psychopharmacology (Berlin) **92:** 180–185.
21. Stephens, D.N. & W. Kehr. 1985. β-Carbolines can enhance or antagonize the effects of punishment in mice. Psychopharmacology (Berlin) **85:** 143–147.
22. Parker, A.J. & K.A. Clarke. 1988. Gait topography in rat locomotion. Physiol. Behav. **48:** 41–47.
23. Ikonomidou, C., F. Bosch, M. Miksa *et al.* 1999. Blockade of NMDA receptors and apoptotic neurodegeneration in the developing brain. Science **283:** 70–74.
24. Engelman, H.S., T.B. Allen & A.B. MacDermott. 1999. The distribution of neurons expressing calcium-permeable AMPA receptors in the superficial laminae of the spinal cord dorsal horn. J. Neurosci. **19:** 2081–2089.
25. Olney, J.W. & L.G. Sharpe. 1969. Brain lesions in infant rhesus monkey treated with monosodium glutamate. Science **166:** 386–388.
26. Petralia, R.S., Y.X. Wang, E. Mayat *et al.* 1997. Glutamate receptor subunit 2–selective antibody shows a differential distribution of Ca^{2+}-impermeable AMPA receptors among populations of neurons. J. Comp. Neurol. **385:** 456–476.
27. Tomiyama, M., R. Rodriguez-Puertas, R. Cortes *et al.* 1996. Differential regional distribution of AMPA receptor subunit messenger RNAs in the human spinal cord as visualized by *in situ* hybridization. Neuroscience **75:** 901–915.
28. Burke, R.E. 1990. *In* The Synaptic Organisation of the Brain, pp. 88–132. Oxford Univ. Press. London/New York.
29. Davis, M. 1997. Neurobiology of fear responses: the role of the amygdala. J. Neuropsychiatr. Clin. Neurosci. **9:** 382–402.
30. Swanson, L.W. & G.D. Petrovich. 1998. What is the amygdala? Trends Neurosci. **21:** 323–331.
31. Schwartz, M.W., S.C. Woods, D. Porte *et al.* 2000. Central nervous system control of food intake. Nature **404:** 661–671.
32. Spencer, P.S., D.N. Roy, A.C. Ludolph *et al.* 1986. Lathyrism: evidence for role of the neuroexcitatory amino acid BOAA. Lancet **2:** 1066–1067.
33. Heath, P.R., J. Tomkins, P.G. Ince *et al.* 2002. Quantitative assessment of AMPA receptor mRNA in human spinal motor neurons isolated by laser capture microdissection. Neuroreport **13:** 1753–1757.
34. Kawahara, Y., K. Ito, H. Sun *et al.* 2004. Glutamate receptors: RNA editing and death of motor neurons. Nature **427:** 801.

35. BERETTA, S., M.T. CARRI, E. BEGHI *et al.* 2003. The sinister side of Italian soccer. Lancet Neurol. **2:** 656–657.
36. LONGSTRETH, W.T., L.M. NELSON, T.D. KOEPSELL *et al.* 1991. Hypotheses to explain the association between vigorous physical activity and amyotrophic lateral sclerosis. Med. Hypotheses **34:** 144–148.
37. SCARMEAS, N., T. SHIH, Y. STERN *et al.* 2002. Premorbid weight, body mass, and varsity athletics in ALS. Neurology **59:** 773–775.
38. KATO, S., M. ODA, H. HAYASHI *et al.* 1994. Participation of the limbic system and its associated areas in the dementia of amyotrophic lateral sclerosis. J. Neurol. Sci. **126:** 62–69.
39. TSUCHIYA, K., M. TAKAHASHI, H. SHIOTSU *et al.* 2002. Sporadic amyotrophic lateral sclerosis with circumscribed temporal atrophy. Neuropathology **22:** 308–316.
40. GALLAGHER, J.P. 1989. Pathologic laughter and crying in ALS: a search for their origin. Acta Neurol. Scand. **80:** 114–117.

Questions and Answers

Session VI: Neuroprotective Agents and Mechanisms

QUESTION FOR XIAOYANG QI

From Ahmet Hoke

Does sapC-PS transfect terminally differentiated neurons?

ANSWER: SapC-PS transfects mouse cortical and hippocampal neurons *in vitro*.

QUESTIONS FOR LECHOSLAW TURSKI

From Moussa Youdim

One major pathological aspect of ALS is the loss of ceruloplasm and accumulation of iron as has been shown in biochemical and MRI studies. Have you looked at abnormal iron metabolism in your novel double-transgenic mice model of ALS, GluR-B(N) and SOD1 [C57BL6Ico-TgN(hSOD1-G93A)]? These studies could shed light on the process of oxidative stress implicated in ALS.

ANSWER: We have not yet studied metabolism of iron in GluR-B(N) mice. We initially focused on overall pathology in the spinal cord and in the brain of these mutants. In addition, it was important to see whether a combination of defects in the function of SOD1 and GluR-B subunit in the AMPA receptor results in a more pronounced pathology in double-transgenic mice. Metabolism of iron may be approached in future studies on these unique mutants.

From Philip Lazarovici

Have you measured the sensory input in the transgenic GluR-B(N)? Have you measured more in detail the mono- and polysynaptic pathways, for example, by injecting tetanus toxin? What happens to the interneurons in the transgenic GluR-B(N) mice during the second year of their life?

ANSWER: We did not specifically address sensory input in GluR-B(N) mice and did not use tetanus toxin in the studies of polysynaptic pathways. However, we investigated interneurons in the spinal cord of GluR-B(N) transgenics and did not detect significant changes in the cell density over a period of two years.

Ann. N.Y. Acad. Sci. 1053: 287–288 (2005).
doi: 10.1196/annals.1344.065

QUESTIONS FOR ITALO MOCCHETTI

From Moussa Youdim

BDNF has been shown to possess antiapoptotic neuroprotective activity via activation of P13-K and ERK-1/2. Presumably, it also activates Akt. In this regard, BDNF behaves similar to the anti-Parkinson drug, rasagiline. This drug has neuroprotective activity and induces BDNF, GDNF, and NGF mRNA. We have shown that its neuroprotective activity is dependent on PKC activation since inhibitors (GF) of PKC prevent this. Have you considered that, in your acute apoptotic studies, BDNF may operate similarly and via PKC activation?

ANSWER: We do not discard the hypothesis that PKC may be involved in the neuroprotective activity of BDNF because previous studies have shown that neuroprotection by BDNF against glutamate toxicity includes this pathway. However, our published data have shown that inhibition of ERK-1/2 prevents BDNF-mediated neuroprotection against gp120. Thus, it is likely that BDNF is neuroprotective against some toxins by PKC activation and others by ERK-1/2.

From Ahmet Hoke

Differences in sensitivity of cortical neurons versus cerebellar granular cells can be due to differences in CXCR versus CCR. Have you looked at chemokine (msp) expression in cortical neurons?

ANSWER: I think that you are right. The different sensitivity of cortical neurons to gp120 versus cerebellar granule cells could be due to the relative levels of chemokine receptors. This should not be surprising because cortical cultures are formed by a variety of neurons, while cerebellar granule cells are homogeneous cultures.

From Philip Lazarovici

NGF was found neuroprotective in the ongoing clinical trial for peripheral neuropathy in AIDS patients. Can you comment on the relevance to the observed BDNF neuroprotective effects in your model?

ANSWER: The models that we are using to test the effects of BDNF are relevant only to BDNF. In fact, both cerebellar granule cells and cortical neurons are sensitive to BDNF, but not to NGF. In previous studies, we failed to observe TrkA expression in either culture. However, we do not discard the hypothesis that NGF may block gp120-mediated neurotoxicity in NGF-responsive neurons such as DRG.

Potentially Neuroprotective and Therapeutic Properties of Nitrous Oxide and Xenon

JACQUES H. ABRAINI,[a,b] HÉLÈNE N. DAVID,[b] AND MARC LEMAIRE[c]

[a]*Centre CYCERON, UMR 6185, Université de Caen–CNRS, 14074 Caen cedex, France*

[b]*NNOXe Pharmaceuticals Incorporated, Québec, QC, G1W 4W5 Canada*

[c]*Air Liquide Research and Development, Claude-Delorme Research Center, 78354 Jouy-en-Josas, France*

ABSTRACT: Despite the beneficial effects of prototypical glutamatergic receptor antagonists in animal models, the pharmacological attempts by the use of such agents have met with very limited clinical success because these compounds produce adverse side effects and possess an intrinsic neurotoxicity at neuroprotective and therapeutic concentrations. Interestingly, nitrous oxide and xenon, which are anesthetic gases with a remarkably safe clinical profile, have been shown to be effective inhibitors of the NMDA receptor. We briefly review accumulating evidence that nitrous oxide and xenon at subanesthetic concentrations may have potentially neuroprotective and therapeutic properties, with a particular focus on their beneficial effects on ischemia-induced neuronal death and amphetamine-induced sensitization. Nitrous oxide at 75-vol% and xenon up to 70-vol% reduce ischemia-induced neuronal death induced by occlusion of the middle cerebral artery in rodents, and decrease NMDA-induced Ca^{2+} influx in neuronal cell cultures, a critical event involved in excitotoxicity. Nitrous oxide at 75-vol% and xenon at 50-vol% further reduced amphetamine-induced locomotor sensitization in rodents. However, at a higher concentration of 75-vol%, xenon shows potentially neurotoxic properties and adverse side effects. Because both agents are rapidly eliminated from the body, it is plausible that their administration at appropriate subanesthetic neuroprotective and therapeutic concentrations may not be associated, in contrast with prototypical NMDA receptor antagonists, with adverse side effects and potentially neurotoxicity. Finally, the possible therapeutic implications in humans are discussed.

KEYWORDS: nitrous oxide; xenon; anesthetic gases; ischemia-induced brain damage; NMDA receptor antagonists; amphetamine sensitization; drug addiction; neuroprotection; neurotoxicity

INTRODUCTION

Glutamate is a neurotransmitter that plays an essential role in many physiological functions. However, under various pathological conditions, neurons can become so sensitive to glutamate that it actually can damage or kill them, mainly through *N*-methyl-D-aspartate (NMDA) receptor–mediated depolarization and/or intraneuronal

Address for correspondence: Professor Jacques H. Abraini, Ph.D., D.Sc., Centre CYCERON, UMR 6185, Université de Caen–CNRS, Boulevard Henri Becquerel, B. P. 5229, 14074 Caen cedex, France. Voice/fax: +33-231-470-102.
abraini@cyceron.fr

**Ann. N.Y. Acad. Sci. 1053: 289–300 (2005). © 2005 New York Academy of Sciences.
doi: 10.1196/annals.1344.025**

calcium influx. Blocking the NMDA receptor and thereby excitotoxicity may therefore help to decrease brain damage and dysfunctions in central nervous system (CNS) disorders, such as stroke, seizures, trauma, amyotrophic lateral sclerosis, and drug addiction.[1] However, despite the beneficial effects of glutamatergic receptor antagonists in animal models of brain diseases and dysfunctions, the pharmacological attempts by the use of such agents have met with very limited clinical success because these compounds produce adverse side effects as well as an intrinsic neurotoxicity at neuroprotective concentrations.[2–5] To avoid or at least to reduce such adverse side effects, the potentially therapeutic interest of low-affinity use-dependent NMDA receptor antagonists, which also possess little to moderate antagonistic action at the cholinergic nicotinic receptor, has been pinpointed.[5,6] Moreover, an additional reason for the failure to translate the neuroprotective potential of NMDA receptor antagonists to clinical use may be the difficulty that most of these agents have in penetrating the blood-brain barrier and reaching the site of brain injury rapidly, especially in the case of acute CNS disorders that require urgent therapeutic action.

Interestingly, parallel to these investigations, nitrous oxide and xenon, which are anesthetics with remarkably safe clinical properties, have been demonstrated, in contrast with volatile anesthetics that mainly act at the $GABA_A$ receptor,[7] to be effective inhibitors of the NMDA receptor[8–10] and to possess a pharmacological profile that resembles that of a low-affinity use-dependent NMDA receptor antagonist.[10] Both gases readily cross the blood-brain barrier, have low blood/gas solubility that is advantageous in terms of rapid inflow and washout (conditions that may favor treatment and reduce risk of neurotoxic side effects), and have been recently shown to possess potentially therapeutic properties. Possible neuroprotection by and therapeutic actions of nitrous oxide and xenon were first addressed by demonstrating that these anesthetic agents reduce neuronal degeneration induced by intraperitoneal administration of *N*-methyl-DL-aspartate (NMDLA)[8,11] and prevent excitotoxic neuronal death in cultured neurons.[11,12] Since then, other studies have shown, as previously hypothesized,[13] that nitrous oxide and xenon reduce cerebral infarct volume induced by middle cerebral artery occlusion (MCAO),[14–16] as well as NMDA-induced Ca^{2+} influxes in cortical cultured neurons,[14] a major critical event involved in excitotoxic neuronal death. In addition, preliminary data suggest that both gases further reduce amphetamine-induced locomotor sensitization.

In the present article, we shortly review these data with a particular focus on the potentially neuroprotective and therapeutic *in vitro* and *in vivo* properties of nitrous oxide and xenon on excitotoxicity and ischemia-induced neuronal death. Finally, possible therapeutic implications in humans are discussed.

NEUROPROTECTIVE AND NEUROTOXIC PROPERTIES OF NITROUS OXIDE AND XENON ON *IN VITRO* AND *IN VIVO* MODELS OF NEURONAL INJURY

The story of nitrous oxide and xenon as possible neuroprotective agents began by the end of the 1990s when it was demonstrated by two independent groups that these anesthetic gases possess antagonistic properties at the NMDA glutamatergic receptor,[8,9] the activation of which is thought to be implicated in both acute and chronic CNS disorders.[1]

Possible neuroprotection by nitrous oxide and xenon was initially demonstrated on *in vitro* and *in vivo* models of neuronal injury. Nitrous oxide was first shown to inhibit excitotoxic neurodegeneration produced by a single intraperitoneal injection of NMDLA (100 mg/kg): cotreatment with nitrous oxide decreased the number of necrotic neurons in the rat arcuate nucleus in a dose-dependent manner (EC_{50} = 55-vol%) that resembles that of MK-801 (EC_{50} = 0.019 mg/kg sc),[8] a well-established NMDA receptor antagonist.[17,18] Then after, such potentially neuroprotective properties were also shown for xenon. This was demonstrated by quantifying c-fos expression in the arcuate nucleus as a marker of neuronal injury induced by subcutaneous administration of NMDLA or ketamine.[19,20] Xenon decreased c-fos expression dose-dependently (EC_{50} = 40-vol%). When used at a volume concentration of 75-vol%, xenon reduced neuronal injury by as much as the prototypical NMDA antagonist MK-801 at the dose of 0.5 mg/kg sc. These potentially neuroprotective properties of xenon were then further demonstrated *in vitro* on neuronal cell cultures,[11,12] and *in vivo* in rats given NMDLA.[11] Xenon exerted a concentration-dependent protection against neuronal injury, assessed by the production of lactate dehydrogenase, induced by oxygen deprivation (xenon EC_{50} = 10-vol%) or exposure to NMDA (xenon EC_{50} = 14-vol%) or glutamate (xenon EC_{50} = 16-vol%). As found for nitrous oxide, xenon dose-dependently reduced the number of degenerated neurons in the arcuate nucleus of rats injected with NMDLA (EC_{50} = 35-vol%). Recent studies have shown that xenon reduced injury in neuronal-glial cocultures[21] as well as hypoxia-induced dopamine release in nerve growth factor–differentiated PC-12 cells used as a model of dopaminergic neurons.[22]

Despite their potentially neuroprotective action in the arcuate nucleus, nitrous oxide and xenon may exhibit neurotoxic properties like prototypical NMDA receptor antagonists do. However, so far as today, such neurotoxic effects have been demonstrated for nitrous oxide, but not for xenon, using *in vitro* and *in vivo* models of neuronal injury. Nitrous oxide was found to produce vacuoles in the posterior cingulated and retrosplenial (PC/RS) cortices (EC_{50} = 117-vol%),[8] where the vacuoles are formed by dilatation of endoplasmic reticulum and swelling of mitochondria and constitute a distinctive cytopathological reaction caused by prototypical NMDA receptor antagonists.[2–4] Similar results were obtained using c-fos expression as a marker of neuronal injury.[11] While xenon inhibited ketamine-induced c-fos expression in the rat PC/RS cortices, nitrous oxide enhanced it.[19] Conversely, ketamine potentiated cerebrocortical damage produced by nitrous oxide.[23] In addition, although neither nitrous oxide at 75-vol% nor xenon at 75-vol% exhibited apoptotic neurodegeneration, it has been recently demonstrated in neonatal rats that nitrous oxide at 75-vol% considerably enhanced isoflurane-induced apoptosis, while xenon at 60-vol% inhibited it.[24]

Altogether, these data have led to the suggestion that xenon, uniquely among compounds with known NMDA receptor antagonist properties, may exhibit neuroprotective action without coexisting neurotoxicity.[11] However, using calcium videomicroscopy in neuronal cell cultures, we found that xenon, under certain conditions, might increase NMDA-induced Ca^{2+} influx,[14] a major critical event involved in excitotoxic neuronal death.[25] As illustrated in FIGURE 1, while xenon at 50-vol%, like nitrous oxide at 75-vol%, decreased NMDA-induced Ca^{2+} influx by 30%, xenon at 75-vol% showed a dual effect, both reducing Ca^{2+} influx produced by low doses (1.25–12.5 μM) of NMDA and potentiating that produced by high doses (50–100 μM) of NMDA. In a similar way, we demonstrate in the present study that posttreatment with xenon at 50-vol% or nitrous oxide at 75-vol%, but not with xenon at 75-vol%, significantly reduced neuronal death induced by intracerebral administration of 75 nmol NMDA (FIG. 1).

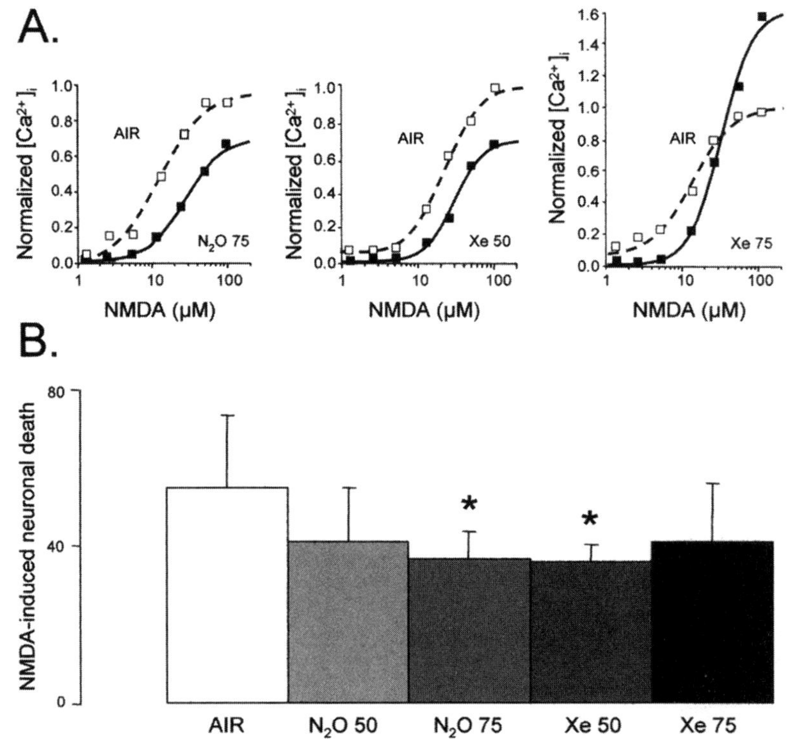

FIGURE 1. **(A)** Effects of nitrous oxide and xenon on NMDA-induced Ca^{2+} influxes in neuronal cell cultures. Intracellular free Ca^{2+} in cortical cultured neurons was measured using fura-2 fluorescence videomicroscopy. The cells were continuously perfused with a HEPES-buffered saline solution; NMDA was applied in a solution previously saturated with nitrous oxide at 75-vol% or xenon at 50- or 75-vol%; controls were given medical air (for further details about the method, see ref. 14). (*Left/Middle*) Both nitrous oxide at 75-vol% and xenon at 50-vol% reduced NMDA-induced Ca^{2+} influxes. (*Right*) Xenon at 75-vol% showed a dual effect, both reducing Ca^{2+} influxes produced by low doses of NMDA (1.25–12.5 μM) and potentiating those produced by high doses of NMDA (50–100 μM). $N = 3$; $n = 105$–150. **(B)** Effects of nitrous oxide and xenon on neuronal death *in vivo* produced by intracerebral administration of 75 nmol NMDA. Nitrous oxide dose-dependently reduced NMDA-induced neuronal death. In contrast, while xenon at 50-vol% significantly reduced NMDA-induced neuronal death in a similar manner to nitrous oxide at 75-vol%, xenon at 75-vol% showed no significant effect. Data are expressed as mean ± SEM of volume of neuronal death (mm^3) produced by intracerebral administration of NMDA. $^*P < 0.05$; $n = 5$–8 per group.

NEUROPROTECTIVE AND ADVERSE PROPERTIES OF NITROUS OXIDE AND XENON ON MODELS OF ISCHEMIA-INDUCED NEURONAL DEATH AND CARDIOPULMONARY BYPASS

Xenon was first shown to attenuate cardiopulmonary bypass–induced neurocognitive and neurologic dysfunction in the rat, a condition that involves risk of cerebral ischemia.[26] In addition, reduction of ischemia-induced infarct volume and neuronal death by nitrous oxide or xenon was also demonstrated in both rats and mice subjected to transient focal cerebral ischemia by MCAO.[14,15]

Attenuation of cardiopulmonary bypass–induced neurocognitive dysfunction was demonstrated as follows.[26] Rats underwent 1 h of cardiopulmonary bypass, during which they were given a gas mixture containing either 30-vol% oxygen + 65-vol% nitrogen + 5-vol% carbon dioxide or 30-vol% oxygen + 60-vol% xenon + 5-vol% nitrogen + 5-vol% carbon dioxide. Then, they were evaluated for neurocognitive outcome on postoperative days 1, 3, 5, and 12 using the Morris water maze. Sham rats (that were cannulated, but did not undergo cardiopulmonary bypass) as well as rats that were given xenon during cardiopulmonary bypass were found to have better significantly neurocognitive outcome compared to control rats on postoperative day 1. Interestingly, this neuroprotective effect of xenon was further found on postoperative days 3, 4, and 12, leading the authors to conclude that cardiopulmonary bypass–induced neurocognitive dysfunction can be attenuated by xenon.

Xenon at 70-vol% was also found to induce neuroprotection compared with nitrous oxide at 70-vol% in a model of transient focal cerebral ischemia.[15] Mice underwent MCAO of 1-h duration during which they were given a gas mixture containing 30-vol% oxygen + 70-vol% xenon, 30-vol% oxygen + 70-vol% nitrous oxide, or 30-vol% oxygen + 35-vol% xenon + 35-vol% nitrous oxide. Then, mice were evaluated for neurologic outcome and cerebral infarct volume, at 24 h after reperfusion. Mice anesthetized with 30-vol% oxygen + 70-vol% xenon showed significantly improved functional outcome on two of the three indices of neurologic scoring used in this study (with the third neurologic scoring nearly significantly different) compared with mice anesthetized with 30-vol% oxygen + 70-vol% nitrous oxide. Animals that received 30-vol% oxygen + 35-vol% xenon + 35-vol% nitrous oxide showed a nonsignificant intermediate neurologic outcome, with one of the third indices of neurologic outcome nearly significantly different. With respect to neurologic outcome, mice that were anesthetized with 30-vol% oxygen + 70-vol% xenon exhibited significantly lower total, cortical, and subcortical infarct volumes compared with mice that were given 30-vol% oxygen + 70-vol% nitrous oxide; mice anesthetized with 30-vol% oxygen + 35-vol% xenon + 35-vol% nitrous oxide showed intermediate neurologic outcome with significantly lower total and cortical, but not subcortical, infarct volumes compared with mice that were given 30-vol% oxygen + 70-vol% nitrous oxide (TABLE 1). Although very interesting as providing both histological and functional data, this study, as stated by the authors themselves, lacks a control awake group of mice that might have actually allowed comparison of neuroprotection between treatments.

We performed MCAO-induced cerebral ischemia of 90-min duration in rats anesthetized with halothane-oxygen and investigated whether nitrous oxide at 75-vol% [this corresponds to 0.6 minimum alveolar anesthetic concentration (MAC) in rats] or xenon at 50-vol% (0.6 MAC in rats) or 75-vol% (0.87 MAC in rats) may reduce

TABLE 1. Infarct volumes in mice treated with nitrous oxide and/or xenon

Infarct volume (mm^3)	Nitrous oxide 70-vol%	Xenon 70-vol%	Nitrous oxide 35-vol% + xenon 35-vol%
Cerebral infarct	59.4 ± 11.5	45.2 ± 17.4*	49.8 ± 14.3*
Cortical infarct	35.5 ± 8.6	24.1 ± 9.9*	26.6 ± 8.9*
Subcortical infarct	23.9 ± 4.8	21.0 ± 8.2‡	23.2 ± 6.0

NOTE: Infarct volumes in mice treated with nitrous oxide at 70-vol%, xenon at 70-vol%, or nitrous oxide at 35-vol% + xenon at 35-vol% during ischemia induced by MCAO ($n = 21$ in each group). *$P < 0.001$, ‡$P < 0.05$ vs. infarct volume in mice treated with nitrous oxide at 70-vol%. From Homi *et al.*[15]

cerebral infarct volume when administered 10–20 min after the MCAO period in freely moving rats (a condition prerequisite for the therapeutic viability of these gases), compared with control rats treated with medical air.[14] During postischemic treatment, animals were placed in an environmentally controlled chamber. No physiologic monitoring or control was performed during postischemic treatment (arterial pressure, blood gases, and rectal temperature were monitored and maintained within their physiologic range throughout MCAO under halothane-oxygen anesthesia) because animals were treated in a closed chamber at subanesthetic concentrations of nitrous oxide or xenon. However, because nitrous oxide and xenon were used at subanesthetic concentrations, this allowed rats to exhibit motor activity and movement during postischemic treatment and probably to self-regulate physiologically. We found that nitrous oxide at 75-vol% and xenon at 50-vol% reduced ischemic neuronal death in the cortex by 70%. In addition, xenon at 50-vol%, but not nitrous oxide at 75-vol%, further decreased by 50% ischemia-induced brain damage in the striatum (a subcortical structure that is notoriously difficult to protect against stroke compared to the cortex because of its lack of collateral vasculature). However, at a higher concentration of 75-vol%, xenon showed no further neuroprotective action and exhibited a dual effect, producing both a trend toward increase in striatal infarction and a trend toward reduction in cortical infarction that did not reach statistical significance. These results, which confirmed what was found on the effects of nitrous oxide at 75-vol% and of xenon at 50- and 75-vol% both *in vitro* on NMDA-induced Ca^{2+} influx in neuronal cell cultures and *in vivo* on neuronal death induced by intracerebral injection of NMDA, are illustrated in FIGURE 2.

However, in contrast with our data demonstrating neuroprotection by postischemic nitrous oxide alone, intraischemic nitrous oxide in rats anesthetized with isoflurane was found to improve neither histologic nor neurologic outcome produced by transient MCAO.[27] Differences in results between both studies might be attributed to differences in models, that is, postischemic treatment with nitrous oxide alone vs. intraischemic treatment with nitrous oxide in the presence of isoflurane.[28] Indeed, as stated above, while xenon inhibited isoflurane-induced apoptotic neurodegeneration, nitrous oxide enhanced it.[24] This may be sufficient to explain differences in neuroprotection between postischemic nitrous oxide alone[14] and intraischemic nitrous oxide in the presence of isoflurane,[27] as well as convergences in neuroprotection between postischemic xenon alone[14] and intraischemic xenon in the presence of isoflurane.[15] In addition, support for neuroprotection by postischemic nitrous oxide alone on histologic outcome is the fact that posttreatment with nitrous oxide (or xenon) alone reduces neuronal death induced by intracerebral injection of NMDA (see above in the present study).

As stated above, both nitrous oxide and xenon readily cross the blood-brain barrier and have low blood/gas solubility that offers advantages in terms of rapid inflow and washout. Therefore, it is likely that the ability of both agents to reduce neuronal death when administered after MCAO accounts for their rapid access to the ischemic core. In this way, the efficacy of xenon at 50-vol%, but not of nitrous oxide at 75-vol%, at reducing neuronal death in the striatum may account at least for the lower blood/gas partition coefficient of xenon compared with nitrous oxide (0.12 vs.

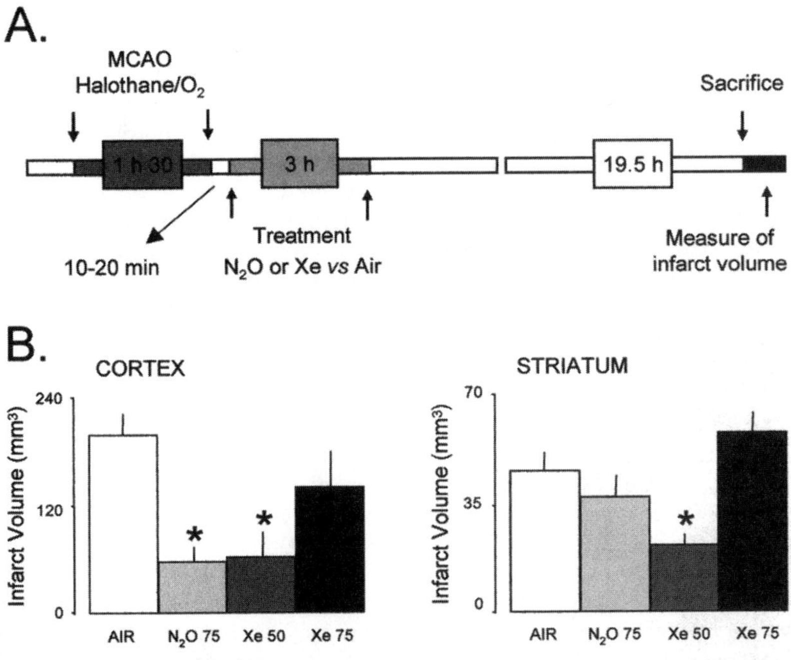

FIGURE 2. **(A)** Experimental protocol for middle cerebral artery occlusion (MCAO): rats were anesthetized with halothane and oxygen (in the absence of nitrous oxide or xenon) and submitted to MCAO for 90 min. Then, 10–20 min after reperfusion, rats were treated for 3 h with nitrous oxide or xenon vs. medical air for control animals. Twenty-four hours after MCAO, the rats were killed, and their brains carefully removed and histologically prepared with cresyl violet in order to measure infarct volume. **(B)** Effects of nitrous oxide and xenon on infarct volume produced by MCAO. (*Left*) Both nitrous oxide at 75-vol% and xenon at 50-vol%, but not xenon at 75-vol%, reduced neuronal death in the cortex by approximately 70%. (*Right*) Xenon at 50-vol%, but not nitrous oxide at 75-vol%, further reduced neuronal death in the striatum by approximately 50%; in contrast, xenon at 75-vol% showed a trend towards an increase in striatal infarction. Data are expressed as mean ± SEM of infarct volume (mm^3). $*P < 0.05$; $n = 5$–6 per group.

0.46).[29] As well as their pharmacologic action, both nitrous oxide and xenon may have physiologic effects on thermoregulation and cerebral circulation and metabolism, which may contribute, at least partly, to their neuroprotective effects. General anesthetics are known to produce hypothermia, a condition that is neuroprotective by itself in various stroke models. However, because temperature was controlled and maintained within normal range in the study performed by Homi *et al.*[15] in anesthetized mice, and probably self-regulated in our freely moving rats,[14] it is highly unlikely that neuroprotection produced by nitrous oxide and xenon might have resulted from an inhibitory action on thermoregulation. With regard to the effects of nitrous oxide and xenon on cerebral blood flow and metabolism, the information obtained from computed tomography studies suggests that xenon may offer advantages over nitrous oxide in terms of vasoreactivity and circulatory and metabolic stability. Indeed, nitrous oxide can increase cerebral blood flow and metabolism and disrupts cerebral vasoreactivity,[30,31] effects that would contraindicate its use for the treatment of clinical situations associated with pathologic increases in intracranial pressure, such as stroke. In contrast, xenon up to 70-vol% produces no significant changes in cerebral blood flow and metabolism,[32–34] and further maintains vasoreactivity.[35] Thus, it is possible that these advantages of xenon over nitrous oxide in terms of circulatory and metabolic stability may have also contributed, at least in part, and in addition to the lower blood/gas partition coefficient of the former, to the neuroprotective action of xenon at 50-vol% in the striatum.

As stated above, xenon at a higher concentration of 75-vol% showed potentially neurotoxic effects.[14] Taken together with the neuroprotective effects of xenon at 50-vol%, this suggests that, depending upon its concentration and the level of the glutamatergic input at the NMDA receptor, xenon may exhibit both neuroprotective and neurotoxic properties, as is known for other NMDA receptor antagonists.[2–5] Interestingly, according to the MAC (an index that allows comparison of inhaled anesthetic potency[36]) of nitrous oxide and xenon as evaluated by loss of the righting reflex,[15] it should be noted that xenon at 75-vol% can be considered equipotent to nitrous oxide at 111-vol%, a concentration that is not far from that of 117-vol%, at which nitrous oxide exhibits neurotoxic properties related to its antagonistic action at the NMDA receptor.[8] This potentially neurotoxic effect of xenon at 75-vol% may appear in contradiction with data obtained from *in vitro* and *in vivo* models of neuronal injury[11,12,19] and further animal models of cardiopulmonary bypass–induced neurocognitive and neurologic dysfunction[26] and transient focal cerebral ischemia,[15] which have suggested that xenon may have neuroprotective properties without coexisting neurotoxicity.[11,19] Such discrepancies may be due to the different models of brain injury used and to their relative severity in terms of excitotoxicity as suggested by the dual effect of xenon at 75-vol% on NMDA-induced Ca^{2+} influx in neuronal cell cultures (e.g., cardiopulmonary bypass[26] < focal cerebral ischemia[14]), as well as to the concentration of xenon used. Indeed, in addition and in contrast with its lack of effects on circulatory functions and metabolism below 70-vol%,[35] xenon at 79-vol% (a concentration equivalent to 117-vol%, at which nitrous oxide shows neurotoxic properties) increases cerebral blood flow that contraindicates its clinical use at high concentrations for the treatment of cerebrovascular diseases.[37] This effect of xenon on circulatory function at concentrations above 70-vol% may also explain, in addition to its dual effect on NMDA-induced Ca^{2+} influx, our finding that xenon at 75-vol% tended to increase cerebral damage in the striatum.

THERAPEUTIC PROPERTIES OF NITROUS OXIDE AND XENON ON AMPHETAMINE-INDUCED LOCOMOTOR SENSITIZATION

A series of clinical trials from a single group have shown that nitrous oxide at analgesic, but not anesthetic, concentrations may be used for the treatment of alcohol and drug addiction,[38–43] although this has been contested[44,45] and yet never been shown by experimental evidence.

In preliminary studies, we investigated the effects of nitrous oxide and xenon on locomotor sensitization to amphetamine in rats, a model for the investigation of the neural mechanisms that underlie the intensification of drug craving, a characteristic of drug addiction in humans.[46] Rats underwent a 3-day period of sensitization from day 1 to day 3 during which they were injected with saline or amphetamine (1 mg/kg ip) and then immediately treated with nitrous oxide, xenon, or medical air for 3 h. This was followed by a 3-day period of reward from day 4 to day 6; finally, on day 7, rats were challenged with amphetamine (1 mg/kg ip) and their locomotor activity was recorded for 90 min. When given concomitantly with amphetamine, we found that nitrous oxide at 75-vol% and xenon at 50-vol%, that is, at equipotent subanesthetic concentrations of 0.6 MAC, prevented the development of locomotor sensitization to amphetamine (while they did not alter the motor response to acute amphetamine). However, although xenon at a higher concentration of 75-vol% corresponding to 0.87 MAC also reduced amphetamine-induced locomotor sensitization, it produced complex and ambivalent additional effects, increasing locomotor response to acute amphetamine in rats pretreated with saline. Taken together, these preliminary data provided the first experimental evidence that nitrous oxide and xenon at appropriate subanesthetic concentrations, but not at higher concentrations not far from their anesthetic concentration, may have potentially therapeutic properties for the treatment of drug addiction.

POSSIBLE THERAPEUTIC IMPLICATIONS IN HUMANS

Based on the data reviewed in the present article, there is accumulating evidence that nitrous oxide and xenon may have potentially neuroprotective and therapeutic properties for the treatment and/or the prevention of brain diseases and dysfunctions. However, xenon at concentrations of 75-vol% further exhibits potentially neurotoxic properties and adverse side effects.

To make interspecies comparisons of inhalation anesthetic potency, a reliable index is the MAC. While the MAC of nitrous oxide is 105-vol% in humans and 128-vol% in the rat,[14,47] that of xenon is 71-vol% in humans and 86-vol% in the rat.[14,48] Thus, if xenon at 86-vol% in rats is equivalent to xenon at 71-vol% in humans, then xenon at 75-vol% in rats will be equivalent to xenon at 62-vol% in humans. Although xenon when used as a general anesthetic under "physiologic" conditions has virtually no side effects,[49,50] accumulating evidence that xenon at 75-vol% in the rat may have potentially neurotoxic properties[14,16,37] suggests that it may not be prudent to use it for treating patients at concentrations higher than 60-vol%. In contrast, neither nitrous oxide at 75-vol% nor xenon at 50-vol% exhibits adverse potentially neurotoxic effects; accordingly, nitrous oxide and xenon at appropriate concentrations (respectively up to 60- and 40-vol%) may be considered for therapeutic applications in humans. Because both agents are rapidly eliminated from the body, it is plausible that their administration at neuroprotective and therapeutic concentrations may not be associated, in contrast with prototypical NMDA receptor antagonists, with adverse CNS side effects and potentially neurotoxicity.

Since nitrous oxide and xenon at appropriate equipotent concentrations produce similar effects, nitrous oxide at first sight could appear as an advantageous solution due to the excessive cost of production of xenon. However, under certain conditions, nitrous oxide can increase cerebral blood flow and metabolism and disrupt cerebral vasoreactivity, effects that contraindicate its use for the treatment of clinical situations associated with pathologic increases in intracranial pressure, such as stroke.[30,31] In addition, in contrast with the clinical treatments of stroke that typically use treatment periods of 1–3 days after the patient is admitted,[6] the treatment of drug addiction necessitates longer therapeutic interventions that could contraindicate the clinical use of nitrous oxide because of its myelotoxic, neuropathotoxic, and hematotoxic effects—mainly caused by inactivation of vitamin B12 and successfully reversed by appropriate pharmacological treatment—when it is used for long periods of time.[51,52] The higher potency of xenon also could allow it being used at lower concentration than nitrous oxide. This may limit the risk of such peripheral toxic effects, which should be noted have not been evidenced so far for xenon. We suggest that combining nitrous oxide and xenon may be a rational formula to obtain optimal beneficial effects, while minimizing the risk of neurotoxicity and adverse side effects and reducing the cost of treatment. However, further investigations are needed to determine what could be the appropriate mixture(s) of nitrous oxide and xenon depending on the type and severity of brain disease and/or dysfunction.

ACKNOWLEDGMENTS

This work was supported by Air Liquide, NNOXe Pharmaceuticals, the University of Caen, and the CNRS. J. H. Abraini and H. N. David are, respectively, CSO and Junior Scientist at NNXOe Pharmaceuticals. M. Lemaire is the Director of the Medical Gas Division at Air Liquide.

REFERENCES

1. Parsons, C.G., W. Danysz & G. Quack. 1998. Glutamate in CNS disorders as a target for drug development: an update. Drug News Perspect. **11:** 523–569.
2. Olney, J.W., J. Labruyere & M.T. Price. 1989. Pathological changes induced in cerebrocortical neurons by phencyclidine and related drugs. Science **244:** 1360–1362.
3. Olney, J.W., J. Labruyere, G. Wang *et al.* 1991. NMDA antagonist neurotoxicity mechanism and prevention. Science **254:** 1515–1518.
4. Fix, A.S., J.W. Horn, K.A. Wightman *et al.* 1993. Neuronal vacuolization and necrosis induced by the noncompetitive *N*-methyl-D-aspartate (NMDA) antagonist MK(+)801 (dizocilpine maleate): a light and electron microscopic evaluation of the rat retrosplenial cortex. Exp. Neurol. **123:** 204–215.
5. Pulvirenti, L. & G.F. Koob. 2002. Being partial to psychostimulant addiction therapy. Trends Pharmacol. Sci. **23:** 151–153.
6. Palmer, G.C. & D. Widzowski. 2000. Low affinity use-dependent NMDA receptor antagonists show promise for clinical development. Amino Acids **19:** 151–155.

7. KRASOWSKI, M.D. & N.L. HARRISON. 1999. General anaesthetic actions on ligand-gated ion channels. Cell. Mol. Life Sci. **55:** 1278–1303.
8. JEVTOVIC-TODOROVIC, V., S.M. TODOROVIC, S. MENNERICK *et al.* 1998. Nitrous oxide (laughing gas) is an NMDA antagonist, neuroprotectant, and neurotoxin. Nat. Med. **4:** 460–463.
9. FRANKS, N.P., R. DICKINSON, S.L.M. DE SOUSA *et al.* 1998. How does xenon produce anesthesia? Nature **396:** 324.
10. YAMAKURA, T. & R.A. HARRIS. 2000. Effects of gaseous anesthetics nitrous oxide and xenon on ligand-gated ion channels: comparison with isoflurane and ethanol. Anesthesiology **93:** 1095–1101.
11. WILHELM, S., D. MA, M. MAZE & N.P. FRANKS. 2002. Effects of xenon on *in vitro* and *in vivo* models of neuronal injury. Anesthesiology **96:** 1485–1491.
12. PETZELT, C., P. BLOM, W. SCHMEHL *et al.* 2003. Prevention of neurotoxicity in hypoxic cortical neurons by the noble gas xenon. Life Sci. **72:** 1909–1918.
13. ALTSCHULER, E.L. 2001. Xenon as neuroprotectant in acute stroke? Med. Hypotheses **56:** 227–228.
14. DAVID, H.N., F. LÉVEILLÉ, L. CHAZALVIEL *et al.* 2003. Reduction of ischemic brain damage by nitrous oxide and xenon. J. Cereb. Blood Flow Metab. **23:** 1168–1173.
15. HOMI, H.M., N. YOKOO, D. MA *et al.* 2003. The neuroprotective effect of xenon administration during transient middle cerebral artery occlusion in mice. Anesthesiology **99:** 876–881.
16. ABRAINI, J.H., H.N. DAVID, O. NICOLE *et al.* 2004. Neuroprotection by nitrous oxide and xenon and its relation to minimum alveolar concentration. Anesthesiology **101:** 260–261.
17. WONG, E.H., J.A. KEMP, T. PRIESTLEY *et al.* 1986. The anticonvulsant MK-801 is a potent *N*-methyl-D-aspartate antagonist. Proc. Natl. Acad. Sci. USA **83:** 7104–7108.
18. OLNEY, J.W., M.T. PRICE, K. SALLES *et al.* 1987. MK-801 powerfully protects against *N*-methyl-D-aspartate neurotoxicity. Eur. J. Pharmacol. **141:** 357–361.
19. NAGATA, A., S. NAKAO, N. NISHIZAWA *et al.* 2001. Xenon inhibits but N(2)O enhances ketamine-induced c-fos expression in the rat posterior cingulate and retrosplenial cortices. Anesth. Analg. **92:** 362–368.
20. MA, D., S. WILHELM, M. MAZE & N.P. FRANKS. 2002. Neuroprotective and neurotoxic properties of the "inert" gas, xenon. Br. J. Anaesth. **89:** 739–746.
21. MA, D., M. HOSSAIN, N. RAJAKUMARASWAMY *et al.* 2003. Combination of xenon and isoflurane produces a synergistic protective effect against oxygen-glucose deprivation injury in a neuronal-glial co-culture model. Anesthesiology **99:** 748–751
22. PETZELT, C., P. BLOM, W. SCHMEHL *et al.* 2005. Xenon prevents cellular damage in differentiated PC-12 cells exposed to hypoxia. BMC Neurosci. **5:** 55.
23. JEVTOVIC-TODOROVIC, V., N. BENSHOFF & J.W. OLNEY. 2000. Ketamine potentiates cerebrocortical damage induced by the common anaesthetic agent nitrous oxide in adult rats. Br. J. Pharmacol. **130:** 1692–1698.
24. WILLIAMSON, P.B., D. MA, M. HOSSAIN *et al.* 2004. Xenon does not cause apoptotic neurodegeneration in the neonatal rat and protects against isoflurane-induced apoptosis. Anesthesiology **101:** A864.
25. GOLDBERG, M.P. & D.W. CHOI. 1993. Combined oxygen and glucose deprivation in cortical cell culture: calcium-dependent and calcium-independent mechanisms of neuronal injury. J. Neurosci. **13:** 3510–3524.
26. MA, D., H. YANG, J. LYNCH *et al.* 2003. Xenon attenuates cardiopulmonary bypass–induced neurologic and neurocognitive dysfunction in the rat. Anesthesiology **98:** 690–698.
27. YOKOO, N., H. SHENG, J. MIXCO *et al.* 2004. Intraischemic nitrous oxide alters neither neurologic nor histologic outcome: a comparison with dizocilpine. Anesth. Analg. **99:** 896–903.
28. ABRAINI, J.H., H.N. DAVID, E.T. MACKENZIE *et al.* 2004. Post-ischemic nitrous oxide alone vs. intra-ischemic nitrous oxide in the presence of isoflurane: what may it change for neuroprotection against cerebral stroke in the rat? Anesth. Analg. In press.
29. GOTO, T., K. SUWA, S. UEZONO *et al.* 1998. The blood-gas partition coefficient of xenon may be lower than generally accepted. Br. J. Anaesth. **80:** 255–256.

30. Field, L.M., D.E. Dorrance, E.K. Krzeminska & L.Z. Barsoum. 1993. Effect of nitrous oxide on cerebral blood flow in normal humans. Br. J. Anaesth. **70:** 154–159.
31. Reinstrup, P., E. Ryding, L. Algotsson *et al.* 1994. Effects of nitrous oxide in human regional blood flow and isolated pial arteries. Anesthesiology **81:** 396–402.
32. Yao, L.P., J. Bandres, E.M. Nemoto *et al.* 1992. Effect of 33% xenon inhalation on whole-brain blood flow and metabolism in awake and fentanyl-anesthetized monkeys. Stroke **23:** 69–74.
33. Whitehurst, S.L., E.M. Nemoto, L. Yao & H. Yonas. 1994. MAC of xenon and halothane in rhesus monkeys. J. Neurosurg. Anesthesiol. **6:** 275–279.
34. Frietsch, T., R. Bogdanski, R. Blobner *et al.* 2001. Effects of xenon on cerebral blood flow and cerebral glucose utilization in rats. Anesthesiology **94:** 290–297.
35. Schmidt, M., T. Marx, C. Papp-Jambor *et al.* 2002. Effect of xenon on cerebral autoregulation in pigs. Anesthesia **57:** 960–966.
36. Eger, E.I., II, L.J. Saidman & B. Brandstater. 1965. Minimum alveolar anesthetic concentration: a standard of anesthetic potency. Anesthesiology **26:** 756–763.
37. Schmidt, M., T. Marx, J. Kotzerke *et al.* 2001. Cerebral and regional organ perfusion in pigs during xenon anesthesia. Anesthesia **56:** 1154–1159.
38. Daynes, G. 1989. The initial management of alcoholism using oxygen and nitrous oxide: a transcultural study. Int. J. Neurosci. **49:** 83–86.
39. Daynes, G. & M.A. Gillman. 1994. Psychotropic analgesic nitrous oxide prevents craving after withdrawal for alcohol, cannabis, and tobacco. Int. J. Neurosci. **76:** 13–16.
40. Gillman, M.A. & F.J. Lichtigfeld. 1991. Placebo and analgesic nitrous oxide for treatment of the alcohol withdrawal state. Br. J. Psychiatry **159:** 672–675.
41. Gillman, M.A. & F.J. Lichtigfeld. 2004. Correct use of analgesic nitrous oxide for the alcohol withdrawal state is essential. J. Clin. Psychopharmacol. **124:** 238–239.
42. Lichtigfeld, F.J. & M.A. Gillman. 1994. Psychotropic analgesic nitrous oxide and neurotransmitter mechanisms involved in the alcohol withdrawal state. Int. J. Neurosci. **76:** 17–33.
43. Ojutkangas, R. & M.A. Gillman. 1994. Psychotropic analgesic nitrous oxide for treating alcohol withdrawal in an outpatient setting. Int. J. Neurosci. **76:** 35–39.
44. Alho, H., T. Methuen, M. Paloheimo *et al.* 2002. Long-term effects of and physiological responses to nitrous oxide gas treatment during alcohol withdrawal: a double-blind, placebo-controlled trial. Alcohol Clin. Exp. Res. **26:** 1816–1822.
45. Alho, H., T. Methuen, M. Paloheimo *et al.* 2003. Nitrous oxide has no effect in the treatment of alcohol withdrawal syndrome: a double-blind placebo-controlled randomized trial. J. Clin. Psychopharmacol. **23:** 211–214.
46. Wolf, M.E. 1998. The role of excitatory amino acids in behavioral sensitization to psychomotor stimulants. Prog. Neurobiol. **54:** 679–720.
47. Hornbein, T.F., E.I. Eger II, P.M. Winter *et al.* 1982. The minimum alveolar concentration of nitrous oxide in man. Anesth. Analg. **61:** 553–556.
48. Cullen, S.C., E.I. Eger II, B.F. Cullen & P. Gregory. 1969. Observations of the anesthetic effect of the combination of xenon and halothane. Anesthesiology **31:** 305–309.
49. Luttropp, H.H., R. Thomasson, S. Dahm *et al.* 1994. Clinical experience with minimal flow xenon anesthesia. Acta Anesthesiol. Scand. **38:** 121–125.
50. Lynch, C., III, J. Baum & R. Tenbrick. 2000. Xenon anesthesia. Anesthesiology **92:** 865–868.
51. Louis-Ferdinand, R.T. 1994. Myelotoxic, neurotoxic, and reproductive adverse effects of nitrous oxide. Adverse Drug React. Toxicol. Rev. **13:** 193–206.
52. Weimann, J. 2003. Toxicity of nitrous oxide. Best Pract. Res. Clin. Anaesthesiol. **17:** 47–61.

Chronic Exposure to Nitrous Oxide Increases [^{3}H]MK801 Binding in the Cerebral Cortex, but Not in the Hippocampus of Adult Mice

NATASCHA SOMMER,[a] CARMELO ROMANO,[b] AND VESNA JEVTOVIC-TODOROVIC[c]

[a]*Friedrich-Alexander-Universität Erlangen-Nürnberg, Erlangen 91054, Germany*

[b]*Department of Ophthalmology, Washington University School of Medicine, St. Louis, Missouri 63110, USA*

[c]*Department of Anesthesiology, University of Virginia Health System, Charlottesville, Virginia 22908, USA*

ABSTRACT: Chronic exposure of adult mice to inhalational anesthetic nitrous oxide (N_2O) results in anesthetic tolerance. N_2O is an NMDA (*N*-methyl-D-aspartate) antagonist. It has been demonstrated that chronic administration of members of the NMDA antagonist class of drugs (e.g., MK801) causes upregulation of NMDA receptors in certain brain regions that could, at least in part, explain the development of tolerance. We sought to determine whether the anesthetic tolerance resulting from chronic exposure to N_2O reflects changes in the number and/or distribution of NMDA receptors. We exposed mice to either a 50- or 75-vol% N_2O atmosphere continuously for 1 or 2 weeks and performed binding studies with [^{3}H]MK801 and NR1 antibodies. Binding studies revealed a significant ($P < 0.05$) increase in [^{3}H]MK801 binding in the cerebral cortex after 2 weeks of N_2O (50- and 75-vol%) exposure. Immunocytochemical binding of NR1 antibodies in selected brain regions showed no changes in distribution pattern. The timing of this increase in [^{3}H]MK801 binding correlates with the time period required for development of tolerance.

KEYWORDS: NMDA receptors; seizures; NMDA antagonists; upregulation; tolerance

INTRODUCTION

Nitrous oxide (laughing gas, N_2O) is an inhalational anesthetic widely used in human medicine and dentistry due to its favorable amnesic and analgesic properties. The mechanism of its anesthetic action had been a mystery for a long time, mainly due to the technical difficulties of working with N_2O *in vitro*, until we showed that N_2O blocks NMDA (*N*-methyl-D-aspartate) receptors both *in vivo* and *in vitro*,

Address for correspondence: Vesna Jevtovic-Todorovic, Department of Anesthesiology, University of Virginia Health System, P. O. Box 800710, Charlottesville, VA 22908. Voice: 434-924-2283; fax: 434-982-0019.
vj3w@virginia.edu

**Ann. N.Y. Acad. Sci. 1053: 301–308 (2005). © 2005 New York Academy of Sciences.
doi: 10.1196/annals.1344.026**

similarly to other NMDA antagonists (e.g., ketamine, MK801).[1] Long-term exposure to N_2O causes anesthetic tolerance, and both long- and short-term use result in withdrawal seizures in animals and humans[2,3] that resemble ethanol-induced tolerance and handling-induced seizures (HIS).[2,4,5] Based on reports that chronic ethanol exposure causes upregulation of different subunits of NMDA receptors[6,7] (especially in cerebral cortex and hippocampus[8,9]), it has been proposed that ethanol-induced tolerance and HIS involve upregulation of NMDA receptors. Since N_2O and ethanol appear to share similar mechanisms of anesthesia tolerance and HIS, our study examines whether the prolonged blockade of NMDA receptors caused by chronic exposure to N_2O results in upregulation of NMDA receptor numbers and/or a changed distribution in the cerebral cortex and hippocampus. We found that the exposure to a subanesthetic N_2O atmosphere containing 50- or 75-vol% for up to 2 weeks (a well-established protocol for studying N_2O-induced tolerance in mice)[10] causes upregulation of NMDA receptors in the cerebral cortex of adult mice.

MATERIALS AND METHODS

Experimental Protocol

A total of 60 adult male mice (C57BL6) (mean weight: 35 g) were used for the experiments. The experiments were approved by the Animal Studies Committee, Washington University School of Medicine, St. Louis, MO, and the Animal Care and Use Committee, University of Virginia Health System, Charlottesville, VA. Gas mixture containing either 75% N_2O/25% oxygen or 50% N_2O/25% oxygen/25% nitrogen was delivered continuously for 1 or 2 weeks to an enclosed Plexiglas chamber from compressed gas cylinders through calibrated gas-specific flowmeters (2–4 L/min) as described by Koblin *et al.*[4,10] For controls, air (75% nitrogen/25% oxygen) was substituted for the N_2O/oxygen mixture. After initial equilibration of the N_2O/oxygen atmosphere inside the chamber, a sample of chamber gas was analyzed by mass spectrometry (Datex-type ULT-I-27-05, Helsinki, Finland).[1] Carbon dioxide accumulation was prevented by maintaining a constant flow of fresh gases using a carbon dioxide absorber containing soda lime. Animals were kept normothermic with unlimited food and water supply in a 12-h light/dark cycle. N_2O, oxygen, and nitrogen were purchased from Praxair Medipure. After either a 1- or 2-week exposure, the animals were taken from the chamber, weighed (to confirm adequate nutritional status), and immediately sacrificed for binding studies.

Binding Studies

For [^{3}H]MK801 binding studies, we used the method described by Williams *et al.*[11] Membranes were prepared using fresh brains kept on ice. Upon removal of cerebellum and brain stem, the cerebral cortex and hippocampus were dissected using dissecting microscope and homogenized with a glass/Teflon homogenizer in 4 mL of 20 mM HEPES buffer with 2 mM EDTA and protein inhibitor. The homogenate was centrifuged for 5 min at 1000*g*; the supernatant was then removed and centrifuged for 30 min at 30,000*g*. The resulting pellet was twice resuspended in 8 mL of 20 mM HEPES with 2 mM EDTA (pH 7.4) and centrifuged at 30,000*g* for 30 min. Binding assays were carried out in polypropylene test tubes containing membranes (70–140 μg) and [^{3}H]MK801 (New England Nuclear–Dupont, Boston, MA). The concentration of [^{3}H]MK801 was 10 nM, in a final incubation volume of 200 μL of 20 mM HEPES and 2 mM EDTA buffer with 100 μM glutamate, 100 μM glycine, and 10 μM spermine. Triplicate samples were incubated at 37°C for 3 h. Nonspecific binding determined in the presence of 10 μM MK801 was less than 10% of total binding. Assays were terminated by the addition of 10 mL of ice-cold buffer (20 mM HEPES, 2 mM EDTA, pH 7.4) followed by rapid filtration (less then 5 s) over glass-fiber filters to avoid dissociation of [^{3}H]MK801. The filters were washed with another 10 mL of buffer and radioactivity was determined by scintillation counting at an efficiency of 40–50% for ^{3}H.

Immunocytochemistry Studies

For immunocytochemistry, the animals were deeply anesthetized with pentobarbital and perfused *via* the heart with 50 mL of heparin solution over 2 min followed by 200 mL of 4% paraformaldehyde in 0.1 M phosphate buffer, pH 7.4, over 5 min. Brains were removed, immersed in fresh fixative, and stored at 4°C. The brains were blocked and serial coronal sections (40 μm thick) were cut on a Vibratome and collected in saline. Floating sections were rinsed 3 times for 5 min with 0.01 M PBS (pH 7.4), incubated for 10 min at room temperature with 3% hydrogen peroxide in 10% methanol in PBS, and subsequently rinsed 3 times with PBS. Sections were then incubated in 0.4% Triton X-100 for 20 min, rinsed again, and incubated in blocking solution (2% bovine serum albumin and 0.2% dry milk in 0.01 M PBS) for 30 min. For primary antibody incubation, the rabbit IgG antibodies were diluted in 2% BSA, 0.05% Triton X-100, and 0.1% sodium azide in PBS. An affinity-purified polyclonal antibody raised against the C-terminus of NR1a (recognizing the major form of NR1, and half the theoretical splice variants) was used for immunostaining. This antibody recognizes the appropriately sized single band on Western blots and immunoprecipitates [^{3}H]MK801 bound to receptors. A commercial antibody (Chemicon, Temecula, CA) against the C2-terminus of the other splice variants was used (NR1v). Optimal dilutions were determined before the experiments and were 1/250 for NR1 and NR1v. Floating sections were incubated in the diluted antibodies for 3 days, rinsed 3 times for 5 min, and incubated in biotinylated goat anti-rabbit IgG for 2 h at room temperature in a 1/200 dilution. They were then rinsed and incubated in avidin-biotin-peroxidase for 1 h. For development, each section was incubated for exactly 10 min in 3,3′-diaminobenzidine with imidazole in TRIS buffer. Each experiment included 2 sections per condition and 2 control sections that were not treated with primary antibodies. The brightness and contrast of each image were consistently enhanced by Adobe PHOTOSHOP Version 2.4.1, and the analysis was done using NIH IMAGE 1.59 software. Background staining values were subtracted from the NR immunoreactive intensities.

Statistics

Statistical analysis was done using *t* test for correlated samples, with statistical significance defined as $P < 0.05$. The *t* test for correlated samples was chosen as each set of control tissue and experimental tissue was treated together during the binding procedure to avoid changes due to time differences (storage time, etc.).

RESULTS

In mice exposed to 50- or 75-vol% N_2O continuously for 1 or 2 weeks, we detected an increase in [^{3}H]MK801 binding in cerebral cortex after the first week of exposure (FIG. 1, top) and that increase became significant after 2 weeks, when compared to the controls ($^*P < 0.05$). In addition, a continuous exposure to 75-vol% N_2O for 2 weeks resulted in a still greater significant increase in [^{3}H]MK801 binding in cerebral cortex, when compared to the 50-vol% N_2O group of mice ($^\dagger P < 0.05$). A small increase in [^{3}H]MK801 binding was also detected in the hippocampus after 2 weeks of exposure (about 10%), but it did not reach statistical significance (FIG. 1, bottom).

To examine the possibility that the upregulation in receptor binding observed in cortical membranes might result from a large change in a small circumscribed region of cortex, we used immunocytochemistry for NMDA receptor subunits, a technique of greater anatomical resolution. Animals were exposed to 75-vol% N_2O for 2 weeks, and cortices were processed for immunostaining utilizing 2 distinct antibodies raised against the major splice variants of the subunit NR1 of NMDA receptors. We obtained antibody distribution in the brain similar to that described by Petralia *et al.*,[12] with intense staining in cerebral cortex and hippocampus. The splice variant detected by antibody "NR1" was located in regions associated with the plasma membrane, while the NR1v splice variant was distributed throughout the cell, with large amounts in the cell interior, as reported by others.[13] Although slight variations in staining intensity were noted between the experimental and control animals (on average, 8–18% higher staining intensity was noted in N_2O-treated animals compared to controls), the differences were not statistically significant and no obvious variations in the cortical distribution of these subunits were detected between treatment groups (FIG. 2).

DISCUSSION

In this study, we demonstrate that continuous exposure of adult mice to 50- or 75-vol% N_2O for 2 weeks resulted in significant increase in [^{3}H]MK801 binding in the cerebral cortex, but not in the hippocampus. We focused our study on the cerebral cortex and the hippocampus because previous studies revealed that [^{3}H]MK801 binding increases in these 2 regions after chronic exposure to NMDA antagonists (e.g., ethanol).[6–9] It is well established that prolonged exposure of mice to subanesthetic concentrations of N_2O (40- to 70-vol%) results in anesthesia tolerance and withdrawal symptoms that develop within 1 week and are significant at 2 weeks of exposure,[10] which coincides with our finding that significant upregulation of NMDA receptors occurs by 2 weeks.

However, it appears less likely that the development of N_2O-induced HIS can be explained by an increased density of NMDA receptors in the cerebral cortex as measured by [^{3}H]MK801 binding. Although a significant increase in the incidence of HIS has been reported after only 60 min of exposure to 75% N_2O,[2] our binding

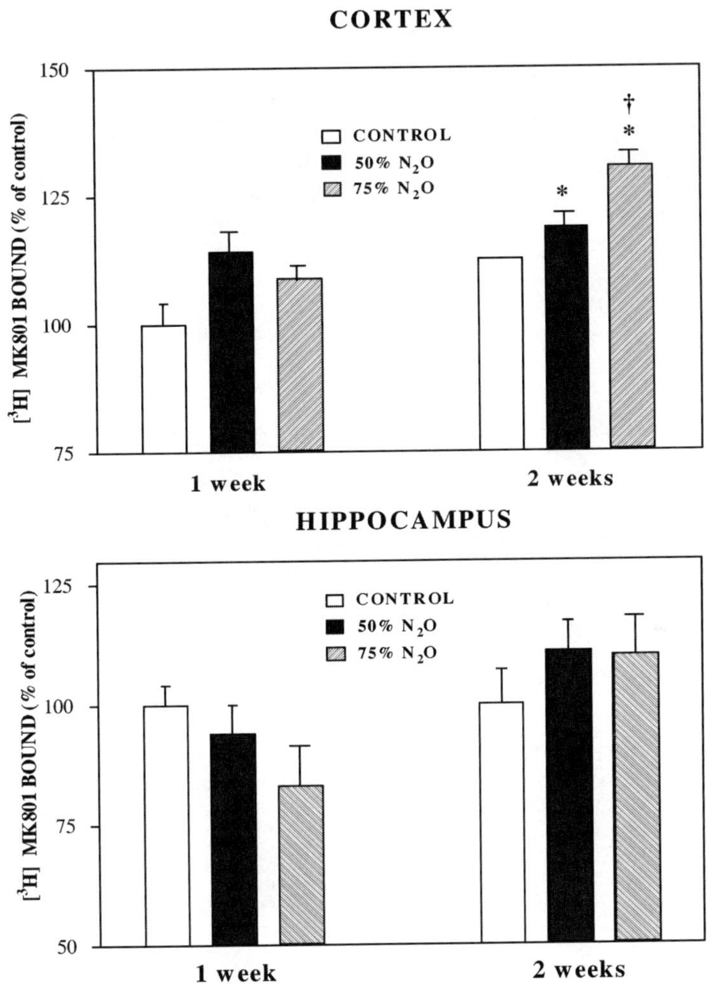

FIGURE 1. [^{3}H]MK801 binding in the cortex (*top*) and the hippocampus (*bottom*) of adult male mice exposed to 50- or 75-vol% N_2O atmosphere for 1 or 2 weeks. [^{3}H]MK801 binding is significantly increased in the cortex after 2 weeks of exposure to 50-vol% [$*t_{(1,8)} = 7.632$, $P < 0.05$] and 75-vol% N_2O [$t_{(1,13)} = 5.37$, $P < 0.05$] compared to control mice. [^{3}H]MK801 binding is significantly [$^{\dagger}t_{(1,17)} = 6.97$, $P < 0.05$] increased in the cortex after 2 weeks of exposure to 75-vol% compared to 50-vol% N_2O. [^{3}H]MK801 binding to NMDA receptors in the cortex and the hippocampus of control animals, when expressed in pmol/mg protein, was 1.05–1.64 and 1.44–1.69, respectively. Each data point represents the mean ± SEM of 5 animals.

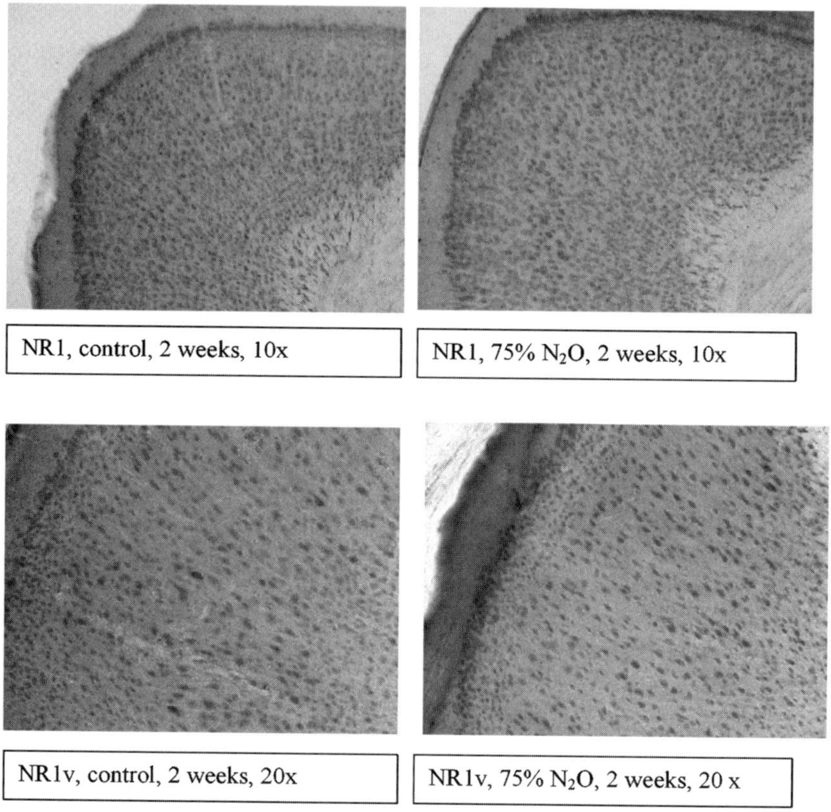

FIGURE 2. NR1 and NR1v immunoreactivity in the cingulate cortex of adult male mice exposed to 75-vol% N_2O atmosphere for 2 weeks. Although NR immunoreactivity is extensive in both control (*left*) and N_2O-treated (*right*) animals, the immunoreactivity is not localized differently within any of the cortical layers of the experimental group in comparison to the controls (magnification: ×10 for NR1 photomicrographs; ×20 for NR1v photomicrographs). However, note that the intensity of the immunostaining is somewhat greater in the experimental group compared to the controls in II cortical layer (8–18% increase on average). [Figure reduced to 80%.]

studies showed no increase in [^{3}H]MK801 binding for any exposure time of a week or less (data not shown).

The upregulation that resulted from N_2O treatment is comparable to the increase in [^{3}H]MK801 binding in adult mice caused by diazepam (7%)[14] and by subanesthetic doses of ethanol (15–30%).[15]

A redistribution of receptors, or a large change in a small, circumscribed subregion, would not be apparent by radioligand binding to membranes prepared from relatively large brain regions. For this reason, we examined the distribution of NR1 subunits in selected cortical brain regions using immunohistochemistry. No changes in the distribution of NR1 subunits were detected.

Our study indicates region-specific changes in [^{3}H]MK801 binding, for example, a significant increase in the number or affinity of binding sites in the cerebral cortex, but not in the hippocampus. Similarly, region-specific upregulation of NMDA receptors in the cerebral cortex, but not in the hippocampus, has been described in studies of tolerance and withdrawal after chronic exposure to ethanol, benzodiazepines, or barbiturates.[14–18] The "peculiar interaction" between $GABA_A$ and NMDA receptors in the cerebral cortex may be responsible for this phenomenon.[19] Although N_2O has a small GABAergic effect in subanesthetic concentrations, it is not clear whether this effect contributes to the region-specific NMDA receptor upregulation resulting from chronic exposure to N_2O.[1,20]

In summary, this study demonstrates for the first time that chronic exposure to N_2O causes an increase in [^{3}H]MK801 binding in the cerebral cortex similar to that caused by chronic exposure to ethanol. However, the functional significance of this upregulation in the development of tolerance to clinical effects of N_2O remains to be determined.

ACKNOWLEDGMENTS

This work was supported in part by the National Institute on Drug Abuse (NIDA) Career Development Award K08-DA00406 (to V. Jevtovic-Todorovic) and the National Institute on Aging (NIA) Grant AG 11355 (to V. Jevtovic-Todorovic). V. Jevtovic-Todorovic is an Established Investigator of the American Heart Association. We wish to thank K. Dikranian for technical assistance.

REFERENCES

1. JEVTOVIC-TODOROVIC, V. *et al.* 1998. Nitrous oxide (laughing gas) is an NMDA antagonist, neuroprotectant, and neurotoxin. Nat. Med. **4**(4): 460–463.
2. BELKNAP, J.K., S.E. LAURSEN & J.C. CRABBE. 1987. Ethanol and nitrous oxide produce withdrawal-induced convulsions by similar mechanisms in mice. Life Sci. **41:** 2033–2040.
3. GILLMAN, M.A. 1992. Nitrous oxide abuse in perspective. Clin. Neuropharmacol. **15:** 297–306.
4. KOBLIN, D.D., D.E. DONG & E.I. EGER II. 1979. Tolerance of mice to nitrous oxide. J. Pharmacol. Exp. Ther. **211**(2): 317–325.
5. VAUGHN, L.K. & R.J. PRUHS. 1995. Strain-dependent variability in nitrous oxide withdrawal seizures frequency. Life Sci. **57**(11): 1125–1130.
6. CHEN, X., M.L. MICHAELIS & E.K. MICHAELIS. 1997. Effects of chronic ethanol treatment on the expression of calcium transport carriers and NMDA/glutamate receptor proteins in brain synaptic membranes. J. Neurochem. **69**(4): 1559–1569.
7. KALLURI, H., A. MEHTA & M. TICKU. 1998. Up-regulation of NMDA receptor subunits in rat brain following chronic ethanol treatment. Mol. Brain Res. **58:** 221–224.
8. DEVAUD, L.L. & A.L. MORROW. 1999. Gender-selective effects of ethanol dependence on NMDA receptor subunit expression in cerebral cortex, hippocampus, and hypothalamus. Eur. J. Pharmacol. **369:** 331–334.
9. TREVISAN, L. *et al.* 1994. Chronic ingestion of ethanol up-regulates NMDAR1 receptor subunit immunoreactivity in rat hippocampus. J. Neurochem. **62**(4): 1635–1638.
10. KOBLIN, D.D. *et al.* 1980. Mice tolerant to nitrous oxide are also tolerant to alcohol. J. Pharmacol. Exp. Ther. **213**(2): 309–312.

11. WILLIAMS, K., C. ROMANO & P.B. MOLINOFF. 1989. Effects of polyamines on the binding of [^{3}H]MK801 to the *N*-methyl-D-aspartate receptor: pharmacological evidence for the existence of a polyamine recognition site. Mol. Pharmacol. **36:** 575–581.
12. PETRALIA, R.S., Y.X. WANG & R.J. WENTHOLD. 1994. The NMDA receptor subunits NR2A and NR2B show histological and ultrastructural localization patterns similar to those of NR1. J. Neurosci. **14**(10)**:** 6102–6120.
13. EHLERS, M.D., W.G. TINGLEY & R.L. HUGANIR. 1995. Regulated subcellular distribution of the NR1 subunit of the NMDA receptor. Science **269**(5231)**:** 1734–1737.
14. TSUDA, M., T. SUZUKI & M. MISAWA. 1998. Region-specific changes in ^{3}H dizocilpine binding in diazepam–withdrawn rats. Neurosci. Lett. **240**(2)**:** 113–115.
15. GULYA, K.A. *et al.* 1991. Brain regional specificity and time-course of changes in the NMDA receptor–ionophore complex during ethanol withdrawal. Brain Res. **547**(1)**:** 129–134.
16. RABBANI, M. *et al.* 1994. Possible involvement of NMDA receptor–mediated transmission in barbiturate physical dependence. Br. J. Pharmacol. **111:** 89–96.
17. SHORT, K.R. & B. TABAKOFF. 1993. Chronic barbiturate treatment increases NMDA receptors, but decreases kainate receptors in mouse cortex. Eur. J. Pharmacol. **230:** 111–114.
18. TSUDA, M. *et al.* 1998. Hypersusceptibility to DMCM-induced seizures during diazepam withdrawal in mice: evidence for up-regulation of NMDA receptors. Naunyn Schmiedeberg's Arch. Pharmacol. **357**(3)**:** 309–315.
19. MATTHEWS, D.B. *et al.* 2000. Chronic blockade of *N*-methyl-D-aspartate receptors alters gamma-aminobutyric acid type A receptor peptide expression and function in the rat. J. Neurochem. **74**(4)**:** 1522–1528.
20. YAMAKURA, T. & R.A. HARRIS. 2000. Effects of gaseous anesthetics nitrous oxide and xenon on ligand-gated ion channels: comparison with isoflurane and ethanol. Anesthesiology **93**(4)**:** 1095–1101.

Systems Biology/Systems Toxicology

Application to Developmental Neurotoxicology/Neuroprotection

WILLIAM SLIKKER, JR., ZENGJUN XU, AND CHENG WANG

Division of Neurotoxicology, National Center for Toxicological Research/FDA, Jefferson, Arkansas 72079, USA

KEYWORDS: systems biology; systems toxicology; ketamine; phencyclidine; NMDA antagonists; neurotoxicity

Systems biology has been defined as the iterative and integrative study of biological systems as systems respond to perturbations. As adapted for toxicology and referred to as systems toxicology, it involves the study of perturbations by chemicals and stressors by monitoring alterations in gene and protein expressions that are linked firmly to toxicological outcome in an iterative and integrative manner. Because of the complexity and temporal features of the manifestations of developmental neurotoxicity, no area of toxicology could benefit more from the systematic application of the systems biology/systems toxicology approach.

In the application of the systems biology/systems toxicology approach to the problem of developmental neurotoxicity produced by ketamine, phencyclidine (PCP), and related NMDA antagonists, the four steps set forth by Hood's group were followed to the extent possible. First, available information on the biological system from *in vitro* and *in vivo* rodent experiments was gathered; a preliminary model of how it functions in descriptive and graphical terms was formulated; and where possible, the genes and proteins expressed in the described pathways were defined. Second, the system was perturbed with chemical agents (PCP and ketamine), and kinetic experiments providing information across developmental time spans were conducted. Third, the model was improved by testing the initial hypothesis and, based on the experimental data, incorporating the new information into the model. Fourth and last, additional perturbations were performed to refine the model by repeating steps 2–4 in an iterative manner.

Although not fully delineated, the working model for NMDA/NMDA antagonist–induced neurodegeneration involves the modulation of the normally occurring brain sculpting mechanisms that control central nervous system development. Exposure of the developing mammal to PCP, ketamine, or other NMDA antagonists perturbs the endogenous NMDA receptor system and results in enhanced neuronal cell death. Upregulation of the NR1 subunit of the NMDA receptor by the presence of an NMDA

Address for correspondence: William Slikker, Jr., Division of Neurotoxicology, National Center for Toxicological Research/FDA, 3900 NCTR Road, Jefferson, Arkansas 72079. Voice: 870-543-7203; fax: 870-543-7745.
wslikker@nctr.fda.gov

**Ann. N.Y. Acad. Sci. 1053: 309–310 (2005). © 2005 New York Academy of Sciences.
doi: 10.1196/annals.1344.056**

antagonist appears critical to the subsequent cell death. Blockade of this NMDA receptor upregulation dramatically diminishes the apoptotic cascade. Another perturbation of the system, the addition of a superoxide dismutase mimetic (M40403), also blocks the apoptotic cascade by decreasing the abundance of the superoxide anion. With the use of a third perturbation, that is, the inhibition of NF-κB translocation by SN50, NMDA/NMDA antagonist–induced neuronal cell death is also prevented. These results indicate that the overall effect of the NF-κB dimer translocation into the cell nucleus is proapoptotic.

The iterative perturbations of the system allowed refinement of the general model and reinforced the selective pathways that represent the whole of the data. Although many more studies will be necessary to achieve a quantitative model, a general pathway has been constructed and discretely perturbed in an iterative manner with carefully selected agents as defined by the systems biology/systems toxicology approach. Precise developmental stage and dose-response experiments with the use of the phenotypic anchor, neuronal cell death, and global gene and protein expression assays remain to be completed. As these data become available for integrative and iterative evaluation, the model will be improved. A well-described model will lead to a better understanding of the potential neurotoxicity of the NMDA antagonists, including many commonly used anesthetic agents, in the developing human.

An Old Story with a New Twist: Do NMDAR1 mRNA Binding Proteins Regulate Expression of the NMDAR1 Receptor in the Presence of Alcohol?

MEENA KUMARI AND ANTJE ANJI

Department of Anatomy and Physiology, College of Veterinary Medicine, Kansas State University, Manhattan, Kansas 66506, USA

ABSTRACT: NMDA receptors not only play a pivotal role in normal physiological processes in the central nervous system (CNS), but have been identified as an important target of ethanol. Chronic exposure to ethanol induces a number of adaptive processes in the CNS, including an upregulation of NMDA receptor number and function. The increase in NMDA receptor number in response to chronic ethanol exposure both *in vivo* and *in vitro* is accompanied by an increase in NMDAR1 and NMDAR2B polypeptide levels. It is widely believed that these adaptive changes play an important role in the development of alcohol dependence and withdrawal syndrome. At the molecular level, chronic ethanol exposure of fetal cortical neurons selectively increases expression of NMDAR1 splice variants lacking exon 5 and exon 22. Chronic ethanol exposure of fetal cortical neurons also increases NMDAR1 mRNA half-life in these neurons. However, when new protein synthesis is inhibited, the half-life of NR1 mRNA in these neurons returns to control values, strongly suggesting that ethanol induces the synthesis of protein(s) that may regulate the decay of NR1 mRNA. In recent years, it has become apparent that regulation of mRNA stability is an important aspect of regulation of gene expression. Changes in mRNA stability can be accomplished by interaction between *cis*-acting sequences in the 3′ untranslated region (3′UTR) of mRNAs and *trans*-acting proteins expressed in cells. Such interactions may protect RNAs from degradation by ribonucleases, thereby increasing the half-life of mRNAs.

KEYWORDS: NMDA receptors; ethanol; splice variants; RNA binding proteins; mRNA stability; fetal cortical neurons

NMDA RECEPTORS

The NMDA receptor, one of the three major subtypes of glutamate receptors, plays a key role in neuronal plasticity that is thought to underlie memory, learning, and development.[1,2] Overstimulation of NMDA receptors can trigger an increase in

Address for correspondence: Meena Kumari, Department of Anatomy and Physiology, College of Veterinary Medicine, Kansas State University, 231 Coles Hall, Manhattan, KS 66506. Voice: 785-532-3115; fax: 785-532-4557.
mkumari@vet.ksu.edu

**Ann. N.Y. Acad. Sci. 1053: 311–318 (2005). © 2005 New York Academy of Sciences.
doi: 10.1196/annals.1344.027**

$[Ca]_i$, resulting in neuronal degeneration and cell death.[3–6] Molecular cloning and functional studies have revealed the existence of multiple receptor subunits that differ in anatomical distribution, properties, and regulation.[7–12] The NMDA receptor forms a heteromeric complex containing combinations of the NMDAR1 (NR1), NMDAR2 (NR2), and the more recently identified NMDAR3 (NR3) subunits.[13,14] The NR1 subunit is expressed ubiquitously in the brain, whereas the NR2 and NR3 subunits are expressed in a more region-specific manner.[7,15,16] Differential splicing

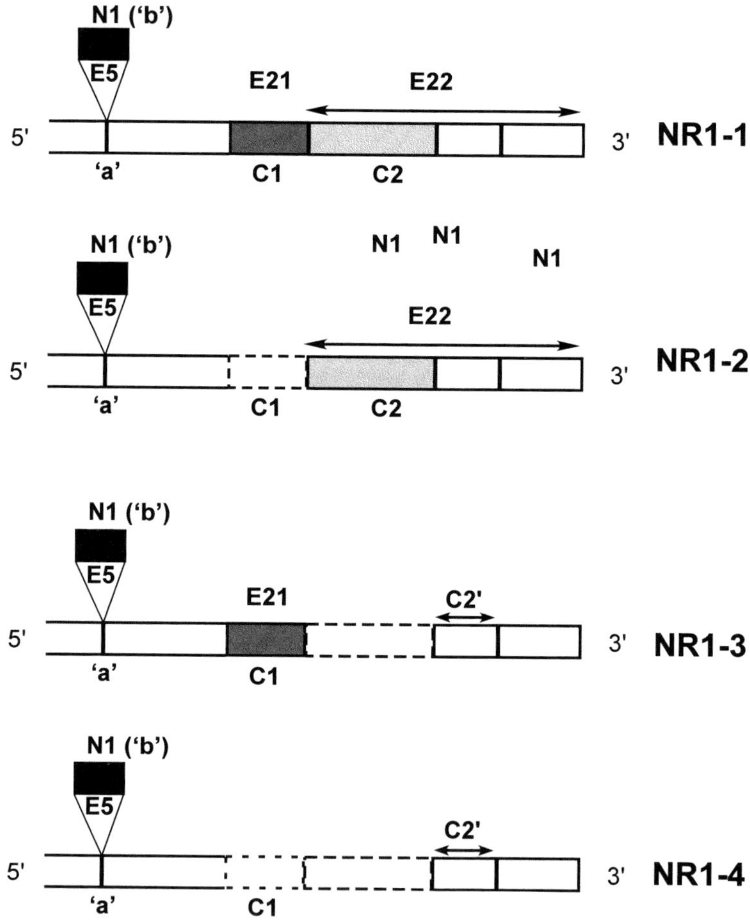

FIGURE 1. Splice variants of the NMDAR1 receptor subunit. NMDAR1 is the product of a single gene. Differential splicing leads to the expression of eight splice variants that are characterized by the inclusion or deletion of one 5′ insert (exon 5) and two 3′ inserts (exons 21 and 22). NMDAR1 splice variants lacking exon 22 or exons 21 and 22 contain an additional cassette, C2′. Inclusion of both exon 21 and exon 22 gives rise to splice variant NR1-1; exclusion of exon 21, but inclusion of exon 22, gives rise to NR1-2. Exclusion of exon 22, but inclusion of exon 21, gives rise to NR1-3; when both exons 21 and 22 are absent, the resulting splice variant is named NR1-4. All these four NR1 splice variants exist in either "b" isoform (inclusion of exon 5) (i.e., NR1-1b, NR1-2b, NR1-3b, NR1-4b) or "a" isoform (exclusion of exon 5) (i.e., NR1-1a, NR1-2a, NR1-3a, NR1-4a).

of the NR1 subunit leads to the expression of eight splice variants that are characterized by the inclusion or deletion of one 5′ insert (exon 5) and two 3′ inserts (exons 21 and 22) (FIG. 1).[17] Exon 5 encodes the N1 splice cassette that lies in the extracellular amino-terminal domain of the NR1 subunit. Exons 21 and 22 encode the carboxyl-terminal splice cassettes, C1 and C2, respectively, and are a part of the intracellular domain of the NR1 subunit. NR1 splice variants lacking exon 22 or exons 21 and 22 contain an additional cassette, C2′, at the carboxyl-terminal end.

Alternate splicing of the NR1 subunit facilitates the generation of NR1 subunits with distinct pharmacological and physiological characteristics. Exon 5 (N1 cassette) regulates the pharmacological properties of the receptor, while splicing of exons 21 (C1 cassette) and 22 (C2 cassette) influences cell surface expression of the NR1 subunit.[17]

EFFECT OF ETHANOL ON NMDA RECEPTORS

NMDA receptors not only play a pivotal role in the normal physiological processes in the central nervous system (CNS), but have been identified as an important target of ethanol. This realization has led to an extensive investigation into the molecular mechanisms by which ethanol affects NMDA receptors. Acute exposure to ethanol inhibits the excitatory action of glutamate at NMDA receptors, contributing to the development of alcohol intoxication. By contrast, chronic exposure to ethanol induces a number of adaptive processes in the CNS, including an upregulation of NMDA receptor number and function.[18,19] The increase in NMDA receptor number in response to chronic ethanol exposure both *in vivo* and *in vitro* is accompanied by an increase in NR1 and NR2B polypeptide levels.[20–23] It is widely believed that these adaptive changes play an important role in the development of alcohol dependence and withdrawal syndrome.

EFFECT OF ETHANOL ON THE NR1 SUBUNIT

RT/PCR and Western blot analyses have recently demonstrated that ethanol has a selective effect on NR1 splice variants. In mouse fetal cortical neurons, chronic ethanol exposure increases mRNA levels of splice variants that lack exon 5. At the polypeptide level, similar ethanol treatment increases expression of splice variants that lack exon 22 or exons 21 and 22 (NR1–3 and NR-4, respectively), but decreases expression of splice variants that contain exon 5. Taken together, in fetal cortical neurons, chronic exposure to ethanol increases the expression of splice variants lacking exon 5 and exon 22. These data suggest that chronic ethanol exposure may alter the pharmacological profile and cell surface expression of NMDA receptors. This notion is supported by the observation made by Rumbaugh and colleagues.[24] These investigators showed that patch-clamp recordings of glutamate responses in human embryonic kidney cells expressing NMDA receptors composed of NR1 splice variants lacking both exons 5 and 22, and the NR2B subunit, exhibit longer deactivation currents as compared to human embryonic kidney cells expressing NR1 splice variants containing exon 5 and lacking exon 22, and the NR2B subunit.[24]

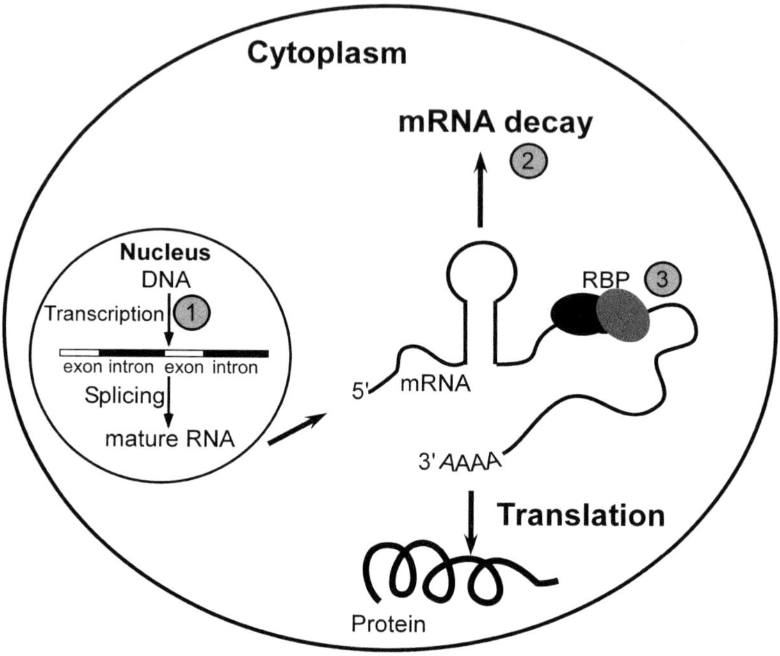

FIGURE 2. Schematic of intracellular sites of action of ethanol on NMDA receptors. Chronic exposure of fetal cortical neurons increases the rate of transcription of the NMDAR2B gene (site 1). Similar treatment increases the half-life of the NMDAR1 receptor mRNA (site 2). Ethanol may also influence the interaction of *trans*-acting factors or RNA binding proteins (RBP) with *cis*-sequences located in the 3′UTR of the NMDAR1 receptor mRNA (site 3).

Further studies in mouse fetal cortical neurons showed that chronic ethanol exposure increases the rate of NR2B gene transcription and, at the same time, increases the half-life of NR1 mRNA in fetal cortical neurons to more than 24 h (FIG. 2).[25]

mRNA STABILITY

Regulation of mRNA turnover or half-life is known to play an important role in regulating gene expression. Changes in mRNA abundance due to alterations in mRNA half-life ultimately affect protein expression of genes.[26] mRNAs exhibit a wide range of half-lives that can be correlated with their functional role in the cell. For instance, β-globin, considered a housekeeping gene, has a half-life of over 20 h, whereas the oncogene *c-myc* has a short half-life of about 10 min.[27,28] It is now appreciated that mRNA decay is a finely tuned process involving *cis*-acting sequence elements residing primarily in the 3′UTR of mRNAs, although in some cases they may be located in the coding region. These stability modifying sequences act in concert with *trans*-acting protein factors regulating mRNA decay.[29,30] To date, most of the *cis*-acting sequences identified destabilize mRNAs. One such sequence element is the well-characterized adenosine uridine–rich (ARE) sequence located in the 3′UTR of some mammalian mRNAs.[31] In some instances, the presence of such an ARE sequence is sufficient to make a normally stable mRNA like β-globin unstable.[32] Recent data have suggested that AREs can be variable in both length and sequence and, as more *cis*-acting sequences are being identified, the complexity of these elements is just being appreciated.[33] The development of assays such as RNA electromobility shift assays and UV cross-link analysis aided the identification of RNA binding proteins or *trans*-acting proteins that target these sequences.

TRANS-ACTING PROTEINS

Data from our lab suggest that RNA binding proteins may also be important regulators of NR1 gene expression. When fetal cortical neurons are cultured in the presence of the protein synthesis inhibitor, cycloheximide, ethanol-induced stabilization of the NR1 mRNA does not occur.[34] Such a requirement for protein synthesis strongly suggests that labile protein factors are necessary for NR1 mRNA stabilization to occur (FIG. 2). Preliminary data from our laboratory further suggest that *cis*-acting regions may be present within the 3′UTR of NR1 mRNA. Taken together, it appears that *cis-trans* interactions play a role in regulating expression of the NR1 subunit in the presence of ethanol. The *trans*-acting proteins are now known to be important regulators of gene expression, and a search for *trans*-acting factors has led to the identification of several proteins, many of which have dual functions.[26] Some of these factors are associated with mRNAs during their transport from the nucleus to the cytoplasm or to their site of translation.[35–38] For instance, renin mRNA is regulated primarily at the level of mRNA turnover. In the search for proteins that mediate the posttranscriptional effects on renin mRNA, Adams and colleagues identified three RNA binding proteins that interact with and regulate the renin mRNA: hydroxyacyl-CoA dehydrogenase/3-ketoacyl-CoA thiolase/enoyl-CoA hydratase β subunit (HADHB), the poly-C binding protein CP1, and HuR.[39] Interestingly, intracellular imaging performed by the same authors revealed a distinct localization of HADHB to the mitochondria, whereas HuR was found in the nucleus and CP1 was distributed throughout the cell. The exact role, however, of this differential cellular localization of these three RNA binding proteins remains to be elucidated. The *trans*-acting proteins play a role in the posttranscriptional regulation of other mRNAs as well. The protein kinase A–induced stabilization of the lactate dehydrogenase-A mRNA is associated with an upregulation of 3′UTR binding activity of three *trans*-acting factors.[40] Similarly, the stabilization of the tyrosine hydroxylase mRNA that occurs when PC12 cells are cultured under hypoxic conditions is accompanied by an increase in formation of the RNA-protein complex.[41]

In the CNS, a number of genes are known to be regulated at the posttranscriptional level and a growing number of RNA binding proteins have been identified in the CNS. Of these, the ELAV-like Hu proteins are best characterized. ELAV-like Hu proteins belong to a small family of RNA binding proteins and are human homologues of *Drosophila* ELAV, an RNA binding protein whose deletion results in embryonic lethal abnormal vision (ELAV) phenotype. So far, four ELAV proteins have been identified: HuB, HuC, HuD, and HuR.[42] The expression of HuB, HuC, and HuD is restricted to the nervous system, whereas HuR is present in most tissues.[43] The Hu proteins bind preferentially to AREs in the 3′UTR of mRNAs, are known to stabilize certain target mRNAs, and influence translation as well as RNA transport. Recent data have demonstrated that HuD is involved in posttranscriptional regulation of the growth-associated protein, GAP-43.[44] Both HuD and GAP-43 are highly expressed in developing neurons and are closely associated with neuronal development and plasticity. Very recent data have solidified the role of Hu proteins in neuronal differentiation. HuD has now been implicated in the posttranscriptional regulation of gene expression that occurs after spatial learning in the hippocampus of rodents. Specifically, a learning-specific increase in HuD is associated with increased expression of GAP-43 mRNA and protein levels.[45,46]

CONCLUSIONS

Ethanol acts on several neurotransmitter systems in the brain, and one of the major targets for this drug is the NMDA receptor. Several laboratories around the world have clearly demonstrated that ethanol affects the NMDA receptor complex at multiple levels. Work in our lab has focused on the regulation of the NR1 subunit at the molecular level. Recent data suggest that the NR1 subunit is regulated at the posttranscriptional level (mRNA stability) in the presence of ethanol. In the last decade, it has become apparent that regulation of mRNA stability is an important regulator of gene expression. Many *cis*-acting sequences and *trans*-acting factors have been identified and prompted questions regarding their physiological role. With a better understanding of the emerging complexity of *cis-trans* interactions on mRNAs, we not only will gain a better understanding of the regulation of gene expression, but also will identify new potential therapeutic targets.

REFERENCES

1. MALENKA, R.C. & R.A. NICOLL. 1993. NMDA-receptor dependent synaptic plasticity: multiple forms and mechanisms. Trends Neurosci. **16:** 521–527.
2. MALENKA, R.C. & R.A. NICOLL. 1999. Long-term potentiation—a decade of progress? Science **285:** 1870–1874.
3. MELDRUM, B. & J. GARTWAITE. 1990. Excitatory amino acid toxicity and neurodegenerative disease. Trends Pharmacol. Sci. **11:** 379–387.
4. DINGLEDINE, R., K. BORGES, D. BOWIE *et al.* 1999. The glutamate receptor ion channels. Pharmacol. Rev. **51:** 7–61.
5. CULL-CANDY, S., S. BRICKLEY & M. FARRANT. 2001. NMDA receptor subunits: diversity, development, and disease. Curr. Opin. Neurobiol. **11:** 327–335.
6. HARDINGHAM, G.E. & H. BADING. 2003. The yin and yang of NMDA receptor signaling. Trends Neurosci. **26:** 81–89.
7. WATANABE, M., Y. INOUE, K. SAKIMURA *et al.* 1992. Developmental changes in distribution of NMDA receptor channel subunit mRNAs. Neuroreport **3:** 1138–1140.
8. LAURIE, D.J. & P.H. SEEBURG. 1994. Regional and developmental heterogeneity in splicing of the rat brain NMDA R1 mRNA. J. Neurosci. **14:** 3180–3194.
9. CIABARRA, A.M., J.M. SULLIVAN, L.G. GAHN *et al.* 1995. Cloning and characterization of chi-1: a developmentally regulated member of a novel class of the ionotropic glutamate receptor family. J. Neurosci. **15:** 6498–6508.
10. DUNAH, A.W., R.P. YASUDA, Y.H. WANG *et al.* 1996. Regional and ontogenic expression of the NMDA receptor subunit NR2D protein in the rat brain using a subunit specific antibody. J. Neurochem. **67:** 2335–2345.

11. PRYBYLOWSKI, K.L. & B.B. WOLFE. 2000. Developmental differences in alternative splicing of the NR1 protein in rat cortex and cerebellum. Brain Res. Dev. Brain Res. **123:** 143–150.
12. AL-HALLAQ, R.A., B.R. JARABEK, Z. FU *et al.* 2002. Association of NR3A with the NMDA receptor NR1 and NR2 subunit. Mol. Pharmacol. **62:** 1119–1127.
13. LUO, J.W., Y. WANG, R.P. YASUDA *et al.* 1997. The majority of NMDA receptor complexes in adult rat cerebral cortex contain at least three different subunits (NR1/NR2A/NR2B). Mol. Pharmacol. **51:** 79–86.
14. DAS, S., Y.F. SASAKI, T. ROTHE *et al.* 1998. Increased NMDA current and spine density in mice lacking the NMDA receptor subunit NR3A. Nature (London) **393:** 377–381.
15. ISHII, T., K. MORIYOSHI, H. SUGIHARA *et al.* 1993. Molecular characterization of the family of the NMDA receptor subunits. J. Biol. Chem. **268:** 2836–2843.
16. SUCHER, N.J., S. AKBARIAN, S.L. CHI *et al.* 1995. Developmental and regional expression pattern of a novel NMDA receptor–like subunit (NMDAR-L) in the rodent brain. J. Neurosci. **15:** 6509–6520.
17. ZUKIN, R.S. & M.V.L. BENNETT. 1995. Alternatively spliced isoforms of the NMDA R1 receptor subunit. Trends Neurosci. **18:** 306–313.
18. SANNA, E., M. SERRA, A. COSSU *et al.* 1993. Chronic ethanol intoxication induces differential effects on $GABA_A$ and NMDA receptor function in the rat brain. Alcohol Clin. Exp. Res. **17:** 115–123.
19. HU, X.J. & M.K. TICKU. 1995. Chronic ethanol treatment upregulates the NMDA receptor function and binding in mammalian cortical neurons. Mol. Brain Res. **30:** 347–356.
20. TREVISAN, L., L.W. FITZGERALD, N. BROSE *et al.* 1994. Chronic ingestion of ethanol upregulates NMDA R1 receptor subunit immunoreactivity in rat hippocampus. J. Neurochem. **62:** 1635–1638.
21. FOLLESA, P. & M.K. TICKU. 1996. Chronic ethanol-mediated up-regulation of the *N*-methyl-D-aspartate receptor polypeptide subunits in mouse cortical neurons in culture. J. Biol. Chem. **271:** 13297–13299.
22. KUMARI, M. 2001. Differential effects of chronic ethanol treatment on *N*-methyl-D-aspartate R1 splice variants in fetal cortical neurons. J. Biol. Chem. **276:** 29764–29771.
23. NAGY, J., S. KOLOK, P. DEZSO *et al.* 2003. Differential alterations in the expression of NMDA receptor subunits following chronic ethanol treatment in primary cultures of rat cortical and hippocampal neurons. Neurochem. Int. **42:** 35–43.
24. RUMBAUGH, G., K. PRYBYLOWSKI, J.F. WANG *et al.* 2000. Exon 5 and spermine regulate deactivation of NMDA receptor subtypes. J. Neurophysiol. **83:** 1300–1306.
25. KUMARI, M. & M.K. TICKU. 1998. Ethanol and regulation of the NMDA receptor subunits in fetal cortical neurons. J. Neurochem. **70:** 1467–1473.
26. TOURRIÈRE, H., K. CHEBLI & J. TAZI. 2002 mRNA degradation machines in eukaryotic cells. Biochimie **84:** 821–837.
27. ROSS, J. & T.D. SULLIVAN. 1985. Half-lives of beta and gamma globulin messenger RNAs and protein synthetic capacity in cultured human reticulocytes. Blood **66:** 1149–1154.
28. DANI, C., J.M. BLANCHARD, M. PIECHACZYK *et al.* 1984. Extreme instability of cmyc mRNA in normal and transformed human cells. Proc. Natl. Acad. Sci. USA **81:** 7046–7050.
29. ZEHNER, Z.E., R.K. SHEPHERD, J. GABRYSZUK *et al.* 1997. RNA-protein interactions with in the 3′ untranslated region of vimentin mRNA. Nucleic Acid Res. **25:** 3362–3370.
30. SELLERS, R.S., C.C. CAPEN & T.J. ROSOL. 2002. Messenger RNA stability of parathyroid hormone–related protein regulated by transforming growth factor-β1. Mol. Cell. Endocrinol. **188:** 37–46.
31. CHEN, C.Y. & B. SHYU. 1995. AU-rich elements: characterization and importance in mRNA degradation. Trends Biochem. Sci. **20:** 465–470.
32. SHAW, G. & R. KAMEN. 1986. A conserved AU sequence from the 3′ untranslated region of GM-CSF mRNA mediates selective mRNA degradation. Cell **46:** 659–667.
33. KUMARI, M., A. ANJI, H. WOODS *et al.* 2003. The molecular effects of alcohol: clues to the enigmatic action of alcohol. Ann. N.Y. Acad. Sci. **993:** 82–94.
34. PESOLE, G., F. MIGNONE, C. GISSI *et al.* 2001. Structural and functional features of eukaryotic mRNA untranslated regions. Gene **276:** 73–81.

35. Lawrence, J.B. & R.H. Singer. 1986. Intracellular localization of mRNAs for cytoskeletal proteins. Cell **45:** 407–415.
36. Fulton, A.B. 1993. Spatial organization of the synthesis of cytoskeletal proteins. J. Cell. Biochem. **52:** 148–152.
37. Fulton, A.B. & T. L'Ecuyer. 1993. Cotranslational assembly of some cytoskeletal proteins: implications and prospects. J. Cell Sci. **105:** 867–871.
38. Morris, E.J. & A.B. Fulton. 1994. Rearrangement of mRNAs for costamere proteins during costamere development in cultured skeletal muscle from chicken. J. Cell Sci. **107:** 377–386.
39. Adams, D.J., D.J. Beveridge, L. van der Weyden *et al.* 2003. HADHB, HuR, and CP1 bind to the distal 3′-untranslated region of human renin mRNA and differentially modulate renin expression. J. Biol. Chem. **278:** 44894–44903.
40. Tian, D., D. Huang, R.C. Brown *et al.* 1998. Protein kinase A stimulates binding of multiple proteins to a U-rich domain in the 3′ UTR of LDH A mRNA that is required for the regulation of mRNA stability. J. Biol. Chem. **273:** 28454–28460.
41. Cyzyk-Krzeska, M.F., Z. Dominski, R. Kole *et al.* 1994. Hypoxia stimulates binding of cytoplasmic protein to pyrimidine rich sequence in the 3′ untranslated region of rat tyrosine hydroxylase mRNA. J. Biol. Chem. **269:** 9940–9945.
42. Good, P.J. 1995. A conserved family of ELAV-like genes in vertebrates. Proc. Natl. Acad. Sci. USA **92:** 4557–4561.
43. Wakamatsu, Y. & J.A. Weston. 1997. Sequential expression and role of Hu RNA binding proteins during neurogenesis. Development **124:** 3449–3460.
44. Perrone-Bizzozero, N. & F. Bolognani. 2002. Role of HuD and other RNA-binding proteins in neural development and plasticity. J. Neurosci. Res. **68:** 121–126.
45. Quattrone, A., A. Pascale, X. Nogues *et al.* 2001. Posttranscriptional regulation gene expression in learning by the neuronal ELAV-like mRNA stabilizing proteins. Proc. Natl. Acad. Sci. USA **98:** 11669–11673.
46. Pascale, A., P.A. Gusev, M. Amadio *et al.* 2004. Increase of the RNA-binding protein HuD and posttranscriptional regulation of the GAP-43 gene during spatial memory. Proc. Natl. Acad. Sci. USA **101:** 1217–1222.

Antioxidative Effect of Vitamin D3 on Zinc-Induced Oxidative Stress in CNS

ANYA M. Y. LIN, K. B. CHEN, AND P. L. CHAO

Department of Medical Research and Education, Veterans General Hospital–Taipei, and Department of Physiology, National Yang-Ming University, Taipei, Taiwan

ABSTRACT: Antioxidative mechanisms of vitamin D3 were evaluated both *in vitro* and *in vivo*. A 4-h incubation of brain homogenates at 37°C increased the formation of Schiff base fluorescent products of malonaldehyde, an indicator of lipid peroxidation. Incubation with vitamin D3 dose-dependently suppressed auto-oxidation. The antioxidative potency for inhibiting zinc-induced lipid peroxidation was as follows: vitamin D3 > Trolox (a water-soluble analogue of vitamin E) ≥ β-estradiol > melatonin. In the presence of high dose of desferrioxamine, a metal chelator, vitamin D3 attenuated auto-oxidation. These *in vitro* data indicate that vitamin D3 may act as a terminator of the lipid peroxidation chain reaction. The antioxidative effect of vitamin D3 on zinc-induced oxidative injury was verified using local infusion of vitamin D3 *in vivo*. Intranigral infusion of zinc elevated lipid peroxidation in the infused substantia nigra and depleted striatal dopamine content at 7 days after infusion. Furthermore, elevated cytosolic cytochrome c and DNA ladder, indicatives of apoptosis, were demonstrated in the infused substantia nigra. Simultaneous infusion of vitamin D3 and zinc prevented oxidative injury and apoptosis induced by zinc alone. The involvement of glia-derived neurotrophic factor (GDNF) expression was excluded since vitamin D3 did not alter GDNF level in the infused substantia nigra at 24 h or 4 days after intranigral infusion of vitamin D3. Our results suggest that vitamin D3, independent of upregulation of GDNF expression, may acutely prevent zinc-induced oxidative injuries via antioxidative mechanisms.

KEYWORDS: vitamin D3; antioxidative action; zinc; transition metal; lipid peroxidation

INTRODUCTION

Vitamin D3, an active metabolite of vitamin D, reportedly possesses a variety of biological functions.[1,2] Recently, a neuroprotective role of vitamin D3 has been suggested. For example, vitamin D3 reportedly reduced neuronal damage induced by H_2O_2 in the ventral mesencephalic neuronal culture.[3] Furthermore, several *in vivo* studies have showed that systemic vitamin D3 attenuated cortical infarction[3] and neurotoxicity induced by 6-hydroxydopamine or iron of rat brain.[4,5] Upregulation of neurotrophic factors, including glia-derived neurotrophic factor (GDNF), has been

Address for correspondence: Anya M. Y. Lin, Department of Medical Research and Education, Veterans General Hospital–Taipei, Taipei 112, Taiwan. Voice: +886-2-28712121, ext. 2688; fax: +886-2-28751562.
myalin@vghtpe.gov.tw

**Ann. N.Y. Acad. Sci. 1053: 319–329 (2005). © 2005 New York Academy of Sciences.
doi: 10.1196/annals.1344.028**

proposed for the vitamin D3–induced neuroprotection.[3–6] Nevertheless, vitamin D3 may also exert its protection via antioxidative actions. In the past decade, several studies have shown that vitamin D3 possesses an antioxidative activity. Vitamin D3 has been demonstrated as a membrane antioxidant that inhibited iron-induced lipid peroxidation of brain liposomes.[7] Systemic vitamin D3 suppressed the elevated lipid peroxidation observed in vitamin D3–deficient rats.[8] A vitamin D3 analogue has been found to inhibit endotoxemia via regulation of free radical formation.[9] Furthermore, vitamin D3 attenuated inducible nitric oxide synthase activity and thus decreased free radical formation in rat primary astrocytes.[10] Moreover, vitamin D3 has been reported to reduce oxidative stress by upregulating antioxidative defense systems, including glutathione content, glutathione peroxidase, and superoxide dismutase in cultured astrocytes[10] and in liver.[11]

Zinc, one of the transition metals, has been reported to induce neurotoxicity in CNS. Indeed, clinical studies have shown accumulation of zinc in the nigrostriatal dopaminergic system in Parkinson's disease patients.[12] Incubation with exogenous zinc has been found to induce cell death in cortical neuronal culture.[13] Furthermore, releases of endogenous zinc were reportedly responsible for the hippocampal neuronal damages induced by kainate[14] or transient forebrain ischemia.[15] Moreover, our previous studies showed that local infusion of zinc induced neurotoxicity in the nigrostriatal dopaminergic system.[16,17] Oxidative stress may be one of the causes for the zinc-induced neurotoxicity. Further, apoptosis and necrosis have been suggested to be responsible for zinc-induced neurotoxicity.[17]

In the present study, the involvement of antioxidative mechanisms in vitamin D3–induced neuroprotection was investigated against zinc-induced oxidative stress. Antioxidative effect of vitamin D3 on both auto-oxidation and zinc-induced lipid peroxidation was performed by incubation of zinc in brain homogenates. The potency of vitamin D3 in suppressing zinc-induced lipid peroxidation was compared with several well-known antioxidants. Desferrioxamine was used as a positive control to study the free radical scavenging property of vitamin D3. Furthermore, the antioxidative effect of vitamin D3 was investigated using local infusion of vitamin D3 in the substantia nigra of anesthetized rats. Several oxidative injuries, including lipid peroxidation in the infused substantia nigra and striatal dopamine content, were evaluated. The effect of intranigral infusion of vitamin D3 on the cytosolic cytochrome c level, an indicator of apoptosis, was investigated using Western blot and immunohistochemical studies.

METHODS

In Vitro *Studies*

Cortical samples were homogenized in chilled Ringer's solution (50 mg/mL) and treated for either auto-oxidation or zinc-induced lipid peroxidation as follows. *Auto-oxidation*: The homogenates were incubated at 37°C for 4 h. Vitamin D3 (Abbot, MI) and desferrioxamine (Sigma, St. Louis, MO) were included in each experiment as described in the results. *Zinc-induced lipid peroxidation*: The homogenates were incubated at 37°C for 4 h following an addition of zinc (200 μM) ± vitamin D3, 6-hydroxy-2,5,7,8-tetramethylchroman-2-carboxylic acid (Trolox, Aldrich, Milwaukee,

WI), β-estradiol, and melatonin (Sigma, St. Louis, MO). A 400-μL sample was transferred to a tube containing 300 μL chloroform and 100 μL methanol. After centrifugation at 8000*g* for 5 min, an aliquot of chloroform extract was transferred to another tube containing 100 μL methanol scanned using a spectrofluorometer. Lipid peroxidation was determined by measuring the levels of malondialdehyde and its dihydropyridine polymers, which emit fluorescence at 426 nm when activated by UV at 356 nm.[18]

In Vivo *Study*

Adult, male Sprague-Dawley rats, weighing 250–350 g, were used. These animals were maintained according to the guidelines established in the "Guide for the care and use of laboratory animals" prepared by the Committee on Care and Use of Laboratory Animals of the Institute of Laboratory Animal Resources Commission on Life Sciences, National Research Council (U.S.A.).

Chronic Surgery and Drug Infusion

To induce oxidative stress in the nigrostriatal system, rats were anesthetized with chloral hydrate (450 mg/kg, ip, Sigma, St. Louis, MO) and placed in a stereotaxic instrument (David Kopf Instruments, Palo Alto, CA). One μL of Krebs-Ringer solution of zinc chloride (zinc, 40 nmol) ± vitamin D3 (0.6 pmol) was infused stereotaxically into substantia nigra (coordinates: 3.2 mm anterior and 2 mm above the interaural zero; 2.1 mm lateral to the midline; 3.5 mm below the incisor bar). Drug solutions were infused at a rate of 0.2 μL/min through a 30-gauge stainless steel needle. The injection needle was held in place for an additional 3 min following drug infusion. After the surgery, rats recovered from anesthesia and were placed in home cages for 7 days.

Fluorescence Assay of Lipid Peroxidation in Substantia Nigra

At the end of each *in vivo* experiment, rats were sacrificed by decapitation. Substantia nigra dissected from both hemispheres was homogenized in chilled 400 μL chloroform and 200 μL methanol. After centrifugation, an aliquot of the chloroform and methanol layer was scanned using a spectrofluorometer. The relative fluorescent intensities of samples in a cuvette were measured as mentioned above.

HPLC-EC Analysis of Striatal Dopamine Content

Rats were decapitated. Regional dissections were performed and striata were immediately frozen in liquid nitrogen and stored at –70°C until analysis. An HPLC with EC detection procedure was used to quantify dopamine content in striatum.[19]

Western Blot Analysis of Cytochrome c

Substantia nigras were dissected and homogenized in 100 μL of ice-cold mitochondrial isolation buffer (70 mM sucrose, 210 mM mannitol, 5 mM Tris-HCl, 1 mM EDTA, 20 mM fluorocitrate, pH 7.4). After homogenization, the suspension was centrifuged at 600*g* for 5 min at 4°C, and the supernatant transferred to a chilled Eppendorf tube and centrifuged at 17,000*g* for 10 min at 4°C. Purity of the cytosolic fraction was determined by measuring cytochrome oxidase. The cytosolic protein samples (50 μg) were run on 15% sodium dodecyl sulfate–polyacrylamide gel electrophoresis and then transferred onto a nitrocellular membrane (Bio-Rad, Richmond, CA) at 80 V for 75 min. Blots were probed with a mouse monoclonal antibody (7H8.2C12, BD Pharmingen, San Diego, CA) against the denatured form of cytochrome c at a dilution of 1:500 at 4°C for 45 min. After primary antibody incubation, the membrane was washed and incubated with horseradish peroxidase–conjugated goat antimouse IgG (Chemicon, Temecula, CA) for 40 min at room temperature. The immunoreaction was visualized using Amersham enhanced chemiluminescence (Amersham Pharmacia Biotech, Buckinghamshire, U.K.). After this detection, the bound primary and secondary antibodies were stripped by incubating the membrane in stripping buffer (100 mM 2-mercaptoethanol, 2% sodium dodecyl sulfate) at 50°C for 30 min. The membrane was reprobed with a mouse cytochrome oxidase subunit IV antibody or β-actin (1:1000) and then visualized with a procedure similar to that for cytochrome c.

Immunostaining of Cytochrome c

Rats were perfused transcardially with chilled saline and followed by 4% paraformaldehyde–PBS solution. Brains were frozen-sectioned coronally at 16 μm using a cryostat. A mouse monoclonal antibody against the native form of cytochrome c (6H2.B4, BD Pharmingen, U.S.A.) was used *in situ*. Sections were then incubated with 0.3% Triton-100 and 1% goat serum, blocked with 3% goat serum, and incubated with mouse anticytochrome c (20 μg/mL) in 1% GS-PBS-T at 4°C overnight. The sections then were incubated with FITC-conjugated secondary antibody for anticytochrome c and visualized under a fluorescence microscope.

Measurement of GDNF by Enzyme-Linked Immunosorbent Assay (ELISA)

Substantia nigra was homogenized in a lysis buffer and centrifuged at 12,000*g* for 20 min. The supernatant was acidified according to the method described.[20] Samples were neutralized to pH 7.4, adjusted to contain the same amount of protein, and assayed for GDNF using GDNF ELISA kits (R&D, Minneapolis, MN). For measurement of GDNF, mouse monoclonal anti-GDNF antibody was used as a capture antibody, and biotinylated goat anti-GDNF antibody was used for detection. A 96-well microplate reader was used to measure the optical densities.

RESULTS

Incubation of brain homogenates at 37°C for 4 h increased the formation of peroxidized lipids compared with those incubated at 0°C (as basal level). Vitamin D3 dose-dependently suppressed the elevated lipid peroxidation (FIG. 1A). Addition of zinc (200 μM) further increased lipid peroxidation. Incubation with vitamin D3 inhibited zinc-induced increase in lipid peroxidation in a concentration-dependent manner (FIG. 1B). Furthermore, the antioxidative capacity of vitamin D3 was compared with that of Trolox (a water-soluble analogue of vitamin E), β-estradiol, and melatonin. Vitamin D3 was found to be about 10^3-fold more potent than Trolox and

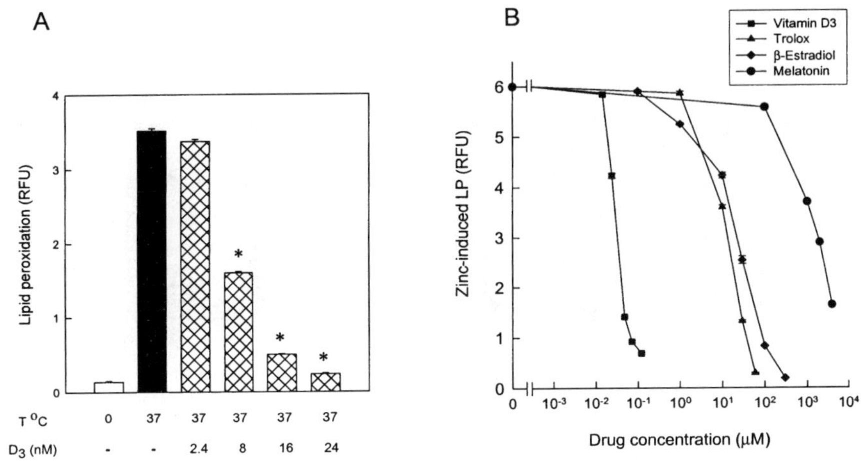

FIGURE 1. Effects of vitamin D3 on auto-oxidation and zinc-induced lipid peroxidation of cortical homogenates. **(A)** A dose-dependent inhibition by vitamin D3 of auto-oxidation of cortical homogenates. Brain homogenates were incubated at 37°C for 4 h with or without addition of vitamin D3. **(B)** Dose-response curves for vitamin D3, Trolox, β-estradiol, and melatonin on zinc-induced lipid peroxidation (LP) of cortical homogenates. Brain LP was reported as relative fluorescence units (RFU). Values are the mean ± SEM (n = 4–5) from a representative experiment that was replicated with similar results. *$P < 0.05$ in vitamin D3 group compared with the control group (37°C) by one-way ANOVA followed by post-hoc analyses.

β-estradiol and 10^5 times more potent than melatonin in preventing the zinc-induced lipid peroxidation (FIG. 1B).

Desferrioxamine was used as a metal ion chelator to study the antioxidative mechanisms of vitamin D3. Both vitamin D3 (24 nM) and desferrioxamine (10 μM) prevented auto-oxidation in a time-dependent manner (FIG. 2). Auto-oxidation was inhibited with a 4-h incubation of vitamin D3 or desferrioxamine. In contrast, no significant inhibition by vitamin D3 or desferrioxamine of auto-oxidation was observed when vitamin D3 or desferrioxamine was included in the brain homogenates for the last hour during a 4-h incubation (FIG. 2). At this time point, auto-oxidation was suppressed when high dose of vitamin D3 (240 nM, FIG. 2A), but not desferrioxamine (100 μM, FIG. 2B), was coincubated. In the presence of high dose of desferrioxamine (100 μM), which did not attenuate auto-oxidation, coincubation of 240 nM vitamin D3 actually suppressed auto-oxidation (FIG. 2B).

To evaluate the antioxidative effect of vitamin D3 on zinc-induced neurotoxicity, zinc with or without vitamin D3 was locally infused in the substantia nigra of anesthetized rats. Seven days after intranigral infusion of zinc, lipid peroxidation was elevated in the infused substantia nigra and the dopamine content was depleted in the ipsilateral striatum (FIG. 3). While intranigral infusion of vitamin D3 alone altered neither basal lipid peroxidation in substantia nigra nor dopamine content in the ipsilateral striatum, coinfusion of vitamin D3 and zinc prevented zinc-induced oxidative injuries (FIG. 3).

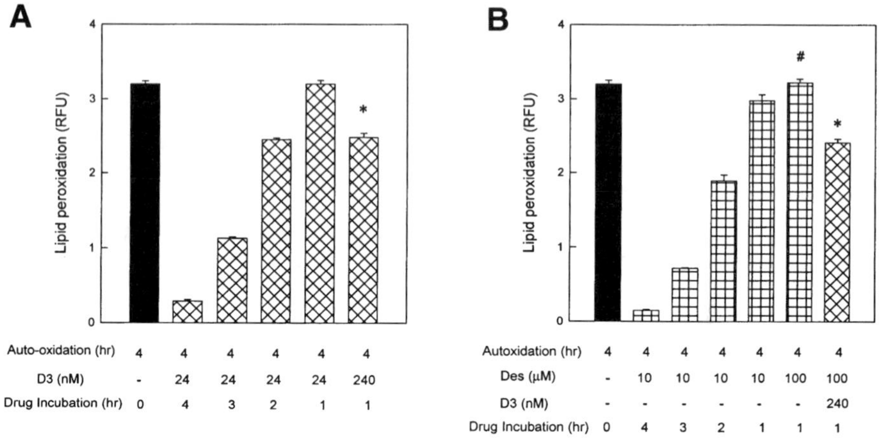

FIGURE 2. The antioxidative action of vitamin D3 on auto-oxidation in the presence of desferrioxamine. **(A)** A time-dependent effect of vitamin D3 on auto-oxidation. $*P < 0.05$ in high vitamin D3 treatment compared with low dose of vitamin D3 at 1 h after drug incubation. **(B)** Desferrioxamine (10 nM) time-dependently inhibited auto-oxidation. No significant inhibition of auto-oxidation was observed when 10 μM or 100 μM desferrioxamine was included in the brain homogenates for the last hour during a 4-h incubation. At this time point, 240 nM vitamin D3 actually attenuated auto-oxidation in the presence of 100 μM desferrioxamine. #Not significant in high dose of desferrioxamine (100 μM) compared with low dose of desferrioxamine (10 μM). $*P < 0.05$ in desferrioxamine (100 μM) + vitamin D3 compared with desferrioxamine (100 μM) alone by one-way ANOVA followed by post-hoc analyses. Brain LP was reported as relative fluorescence units (RFU). Values are the mean ± SEM ($n = 3$) from a representative experiment that was replicated with similar results.

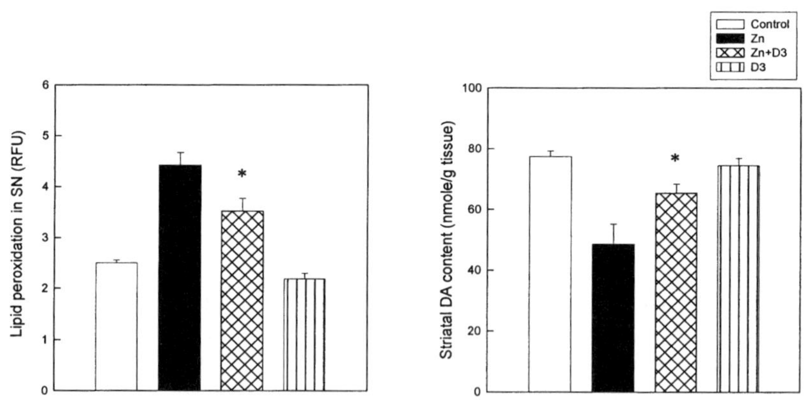

FIGURE 3. Effects of vitamin D3 on zinc-induced oxidative injuries in the nigrostriatal dopaminergic system at 7 days after an intranigral infusion of zinc. LP in the microdissected substantia nigra was measured and reported as relative fluorescence units (RFU). Striatal dopamine content was determined using HPLC-EC detection. Values are the mean ± SEM (n = 4–6). $*P < 0.05$ in vitamin D3 + zinc group compared with zinc group by one-way ANOVA followed by post-hoc analyses.

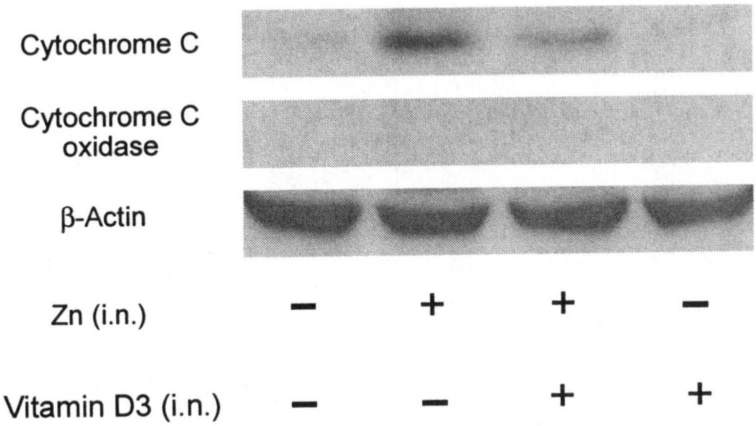

FIGURE 4. Effects of vitamin D3 on zinc-induced elevation in cytosolic cytochrome c level of substantia nigra at 4 h after an intranigral infusion of zinc. A representative result of cytochrome c in the cytosolic fraction of substantia nigra was detected by Western blotting at 4 h after an intranigral infusion of zinc ± vitamin D3. Cytochrome oxidase was not detected, indicating the purity of the cytosolic fraction. Fifty μg of protein was loaded in each lane in all experiments. Similar results were obtained from three independent experiments.

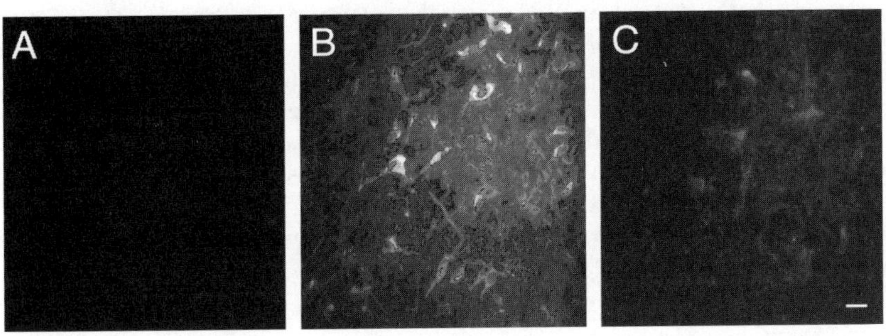

FIGURE 5. Fluorescent microscopic images show reduction in cytosolic cytochrome c immunofluorescence in the substantia nigra infused with zinc and vitamin D3 mixture. Four hours after intranigral infusion, a strong immunofluorescence was obtained in the zinc-infused substantia nigra (**B**) compared with the intact control (**A**). The cytoplasmic cytochrome c fluorescence was attenuated in the substantia nigra receiving zinc and vitamin D3 mixture (**C**). Scale bar: 20 μm.

To evaluate the effect of local vitamin D3 on zinc-induced apoptosis, the cytosolic cytochrome c of substantia nigra was examined using Western blot analysis and immunofluorescent staining. Four hours after intranigral infusion of zinc, cytosolic cytochrome c levels were increased in the infused substantia nigra, whereas cytochrome c oxidase (subunit IV) was nearly absent (FIG. 4). The absence of cytochrome c oxidase in the cytosolic extract indicated that the cytosolic extracts were free of mitochondrial contamination. While vitamin D3 alone did not elevate the cytochrome c in the cytosolic extracts of the zinc-infused substantia nigra, infusion

TABLE 1. GDNF levels in intact SN or SN receiving zinc, vitamin D3, or zinc plus vitamin D3 mixture

GDNF level (pg/mg tissue)	Intact SN	Zn	Zn + D3	D3
24 h after intranigral infusion	29.9 ± 3.3 (4)	37.0 ± 3.5 (4)	32.2 ± 4.1 (4)	34.9 ± 5.3 (4)
4 days after intranigral infusion	24.6 ± 1.9 (4)	28.6 ± 4.6* (4)	25.1 ± 3.7 (4)	30.7 ± 3.1 (4)

NOTE: Local vitamin D3 had no effect on basal GDNF levels measured by ELISA assay. Values are the mean ± SEM. Numbers in parentheses represent sample size. Similar results were obtained in duplicates. *$P < 0.05$ in zinc-infused substantia nigra at 4 days after infusion compared with substantia nigra at 24 h after the infusion by one-way ANOVA followed by post-hoc analysis.

of vitamin D3 and zinc mixture inhibited zinc-induced increase in cytosolic cytochrome c in the infused substantia nigra (FIG. 4). The distribution of cytosolic cytochrome c was confirmed using immunofluorescent staining. A less intensive cytoplasmic distribution of cytochrome c fluorescence in the substantia nigra infused with zinc and vitamin D3 mixture was observed compared with that with zinc (FIG. 5).

Using the technique of ELISA, the basal GDNF level in the intact substantia nigra averaged 29.9 ± 3.3 pg/mg tissue (n = 4). Twenty-four hours after intranigral infusion, the GDNF level was not significantly changed in the zinc-infused substantia nigra. Intranigral infusion of vitamin D3 alone did not elevate GDNF level in the infused substantia nigra. Furthermore, the GDNF level was not increased in the substantia nigra receiving local infusion of vitamin D3 and zinc mixture. Four days after intranigral infusion, the GDNF level in the zinc-infused substantia nigra was insignificantly decreased compared with that after 24 h. At the same time, the GDNF level was not increased in the substantia nigra receiving the zinc and vitamin D3 mixture (TABLE 1).

DISCUSSION

Due to the pathophysiology of oxidative stress in the CNS neurodegenerative diseases,[21–23] several neuroprotective strategies have been proposed,[24–28] including supplementation with antioxidants,[26,27] upregulation of antioxidative defensive enzymes,[27] and intermittent hypoxia.[28] In the past decade, vitamin D3 has been found to be antioxidative[6–10] and may be neuroprotective. Our present study further supports this notion in that D3 dose-dependently suppressed auto-oxidation and zinc-induced lipid peroxidation in cortical homogenates. Moreover, our data showed a time-dependent inhibition of auto-oxidation by vitamin D3. In the presence of 100 μM desferrioxamine, which chelated metal ion and had no effect on the elevated lipid peroxidation, 240 nM vitamin D3 significantly attenuated auto-oxidation. These data indicate that vitamin D3 may be a terminator of the lipid peroxidation chain reaction.

Compared with several well-known antioxidants, vitamin D3 may be one of the most powerful antioxidants in biological organisms as shown in the present study.

The antioxidative potencies of vitamin D3 and vitamin E have been compared and the results varied. Vitamin D3 has been found equally potent as that of vitamin E in suppressing lipid peroxidation in liver.[11] However, our *in vitro* study demonstrated that vitamin D3 was 10^3-fold more potent than Trolox (a water-soluble analogue of vitamin E) in inhibiting zinc-induced lipid peroxidation. Similar results were observed in suppressing iron-induced lipid peroxidation in the cortical homogenates (unpublished observation). The reasons for the discrepancy may be due to different tissues and/or the different routes of drug administration used in our studies and Sardar's study.[11] In Sardar's study, vitamin E was supplied in diet, while vitamin D3 was orally applied, and bioavailabilities[11] of vitamins D3 and E may result in different dose responses. In contrast, our *in vitro* study used the exact doses of vitamin D3 and vitamin E and these drugs were incubated in identical conditions. Melatonin, which has been used as a lipid-soluble antioxidant,[26,27] was found to be 10^5 times less potent than vitamin D3 in our study. β-Estradiol, a well-known steroid, possessing antioxidative actions via metal-chelating activity and radical scavenging activity, was used as a positive control.[29,30] Our data showed that vitamin D3 is antioxidative, with similar mechanisms as, but 10^3 times more potent than, β-estradiol in inhibiting zinc-induced lipid peroxidation.

Two well-known pathways participate in activation of vitamin D3 receptors. One is a nuclear receptor–mediated genomic pathway that regulates gene transcription and the other is a membrane receptor–mediated nongenomic pathway that rapidly opens calcium channels.[1] Upregulation of GDNF levels has been reported in the neuroprotection by chronic administration of vitamin D3 (ip) in our previous study[5] and others.[3,4] These data suggest that receptor activation through genomic and nongenomic pathways[1] may be involved in this vitamin D3–induced neuroprotection.[3–5] In contrast, cortical homogenates in which cellular integrity was disrupted were used in the present study to rule out the possibility of receptor activation, and our *in vitro* data showed an inhibition by vitamin D3 of auto-oxidation and zinc-induced lipid peroxidation. Furthermore, our *in vivo* data demonstrated no upregulation of GDNF expression when local infusion of vitamin D3 diminished the elevation in cytosolic cytochrome c and the subsequent oxidative injuries induced by zinc alone in the nigrostriatal dopaminergic system. These data directly exclude the involvement of GDNF in the vitamin D3–induced neuroprotection observed in the present study. While vitamin D3 reportedly activated the receptor-mediated calcium translocation[1,31,32] that may further induce apoptosis,[33,34] local infusion of vitamin D3 (0.6 pmol) alone did not increase the cytosolic cytochrome c in the infused substantia nigra. Moreover, vitamin D3 altered neither lipid peroxidation in the infused substantia nigra nor striatal dopaminergic content at 7 days after the infusion. These data indicate that vitamin D3 may attenuate zinc-induced oxidative injury via antioxidative mechanisms instead of through genomic and/or nongenomic activation.[1]

So far, our study has shown neuroprotection by vitamin D3; however, vitamin D3 has been reported to reduce cell proliferation and increase apoptosis in response to oxidative stress.[35] One of the possibilities may be due to vitamin D3–induced production of thioredoxin-binding protein-2/vitamin D3 upregulated protein-1 (TBP-2/VDUP-1),[36] which suppresses thioredoxin function,[35,37] an antioxidative defense system in biological organisms. The dose of vitamin D3 required to upregulate the TBP-2/VDUP-1 was 1 μM and a significant upregulation of TBP-2/VDUP-1 was observed 16 h after the incubation.[35] In contrast, the doses of vitamin D3 were 24 nM in our *in vitro* study or 0.6 pmoles in our animal study, and both treatments significantly reduced zinc-induced lipid peroxidation at 4 h after incubation or local infusion of zinc. Thus, TBP-2/VDUP-1 may not be involved in the neuroprotection of vitamin D3 in the present study.

In conclusion, our *in vitro* data showed that vitamin D3 possesses a very powerful antioxidative property and is capable of suppressing auto-oxidation and zinc-induced lipid peroxidation. Furthermore, the *in vivo* study showed that local vitamin D3 alone did not cause deleterious effects, but efficiently prevented zinc-induced oxidative injuries. These data suggest that, in addition to upregulation of neurotrophic factors, antioxidative mechanisms of vitamin D3 may be considered in counteracting oxidative injuries in the CNS.[1]

ACKNOWLEDGMENTS

This study was supported by Grant Nos. NSC90-2420-B-075-017 and VGH92-338 (Taipei, Taiwan).

REFERENCES

1. NORMAN, A.W. *et al.* 1992. 1,25(OH)$_2$-Vitamin D3, a steroid hormone that produces biological effects via both genomic and nongenomic pathway. J. Steroid Biochem. Mol. Biol. **41:** 231–240.
2. REICHEL, H. *et al.* 1989. The role of the vitamin D endocrine system in health and disease. N. Engl. J. Med. **320:** 980–991.
3. WANG, J.Y. *et al.* 2001. Vitamin D3 attenuated 6-OHDA-induced neurotoxicity in rats. Brain Res. **904:** 67–75.
4. WANG, Y. *et al.* 2000. Vitamin D3 attenuates cortical infarction induced by middle cerebral arterial ligation in rats. Neuropharmacology **39:** 873–880.
5. CHEN, K.B. *et al.* 2003. Systemic vitamin D3 attenuated oxidative injuries in the locus coeruleus of rat brain. Ann. N.Y. Acad. Sci. **993:** 313–324.
6. NAVEILHAN, P. *et al.* 1996. 1,25(OH)$_2$-Vitamin D3, an inducer of glial cell-line–derived neurotrophic factor. Neuroreport **7:** 2171–2175.
7. WISEMAN, H. 1993. Vitamin D is a membrane antioxidant: ability to inhibit iron-dependent lipid peroxidation in liposomes compared to cholesterol, ergosterol, and tamoxifen and relevance to anticancer action. FEBS J. **326:** 285–288.
8. KUZMENKO, A.I. *et al.* 1997. Effects of vitamin D3 and ecdysterone on free-radical lipid peroxidation. Biochemistry (Mosc.) **62:** 609–612.
9. HORIUCHI, H. *et al.* 1999. Protective effect of vitamin D3 analogues on endotoxin shock in mice. Agents Actions **33:** 343–348.
10. GARCION, E. *et al.* 1999. 1,25-Dihydroxyvitamin D3 regulates the synthesis of γ-glutamyl transpeptidase and glutathione levels in rat primary astrocytes. J. Neurochem. **73:** 859–866.
11. SARDAR, S. *et al.* 1996. Comparative effectiveness of vitamin D3 and dietary vitamin E on peroxidation of lipids and enzymes of the hepatic antioxidants system in Sprague-Dawley rats. Int. J. Vitamin Nutrition Res. **66:** 39–45.
12. DEXTER, D.T. *et al.* 1989. Increased nigral iron content and alteration in other metal ions occurring in brain in Parkinson's disease. J. Neurochem. **52:** 1830–1836.
13. MANEV, H. *et al.* 1997. Characterization of zinc-induced neuronal death in primary cultures of rat cerebellar granule cells. Exp. Neurol. **146:** 171–178.
14. ASSAF, S.Y. & S.H. CHUNG. 1984. Release of endogenous Zn from brain tissue during activity. Nature **308:** 734–736.
15. KOH, J.Y. *et al.* 1996. The role of zinc in selective neuronal death after transient global cerebral ischemia. Science **272:** 1013–1016.

16. LIN, A.M.Y. 2001. Coexistence of zinc and iron augmented oxidative injuries in the nigrostriatal dopaminergic system of SD rats. Free Radical Biol. Med. **30:** 225–231.
17. LIN, A.M.Y. *et al.* 2003. Zinc-induced apoptosis in substantia nigra of rat brain: neuroprotection by vitamin D3. Free Radical Biol. Med. **34:** 1416–1425.
18. KIKUGAWA, K. *et al.* 1989. Fluorescent and crosslinked protein formed by free radical and aldehyde species generated during lipid peroxidation. Adv. Exp. Med. Biol. **266:** 345–356.
19. CHIUEH, C.C. *et al.* 1983. 6-Fluorocatecholamines as false adrenergic neurotransmitters. J. Pharmacol. Exp. Ther. **225:** 529–533.
20. OKRAGKY, A.J. & M. HAAK-FRENDSCHO. 1997. An acid treatment method for enhanced detection of GDNF in biological samples. Exp. Neurol. **145:** 592–596.
21. HALLIWELL, B. & J.M. GUTTERIDGE. 1984. Oxygen toxicity, oxygen radicals, transition metals, and neurodegenerative diseases. Biochem. J. **219:** 1–14.
22. KOUTSILIERI, E. *et al.* 2002. Free radicals in Parkinson's dieease. J. Neurol. **249**(S2): II1–II5.
23. COHEN, G. & P. WERNER. 1994. Free radicals, oxidative stress, and neurodegeneration. *In* Neurodegenerative Diseases, pp. 139–162. Saunders. Philadelphia.
24. BEAL, M.F. 2003. Bioenergetic approaches for neuroprotection in Parkinson's disease. Ann. Neurol. **53**(suppl. 3): S39–S47.
25. ALLEGRA, M. *et al.* 2003. The chemistry of melatonin's interaction with reactive species. J. Pineal Res. **34:** 1–10.
26. REITER, R.J. 1998. Oxidative damage in the central nervous system: protection by melatonin. Prog. Neurobiol. **56:** 359–384.
27. LIN, A.M.Y. & L.T. HO. 2000. Melatonin suppresses iron-induced neurodegeneration in rat brain. Free Radical Biol. Med. **28:** 904–911.
28. LIN, A.M.Y. *et al.* 2002. Neuroprotective effect of intermittent hypoxia on iron-induced oxidative injury in rat brain. Exp. Neurol. **176:** 328–335.
29. MERCE, A.L.R. *et al.* 1996. Potentiometric study of vitamin D3 complexes with manganese (II), iron (II), iron (III), and zinc (II) in water-ethanol medium. J. Inorganic Biochem. **73:** 167–172.
30. ROMER, W. *et al.* 1997. Novel "scavestrogens" and their radical scavenging effects, iron-chelating, and antioxidative activities and total antioxidative activities. Steroids **62:** 304–310.
31. BOLAND, R.L. *et al.* 1991. Single cell analysis of changes in cytosolic calcium induced by vitamin D3 metabolites in cultured rat mesangial cells. Biochem. Biophys. Res. Commun. **180:** 833–840.
32. TASAKA, T. *et al.* 1991. Mechanism of transient increase in intracellular concentration of free calcium ions in HL-60 cell differentiation induced by vitamin D3 and phorbol ester. Biochem. Int. **23:** 137–143.
33. BUDD, S.L. 1998. Mechanism of neuronal damage in brain hypoxia/ischemia focus on the role of mitochondrial calcium accumulation. Pharmacol. Ther. **80:** 203–229.
34. VIRAG, L. *et al.* 1999. Requirement of intracellular calcium mobilization for peroxynitrite-induced poly(ADP-ribose) synthetase activation and cytotoxicity. Mol. Pharmacol. **56:** 824–833.
35. JUNN, E. *et al.* 2000. Vitamin D3 upregulated protein 1 mediates oxidative stress via suppressing the thioredoxin function. J. Immunol. **164:** 6287–6295.
36. CHEN, K.S. *et al.* 1993. Isolation and expression of human 1,25-dihydroxyvitamin D3 24-hydroxylase cDNA. Proc. Natl. Acad. Sci. USA **90:** 4543–4547.
37. NISHIYAMA, A. *et al.* 1999. Identification of thioredoxin-binding protein-2/vitamin D3 upregulated protein 1 as a negative regulator of thioredoxin function and expression. J. Biol. Chem. **274:** 21645–21650.

Questions and Answers

Session VII: The NMDA Receptor as a Target for Neurotoxicity and Neuroprotection

QUESTIONS FOR VESNA JEVTOVIC-TODOROVIC

From Hari Shanker Sharma

You have shown anesthetic-induced changes in rats that are 1 to 14 days old. You found changes at 7 days, but not at 14 days. Since the BBB (blood-brain barrier) is not matured before 21–35 days, what is the role of BBB in your studies? Another question is about the technical identification about apoptotic cell death at the EM level. How can one differentiate apoptotic cell death at EM as normal (physiological) versus that induced by anesthetic agents?

ANSWER: All general anesthetics that are commonly used in clinical practice easily cross the BBB regardless of age. Thus, the maturity of the BBB does not play a crucial role in determining the neurotoxic and/or neurotherapeutic effects of general anesthetics. As for the differentiation between the "physiological" apoptotic cell death and the apoptotic cell death induced by the anesthetic agents, these two processes are indistinguishable and there are no ultrastructural differences that could be detected with EM. The main difference is in the intensity and the severity of the apoptotic reaction. Normally, $<0.5\%$ of the developing neurons undergo this type of cell death; in contrast, in the presence of general anesthetics, many more developing neurons succumb to it (as much as 25% in some vulnerable brain regions).

From Philip Lazarovici

The blood anesthetic concentration is affecting the extracellular and intracellular O_2 partition coefficient. Have you measured "precisely" the normal intracellular O_2 concentration?

ANSWER: We have not measured the normal intracellular O_2 concentration. Our data concerning the adequacy of oxygenation while under anesthesia pertain to the measurements of the partial pressure of oxygen in the arterial blood.

From Chia-Yi Kuan

Why are postnatal day 7 rat pups particularly vulnerable to anesthesia-induced apoptosis? Why not postnatal day 3 or postnatal day 10? Is there any biological process that you can correlate to the effect? Have you examined Bax knockout or transgenic Bcl-2 mice to see whether they are less vulnerable to anesthesia-induced apoptosis? Do you see neuron apoptosis when you apply isoflurane or nitrous oxide alone?

Ann. N.Y. Acad. Sci. 1053: 330–333 (2005). © 2005 New York Academy of Sciences.
doi: 10.1196/annals.1344.066

ANSWER: We believe that 7-day-old rat pups are most vulnerable because this is at the peak of their brain development when they are most sensitive to general inhibition caused by the anesthetics. We have not done any work with Bax knockout mice, but we did determine using Western blot studies that general anesthetics activate the intrinsic (Bcl-2-dependent) apoptotic pathway early on. Isoflurane alone, but not nitrous oxide, causes dose-dependent apoptotic neurodegeneration.

From Karl Sanzenbacher

A pup that is 1–7 days old corresponds to the last trimester of the human fetus. In the neonatal intensive care unit (NICU), the conceptual age is the beginning of an EEG interpretation of what is to be considered normal or abnormal. There are weekly changes that occur. Is there any neurophysiology that could help us in the NICU? To what degree does ketamine cross the placenta?

ANSWER: It remains to be determined whether any neurophysiology testing could be of practical use in the NICU. If the degree of neuronal inhibition during the development is directly related to the severity of the neuronal damage, then it may be potentially beneficial to determine the degree of the neuronal inhibition in sedated children (neonates in particular) so that the anesthetic drugs could be administered in only minimally needed doses.

From Lars Wiklund

I am extremely alarmed by the facts in your presentation on the anesthesia effects on the developing brain. As a responsible anesthesiologist in my home country, I have to react to your findings as regards advice to colleagues and parents when an anesthetic is needed during the first few years of life. I simply do not know yet and have to reconsider the situation. Can you comment on this?

ANSWER: I feel the same way. We will have a lot of work to do to determine the practical implications of these findings. It is certainly very intriguing. General anesthesia is a necessity that sometimes cannot be avoided when pregnant mothers and newborn infants present with life-threatening conditions requiring surgery and/or prolonged stay in the ICU. Based on presently available data, it seems prudent to assume a defensive and very critical approach in weighing all the risks and benefits of exposing a very young child (younger than 2 years of age) to general anesthesia.

QUESTION FOR JACQUES ABRAINI

From Lars Wiklund

The neuroprotective effect of xenon was present at 50%, but not at 75%. The lack of effect or rather the adverse effect was said to be due to toxicity of the gas. The greater concentration (i.e., 75%) might be used for inhalational anesthesia. The therapeutic window thus seems very narrow. Have I understood what you said correctly?

ANSWER: In fact, xenon's toxicity depends on whether or not this gas is used under physiologic or excitotoxic conditions. When used as a general anesthetic under physiologic, nonexcitotoxic conditions, xenon has virtually no side effects. However, there is accumulating evidence mainly in rodents that xenon at 75-vol% when used as a treatment for excitotoxic injury may have potentially neurotoxic properties. Thus, considering comparison of xenon's anesthetic potency in humans and rodents, these data suggest that it may be not prudent to use xenon for treating patients with excitotoxic injury at concentrations higher than 60-vol%. In addition, xenon at 50-vol% in the rat subjected to excitotoxic injury shows no potentially neurotoxic properties. This suggests that xenon at 40-vol% may be the "ideal" xenon concentration for treating patients suffering diseases with an excitotoxic component, leading to maximal effect with no concomitant neurotoxicity. However, depending on the severity and the type of disease, for example, acute vs. chronic, and on the duration of treatment required, the therapeutic concentration of xenon may be adjusted between 20- and 50-vol% in humans.

QUESTIONS FOR WILLIAM SLIKKER, JR.

From Gregory Oxenkrug

Ketamine is an exogenous NMDA antagonist. There are known endogenous NMDA antagonists, such as kynurenine derivatives (quinoline, etc.), whose production is activated by stress. What might be the role of these endogenous NMDA antagonists in development?

ANSWER: Acute stress or oxidative stress elevates the levels of kynurenine in the plasma and most parts of the brain during development and in adulthood. A pathologic overabundance of the endogenous excitotoxin, quinolinic acid, or a hypofunction of kynurenic acid has been hypothetically linked to the occurrence of seizures and neuronal cell death. Kynurenic acid (a metabolite of the kynurenine pathway) has a broad spectrum of antagonist activities for the three ionotropic excitatory amino acid receptors. At low concentrations, it may block the glycine coagonist site of the NMDA receptor. In general, some metabolites of the kynurenine pathway such as 3-hydroxykynurenine are neurotoxic, and the other metabolites such as kynurenic acid may be neuroprotective. However, the underlying mechanisms are still largely unknown, especially during development.

In contrast to the endogenous NMDA antagonists, ketamine is a specific NMDA receptor channel blocker. Ketamine administration results in an upregulation of the NMDA receptor NR1 subunit protein. Coadministration of antisense of NR1 specifically prevents the synthesis of NR1 protein and subsequently blocks the ketamine-induced neuronal cell death.

From Syed Imam

Does NR1 antisense get into the cell? How do you know that 8-oxoG staining is a real damage effect since you do not have a nuclear marker?

ANSWER: Yes, 18-mer NR1 antisense oligonucleotide is membrane-permeable. NR1 antisense can get into the cells and can block the process of NR1 subunit protein synthesis. This effect has also been observed in other similar experiments. Coadministration of NR1 antisense with PCP prevents PCP-induced neuronal cell death.

8-OxoG is a modification of guanine induced by endogenous or extraneous ROS. 8-OxoG is used as a biomarker for oxidative DNA damage. To detect and localize oxidative DNA damage associated with ketamine, double-immunofluorescence analyses were performed by using monoclonal anti-8-oxoG and polyclonal anti-NCAM (neural cell adhesion molecule) antibodies. Our data revealed that 8-oxoG was primarily localized in the nucleus as well as in mitochondria (mitochondrial DNA), and in neurons (colocalized with NCAM) and glial cells. Ketamine (10 μM) remarkably upregulated the 8-oxoG expression in nuclei and mitochondria (intense staining) after 6-h withdrawal compared with controls. In the immunocytochemical photomicrographs, the nuclei and cytoplasm can easily be distinguished. In addition, the nuclear proteins and mitochondria have been extracted and are ready for undergoing Western blot assays with 8-oxoG antibody. The Western blot data will be helpful to verify the immunocytochemical results.

Antioxidant Effects of *N*-Acetylserotonin

Possible Mechanisms and Clinical Implications

GREGORY OXENKRUG

Melatonin Clinic and Pineal Research Laboratory, Department of Psychiatry, Tufts University School of Medicine, Boston, Massachusetts, USA

ABSTRACT: This paper will review our recent data relevant to the antioxidant effects of *N*-acetylserotonin (NAS), the immediate precursor of melatonin, the pineal gland indole. Mechanisms of the antioxidant effects of NAS might involve interaction with melatonin type 3 receptors and nonreceptor mechanisms such as stimulation of glutathione peroxidase, an antioxidant enzyme; inhibition of lipid peroxidation; suppression of phospholipase A2 activation; attenuation of tumor necrosis factor-α production; prevention of pathological opening of the mitochondrial permeability transition pores; and inhibition of sepiapterin reductase, the key enzyme of biosynthesis of tetrahydrobiopterin, the essential cofactor of nitric oxide synthase. NAS actions on some of these enzymes might be receptor-mediated. Protective effects of NAS against oxidative damage are independent from the effect of melatonin and, depending on the model, are 5 to 20 times stronger than that of melatonin. Antioxidant effect of NAS might underpin its cognition-enhancing, antiaging, antidepressant, antihypertensive, and antitumor effects. NAS and its derivatives might be useful in protection against oxidative stress–related disorders (cell death, mutagenesis, aging) and diseases (sepsis, cancer, postischemic trauma, Alzheimer's disease, parkinsonism).

KEYWORDS: *N*-acetylserotonin; TNF-α; lipid peroxidation; lipopolysaccharide; sepiapterin reductase; PLA2

INTRODUCTION

N-Acetylserotonin (NAS) is synthesized (mainly in the pineal gland) from serotonin (5-HT) via *N*-acetylation of 5-HT. NAS, then, is methylated into melatonin. Until recently, NAS was considered only as the precursor of melatonin in the process of melatonin biosynthesis from serotonin. Very few researchers pointed out the possible effects of NAS, independent from melatonin, that is, its memory-facilitating,[1] hypothermic,[2] analgesic,[3] and (most recently) antioxidative action.[4] Furthermore, about 15% of melatonin is demethylated *in vivo* "back" into NAS,[5,6] suggesting that *in vivo* effects of supraphysiological concentrations of melatonin might be partially mediated by NAS formed from melatonin:

Address for correspondence: Dr. Gregory Oxenkrug, Melatonin Clinic and Pineal Research Laboratory, Department of Psychiatry, Tufts University School of Medicine, Boston, MA 02135. Voice: 617-636-0219; fax: 617-636-8442.
goxenkrug@tufts-nemc.org

Ann. N.Y. Acad. Sci. 1053: 334–347 (2005). © 2005 New York Academy of Sciences.
doi: 10.1196/annals.1344.029

SEROTONIN ⟶ NAS ⇄ MELATONIN

The present paper will review our recent data on the possible mechanisms of the antioxidant effects of NAS and discuss the possible clinical applications of NAS and its derivatives.

MECHANISMS OF NAS EFFECTS

Literature and our data suggest that NAS effects might be mediated via receptors and nonreceptor-related mechanisms. The action of NAS on some enzymes might be receptor-mediated (TABLE 1).

Receptor-Mediated Mechanisms of the Antioxidant Effects of NAS

Melatonin Type 3 Receptor

The possibility of the receptor-related mechanism(s) of NAS effects has been supported by the recent discovery of melatonin type 3 (MT3) receptor.[7] Melatonin involvement in the regulation of circadian rhythms and some other functions is mediated via membrane G protein–coupled receptors of two types: MT1 and MT2.[8] MT3 receptor is different from MT1 and MT2 receptors: it is possible that MT3 receptor is not G protein–coupled and represents a binding site for quinone reductase 2.[7] While melatonin is a full agonist of MT1 and MT2 receptors, the MT3 receptor has higher affinity to NAS than to melatonin. The pharmacological profile of MT3 receptor (order of affinities: 2-iodomelatonin > NAS > melatonin) is clearly distinct from that of the cloned mammalian receptors MT1 and MT2 (2-iodomelatonin > melatonin >>>> NAS). NAS and 5-methoxycarbonylamino-*N*-acetyltryptamine (5-MCA-NAT) are selective agonists, while prazosin and *N*-acetyltryptamine are selective antagonists for the MT3 melatonin receptor.[8] One might suggest that MT3 receptor should be more appropriately designated as the NAS receptor.

Phospholipase A2 and MT3 Receptor

Phospholipase A2 (PLA2) enzymes are responsible for the hydrolysis of neuronal membrane phospholipids. Cytosolic phospholipase A2 (cPLA2) catalyzes arachidonic acid (AA) release from membrane phospholipids. Enhanced activity of cPLA2 is associated with oxidative stress and aging.[9] The selective MT3 receptor agonist, 5-MCA-NAT, reduced rat pineal cPLA2 protein and mRNA expression, suggesting that downregulation of cPLA2 expression is mediated by MT3 receptor.[10] Inhibition of cPLA2 might contribute to the antioxidant effect of NAS since AA is the primary substrate for lipid peroxidation.[11] It is noteworthy that, besides MT3 receptor, cPLA2 might be activated by nonreceptor mechanisms, such as end products of lipid peroxidation (see subsection on LIPID PEROXIDATION below).

Leukocyte Adhesion and MT3 Receptor

The recruitment of circulating blood cells to specific sites plays an important role in inflammation, immune response, tumorigenesis, and atherosclerosis.[12] The study

TABLE 1. Possible mechanisms of the antioxidant effect of NAS

Target	Effect	Receptor	Nonreceptor	Ref.
In Vitro				
Arachidonic acid cascade				
PLA2	↓	MT3	Yes	10
Lipid peroxidation	↓		Yes	18–23
LPS-induced lipid peroxidation	↓		Yes	17
NO synthesis				
SPR	↓		Yes	31, 32
BH4 synthesis	↓		Yes	27
iNOS	↓		Yes	34
TNF-α	↓		Yes	34; Perianayagam *et al.*, this volume
NF-κB	↓		Yes	4
Other targets				
Free radical scavenging	↓		Yes	41
NO scavenging	↓		Yes	40
MTP-induced opening	↓		Yes	38
β-Amyloid toxicity	↓		Yes	39
Glutathione peroxidase	↑		Yes	16
Superoxide production	↓		Yes	Perianayagam *et al.*, this volume
Leukocyte adhesion	↓	MT3		13
In/Ex Vivo				
Lipid peroxidation	↓		Yes	16
Angiogenesis	↓		Yes	71
Tumorigenesis	↓	MT3	Yes	66–70
Immobilization time (tail suspension test)	↓	MT3		53, 54
Hypertension (SHR)	↓	MT1, MT2		58
Hypotension (LPS)	↑		Yes	34
LPS lethality	↓		Yes	17, 34
Life span	↑		Yes	16
"Cognition": active avoidance	↑		Yes	1, 39
"Cognition": water maze	↑		Yes	39

ABBREVIATIONS: PLA2, phospholipase A2; LPS, lipopolysaccharide; NO, nitric oxide; SPR, sepiapterin reductase; BH4, tetrahydrobiopterin: iNOS, inducible nitric oxide synthase; TNF-α, tumor necrosis factor-α; NF-κB, nuclear factor kappa B; MTP, mitochondrial transition pores; SHR, spontaneously hypertensive rats.

of the effect of NAS and melatonin on the microcirculation during acute inflammation revealed that melatonin inhibits both leukocyte rolling and adhesion, while NAS inhibits only leukocyte adhesion. The rank order of potency of agonists and antagonist receptor selective ligands suggested that the activation of MT2 and MT3 melatonin binding site receptors modulates leukocyte rolling and adhesion, respectively.[13]

Nonreceptor-Mediated Mechanisms of the Antioxidant Effects of NAS

Lipid Peroxidation

Oxidative damage occurs when free radicals produced within an organism are not completely destroyed by the appropriate endogenous defense systems. Because lipids are a major component of living organisms and probably the first easy target of free radicals once they are produced, lipid peroxidation might play an important role in initiating and/or mediating some aspects of the aging process.[11]

Malondialdehyde and 4-hydroxyalkenals (MDA + HAE) are the end products of lipid peroxidation, and evaluation of their levels is used to determine the activity of lipid peroxidation. It is noteworthy that MDA + HAE are not only the commonly used indices of lipid peroxidation activity, but by themselves are toxic products perpetuating further chromosomal damage to living cells[14] and facilitating PLA2-induced hydrolysis of the membrane phospholipids:[15]

$$\text{phospholipids} \rightarrow \text{cPLA2} \rightarrow \text{AA} \rightarrow \text{lipid peroxidation} \rightarrow \text{MDA} + \text{HAE}.$$

Administration of NAS (30 mg/kg, sc, 4 weeks) resulted in a drastic decrease of lipid peroxidation (MDA + HAE) and an increase of glutathione peroxidase in brain and kidney tissues of 11-month-old C3H mice,[16] and protected against the lethal effect of lipopolysaccharide (LPS) *in vivo*.[17] In the *in vitro* experiments, NAS was 16 times stronger than melatonin against iron- and LPS-induced lipid peroxidation in rat brain tissue (Oxenkrug and Requintina, this volume).

The protective effect of NAS against oxidative damage induced by various agents, such as linoleic acid, iron, and copper, is independent from the effect of melatonin.[18–20] It is noteworthy that literature data consistently indicated up to 5, 10, and 20 times stronger antioxidant effect of NAS in comparison with melatonin (see refs. 21–23, respectively). Melatonin and NAS might exert even opposite effects on lipid peroxidation[24] (TABLE 2).

Inhibition of lipid peroxidation by NAS is unlikely to be mediated by MT3 receptor since the selective MT3 agonist, 5-MCA-NAT, did not affect iron- and LPS-induced rat brain lipid peroxidation (Requintina and Oxenkrug, this volume). This observation is consistent with the reports that melatonin exerted antioxidant effect in membrane systems and in cell types free of melatonin receptors[25] and that melatonin agonists did not mimic the neuroprotective action of melatonin against β-amyloid in rat hippocampal cells.[26]

Nitric Oxide Pathway of Reactive Oxygen Species Formation

Nitric oxide (NO) synthesis is catalyzed by nitric oxide synthase (NOS), which exists in three isoforms: neuronal, endothelial, and inducible. Activation of the inducible nitric oxide synthase (iNOS) resulted in the overproduction of NO, which (in excessive quantity) has a strong pro-oxidant effect.[11] 5,6,7,8-Tetrahydrobiopterin

TABLE 2. Comparison of the antioxidative efficacy of NAS and melatonin

Experimental conditions	Melatonin	NAS	Ratio	Ref.
Sepiapterin Reductase				
Sprague-Dawley rats, brain enzyme, K_i	30 μM	0.20 μM	150	32
Sprague-Dawley rats, RBC enzyme, K_i	25 μM	0.17 μM	147	32
Bovine adrenal medulla, K_i	10 μM	0.12 μM	83	31
Lipid Peroxidation				
Rat brain (LPS-induced), 50% inhibition	800 μM	50 μM	16	Oxenkrug and Requintina, this volume
Bovine retina (induced by ascorbate-Fe^{2+}), IC_{50}	9.82 μM	0.43 μM	22	23
LDL oxidation (copper-induced), minimal effective concentration	10 μM	1 μM	10	22
Rat retina (NO-induced), % inhibition by 4 mM	40%	60%		20
Hamster, testes (Fe^{2+}), minimal effective concentration	0.25 mM	0.05 mM	5	21
Vitamin E consumption in human RBC induced by:				
Cumene hydroperoxide	↑	↓		24
H_2O_2	↑	↓		24
ROS formation in human PBL	10% inhibition	80% inhibition		41

NOTE: Ratio is that of melatonin to NAS; RBC, red blood cells; PBL, peripheral blood lymphocytes; ROS, reactive oxygen species; LDL, low-density lipoprotein.

(BH4) is an essential cofactor of NOS. Biosynthesis of BH4 occurs via two distinct pathways:

(*a*) A *de novo* synthesis from guanosine triphosphate (GTP) that involves three enzymes—GTP cyclohydrolase I (GTPCH), the first and rate-limiting enzyme in the *de novo* synthesis of BH4 (EC 3.5.4.16); pyruvoyltetrahydropterin synthase; and sepiapterin reductase (SPR):

De novo synthesis: GTP → GTPCH → sepiapterin → SPR → BH4.

(*b*) A salvage pathway, that is, BH4 synthesis from sepiapterin, which is catalyzed by SPR:

Salvage pathway: sepiapterin → SPR → BH4.

Therefore, in both pathways, sepiapterin serves as the immediate precursor of BH4.[27] The importance of SPR is stressed by the fact that GTP cyclohydrolase I is not a rate-limiting step of BH4 biosynthesis in humans.[28] The human SPR gene was mapped to chromosome band 2p13.[29] Crystal structure of mouse SPR reveals two very specific binding motifs for competitive inhibition of the enzyme.[30] NAS is optimally able to occupy both of these two motifs.[31]

NAS is a selective inhibitor of SPR, the key enzyme of BH4 synthesis. NAS is a much stronger SPR inhibitor than melatonin (K_i: 0.17 vs. 25 μM, respectively)[31,32] (TABLE 2). Inhibition of SPR by NAS blocks BH4 biosynthesis.[27] Since BH4 is a cofactor of all known isoforms of the NOS, NAS might prevent excessive production of NO, which has powerful pro-oxidant effects.[11] Excessive NO is toxic by itself, and interacts with superoxide radical to form the peroxynitrite anion, which in its turn might trigger lipid peroxidation.[20]

Tumor Necrosis Factor-α

Tumor necrosis factor-α (TNF-α) is one of the inflammatory cytokines and the key mediator of the systemic inflammatory response. TNF-α is released mainly by mononuclear phagocytes in response to LPS. Activation of TNF-α receptor 1 leads to the generation of reactive oxygen species (ROS).[33]

The effect of NAS on TNF-α was evaluated in two studies with contradictory results.[34,35] We found that NAS strongly inhibited LPS-induced TNF-α formation in differentiated THP-1 cells (Perianayagam *et al.*, this volume).

Since TNF-α causes an up to 30-fold induction of GTP cyclohydrolase I[36] and stimulates expression of iNOS,[37] NAS-induced suppression of TNF-α production might contribute to inhibition of BH4 synthesis and activation of the iNOS.

Therefore, NAS might suppress both key enzymes of BH4 synthesis—SPR (directly) and GTPCH (indirectly via TNF-α):

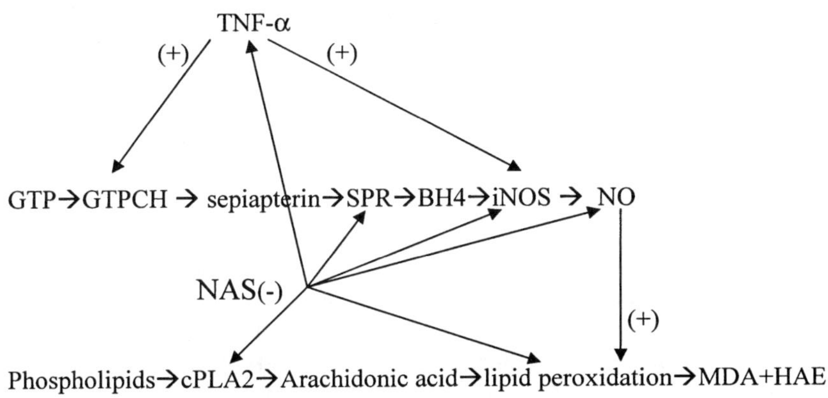

(+) activation; (-) inhibition

Mitochondrial Permeability Transition Pores

Mitochondrial permeability transition pores (PTPs) regulate transport of calcium ions and proteins with molecular weights up to 1.5 kDa. Pathological activation of PTP (and irreversible opening of pores) represents a major step in the development of neurotoxicity and neurodegeneration. NAS in physiological concentrations (5 to 50 nM) suppressed PTP openings induced by calcium and MPP+.[38] This effect of NAS might be related to NAS neuroprotective action.[39]

Clinical Implications

Our data suggest that NAS might interfere with the two major pathways of free radical formation: PLA2–lipid peroxidation cascade (Oxenkrug and Requintina, this volume) and iNOS-dependent NO production (Perianayagam *et al.*, this volume). It also stimulates antioxidant enzymes[16] and inhibits MPP+ induced opening of the mitochondrial PTPs.[38]

Literature data pointed to additional mechanisms of the antioxidant effects of NAS: suppression of NF-κB activation,[4] scavenging of NO[40] and of free radicals,[41] and inhibition of iNOS expression.[34]

These effects of NAS might provide biological underpinning for the cognition-enhancing, antiaging, antidepressant, and antihypertensive effects of NAS. NAS and its derivatives might be useful in protection against oxidative stress–related disorders (cell death, mutagenesis, aging) and diseases (sepsis, cancer, postischemic trauma, Alzheimer's disease, and parkinsonism).

NAS and Cognition

The very first observation of the cognition-enhancing effect of NAS demonstrated that administration of "memory peptide", scotophobin A, resulted in accumulation of NAS since scotophobin was, in fact, the inhibitor of hydroxy-indole-*O*-methyl-transferase, the enzyme facilitating NAS conversion into melatonin.[1] In our studies, the 3 weeks of NAS treatment reversed the impairment of performance induced in Wistar rats by cholinergic toxin (AF64A) in active avoidance and water maze tests.[39] The cognition-enhancing effect of NAS might be further supported by observations of NAS protective effect against β-amyloid toxicity in cultured rat cerebellar granule cells;[39] against MPP+ and β-amyloid–induced pathological activation of mitochondrial PTPs;[38] and against LPS-induced lipid peroxidation in rat brain, liver, and kidney tissues.[17]

NAS and Aging

Aging is characteristically accompanied by a shift within innate immunity towards a proinflammatory status. TNF-α, a proinflammatory mediator, can trigger chronic inflammatory processes in microglial cells and astrocytes.[42]

We were first to report that NAS administered in drinking water starting at 4 weeks of age delayed the occurrence of first death from the 11th to 15th month of age, and prolonged the life span by more than 20% in C3H male mice.[16] The index of oxidative damage, lipid peroxidation (MDA + HAE), increased in liver (from 3- to 6- to 12-month-olds), and kidney (from 3- to 6-month-olds, without further increase in 12-month-olds) of C57BL/6J male mice.[43] Inhibition of lipid peroxidation might contribute to the antiaging action of NAS. We have observed that NAS (4 weeks, 30 mg/kg/day, and 1 mg/kg, respectively, sc) decreased levels of brain (2.2-fold) and kidney MDA + HAE in 11-month-old male C57BL/6J mice.[16]

NAS might contribute to the antiaging effect of (–)deprenyl, an irreversible selective MAO-B inhibitor with well-documented antiaging effect,[44] since 6-month administration of (–)deprenyl (0.25 mg/kg, sc) increased rat pineal NAS levels during the dark period.[45,46]

Antidepressant-like Effect of NAS in the Mouse Tail Suspension Test

Melatonin revealed antidepressant-like activity in the two modifications of the "frog" test,[47] that is, suppression of righting reflex in frogs pretreated by non-selective[48] and selective MAO-A inhibitors.[49] NAS did not exert any antidepressant-like activity in the frog test (our unpublished data). It is not uncommon for the tested drugs to reveal antidepressant-like activity in some (but not all) tests since screening tests are not models of depression, but methods for revealing some characteristics shared by different antidepressants.[50]

To assess the antidepressant potential of NAS, we have used the mouse tail suspension test. The tail suspension test is a variant of the "behavioral despair" forced swimming test in which immobility is induced by suspending an animal by the tail. Many clinically effective tricyclic, heterocyclic, and atypical antidepressants reduce the immobility that mice display after active and unsuccessful attempts to escape when suspended by the tail.[50]

To evaluate the effect of NAS, we have used C57BL/6 mice since this strain of mice combines the presence of 2-[I-125]iodomelatonin binding sites[8] with the virtual absence of the enzymes of pineal melatonin biosynthesis from serotonin.[51] Although nighttime increase of pineal melatonin has been recently described in C57BL/6 mice, its physiological significance is questionable since its amplitude was very low and duration of the peak was only about 15 min. Thus, the C57BL/6 strain of mice allows for the evaluation of the effects of NAS itself without any confounding effect of melatonin synthesized from the injected NAS.[52] NAS decreased the duration of immobility similar to known antidepressants. The effect was dose-dependent: low dose of NAS (5 mg/kg) did not affect the duration of immobility, while higher doses (15, 30, and 45 mg/kg) decreased the duration of immobility.[53] Although melatonin decreased the duration of immobility as well, the effect of NAS most likely did not depend on NAS conversion into melatonin (see above). Our preliminary results suggest that NAS and melatonin effects in the mouse tail suspension test might be mediated by the different melatonin and/or serotonin receptors.

A selective agonist of the MT3 receptor, 5-MCA-NAT, decreased the immobilization time, while a selective antagonist of MT3 receptors, prazosin, prevented antidepressant-like effects of NAS and 5-MCA-NAT. The selective MT2 receptor antagonist, 4P-PDOT, had no effect on NAS-induced decrease of the duration of immobility.[54] Therefore, antidepressant-like effect of NAS in mouse tail suspension test might be mediated by MT3 receptors.

NAS influence on TNF-α production and NO formation might contribute to its antidepressant effect. The macrophage theory of depression proposes that an excessive secretion of monocyte/macrophage cytokines causes symptoms of depression.[55] Elevated levels of TNF-α and cortisol concomitant with decreased levels of ACTH were found in the patients suffering from depression, in comparison to healthy controls.[56] It is noteworthy that blood platelet levels of endothelial NOS and plasma NO metabolite were much lower in patients with major depression than in healthy controls.[57]

NAS in Spontaneously Hypertensive Rats

In the psychiatric clinic, the hypotensive effect of MAO-A inhibitors is an unwanted side effect of antidepressant treatment, setting a limit on their use, particularly among the elderly population. The mechanism of this hypotensive effect of MAO inhibitors is not clear. Since pinealectomy produces hypertension in normotensive rats, it has been proposed that melatonin is an endogenous hypotensive factor.[58]

Considering that MAO-A inhibitors produce both hypotension and elevations of pineal melatonin levels, we proposed that the two are linked. Our observation that pinealectomy attenuated the hypotensive effect of the selective MAO-A inhibitor, clorgyline, in Sprague-Dawley rats supported this suggestion.[59] However, our further studies suggested that NAS rather than melatonin mediated the hypotensive effect of MAO-A inhibition in spontaneously hypertensive (SHR) rats. SHR rats are the most accepted experimental model of human essential hypertension. Born normotensive, SHR rats developed hypertension at 12 weeks of age, while their genetic counterparts, Wistar-Kyoto (WKY) rats, remained normotensive.[60]

Thus, comparison of pineal NAS and melatonin basal levels revealed age-associated (and hypertension-associated) changes in NAS, but not melatonin, in SHR rats. The nighttime pineal NAS (but not melatonin) levels in 4-week-old, normotensive, SHR rats were higher than in the 12-week-old, hypertensive, SHR rats. There were no age-associated changes of pineal NAS in WKY rats (Oxenkrug and Requintina, unpublished data). Isoproterenol, an agonist of β1-adrenoceptors, induced higher pineal NAS levels in 4-week-old, normotensive, SHR rats than in 12-week-old, hypertensive, SHR rats.[58] What is more, the circadian rhythm of the pineal NAS and melatonin was phase-advanced in 12-week-old, hypertensive, SHR rats in comparison with the 12-week-old, normotensive, WKY rats.[61] The additional indication of association of NAS, rather than melatonin, with hypertension in SHR rats came from our studies of the effect of cold-immobilization stress on pineal gland. We previously observed that cold-immobilization stress, which increased the brain level of tribulin (the "endogenous MAO-A inhibitor"), dramatically elevated pineal levels of NAS and melatonin in Sprague-Dawley rats.[62] Our further studies indicated that cold-immobilization stress induced higher pineal NAS levels in SHR than in WKY rats. However, the higher elevation of pineal NAS levels in SHR than in WKY rats did not result in higher melatonin levels in SHR rats. In fact, pineal melatonin levels after cold-immobilization stress were of the same value in SHR and WKY rats.[63]

The linkage between age, hypertension, and basal, isoproterenol-, and cold-immobilization stress–induced pineal NAS levels in SHR rats suggested that NAS might be the endogenous factor protecting rats from the development of hypertension.[58] It is noteworthy that the basal brain MAO-A inhibitory activity of tribulin was three times higher in SHR than in WKY rats, while no difference was found in brain MAO-B inhibitory activity of tribulin.[64] One might suggest that the development of hypertension in SHR is influenced by the MAO-A inhibiting activity (tribulin) since the increase of this activity would facilitate formation of NAS, the alleged endogenous antihypertensive factor. Thus, the higher basal MAO-A inhibiting activity in SHR vs. WKY rats might be considered as the protective mechanism (although eventually insufficient) against the development of hypertension in SHR rats.[64]

NAS Effect on Blood Pressure

NAS attenuated phenylephrine-induced contractions of rat aortic rings[65] and decreased blood pressure in SHR rats. The rapid conversion of subcutaneously injected NAS into melatonin[52] might account for the rather weak hypotensive effect of NAS in the intact SHR rats. Hypotensive effect of NAS was augmented under conditions precluding NAS transformation into melatonin, that is, in pinealectomized rats and in rats pretreated with *S*-adenosylhomocysteine, the inhibitor of NAS methylation into melatonin.[58] The mechanism(s) of antihypertensive effect of NAS is not clear. It might be related to NAS antioxidant effects, inhibition of SPR, PLA2, or interaction with the melatonin receptors.[8]

NAS and Antitumor Effect

NAS was as potent as melatonin in decreasing growth and increasing tyrosinase activity of human melanoma cells. Prazosin, a selective antagonist of MT3 receptors, exhibited no effect per se, but reversed both responses to melatonin, suggesting the involvement of MT3 receptors.[66]

Nonreceptor-dependent mechanisms of antitumor effects of NAS might be related to its effects on NO synthesis. BH4 caused a concentration-dependent increase in proliferation of rat pheochromocytoma (PC12) cells, rat C6 glioma cells, and SV40-transformed human fibroblasts. NAS blocked the BH4-induced increase in proliferation of PC12 cells. This effect was attributed to NAS ability to inhibit BH4 formation from sepiapterin via inhibition of SPR.[67] It is noteworthy that SHR rats with higher NAS levels than WKY rats (see subsection NAS IN SPONTANEOUSLY HYPERTENSIVE RATS) have lower susceptibility to tumorigenesis induced by nickel[68] or quinoline,[69] and DMBA-induced mammary cancers.[70] Antiangiogenesis effect of NAS mediated via inhibition of SPR[71] might also contribute to the antitumor effects of NAS.

NAS and Septic Shock

Pathogenic mechanisms of septic shock involve the release of the bacterial membrane component LPS, which triggers the production of inflammatory cytokines (such as TNF-α), and of iNOS, resulting in extensive oxidative damage with the formation of ROS.[72] NAS protected against LPS-induced hypotensive shock in rats[34] and LPS lethal effect in mice.[17] NAS protective effect against LPS might be attributed to NAS ability to inhibit SPR activity, iNOS and TNF-α production, and LPS-induced lipid peroxidation.

NAS and Oxidative Stress–Related Conditions

The above-discussed NAS effects (see sections RECEPTOR-MEDIATED MECHANISMS OF THE ANTIOXIDANT EFFECTS OF NAS and NONRECEPTOR-MEDIATED MECHANISMS OF THE ANTIOXIDANT EFFECTS OF NAS) might be useful for the treatment of conditions involving oxidative damage such as carcinogenesis, mutation, degenerative disorders (Parkinson's and Alzheimer's disorders), toxic effects of chemotherapy and radiation therapy, demyelination disorders (multiple sclerosis),[11] psychoses,[73] and severe burns,[74] and as an antiaging intervention.[16]

CONCLUSIONS

Literature and our studies revealed antidepressant, antiaging, antitumor, and antihypertensive effects of NAS, one of the indoles of the pineal gland. Mechanisms of

NAS action might involve interaction with MT3 receptors and nonreceptor mechanisms such as inhibition of lipid peroxidation, PLA2, TNF-α, and SPR, the key enzyme of biosynthesis of BH4, the essential cofactor of NO synthase. It is noteworthy that inhibition of PLA2 by NAS is MT3-mediated via MT3 receptor. Antidepressant effect of NAS might be mediated by MT3 receptor and by TNF-α inhibition. NAS effects on lipid peroxidation and PLA2 might be responsible for its antiaging effects. Antihypertensive effect of NAS might depend upon NAS interaction with MT3 receptors, SPR, and PLA2. Antitumor action of NAS might involve PLA2, TNF-α, SPR, and MT3 receptors. NAS and its derivatives might be useful in the treatment of the conditions associated with oxidative stress.

REFERENCES

1. SATAKE, N. & B.E. MORTON. 1979. Scotophobin A causes dark avoidance in goldfish by elevating pineal *N*-acetylserotonin. Pharmacol. Biochem. Behav. **10:** 449–456.
2. MORTON, D.J. 1987. Both hydroxy- and methoxyindoles modify basal temperature in the rat. J. Pineal Res. **4:** 1–5.
3. PSARAKIS, S., G. BROWN & L.J. GROTA. 1988. Analgesia induced by *N*-acetyl-serotonin in the central nervous system. Life Sci. **42:** 1109–1116.
4. LEZOUALC'H, F., M. SPARAPANI & C. BENI. 1998. *N*-Acetylserotonin (normelatonin) and melatonin protect neurons against oxidative challenges and suppress the activity of the transcription factor NF-κB. J. Pineal Res. **24:** 168–178.
5. LEONE, R.M. & R.E. SILMAN. 1984. Melatonin can be differentially metabolized in the rat to produce *N*-acetyl-serotonin in addition to 6-hydroxy-melatonin. Endocrinology **114:** 1825–1832.
6. YOUNG, I.M., R.M. LEONE, P. FRANCIS *et al.* 1985. Melatonin is metabolized to *N*-acetyl serotonin and 6-hydroxymelatonin in man. J. Clin. Endocrinol. Metab. **60:** 114–119.
7. NOSJEAN, O., M. FERRO, F. COGE *et al.* 2000. Identification of the melatonin-binding site Mt3 as the quinone reductase 2. J. Biol. Chem. **275:** 31311–31317.
8. DUBOCOVICH, M.L., M.A. RIVERA-BERMUDEZ, M.J. GERDIN & M.I. MASANA. 2003. Molecular pharmacology, regulation, and function of mammalian melatonin receptors. Front. Biosci. **8:** 1093–1098.
9. SESTINI, E.A., J.C. CARLSON & R. ALLSOPP. 1991. The effects of ambient temperature on life span, lipid peroxidation, superoxide dismutase, and phospholipase A2 activity in *Drosophila melanogaster*. Exp. Gerontol. **26:** 385–395.
10. LI, B., H. ZHANG, M. AKBAR & H.Y. KIM. 2000. Negative regulation of cytosolic phospholipase A(2) by melatonin in the rat pineal gland. Biochem. J. **351**(part 3)**:** 709–716.
11. KOHEN, R. & A. NYSKA. 2002. Oxidation of biological systems: oxidative stress phenomena, antioxidants, redox reactions, and methods for their quantification. Toxicol. Pathol. **30:** 620–650.
12. CELI, A., R. LORENZET, B. FURIE & B.C. FURIE. 1997. Platelet–leukocyte–endothelial cell interaction on the blood vessel wall. Semin. Hematol. **34:** 327–335.
13. LOTUFO, C.M., C. LOPES, M.L. DUBOCOVICH *et al.* 2001. Melatonin and *N*-acetyl-serotonin inhibit leukocyte rolling and adhesion to rat microcirculation. Eur. J. Pharmacol. **430:** 351–357.
14. KARLHUBER, G.M., H.C. BAUER & P.M. ECKL. 1997. Cytotoxic and genotoxic effects of 4-hydroxynonenal in cerebral endothelial cells. Mutat. Res. **381:** 209–216.
15. AKIBA, S., R. NAGAMOTO, M. HAYAMA & T. SATO. 1997. Lipid peroxide overcomes the inability of platelet secretory phospholipase A2 to hydrolyze membrane phopholipids in rabbit platelets. J. Biochem. (Tokyo) **122:** 859–864.
16. OXENKRUG, G.F., P.J. REQUINTINA & S. BACHURIN. 2001. Antioxidant and anti-aging activity of *N*-acetylserotonin in the *in vivo* and *in vitro* models. Ann. N.Y. Acad. Sci. **939:** 190–199.

17. REQUINTINA, P.J. & G.F. OXENKRUG. 2003. Differential effects of lipopolysaccharide on lipid peroxidation in F344N, SHR rats and BALB/C mice, and protection of melatonin and NAS against its toxicity. Ann. N.Y. Acad. Sci. **993:** 325–333.
18. LONGONI, B., W.A. PRYOR & P. MARCHIAFAVA. 1997. Inhibition of lipid peroxidation by *N*-acetylserotonin and its role in retinal physiology. Biochem. Biophys. Res. Commun. **233:** 778–780.
19. GARCIA, J.J., R.J. REITER, M. KARBOWNIK *et al.* 2001. *N*-Acetylserotonin suppresses hepatic microsomal membrane rigidity associated with lipid peroxidation. Eur. J. Pharmacol. **428:** 169–175.
20. SIU, A.W., R.J. REITER & C.H. TO. 1999. Pineal indoleamines and vitamin E reduce nitric oxide–induced lipid peroxidation in rat retinal homogenates. J. Pineal Res. **27:** 122–128.
21. KARBOWNIK, M., E. GITTO, A. LEWINSKI & R.J. REITER. 2001. Relative efficacies of indole antioxidants in reducing autoxidation and iron-induced lipid peroxidation in hamster testes. J. Cell. Biochem. **81:** 693–699.
22. SEEGAR, H., A.O. MUECK & T.H. LIPPERT. 1997. Effect of melatonin and metabolites on copper-mediated oxidation of low density lipoprotein. Br. J. Clin. Pharmacol. **44:** 283–284.
23. GUAJARDO, M.H., A.M. TERRASA & A. CATALA. 2003. Protective effect of indoleamines on *in vitro* ascorbate-Fe^{2+} dependent lipid peroxidation of rod outer segment membranes of bovine retina. J. Pineal Res. **35:** 276–282.
24. BARSACCHI, R., C. KUSMIC, E. DAMIANI *et al.* 1998. Vitamin E consumption induced by oxidative stress in red blood cells is enhanced by melatonin and reduced by *N*-acetylserotonin. Free Radical Biol. Med. **24:** 1187–1192.
25. REITER, R.J., B. POEGGELER, D-X. TAN *et al.* 1993. Antioxidant capacity of melatonin: a novel function not requiring a receptor. Neuroendocrinol. Lett. **32:** 103–116.
26. PAPPOLLA, M.A., M.J. SIMOVICH, T. BRYANT-THOMAS *et al.* 2002. The neuroprotective activities of melatonin against the Alzheimer beta-protein are not mediated by melatonin membrane receptors. J. Pineal Res. **32:** 135–142.
27. THONY, B., G. AUERBACH & N. BLAU. 2000. Tetrahydrobiopterin biosynthesis, regeneration, and functions. Biochem. J. **347**(part 1)**:** 1–16.
28. SCHOEDON, G., M. SCHNEEMANN, S. HOFER *et al.* 1993. Regulation of the L-arginine-dependent and tetrahydrobiopterin-dependent biosynthesis of nitric oxide in murine macrophages. Eur. J. Biochem. **213:** 833–839.
29. OHYE, T., T.A. HORI, S. KATOH *et al.* 1998. Genomic organization and chromosomal localization of the human sepiapterin reductase gene. Biochem. Biophys. Res. Commun. **251:** 597–602.
30. AUERBACH, G., A. HERRMANN, M. GUTLICH *et al.* 1997. The 1.25 A crystal structure of sepiapterin reductase reveals its binding mode to pterins and brain neurotransmitters. EMBO J. **16:** 7219–7230.
31. SMITH, G.K., D.S. DUCH, M.P. EDELSTEIN & E.C. BIGHAM. 1992. New inhibitors of sepiapterin reductase: lack of an effect of intracellular tetrahydrobiopterin depletion upon *in vitro* proliferation of two human cell lines. J. Biol. Chem. **267:** 5599–5607.
32. KATOH, S., T. SUEOKA & S. YAMADA. 1982. Direct inhibition of brain sepiapterine reductase by catecholamine and indoleamine. Biochem. Biophys. Res. Commun. **105:** 75–81.
33. DING, W.X., H.M. NI, D. DIFRANCESCA *et al.* 2004. Bid-dependent generation of oxygen radicals promotes death receptor activation–induced apoptosis in murine hepatocytes. Hepatology **40:** 403–413.
34. KLEMM, P., M. HECKER, H. STOCKHAUSEN *et al.* 1995. Inhibition by *N*-acetyl-5-hydroxytryptamine of nitric oxide synthase expression in cultured cells and in the anaesthetized rat. Br. J. Pharmacol. **115:** 1175–1181.
35. SACCO, S., L. AQUILINI, P. GHEZZI *et al.* 1998. Mechanism of the inhibitory effect of melatonin on tumor necrosis factor production *in vivo* and *in vitro*. Eur. J. Pharmacol. **343:** 249–255.
36. WERNER, E.R., G. WERNER-FELMAYER, D. FUCHS *et al.* 1991. Impact of tumour necrosis factor-alpha and interferon-gamma on tetrahydrobiopterin synthesis in murine fibroblasts and macrophages. Biochem. J. **280**(part 3)**:** 709–714.

37. MURTHY, K.G., C. SZABO & A.L. SALTZMAN. 2004. Cytokines stimulate expression of inducible nitric oxide synthase in DLD-1 human adenocarcinoma cells by activating poly (A) polymerase. Inflamm. Res. **53:** 604–608.
38. BACHURIN, S.O., E.P. SHEVTSOVA, E.G. KIREEVA *et al.* 2003. Mitochondria as a target for neurotoxins and neuroprotective agents. Ann. N.Y. Acad. Sci. **993:** 334–344.
39. BACHURIN, S., G. OXENKRUG, N. LERMONTOVA *et al.* 1999. *N*-Acetylserotonin, melatonin, and their derivatives improve cognition and protect against β-amyloid-induced neurotoxicity. Ann. N.Y. Acad. Sci. **890:** 155–166.
40. NODA, Y., A. MORI, R. LIBURDY & L. PACKER. 1999. Melatonin and its precursors scavenge nitric oxide. J. Pineal Res. **27:** 159–163.
41. WOLFLER, A., P.M. ABUJA, K. SCHAUENSTEIN & P.M. LIEBMANN. 1999. *N*-Acetylserotonin is a better extra- and intracellular antioxidant than melatonin. FEBS Lett. **449:** 206–210.
42. BLASKO, I., M. STAMPFER-KOUNTCHEV, P. ROBATSCHER *et al.* 2004. How chronic inflammation can affect the brain and support the development of Alzheimer's disease in old age: the role of microglia and astrocytes. Aging Cell **3:** 169–176.
43. OXENKRUG, G.F. & P.J. REQUINTINA. 2003. Mating attenuates aging-associated increase of lipid peroxidation activity in C57BL/6J mice. Ann. N.Y. Acad. Sci. **993:** 161–167.
44. KNOLL, J. 1998. The striatal dopamine dependency of life span in male rats: longevity study with (–)deprenyl. Mech. Aging Dev. **46:** 237–262.
45. OXENKRUG, G.F., P.J. REQUINTINA, R.M. CORREA & A. YUWILER. 1994. The effect of 6-months *l*-deprenyl administration on pineal MAO-A and MAO-B activity and on the content of melatonin and related indoles in aged female Fisher 344N rats. J. Neural Transm. Suppl. **41:** 249–252.
46. OXENKRUG, G.F. 2004. Anti-aging effect of (–)deprenyl and inhibition of lipid peroxidation by *N*-acetylserotonin and mating (a mini-review). *In* Monoamine Oxidase Inhibitors and Their Role in Neurotransmission (Drug Development), pp. 307–317. Medicina. Budapest.
47. LAPIN, I.P., G.F. OXENKRUG, S.V. OSIPOVA & N.V. USKOVA. 1970. The frog as a subject for screening thymoleptic drugs. J. Pharm. Pharmacol. **22:** 781–782.
48. SKENE, D. & B. POTGIETER. 1981. Investigation of two animal models of depression. S. Afr. J. Sci. **77:** 180–182.
49. REQUINTINA, P.J., G.F. OXENKRUG, A. YUWILER & A.J. OXENKRUG. 1994. Synergistic sedative effect of selective MAO-A (but not B) inhibitors and melatonin in frogs. J. Neural Transm. Suppl. **41:** 141–144.
50. POURSOLT, R.D., R.A. MCARTUR & A. LENEGRE. 1993. Psychotropic screening procedures. *In* Models in Behavioral Pharmacology, pp. 23–50. Elsevier. Amsterdam/New York.
51. ROSEBOOM, P.H., M.A. NAMBOODIRI, D.B. ZIMONJIC *et al.* 1998. Natural melatonin "knockdown" in C57BL/6J mice: rare mechanism truncates serotonin *N*-acetyltransferase. Brain Res. Mol. Brain Res. **63:** 189–197.
52. OXENKRUG, G.F. & P.J. REQUINTINA. 1994. Stimulation of rat pineal melatonin biosynthesis by *N*-acetylserotonin. Int. J. Neurosci. **77:** 237–241.
53. PRAKHIE, I.V. & G.F. OXENKRUG. 1998. The effect of nifedipine, Ca^{++} antagonist, on activity of MAO inhibitors, *N*-acetylserotonin and melatonin, in the mouse tail suspension test. Int. J. Neuropsychopharmacol. **1:** 35–40.
54. OXENKRUG, G.F. & I.V. PRAKHIE. 2001. Melatonin (MT-3) receptor mediates depressive-/antidepressant-like behavior in the mouse tail suspension test. Biol. Psychiatry **49:** 168S.
55. MIDDLE, F., I. JONES, E. ROBERTSON *et al.* 2000. Tumour necrosis factor alpha and bipolar affective puerperal psychosis. Psychiatr. Genet. **10:** 195–198.
56. TRZONKOWSKI, P., J. MYSLIWSKA, B. GODLEWSKA *et al.* 2004. Immune consequences of the spontaneous pro-inflammatory status in depressed elderly patients. Brain Behav. Immun. **18:** 135–148.
57. CHRAPKO, W.E., P. JURASZ, M.W. RADOMSKI *et al.* 2004. Decreased platelet nitric oxide synthase activity and plasma nitric oxide metabolites in major depressive disorder. Biol. Psychiatry **56:** 129–134.
58. OXENKRUG, G.F. 1999. Antidepressive and antihypertensive effects of MAO-A inhibition: role of *N*-acetylserotonin (a review). Neurology **792:** 213–224.
59. OXENKRUG, G.F., R.B. MCCAULEY, D.J. FONTANA *et al.* 1986. Possible melatonin involvement in the hypotensive effect of MAO inhibitors. J. Neural Transm. **66:** 271–280.

60. OKAMOTO, K. & K. AOKI. 1963. Development of a strain of spontaneously hypertensive rats. Jpn. Circ. J. **27:** 282–293.
61. OXENKRUG, G.F. & P.J. REQUINTINA. 1992. Phase advanced circadian rhythm of the pineal melatonin biosynthesis in spontaneously hypertensive rats. Biol. Psychiatry **31:** 37S.
62. OXENKRUG, G.F. & I.M. MCINTYRE. 1985. Stress induced synthesis of melatonin: possible involvement of the endogenous inhibitor (tribulin). Life Sci. **37:** 1743–1746.
63. OXENKRUG, G.F. & P.J. REQUINTINA. 1998. The effect of MAO-A inhibition and cold-immobilization stress on *N*-acetylserotonin and melatonin in SHR and WKY rats. J. Neural Transm. Suppl. **52:** 333–336.
64. OXENKRUG, G.F., A.E. MEDVEDEV, P.J. REQUINTINA & V. GLOVER. 2000. The effect of cold immobilization stress on brain MAO-A inhibitory activity and pineal *N*-acetylserotonin and melatonin in spontaneously hypertensive rats. Stress Med. **16:** 239–241.
65. JOLY, G.A. & R.G. KILBOURN. 1997. Tetrahydrobiopterin synthesis inhibitors induce nitric oxide synthesis in rat aorta. Gen. Pharmacol. **28:** 475–480.
66. SOUZA, A.V., M.A. VISCONTI & A.M. CASTRUCCI. 2003. Melatonin biological activity and binding sites in human melanoma cells. J. Pineal Res. **34:** 242–248.
67. ANASTASIADIS, P.Z., J.C. STATES, B.A. IMERMAN *et al.* 1996. Mitogenic effects of tetrahydrobiopterin in PC12 cells. Mol. Pharmacol. **49:** 149–155.
68. OHMORI, T., K. OKADA, M. TERADA & R. TABEI. 1999. Low susceptibility of specific inbred colonies of rats to nickel tumorigenesis in soft tissue. Cancer Lett. **136:** 53–58.
69. FUTAKUCHI, M., R. HASEGAWA, A. YAMAMOTO *et al.* 1996. Low susceptibility of the spontaneously hypertensive rat (SHR) to quinoline-induction of hepatic hemangioendothelial sarcomas. Cancer Lett. **104:** 37–41.
70. HARRIS, S.R., R.S. MEHTA, D.K. HARTLE *et al.* 1994. Failure of high fat diets to promote mammary cancers in spontaneously hypertensive rats. Cancer Lett. **87:** 9–15.
71. SHIMIZU, S., M. YASUDA, M. ISHII *et al.* 1999. Stimulation of *in vitro* angiogenesis by tetrahydrobiopterin in bovine aortic endothelial cells. Jpn. J. Pharmacol. **80:** 177–180.
72. FAURE, E., L. THOMAS, H. XU *et al.* 2001. Bacterial lipopolysaccharide and IFN-gamma induce Toll-like receptor 2 and Toll-like receptor 4 expression in human endothelial cells: role of NF-kappaB activation. J. Immunol. **166:** 2018–2024.
73. ROSENBERGER, T.A., N.E. VILLACRESES, J.T. HOVDA *et al.* 2004. Rat brain arachidonic acid metabolism is increased by a 6-day intracerebral ventricular infusion of bacterial lipopolysaccharide. J. Neurochem. **88:** 1168–1178.
74. DAVIS, K.A., J.M. SANTANIELLO, L.K. HE *et al.* 2004. Burn injury and pulmonary sepsis: development of a clinically relevant model. J. Trauma **56:** 272–278.

Novel Neuroprotective Mechanism of Action of Rasagiline Is Associated with Its Propargyl Moiety: Interaction of Bcl-2 Family Members with PKC Pathway

ORLY WEINREB, TAMAR AMIT, ORIT BAR-AM, ORLY CHILLAG-TALMOR, AND MOUSSA B. H. YOUDIM

Eve Topf and USA National Parkinson Foundation Centers of Excellence for Neurodegenerative Diseases Research, Department of Pharmacology, Rappaport Family Research Institute, Technion–Faculty of Medicine, 31096 Haifa, Israel

ABSTRACT: Our studies have provided new insights into the biological mechanism of neuroprotection of the anti-Parkinson drug, rasagiline [*N*-propargyl-(1*R*)-aminoindan], involving the association of Bcl-2 family proteins with protein kinase C (PKC) pathway. In a model of serum withdrawal–induced apoptosis of rat pheochromocytoma PC12 cells, rasagiline and its propargyl moiety, *N*-propargylamine, decreased cell death via multiple neuroprotective pathways that include the stimulation of PKC phosphorylation; upregulation of PKCϵ mRNA; induction of Bcl-X_L, Bcl-w, and brain-derived neurotrophic factor (BDNF) mRNAs; and downregulation of PKCγ, Bad, and Bax mRNAs. Moreover, these drugs inhibited the cleavage and activation of pro-caspase-3 and poly(ADP-ribose) polymerase (PARP), while PKC inhibitor, GF109203X, reversed these actions. In addition, rasagiline decreased serum-free-induced levels of the important regulator of cell death, Bad, which was also blocked by GF109203X, indicating the involvement of PKC-dependent cell survival activity of rasagiline. Structure activity studies have established that *N*-propargylamine is essential for the novel neuroprotective and the neuronal cell survival activity of rasagiline since this moiety itself revealed similar protective effects and mechanisms of action. These results have led us to develop several multifunctional neuroprotective drugs containing the propargyl moiety and iron-chelating property for the treatment and/or prevention of neurodegenerative diseases.

KEYWORDS: rasagiline; *N*-propargylamine; neuroprotection; protein kinase C; Bcl-2 family members; caspase-3

Address for correspondence: Prof. M. B. H. Youdim, Department of Pharmacology, Technion–Faculty of Medicine, P. O. Box 9697, 31096 Haifa, Israel. Voice: +972-4-8295290; fax: +972-4-8513145.

youdim@tx.technion.ac.il

Ann. N.Y. Acad. Sci. 1053: 348–355 (2005). © 2005 New York Academy of Sciences. doi: 10.1196/annals.1344.030

Rasagiline **N-Propargylamine**

FIGURE 1. The chemical structures of the anti-Parkinson drug/monoamine oxidase B (MAO-B) inhibitor, rasagiline (Agilect), and its propargyl moiety, *N*-propargylamine.

INTRODUCTION

The anti-Parkinson drug, rasagiline (FIG. 1) [*N*-propargyl-(1*R*)-aminoindan],[1] a selective irreversible monoamine oxidase B (MAO-B) inhibitor,[2] has neuroprotective activity against a variety of neurotoxins in cell cultures,[3–5] in animal models of head trauma,[6] and in *N*-methyl-4-phenyl-1,2,3,6-tetrahydropyridine (MPTP)–induced neurotoxicity.[7] In light of recently reported benefits in patients with early illness, rasagiline (Agilect) is a promising new treatment for Parkinson's disease (PD) and may have disease-modifying properties.[8] The mechanism underlying the neuroprotection by rasagiline has been studied in human neuroblastoma SH-SY5Y and rat pheochromocytoma PC12 cells in culture against apoptosis induced by *N*-methyl-(*R*)salsolinol; the peroxynitrite donor, SIN-1; 6-hydroxydopamine; and serum and nerve growth factor (NGF) withdrawal.[9] We have previously shown that rasagiline and related propargylamines suppressed the apoptotic cell death cascade initiated by the mitochondria.[2,10] These drugs prevented proapoptotic decline in mitochondrial membrane potential due to permeability transition pores and the activation of the following apoptotic processes: activation of caspase-3; nuclear translocation of glyceraldehyde-3-phosphate dehydrogenase; and nucleosomal DNA fragmentation.[5,11] In addition, rasagiline increased the expression of antiapoptotic Bcl-2 and Bcl-X_L in SH-SY5Y cells.[12] Structure activity studies have indicated that the propargyl moiety is essential for the antiapoptotic function of cyclic benzyl-(rasagiline)[13] and aliphatic [*N*-(2-heptyl)-*N*-propargylamine] propargylamines.[14] Further, we have recently shown that rasagiline, as well as its anti-Alzheimer drug derivatives, ladostigil (TV3326) and TV3279, induce the release of the nonamyloidogenic α-secretase form of soluble APP (sAPPα) from SH-SY5Y neuroblastoma and PC12 cells by the mitogen-activated protein kinase (MAPK) and PKC-dependent mechanisms.[15]

This review describes the effect of rasagiline-induced neuroprotection in a model of serum withdrawal–induced cell death[16,17] of PC12 cells, and the possible association between Bcl-2 family members and PKC in neuronal cell survival. Studies on the structure-activity relationship[18,19] demonstrated the essentiality of the propargyl moiety of rasagiline, *N*-propargylamine (FIG. 1), in the novel neuroprotective mechanism.

THE MECHANISM UNDERLYING NEUROPROTECTIVE ACTIVITY OF RASAGILINE

Prevention of Serum Deprivation–Induced Cell Death by Rasagiline Associating with PKC Pathway and Bcl-2 Family Proteins

Previous study illustrated that the neuroprotective and antiapoptotic activity of rasagiline in SH-SY5Y cells is associated with the induction of antiapoptotic Bcl-2 and Bcl-X_L, which results in the prevention of the fall in mitochondrial membrane potential and inhibition of mitochondrial permeability transition.[20] In addition, our recent data[18] provide evidence whereby activation/regulation of PKC in association with the Bcl-2 protein family promotes neuronal survival by rasagiline, and this is related to its propargyl moiety, as summarized in the schematic model (FIG. 2).

The role of PKC activation in the mechanism of rasagiline neuroprotection is supported by the results that rasagiline can activate the essential PKC isoforms involved in cell survival pathways, PKCα and PKCε, and the blocking of its neuroprotective action by inhibition of PKC activity.[18] Furthermore, gene expression analysis revealed that exposure of serum-deprived PC12 cells to rasagiline markedly increased PKCε mRNA expression. By contrast, rasagiline prevented the increase in PKCγ mRNA level, which occurred in serum-deprived PC12 cells.[18] These findings are also in line with our previous data indicating an involvement of PKC in the release of the neuroprotective/neurotrophic, nonamyloidogenic sAPPα by rasagiline *in vitro*.[21] Evidence has shown that rasagiline upregulates p-PKC levels and the expression of PKCα and PKCε isoenzymes in mice hippocampus,[22] and complements previous observations showing that certain PKC isoforms are intimately involved in cell survival/death signals that protect against cell death. Thus, PKCα is known to phosphorylate Bcl-2 in a site that increases its antiapoptotic function,[23] and overexpression of PKCε results in increased expression of Bcl-2.[24] Moreover, suppression of PKCα triggers apoptosis through downregulation of Bcl-X_L.[25] In addition, MAPK/ERK cascades, which have been shown to inhibit cell death in a number of systems, can be activated by PKC. Hence, PKCα phosphorylates and activates raf-1, an upstream kinase in the MAPK/ERK pathway;[26] PKCε regulates ERK-1 and -2 activation; and pharmacological inhibition of MAPK/ERK signaling blocks phorbol ester–induced protection of neuronal cells against glutamate toxicity.[27] Also, the MAPK/ERK cascade has been recently found to be upregulated by rasagiline.[15,21] Rasagiline directly activates the PKC-MAPK pathway by concentration- and time-dependent phosphorylation of p42 and p44 MAPK since the ERK1/ERK2 inhibitor, PD98059, and the PKC inhibitor, GF109203X, prevented the neuroprotective effect of rasagiline in the serum-deprived cell culture.

In addition to the activation/regulation of the prosurvival PKC pathway by rasagiline, our study provided evidence that the neuroprotection effect of this drug is mediated by gene regulation of the Bcl-2-related protein family.[18] Gene expression analysis has revealed a decrease in mRNA of the proapoptotic members, Bax and Bad, and an increase in mRNA of the cell survival members, Bcl-w and Bcl-X_L.[12] These results are relevant to the fact that the Bcl-2-related protein family regulates the mitochondrial membrane permeability transition (PT) pore, and triggers dissipation of mitochondrial membrane potential ($\Delta\Psi m$) and release of cytochrome *c*–inducing

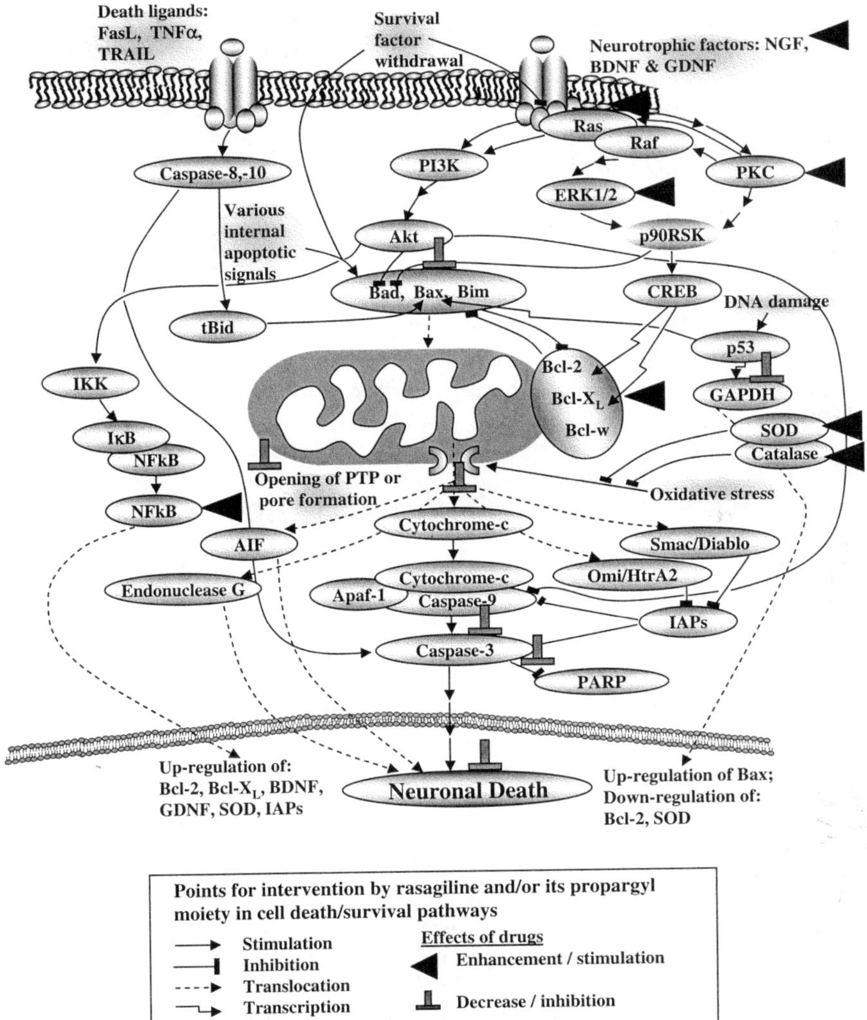

FIGURE 2. Proposed schematic model for the neuroprotective effect of rasagiline and *N*-propargylamine.

downstream events, including caspase-3 activation, resulting in neuronal cell death.[10,28]

In line with the impact of rasagiline on cell death, we have previously demonstrated that rasagiline prevented the effect of serum-free-induced cleavage and activation of caspase-3 and poly(ADP-ribose) polymerase (PARP).[18] The PKC inhibitor, GF109203X, reversed these suppressive effects of rasagiline. In addition, the involvement and importance of the PKC pathway in rasagiline-induced inactivation of the BH3-only proapoptotic Bcl-2 family members, Bad, were further demonstrated by using the PKC inhibitor, GF109203X. Rasagiline decreased serum-free-induced levels of Bad, while GF109203X blocked this effect. These former studies with rasagiline are consistent with PKC-dependent promotion of cell survival via phosphorylation and inactivation of Bad-mediated cell death,[29] and suggest the involvement of Bcl-2 and PKC-MAPK pathway in the neuroprotective activity of rasagiline.

Effect of Rasagiline on Neurotrophic Factors

Rasagiline and its propargyl moiety have been demonstrated to upregulate the gene expression of the neurotrophic factor, brain-derived neurotrophic factor (BDNF),[18] suggesting a possible association between the neuroprotective mechanism of action of these compounds and upregulation of BDNF gene expression. BDNF has been shown to be involved in neuroprotection and neurorescue of several neurons, including dopaminergic and cholinergic, and promote survival of major neuronal types affected in Alzheimer's disease (AD) and PD.[30] Thus, reduced expression of BDNF was demonstrated in the substantia nigra of individuals with PD,[31] and BDNF prevented the spontaneous death of dopaminergic neurons in rat primary mesencephalic culture,[32] as well as the reduction in striatal dopamine content induced by MPTP in mice. Interestingly, BDNF was also reported to regulate PKC activation[33] and affect Bcl-w and Bcl-X_L expression.[34] Rasagiline was recently reported to enhance gene expression of β-NGF and its downstream transcription factors—NGF-1A binding protein (EGR1) and the early growth response protein-3 (EGR3)—in response to the proapoptotic action of MPTP *in vivo*.[35] An *in vitro* study, in neuronal cells, described that rasagiline increased the expression of the glial cell line–derived neurotrophic factor (GDNF), suggesting that this induction may suppress the death process and promote the survival of dopaminergic neurons.[36]

MECHANISM OF ACTION OF *N*-PROPARGYLAMINE

It was recently shown that free *N*-propargylamine, similar to rasagiline, exerts neuroprotective activity against apoptosis induced by serum withdrawal[18] and the endogenous neurotoxin, *N*-methyl(*R*)salsolinol.[10,19] *N*-Propargylamine has a potent neuroprotective activity via downregulation of Bax and Bad and induction of Bcl-2 and Bcl-X_L, as well as the neurotrophic factors, GDNF and BDNF.[19,36] In addition, the ability of *N*-propargylamine to augment the viability of serum-deprived cells, activate PKC phosphorylation, increase PKCε mRNA expression, and reduce PKCγ mRNA expression[18] strengthens its crucial role in the neuroprotective activity of rasagiline and other rasagiline-related derivatives. Consistent with these studies, *N*-propargylamine, similar to rasagiline, induced the secretion of sAPPα and increased

MAPK phosphorylation.[21] Structure activity studies have established that the PKC-Bcl-2 interaction–induced neuroprotection is the property of the propargyl moiety of rasagiline.

CONCLUSIONS AND PERSPECTIVES FOR THE FUTURE

In conclusion, the neuroprotection described for rasagiline, its derivatives, and the novel propargylamine-containing iron chelators does not depend on inhibition of MAO-B,[20] but rather is associated with some intrinsic pharmacological action of the propargyl moiety in these compounds, acting on the mitochondrial cell survival proteins. The activation of PKC related to Bcl-2 family members, the regulation of neurotrophic factors, and the stimulation of MAPK pathway by rasagiline and its propargyl moiety is a novel mechanism of action, which might be considered in developing new neuroprotective drugs to halt the decline of neurons in neurodegenerative diseases.

Iron may have a primary or pivotal role in neurodegenerative processes[37] since animal models of PD have shown that iron chelators are neuroprotective.[38,39] Recently, we have developed several novel multifunctional iron-chelating drugs from our prototype neuroprotective iron chelator, VK-28, possessing propargyl moiety for the treatment and/or prevention of neurodegenerative diseases. We are currently investigating whether their mechanism of neuroprotection is similar to that of rasagiline and *N*-propargylamine, as described in this review.

ACKNOWLEDGMENTS

We acknowledge the support of Teva Pharmaceutical (Netanya, Israel); the National Parkinson Foundation (Miami, FL); the Stein Foundation (Philadelphia, PA); and the Rappaport Family Research Institute, Technion–Israel Institute of Technology, and Golding Parkinson Research Fund (Technion, Haifa, Israel).

REFERENCES

1. PARKINSON STUDY GROUP. 2002. A controlled trial of rasagiline in early Parkinson disease: the TEMPO Study. Arch. Neurol. **59:** 1937–1943.
2. YOUDIM, M.B.H. *et al.* 2001. The anti-Parkinson drug rasagiline and its cholinesterase inhibitor derivatives exert neuroprotection unrelated to MAO inhibition in cell culture and *in vivo*. Ann. N.Y. Acad. Sci. **939:** 450–458.
3. FINBERG, J.P. *et al.* 1998. Increased survival of dopaminergic neurons by rasagiline, a monoamine oxidase B inhibitor. Neuroreport **9:** 703–707.
4. MARUYAMA, W., M.B.H. YOUDIM & M. NAOI. 2000. Antiapoptotic function of *N*-propargylamine-1(*R*)- and (*S*)-aminoindan, rasagiline, and TV1022. Ann. N.Y. Acad. Sci. **939:** 320–329.
5. MARUYAMA, W. *et al.* 2001. Transfection-enforced Bcl-2 overexpression and an anti-Parkinson drug, rasagiline, prevent nuclear accumulation of glyceraldehyde-3-phosphate dehydrogenase induced by an endogenous dopaminergic neurotoxin, *N*-methyl-(*R*)salsolinol. J. Neurochem. **78:** 727–735.
6. HUANG, W. *et al.* 1999. Neuroprotective effect of rasagiline, a selective monoamine oxidase–B inhibitor, against closed head injury in the mouse. Eur. J. Pharmacol. **366:** 127–135.

7. Sagi, Y., M. Weinstock & M.B.H. Youdim. 2003. Attenuation of MPTP-induced dopaminergic neurotoxicity by TV3326, a cholinesterase–monoamine oxidase inhibitor. J. Neurochem. **2:** 290–297.
8. Group, P.S. 2005. A randomized placebo-controlled trial of rasagiline in levodopa-treated patients with Parkinson disease and motor fluctuations: the PRESTO study. Arch. Neurol. **62:** 241–248.
9. Naoi, M. & W. Maruyama. 2001. Future of neuroprotection in Parkinson's disease. Park. Relat. Disord. **8:** 139–145.
10. Akao, Y. *et al.* 2002. Mitochondrial permeability transition mediates apoptosis induced by *N*-methyl(*R*)salsolinol, an endogenous neurotoxin, and is inhibited by Bcl-2 and rasagiline, *N*-propargyl-1(*R*)-aminoindan. J. Neurochem. **82:** 913–923.
11. Youdim, M.B.H. & M. Weinstock. 2002. Molecular basis of neuroprotective activities of rasagiline and the anti-Alzheimer drug, TV3326, [(*N*-propargyl-(3*R*)aminoindan-5-yl)-ethyl methyl carbamate]. Cell. Mol. Neurobiol. **21:** 555–573.
12. Akao, Y. *et al.* 2002. An anti-Parkinson's disease drug, *N*-propargyl-1(*R*)-aminoindan (rasagiline), enhances expression of anti-apoptotic Bcl-2 in human dopaminergic SH-SY5Y cells. Neurosci. Lett. **326:** 105–108.
13. Maruyama, W. *et al.* 2000. Neurotoxin induced apoptosis in dopamine neurons: protection by propargylamine derivatives, rasagiline, and TV 1022. *In* Advances in Research on Neurodegeneration. Vol. 8. Springer-Verlag. Berlin/Wien/New York.
14. Maruyama, W. *et al.* 2001. Enantio-specific induction of apoptosis by an endogenous neurotoxin, *N*-methyl(*R*)salsolinol, in dopaminergic SH-SY5Y cells: suppression of apoptosis by *N*-(2-heptyl)-*N*-methylpropargylamine. J. Neural Transm. **108:** 11–24.
15. Yogev-Falach, M. *et al.* 2002. The involvement of mitogen-activated protein (MAP) kinase in the regulation of amyloid precursor protein processing by novel cholinesterase inhibitors derived from rasagiline. FASEB J. **16:** 1674–1676.
16. Rukenstein, A., R.E. Rydel & L.A. Greene. 1991. Multiple agents rescue PC12 cells from serum-free cell death by translation- and transcription-independent mechanisms. J. Neurosci. **11:** 2552–2563.
17. Maroto, R. & J.R. Perez-Polo. 1997. Bcl-2-related protein expression in apoptosis: oxidative stress versus serum deprivation in PC12 cells. J. Neurochem. **69:** 514–523.
18. Weinreb, O. *et al.* 2004. Neuroprotection via pro-survival protein kinase C isoforms associated with Bcl-2 family members. FASEB J. **18:** 1471–1473.
19. Yi, H. *et al.* 2005. *N*-Propargylamine protects SH-SY5Y cells from apoptosis induced by an endogenous neurotoxin, *N*-methyl(*R*)salsolinol, through stabilization of mitochondrial membrane and induction of anti-apoptotic Bcl-2. J. Neural Transm. In press.
20. Youdim, M.B.H. *et al.* 2003. The essentiality of Bcl-2, PKC, and proteasome-ubiquitin complex activations in the neuroprotective-antiapoptotic action of the anti-Parkinson drug, rasagiline. Biochem. Pharmacol. **66:** 1635–1641.
21. Yogev-Falach, M. *et al.* 2003. The importance of propargylamine moiety in the anti-Parkinson drug rasagiline and its derivatives for MAPK-dependent amyloid precursor protein processing. FASEB J. **17:** 2325–2327.
22. Bar-Am, O. *et al.* 2004. Regulation of protein kinase C by the anti-Parkinson drug, MAO-B inhibitor, rasagiline and its derivatives, *in vivo*. J. Neurochem. **89:** 1119–1125.
23. Ruvolo, P.P. *et al.* 1998. A functional role for mitochondrial protein kinase Cα in Bcl2 phosphorylation and suppression of apoptosis. J. Biol. Chem. **273:** 25436–25442.
24. Gubina, E. *et al.* 1998. Overexpression of protein kinase C isoform epsilon, but not delta in human interleukin-3-dependent cells suppresses apoptosis and induces bcl-2 expression. Blood **91:** 823–829.
25. Hsieh, Y.C. *et al.* 2003. Suppression of protein kinase Cα triggers apoptosis through down-regulation of Bcl-X_L in a rat hepatic epithelial cell line. Shock **19:** 582–587.
26. Kribben, A. *et al.* 1993. AVP-induced activation of MAP kinase in vascular smooth muscle cells is mediated through protein kinase C. Am. J. Physiol. **265:** C939–C945.
27. Maher, P. 2001. How protein kinase C activation protects nerve cells from oxidative stress–induced cell death. J. Neurosci. **21:** 2929–2938.
28. Tsujimoto, Y. & S. Shimizu. 2000. Bcl-2 family: life-or-death switch. FEBS Lett. **466:** 6–10.

29. TAN, Y. *et al.* 1999. p90(RSK) blocks bad-mediated cell death via a protein kinase C–dependent pathway. J. Biol. Chem. **274:** 34859–34867.
30. MURER, M.G., Q. YAN & R. RAISMAN-VOZARI. 2001. Brain-derived neurotrophic factor in the control human brain, and in Alzheimer's disease and Parkinson's disease. Prog. Neurobiol. **63:** 71–124.
31. PARAIN, K. *et al.* 1999. Reduced expression of brain-derived neurotrophic factor protein in Parkinson's disease substantia nigra. Neuroreport **10:** 557–561.
32. HYMAN, C. *et al.* 1991. BDNF is a neurotrophic factor for dopaminergic neurons of the substantia nigra. Nature **350:** 230–232.
33. TREMBLAY, R. *et al.* 1999. Evidence that brain-derived neurotrophic factor neuroprotection is linked to its ability to reverse the NMDA-induced inactivation of protein kinase C in cortical neurons. J. Neurochem. **72:** 102–111.
34. MIDDLETON, G. *et al.* 2001. Reciprocal developmental changes in the roles of Bcl-w and Bcl-x(L) in regulating sensory neuron survival. Development **128:** 447–457.
35. SAGI, Y., S. MANDEL & M.B.H. YOUDIM. 2003. Genomic and proteomic profiling of the neuroprotective mechanisms of rasagiline in the mouse MPTP model of PD. Neural Plas. **10:** 227.
36. MARUYAMA, W. *et al.* 2004. *N*-Propargyl-1(*R*)-aminoindan, rasagiline, increases glial cell line–derived neurotrophic factor (GDNF) in neuroblastoma SH-SY5Y cells through activation of NF-kappaB transcription factor. Neurochem. Int. **44:** 393–400.
37. ZECCA, L. *et al.* 2004. Iron, brain ageing, and neurodegenerative disorders. Nat. Rev. Neurosci. **5:** 863–873.
38. BEN-SHACHAR, D. *et al.* 2004. Neuroprotection by a novel brain permeable iron chelator, VK-28, against 6-hydroxydopamine lesion in rats. Neuropharmacology **46:** 254–263.
39. YOUDIM, M.B.H., G. STEPHENSON & D. BEN-SHACHAR. 2004. Ironing iron out in Parkinson's disease and other neurodegenerative diseases with iron chelators: a lesson from 6-hydroxydopamine and iron chelators, desferal and VK-28. Ann. N.Y. Acad. Sci. **1012:** 306–325.

Gene Expression Profiling of Sporadic Parkinson's Disease Substantia Nigra Pars Compacta Reveals Impairment of Ubiquitin-Proteasome Subunits, SKP1A, Aldehyde Dehydrogenase, and Chaperone HSC-70

SILVIA MANDEL,[a] EDNA GRUNBLATT,[b] PETER RIEDERER,[b] NINETTE AMARIGLIO,[c] JASMINE JACOB HIRSCH,[c] GIDEON RECHAVI,[c] AND MOUSSA B. H. YOUDIM[a]

[a]*Eve Topf and USA National Parkinson Foundation Centers of Excellence and Department of Pharmacology, Technion–Rappaport Family Faculty of Medicine, Haifa, Israel*

[b]*Institute of Clinical Neurochemistry and National Parkinson Foundation Center of Excellence Laboratories, Clinic and Polyclinic for Psychiatry and Psychotherapy, Bayerische Julius-Maximilians-University of Würzburg, Würzburg, Germany*

[c]*Functional Genomics Unit, Institute of Hematology, Sheba Medical Center, Tel-Aviv, Israel*

ABSTRACT: Sporadic Parkinson's disease (PD) constitutes 99% of the disorder, while the remaining 1% of the cases is of familial (genetic) origin. The mutations reported to be associated with familial PD indicate impairment in protein processing and misfolding, as is handled by the ubiquitin-proteasome system (UPS), and in mitochondrial function. For these reasons, we have recently applied, for the first time, Affymetrix oligonucleotide microarray technique in the substantia nigra pars compacta of sporadic parkinsonian patients for studying global gene expression analysis and comparison to the alterations identified in inherited PD. This study identified decreased expression of 68 genes and elevation of 69 genes. Classification into functional groups revealed that the downregulated genes are related to signal transduction, protein degradation (e.g., ubiquitin-proteasome subunits), dopaminergic transmission/metabolism, iron transport, protein modification/phosphorylation, and energy pathways/glycolysis functional classes. A major finding is the decreased expressions of 5 subunits of the UPS, SKP1A, a member of the SCF (E3) ubiquitin ligase complex, and chaperone HSC-70, which can lead to a wide impairment in the function of an entire repertoire of proteins. The upregulated genes are clustered in cell adhesion/cytoskeleton, extracellular matrix components, cell cycle, protein modification/phosphorylation, protein metabolism and tran-

Address for correspondence: Prof. Moussa B. H. Youdim, Eve Topf and NPF Centers, Technion–Faculty of Medicine, Efron St., P. O. Box 9697, 31096 Haifa, Israel. Voice: +972-4-8295289; fax: +972-4-8513145.
youdim@tx.technion.ac.il

Ann. N.Y. Acad. Sci. 1053: 356–375 (2005). © 2005 New York Academy of Sciences.
doi: 10.1196/annals.1344.031

scription, and inflammation/hypoxia (e.g., key iron and oxygen sensor EGLN1) classes. The study shows, for the first time, a convergence in the pathogenic processes that are observed in hereditary (familial) and sporadic PD, where abnormal iron metabolism, oxidative stress, and aggregation of proteins occur. An additional breakthrough in this research is the identification of a number of previously unsuspected crucial gene players that are also involved in the process of neurodegeneration, which can serve as specific biomarkers for PD and novel drug development.

KEYWORDS: Affymetrix; microarray; Parkinson's disease (PD); substantia nigra pars compacta; cerebellum; gene expression; quantitative real-time PCR; ubiquitin-proteasome system; α-synuclein; SKP1A; HSC-70; iron; MPTP; hypoxia; oxidative stress; inflammatory process; apoptosis

INTRODUCTION

Neuropathological and neurochemical studies on substantia nigra (SN) from Parkinson's disease (PD) brains and its animal models have established several pathogenic processes at the time of neuronal death, although the etiology of the disease remains elusive. Potential contributing factors include ongoing selective oxidative stress (OS) resulting from mitochondrial dysfunction, auto-oxidation, or enzymatic (monoamine oxidase, MAO) oxidation of dopamine (DA), and excessive iron accumulation in the SN pars compacta (pc).[1–5] Specifically, redox-active iron has been observed within the melanin-containing neurons that selectively die and in the rim of Lewy bodies (LB), the morphological hallmark of PD. LB are composed of lipids, aggregated α-synuclein (concentrating in its peripheral halo), and ubiquitinated, hyperphosphorylated neurofilament proteins.[6] A number of recent studies[7–9] have shown that α-synuclein forms toxic aggregates in the presence of iron and this is considered a contributing factor to the formation of LB via OS. Dysregulation of brain iron metabolism has taken center stage in neurodegenerative diseases since a significant number of mutated iron metabolism genes have now been shown to be directly involved in neurodegeneration[10–12] (FIG. 1). Thus, iron redox status may constitute a pivotal factor contributing to the extent of protein misfolding and aggregation in the aging and disease-affected brain. The MPTP and 6-OHDA animal models and cellular models of PD, regardless of their intrinsic limitations (e.g., lack of neuronal inclusion bodies and progressive nature), have to a large extent replicated many of the neurochemical and anatomical characteristics of the parkinsonian syndrome in rodents, primates, and other species.[13,14]

CURRENT MOLECULAR BASIS OF PD DOPAMINERGIC DEGENERATION

Ubiquitination and proteasomal-mediated protein handling defects are thought to be common features in PD and other chronic neurodegenerative diseases such as Alzheimer's disease (AD), amyotrophic lateral sclerosis (ALS), and Huntington's disease and in aging.[15,16] This is suggested to lead to impairment of several cellular processes associated with ubiquitination such as cell cycle, processing and regulation of transcription, intracellular trafficking, signaling pathways, degradation, and

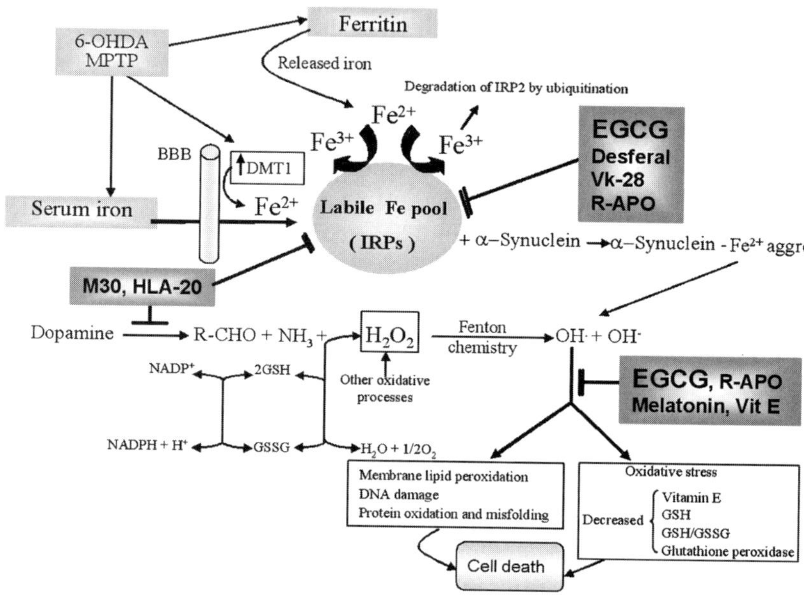

FIGURE 1. Possible mechanism of neurotoxin-induced iron uptake, release, and interaction with α-synuclein resulting in OS-initiated neurodegeneration and its prevention by iron chelators/antioxidants. The mechanism by which 6-hydroxydopamine (6-OHDA) and 1-methyl-4-phenyl-1,2,3,6-tetrahydropyridine (MPTP) induce an increase of iron in SNpc and within the melanin-containing neurons is not known. These neurotoxins (a) may activate the divalent metal transporter 1 (DMT1), which is responsible for iron transport into the brain across the cell membrane; (b) may alter the blood-brain barrier (BBB), thereby allowing iron access to the brain; or (c) may induce release of iron from ferritin, which enters the labile (redox-active) pool of iron. It is the labile pool of iron that can initiate the Fenton chemistry in response to the presence of hydrogen peroxide, thus generating the highly reactive hydroxyl radical ($OH^{\bullet}$). The resultant effect is the depletion of cell-reduced glutathione (GSH), the rate-limiting cofactor of glutathione peroxidase, the main enzymatic pathway in the brain, to eliminate hydrogen peroxide. The labile pool of iron can also cause aggregation of α-synuclein to the neurotoxic form, which can also generate $OH^{\bullet}$. The net effect is OS-dependent damage to neuron antioxidant mechanisms, membrane lipid peroxidation, demise of cell and mitochondrial membranes, protein misfolding, and ultimately cell death. Neuroprotective agents that can be used to prevent iron-induced neurodegeneration include M30 and HLA-20 (bifunctional iron chelator–MAO inhibitors); desferal, VK-28, R-APO (*R*-apomorphine), and EGCG (iron chelators); and R-APO, EGCG, melatonin, and vitamin E (radical scavengers). *Sharp arrows* indicate positive inputs, whereas *blunt arrows* are for inhibitory inputs. Reproduced with minor modifications from ref. 87.

aggregation of normal and damaged intracellular proteins.[15] A significant body of evidence points to a crucial role for protein misfolding and aggregation in the formation of protein inclusion bodies (LB) in sporadic PD. A loss of 20S proteasome α-subunits[17,18] and a reduction in the activity of the 26/20S proteasome system in SNpc of sporadic PD have also been reported.[18]

Impairment of protein handling and catabolism together with an ongoing state of OS and highly significant accumulation of iron are considered common hallmarks, not only of sporadic, but also of inherited forms of PD, especially the mutation in the gene encoding parkin.[19] The discovery of three apparently independent gene mutations in α-synuclein, parkin, and ubiquitin C-terminal hydrolase-L1 (UCHL-1), which are thought to impair the activity of the ubiquitin-proteasome system (UPS) in rare forms of genetic PD, has highlighted the importance of protein handling processes in PD neurodegeneration (for review, see ref. 14). The proteins coded by these genes accumulate in LB[20] together with iron.[21] However, parkin mutant patients, unlike sporadic PD, do not exhibit LB, questioning the alleged deleterious role of LB in the process of DA neurotoxicity and neurodegeneration. In fact, recent studies indicate that LB may represent a neuroprotective compensatory reaction by the brain to protect itself from oxidative and proteotoxic insults.[22,23] Thus, it can be speculated that the early age onset of PD associated with parkin mutation might partly result from a lack of these protective inclusion bodies, thereby promoting a premature appearance of the disease.

Recently, recessive mutations in DJ-1[24] and PINK1 (PTEN-induced kinase 1)[25] were proposed to play a protective role in cellular response to OS. This and their presumed localization in the mitochondria suggest a common pathogenic role in idiopathic and genetic forms of PD, incriminating the demise of mitochondria as the culprit in neurodegeneration. Thus, it can be hypothesized that the vulnerability of the dopaminergic neurons of SNpc to OS and high free-iron levels, and the failure of the UPS to adequately remove abnormal proteins, may constitute the basis for the etiopathology of sporadic PD. More recently, mutations in the LRRK2 gene, encoding a large multifunctional protein including a protein kinase domain, and several other major functional domains, have been identified in families with autosomal dominant parkinsonism.[26,27] These findings demonstrate association of LRRK2 with the pathogenesis of several major neurodegenerative disorders associated with parkinsonism.

GENE EXPRESSION PROFILING OF PARKINSONIAN SUBSTANTIA NIGRA PARS COMPACTA

We have performed the first, large-scale analysis of gene expression profiles of postmortem SNpc of parkinsonian brains and compared them to matched controls and unaffected brain regions [cerebellum and SN pars reticulate (SNr)].[28,d] All experiments were performed using Affymetrix HG-FOCUS oligonucleotide arrays (www.affymetrix.com/support/technical/datasheets/human_datasheet.pdf). Total

[d]During the proofreading of the present paper, three articles on gene expression profiling of parkinsonian substantia nigra appeared that partially substantiated our own data. See refs. 89–91. These articles were not aware of our earlier paper (ref. 28).

RNA from each sample was used to prepare biotinylated target RNA, with minor modifications from the manufacturer's recommendations (www.affymetrix.com/support/technical/manual/expression_manual.affx). *In vitro* transcription was performed with biotinylated UTP and CTP (Enzo Diagnostics), resulting in ~100-fold amplification of RNA. For a complete description of procedures, see http://bioinf.-picr.man.ac.uk/mbcf/downloads/GeneChip_Target_Prep_Protocol_CRUK_v_2.pdf//. A total of 17 gene chips were employed (12 for the SNpc and 5 for the cerebellum of PD patients and age-matched controls). For statistical analysis, genes were filtered using MAS 5 algorithm results. One expected difficulty when working with postmortem samples is the various degrees of degradation in the RNA preparations. Therefore, cRNAs originating from these samples contain more 3′ ends than 5′ ends. Since the Affymetrix array probe sets are designed so that the 3′ ends are selected whenever possible (www.affymetrix.com/support/technical/technotes/hgu133_design_technote.pdf), the analysis of relatively high 3′ content samples becomes feasible. Probe sets detected by MAS 5 as present (P) have a signal with a p value lower than 0.04 (determined from the probes contained in the probe set). This allows the use of present call with confidence. Samples that are partially degraded may hybridize to part of the probes in the probe sets, leading to a high p value (and detected as absent). If the probe set in at least 4 out of 6 samples was detected as present and all of the signals were greater than 20, we determined this probe set to be present. A list of 3517 probe sets representing genes with signals higher than 20 and detected as present (P) in all control samples, or with signals higher than 20 in all PD samples and detected as present in 4 out of the 6 samples, was generated from the 8763 probe sets contained on the array (supplementary data, http://eng.sheba.co.il/genomics). Two hundred sixty-two probe sets differentiated between patient and control samples as determined by the Wilcoxon rank-sum test ($p < 0.05$) (supplementary data, http://eng.sheba.co.il/genomics). Probe sets were further filtered, selecting those where the ratio of the average (geomean) signals of the PD samples and the average signals of the control samples exceeded 1.5 or was lower than 0.66. The use of the aforementioned cutoffs together with the statistical test provide a high stringency analysis and the possibility to focus on defined subsets of genes engaged in a common biological process (or processes). Confirmation of gene expressions was made by analysis with quantitative real-time PCR. We used the geNorm program (http://medgen31.ugent.be/jvdesomp/genorm) to determine the most stable housekeeping genes from a set of tested genes in a given cDNA sample panel, calculating a gene expression normalization factor for each tissue sample based on the geometric mean of a user-defined number of housekeeping genes.

One hundred thirty-seven differentially expressed genes compared to age-matched controls were identified out of 3517 valid probe sets. Of these, 68 were transcriptionally downregulated and 69 were upregulated. The genes were classified into functional groups according to Gene Ontology annotation tools.[29] The downregulated genes in PD were observed in signal transduction, protein degradation, dopaminergic transmission and metabolism, ion transport, protein modification/phosphorylation, and energy pathways/glycolysis functional classes (TABLE 1). Within the proteolytic group, decreased expression was observed of both catalytic and regulatory subunits of the UPS such as 20S proteasome subunits α-5 (PSMA5), α-3 (PSMA3), and α-2 (PSMA2), two subunits of the 19S regulatory complex of the 26S proteasome, the non-ATPase subunit 8 (PSMD8/Rpn12), and the ATPase subunit 4 (PSMC4/TBP7/

TABLE 1. Major downregulated genes in SNpc of PD

GenBank	Symbol	Gene name	Fold of control
		Proteolysis and peptidolysis*	
NM_006503.1	PSMC4	Proteasome (prosome, macropain) 26S subunit, ATPase, 4	0.52
NM_002790.1	PSMA5	Proteasome (prosome, macropain) subunit, alpha type, 5	0.47
NM_002787.1	PSMA2	Proteasome (prosome, macropain) subunit, alpha type, 2	0.65
NM_002788.1	PSMA3	Proteasome (prosome, macropain) subunit, alpha type, 3	0.42
NM_005339.2	HIP2	Huntingtin interacting protein 2	0.54
NM_002570.1	PACE4	Paired basic amino acid cleaving system 4	0.59
NM_006930.1	SKP1A	S-phase kinase-associated protein 1A (p19A)	0.51
AB034951.1	HSPA8	Chaperone: isoform 2 may function as an endogenous inhibitory regulator of HSC-70 by competing for cochaperones	0.55
		Dopamine transport/transmission/metabolism	
AI269290	SLC18	Solute carrier family 18 (vesicular monoamine), member 2	0.47
M30471.1	ADH5	Alcohol dehydrogenase 5 (class III), chi polypeptide	0.62
NM_000689.1	ALDH1A1	Aldehyde dehydrogenase 1 family, member A1	0.35
NM_016300.1	ARPP-21	Cyclic AMP–regulated phosphoprotein, 21 kDa	0.51
		Protein modification/phosphorylation	
NM_003138.1	SRPK2	SFRS protein kinase 2	0.46
		Energy pathways/glycolysis	
NM_004373.1	COX6A1	Cytochrome c oxidase subunit VIa polypeptide 1	0.58
NM_002627.1	PFKP	Phosphofructokinase, platelet	0.66
NM_000436.1	OXCT	3-Oxoacid CoA transferase	0.57
NM_000158.1	GBE1	Glucan (1,4-alpha), branching enzyme 1 (glycogen branching enzyme, Andersen's disease, glycogen storage disease type IV)	0.45
AV727381	UQCRC2	Ubiquinol–cytochrome c reductase core protein II	0.59

TABLE 1. (*continued*) Major downregulated genes in SNpc of PD

GenBank	Symbol	Gene name	Fold of control
		Signal transduction	
NM_006055.1	LANCL1	LanC lantibiotic synthetase component C–like 1 (bacterial)	0.57
NM_006218.1	PIK3CA	Phosphoinositide-3-kinase, catalytic, alpha polypeptide	0.50
NM_006226.1	PLCL1	Phospholipase C–like 1	0.48
NM_005274.1	GNG5	Guanine nucleotide binding protein (G protein), gamma 5	0.66
AL049933.1	GNAI1	Guanine nucleotide binding protein (G protein), alpha inhibiting activity polypeptide 1	0.64
AF022375.1	VEGF	Vascular endothelial growth factor	0.49
AI263909	RHOB	Ras homologue gene family, member B	0.61

NOTE: Genes are clustered into groups by biological function. The mean fold-change of each gene in PD samples relative to control samples as well as the gene symbol and GenBank accession numbers are indicated. The genes shown are taken out of 68 downregulated genes. Specific categories determined to be significantly overrepresented using the statistical clustering program EASE are indicated by an asterisk.

Rpt3). Also, two genes related to protein handling were prominently decreased in PD brains: S-phase kinase-associated protein 1A (p19A) (SKP1A) and the heat-shock 70-kDa protein 8 (HSPA8), coding for HSC-70, a member of the HSP70 chaperone family. Regarding DA neurotransmission and metabolism, major decreases were reported for cyclic AMP–regulated phosphoprotein (ARPP-21), solute carrier family 18 (vesicular monoamine member 2, VMAT2), and aldehyde dehydrogenase 1 family member A1 (ALDH1A1).

The upregulated genes in PD are clustered mainly in biological processes involving cell adhesion/cytoskeleton, extracellular matrix components, cell cycle, protein modification/phosphorylation, protein metabolism, transcription, and inflammation/stress (TABLE 2). The most prominent gene alterations include PARVA (parvin, alpha), LGALS9 [lectin, galactoside-binding, soluble, 9 (galectin 9)], and SELPLG (selectin P ligand), belonging to the cell adhesion functional group. PENK (proenkephalin) and LRP6 (low density lipoprotein receptor–related protein 6) are related to the cell signaling class. EGLN1 [egl nine homologue 1 (*C. elegans*)], EIF4G1 (eukaryotic translation initiation factor 4 gamma, 1), MAN2B1 (mannosidase, alpha, class 2B, member 1), and SPHK1 (sphingosine kinase 1) are from the protein and lipid metabolism and phosphorylation categories. LOC56920 (semaphorin sem2) is involved in cell development, and ZSIG11 (putative secreted protein ZSIG11) and SRRM2 (a serine/arginine repetitive matrix 2) both have unknown functions.

Real-time PCR analysis corroborated the oligonucleotide array results, showing a significant decreased expression of SKP1A, VMAT2, and HSP8 in the SNpc of PD. These alterations are specific to the compacta area since no difference in expression levels was detected in either the SNr or cerebellum between PD and matched control.

TABLE 2. Major upregulated genes in SNpc of PD

GenBank	Symbol	Gene	Fold-change
		Cell adhesion*	
NM_014288.1	ITGB3BP	Integrin beta 3 binding protein (beta 3 endonexin)	1.67
NM_000632.2	ITGAM	Integrin, alpha M [complement component receptor 3, alpha; also known as CD11b (p170), macrophage antigen alpha polypeptide]	1.54
AF018081.1	COL18A1	Collagen, type XVIII, alpha 1	1.57
AI741056	SELPLG	Selectin P ligand	2.10
AF065389.1	TM4SF9	Transmembrane 4 superfamily member 9	1.60
AK022316.1	PARVA	Parvin, alpha	1.80
X79683.1	LAMB2	Laminin, beta 2 (laminin S)	1.76
NM_006043.1	HS3ST2	Heparan sulfate (glucosamine) 3-*O*-sulfotransferase 2	1.84
U58766	TSTA3	Tissue-specific transplantation antigen P35B	1.60
AI984221	COL5A3	Collagen, type V, alpha 3	1.68
		Cell motility/cytoskeleton	
NM_002579.1	PALM	Paralemmin	1.59
NM_003803.1	MYOM1	Myomesin 1 (skelemin) 185 kDa	2.13
M62994.1	FLNB	Filamin B, beta (actin binding protein 278)	1.75
		Development	
NM_000190.1	HMBS	Hydroxymethylbilane synthase	1.65
NM_000423.1	KRT2A	Keratin 2A (epidermal ichthyosis bullosa of Siemens)	2.04
NM_020163.1	LOC56920	Semaphorin sem2	1.98
		Protein biosynthesis	
BE966878	EIF4G1	Eukaryotic translation initiation factor 4 gamma, 1	1.69
BC005057.1	EIF4EBP2	Eukaryotic translation initiation factor 4E binding protein 2	1.75
BC005369.1	EGLN1	Egl nine homologue 1 (*C. elegans*)	2.37
		Cell cycle	
NM_004383.1	CSK	C-src tyrosine kinase	1.59
AF241788.1	NUDC	Nuclear distribution gene C homologue (*A. nidulans*)	1.52
NM_007076.1	HYPE	Huntingtin interacting protein E	1.54
D88435	GAK	Cyclin G–associated kinase	1.54

TABLE 2. (*continued*) Major upregulated genes in SNpc of PD

GenBank	Symbol	Gene	Fold-change
		Immune response	
AI743792	SIAT1	Sialyltransferase 1 (beta-galactoside alpha-2,6-sialyltransferase)	1.79
NM_005211.1	CSF1R	Colony stimulating factor 1 receptor, formerly McDonough feline sarcoma viral (v-fms) oncogene homologue	1.57
AI073984	ICSBP1	Interferon consensus sequence binding protein 1	1.88
X59350	CD22	CD22 antigen	1.60
		Response to stress	
NM_001983.1	ERCC1	Excision repair cross-complementing rodent repair deficiency, complementation group 1 (includes overlapping antisense sequence)	1.61
AK023253.1	DNAJB5	DnaJ (HSP40) homologue, subfamily B, member 5	1.73
		Apoptosis	
AI721219	TRAF3	TNF receptor–associated factor 3	1.63

NOTE: The genes shown are taken out of 69 upregulated genes. Specific categories determined to be significantly overrepresented using the statistical clustering program EASE are indicated by an asterisk.

IMPAIRMENT IN UPS: DECREASE IN SKP1A AND PROTEASOME SUBUNITS

The global gene expression changes in the SNpc of postmortem parkinsonian brains as compared to age-matched controls[28] shows, for the first time, diminished expression of an essential component of protein catabolism, the SKP1A gene. Its decline was accompanied by decreased expression in various subunits of the 26S proteasome, in energy pathways, and in signal transduction. SKP1 is part of the Rbx family of RING proteins[30] functioning within modular multiprotein Skp1, Cullin, and a substrate-recognizing F-box protein (SCF). This unit allows the formation of multiple E3 complexes, which in turn are able to recognize a wide spectrum of different protein substrates. SCF complexes are modular: SKP1 can interact with several F-box proteins, which are responsible for specific target recognition, thereby providing functional diversity and increasing the repertoire of proteins processed by this complex. Humans express only one functional SKP1 isoform.[31] The decrease in its expression may constitute a rate-limiting factor and may account for the accumulation of a wide spectrum of ubiquitinated protein aggregates in brains of PD patients, including tyrosine hydroxylase, synphilin-1, α-synuclein, and phosphorylated tau.[32–34] The particular susceptibility of the SNpc to different types of stress, such as increased iron concentration, enzymatic (MAO) and nonenzymatic (auto-oxidation) DA metabolism, abnormal protein accumulation, proteasomal inhibition, and neurotoxin-induced OS, may be associated with progressive reduction in SKP1A. In this context, the PA28 multisubunit proteasome activator (a component of the 26S proteasome) protein levels were shown to be very low in the SNpc of both normal and idiopathic PD subjects compared to other brain areas,[18] possibly exacerbating the already compromised DA-containing neurons to the various stress insults. Parkin may also function within a novel SCF-like complex, along with the F-box/WD repeat protein hSel-10, responsible for substrate recognition, and Cullin1, which however does not include SKP1.[35] Thus, parkin may associate with adaptor proteins other than hSel-10. Such complexes would likely display diverse substrate specificity and may explain the several targets that have been reported for parkin.[36]

The concomitant decrease in 3 subunits of the 20S proteasome mRNA and in 2 subunits of the 19S regulatory complex of the 26S proteasome in the SN of PD brains, together with reduction in SKP1, may further contribute to dopaminergic neurodegeneration. The 19S complexes are located at one or both extremities of the 20S proteolytic core of the proteasome[37,38] and comprise at least 18 subunits.[39] They are subdivided into 2 subcomplexes, the "base" and the "lid", which form the portions proximal and distal to the 20S proteolytic core, respectively, and all together form the 26S complex. The lid consists of 8 regulatory particle non-ATPase (Rpn) subunits, including PSMD8/Rpn12. One important function of the lid is to recognize multi-ubiquitinated proteins and other potential substrates of the proteasome.[40] The base contains 3 non-ATPase subunits (Rpn1, Rpn2, and Rpn10, this last common to both base and lid) and 6 putative ATPase subunits (Rpt1–6), including PSMC4/TBP7. These interact with nonnative conformations of nonubiquitinated target proteins[40–42] and one of them, S6′/TBP1, was found to bind aggregated or monomeric α-synuclein.[43,44] In the same context, it has been recently reported that PSMC4, also called regulatory proteasomal protein S6, specifically interacts with both wild-type and mutant synphilin-1,[45] another presynaptic protein, associated with synaptic vesicles.[46] Synphilin-1 was found associated with α-synuclein and, similarly, it accumulates in LB.[47] Thus, the decreased levels of PSMC4 found by us, together with the progressive inhibition of the UPS by the slow, but persistent aggregation of α-synuclein, may cause the accumulation in LB.[6,32] The observed increase in the expression of the glycosaminoglycan heparan-sulfate gene in PD samples may possibly contribute as well to fibrillation and aggregation of α-synuclein, as suggested.[48]

Each of the 6 ATPases is essential and they account for the ATP requirement for proteolysis and for association of the 20S and 19S complexes to form the 26S complex.[49,50] Thus, the decline in the expression of PSMC4/TBP7 in brains of parkinsonian patients may contribute to decreased levels of 26S proteasome complex, abnormal accumulation of ubiquitinated proteins, and reduced rates of degradation of short-lived proteins such as cyclins, which in turn may induce cell defects (for review, see refs. 37 and 38). Accumulation of cyclins and cyclin-dependent kinases has been reported in postmitotic neurons undergoing apoptosis[51,52] and in the MPTP model of PD.[53] It has been suggested that this event may represent an attempt at cell cycle reentry.[54]

These findings are in line with a previous report of decreased expression of the 20S proteasome α-subunits, but not β-subunits; decreased protein expression levels of some 19S subunits; and functional deficits in the 26/20S proteasome activity in the SNpc of patients with sporadic PD.[18] In this study, however, the exact nature of the different subunits affected was not established as the antibodies employed in the Western blot analyses recognize sequences that are common to the various proteasome subunits and because of possible protein dimerization, leading to over-estimation of the molecular weight. Thus, our study provides a wider view, revealing gene changes in the expression of specific proteasome components.

HEAT-SHOCK PROTEIN CHAPERONE HSC-70

Neurodegenerative diseases are considered, at present, OS-dependent protein conformational disorders, characterized by misfolding and aggregation of proteins including α-synuclein, amyloid β-peptide, and phosphorylated tau. Recent evidence indicates that molecular chaperones are among the most potent suppressors of neurodegeneration known for animal models of human disease.[55] Proteotoxic insults to cells or several stress conditions can induce upregulation of molecular chaperones aimed at protecting cells by assisting in correct folding of wild-type and mutated proteins. One example is the 70-kDa heat-shock cognate protein (HSC-70),[56] a member of the heat-shock protein 70 (HSP70) family. It is suggested that HSC-70 normally mediates cellular processes such as protein folding, refolding, assembly, disassembly, and protein translocation via biological membranes. It has been shown that overexpression of HSP70 reduces the amount of misfolded, aggregated α-synuclein species *in vivo* and *in vitro*;[57] prevents the loss of dopaminergic neurons in a model of PD in transgenic flies expressing either the wild-type α-synuclein or the mutant forms A30P and A53T;[58] and suppresses the degeneration associated with polyglutamine pathogenicity.[59] We have found significant decreased gene expression of HSP8, coding for HSC-70, specifically in the SNpc of 5 out of 6 parkinsonian patients, as further confirmed by real-time quantitative PCR, whereas no significant alterations were observed between SNr or cerebellum from PD patients and controls, suggestive of tissue specificity.[28] Recently, a functional polymorphism in the 5′ promoter region of HSP70-1 has been reported in 274 PD patients, which may increase susceptibility to PD.[60]

In addition to the involvement of HSC-70 in vesicular and nuclear trafficking, it may play a role in protein ubiquitination through recognition of unfolded or aberrant proteins and delivery to a cochaperone, E3 ligase enzyme CHIP (carboxyl-terminus of HSC-70 interacting protein).[61] CHIP can cooperate with HSP90 and/or HSP70/HSC-70 and ubiquitinate their attached misfolded substrates. Thus, the HSC-70/CHIP pair represents an E3 ligase for specifically recognizing unfolded proteins presented by the chaperones. This molecular chaperone-UPS quality-control system is of extreme importance in neurodegenerative diseases since proteins that evade refolding or degradation by the UPS form aggregates that accumulate into inclusion bodies. Indeed, molecular chaperones, as well as ubiquitin and proteasome, are recruited to inclusion bodies and LB,[62,63] indicating the attempt of the quality-control system to degrade damaged proteins or prevent their removal. In fact, a number of neurodegenerative diseases appear to result from failure of the protein quality-control system.[55,62]

CELL ADHESION MOLECULES, IRON, AND OXIDATIVE STRESS

An association between genes playing essential roles in neuronal development, such as cell migration and axonal elongation, as well as components of the cytoskeleton and AD, has recently been suggested.[64] A similar hypothesis can be assigned to PD where abnormal phosphorylation of cytoskeleton components (e.g., neurofilaments, microtubule-associated proteins) and ubiquitination of synaptic and other proteins are encountered within the LB.[6] Our findings, showing abnormal up-regulation of genes with structural and phosphorylative molecular functions integral to membrane and extracellular matrix (cell adhesion process), support this assumption and extend our knowledge, revealing potential new gene targets for future therapeutics. During brain inflammations such as those reported in PD, AD, and multiple sclerosis, the breakdown in the organization of key cell adhesion molecules and reduction in their signal transduction pathways may generate brain pathology, probably related to the recruitment of glial cells and macrophages and to the elevation in cytokines and OS. In addition, in 5 out of the 6 patients, we observed a striking induction by more than 1.5-fold of the EGLN1 gene,[28] a recently described proline hydroxylase enzyme belonging to the iron- and 2-oxoglutarate-dependent dioxygenase superfamily.[65] These enzymes act as key iron and oxygen sensors controlling the expression of the transcription factor, hypoxia-inducible factor-1 alpha (HIF), a master regulator orchestrating the coordinated induction of an array of hypoxia-sensitive genes. The target genes of HIF are especially related to angiogenesis, cell proliferation/survival, and glucose/iron metabolism.[66] Upon high oxygen levels or iron overload, the EGLN hydroxylases target HIF to proteasomal degradation. Interestingly, the free iron–induced proteasome-mediated degradation of iron regulatory protein (IRP2) also involves activation of 2-oxoglutarate-dependent dioxygenases and is inhibited by iron chelators.[67,68] Thus, it is possible that IRP2 is a substrate of EGLN1, which causes posttranslational modification, signaling it for protein degradation. Excessive production of EGLN1 in the SNpc may lead to a fall in IRP2 and subsequent decrease in transferrin receptor (TfR) mRNA and an increase in ferritin levels, both subjected to positive and negative transcriptional regulation by IRP2, respectively.[69,70] Recent studies in knockout mice for IRP2 have revealed accumulation of iron in the striatum with substantial bradykinesia and tremor.[71]

Increased expression of the iron and OS sensor protein may be directly responsible for the observed reduction in phosphofructokinase and also the angiogenic factor VEGF, both regulated by the HIF proteins.[72] Phosphofructokinase is the key regulatory enzyme that controls the glucose flux through the glycolytic pathway. Similarly, VEGF activates genes involved in glucose transport and metabolism via activation of the PI3K and ras pathways. This finding supports previous reports in human PD patients using positron emission tomography (PET) analysis, demonstrating a decrease in glucose uptake into the SN,[73] and gives a wider view of major survival pathways affected by the disease. These observations, together with the additional decrease in a number of energy pathways/glycolysis-related genes, as well as increases in iron/OS and inflammatory genes, is consistent with the hypothesis that mitochondrial dysfunction and reactive oxygen and nitrogen species contribute to the pathogenesis of PD. In line with this, a recent study linked a recessive mutation in the putative free radical sensor DJ-1 gene, with early-onset parkinsonism.[24] To our surprise, apoptosis-related genes constituted the smallest functional class in PD samples, questioning the relevance of programmed cell death in the neurodegenerative cascade of events occurring in the disease. The role of apoptosis in PD is highly controversial since the evidence for it does not correlate with the pathological findings and the rate of neurodegeneration. We cannot exclude the possibility that apoptotic changes occurred at earlier stages and then declined with disease progression.

DA NEUROTRANSMISSION AND METABOLISM

The disruption in the neuronal processes described earlier may be exacerbated by the observed reduction in the expression of cell signaling genes, which may be coupled to cell adhesion protein complexes and in genes belonging to the vesicle secretory pathway and dopaminergic neurotransmission and metabolism in the parkinsonian SN.[28] Real-time PCR confirmatory analysis revealed a specific reduction of vesicular monoamine transporter VMAT2 (SCL18A2) mRNA in the SNpc, while the changes in the SNr were less pronounced. This finding is in agreement with previous reports on postmortem SN of controls and PD showing a marked reduction of VMAT2 mRNA in PD that was associated with marked reductions in both DA transporter and VMAT2 signal per cell in the remaining pigmented neurons.[74,75] Three other striking changes, also related to DA transmission and metabolism, are the reduced expression of ALDH1A1, ADH5, and ARPP-21 mRNAs coding for aldehyde dehydrogenase (ALDH), alcohol dehydrogenase (ADH), and cAMP-regulated phosphoprotein, respectively. ARPP-21 is specifically enriched in DA-innervated brain regions of the basal ganglia (e.g., caudate-putamen) and in the SN.[76,77] Similar to DARPP-32 (DA and adenosine 3′,5′-monophosphate–regulated phosphoprotein-32K), ARPP-21 is activated by DA receptor D1 and thus may represent an index of functional activity of D1 neurotransmission. To our knowledge, this is the first report of decreased ARPP-21 mRNA levels in PD SN. ALDH1 has been found to be highly expressed and specifically in DA cells of the SN and ventral tegmental area (VTA), and to be markedly reduced in dopaminergic neurons of the SNpc (but not in those of the VTA) of PD brains.[78] In our analysis, we have found that it is the isoform ALDH1A1 that is specifically reduced in the SN of PD. This isoform has been recently identified as being expressed selectively in the DA-containing neurons of the rat SN and VTA, while the dopaminergic neurons of the hypothalamus express the ALDH1A3 isozyme.[79] This is supported by *in vivo* studies showing that striatal ALDH activity in 6-hydroxydopamine-treated rats,[80] or in cats after an electrical induced lesion,[81] was significantly reduced. DA is equally well metabolized in human brain striatum by MAO A and B[82,83] to very reactive aldehyde derivatives (3,4-dihydroxyphenylacetaldehyde and 4-hydroxy-3-methoxyphenylacetaldehyde) that rarely accumulate in the striatum.

ALDHs and ADHs are involved in the degradation of these aldehyde derivatives,[84] which are then metabolized to homovanillic acid and 3,4-dihydroxyphenylacetic acid, and in detoxification of aldehydes that are highly reactive and neurotoxic[85] (see FIG. 2). Thus, alteration in DA transmission may alter ALDH and ADH activities; conversely, changes in ALDH-ADH-mediated metabolism may affect DA levels in nerve cell bodies and terminal fields in basal ganglia and the limbic system. This is of major relevance in light of recent evidence for mutations in genes encoding ADHs as genetic risk factors for PD.[86] These proteins (ALDH, ADH, and ARPP-21), in

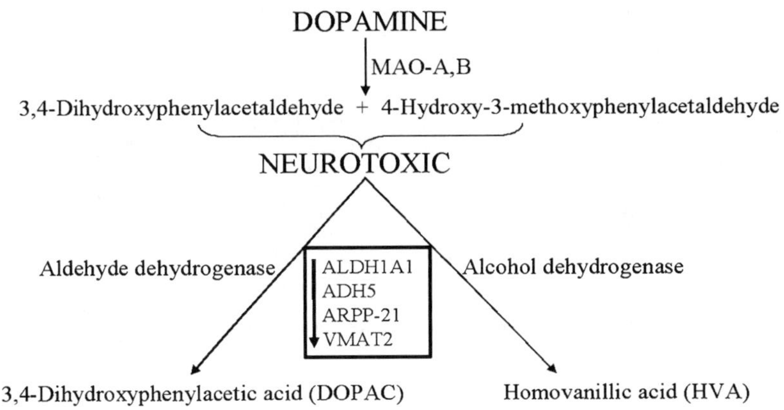

FIGURE 2. The pathway of DA metabolism and its abnormality in SNpc of PD. The reduction in ALDH1A1 and ADH5 gene expression can contribute to the process of neurodegeneration. Similar results have been obtained in 6-OHDA and electrical lesions in animal models of PD.[80,81] The consequential effect can be accumulation of neurotoxic aldehydes and alcohol metabolites generated from DA. The decrease in the levels of DA metabolism and neurotransmission–related genes (VMAT2 and ARPP-21) may seriously compromise neurotransmitter storage and correlate with DA neuron dysfunction.

conjunction with VMAT2, may now be considered new markers for PD. The overall decrease in the levels of these DA neurotransmission and metabolism–related genes observed in this study may seriously compromise neurotransmitter storage and may correlate with DA neuron dysfunction. Impairment of cell transport and vesicle trafficking, carrying a wide repertoire of intracellular and membrane proteins, may well account for their aggregation and cell deposition into cytoplasmic inclusions (aggresomes) and in LB.

One simple hypothesis explaining our observations is that loss of DA-containing neuronal bodies and neuronal synapses may account for the reduced levels of the gene products. This assumption would predict similar gene expression changes in a vast repertoire of vesicle traffic or synapse-related genes. However, as emerged from our microarray and real-time PCR confirmations, the expression of many genes related to these categories such as Rab3b, syntaxin 6, and COP zeta 2, was not altered in PD. Also, the invasion by microglia and astrocytes of the SNpc from PD afflicted individuals may mask or "dilute" in part the extent of the changes that occur specifically in the remaining melanin-containing dopaminergic neurons. This is why we are currently analyzing the protein expression levels of the major gene alterations observed in PD patients, specifically in the melanized neurons. For instance, SKP1 and ALDH1 protein levels are extremely low within the TH-positive dopaminergic neurons of the ventral-caudal SNpc (the major affected area in PD) from PD subjects (data not shown), confirming the gene expression results.

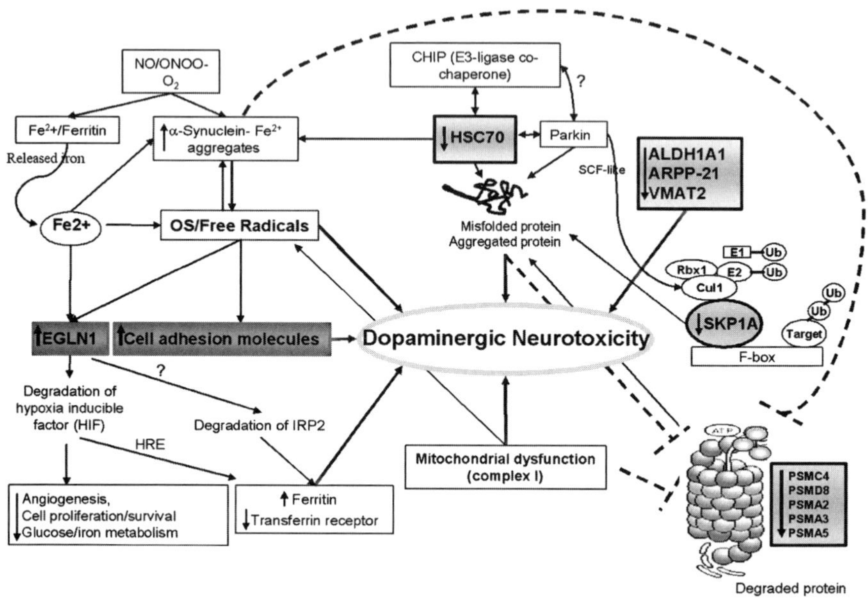

FIGURE 3. Schematic diagram of major gene and neurochemical alterations in human SNpc of PD. Gene expression analysis of SNpc of PD has confirmed and extended the previously established complexities by which DA neurons degenerate. These findings do not allow a conclusion to be reached regarding the primary biochemical event(s) that induces the "domino" death cascade. OS, resulting from excessive generation of nitric oxide/peroxynitrite ($NO/ONOO^-$), O_2, or hydroxyl radicals, can lead to dysregulation of iron metabolism, induction of α-synuclein aggregation, and mitochondrial dysfunction. Free (labile) iron itself can cause OS, aggregation of α-synuclein, and degradation of iron regulatory protein 2 (IRP2) via activation of egl nine homologue 1 (*C. elegans*) (EGLN1), which is a key iron and OS sensor. This in turn results in proteasomal degradation of hypoxia-inducible factor (HIF) and IRP2, with subsequent decreases in cell survival/proliferation, glucose, and iron metabolism genes. Increases in the expression of cell adhesion molecules and components of the extracellular matrix in response to OS/free radicals can result in cell assembly disruption. Aldehyde derivatives of DA metabolism are highly neurotoxic, and aldehyde dehydrogenase (ALDH) is the key enzyme for their metabolism to inert acidic metabolites (homovanillic acid and dihydroxyphenylacetic acid). The reduction in gene expression of ALDH1A1, ARPP-21, and VMAT2, which are located within DA-containing neurons of SNpc, may contribute to a failure in DA transmission and metabolism. Significant evidence has been provided for involvement of protein misfolding in DA neuron death. SKP1A is part of the SCF (SKP, Cullin, F-box protein) ubiquitin ligase component (E3) that regulates normal degradation of a wide arrays of proteins, which may include α-synuclein, parkin, IRP2, HIF, etc. Its decline can cause evasion of proteins subjected to SCF/26S proteasome complex degradation. This protein processing is exacerbated if some of the 26S proteasome subunits are downregulated, as observed in the present study, since they are an integral part of the regulatory and catalytic activity of the proteasome. The decreased expression of the chaperone HSC-70 may affect the correct folding of several proteins that are specifically ubiquitinated by the cochaperone carboxyl-terminus of HSC-70 interacting protein (CHIP), as well as parkin-CHIP-mediated ubiquitination,[88] and may increase aggregation of α-synuclein and iron-induced OS. *Red boxes* are for upregulated genes and *blue boxes* are for downregulated genes [color shown only for the online Web version]. *Sharp arrows* indicate positive inputs, whereas *blunt arrows* are for inhibitory inputs. (From ref. 28.)

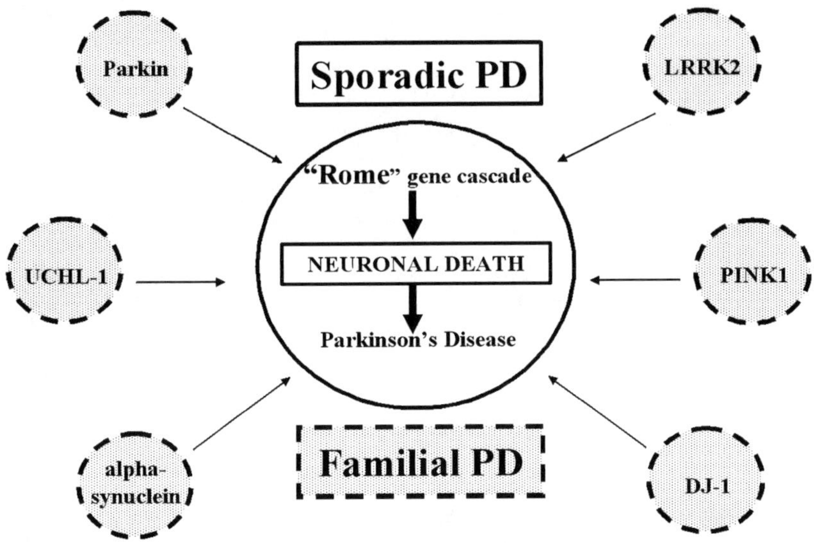

FIGURE 4. All roads lead to Rome. The cluster of gene expression changes demonstrated in sporadic parkinsonian SNpc may very well represent the central core ("Rome" gene cascade) by which DA neurons degenerate in SNpc of sporadic as well as familial PD. This is evidenced by the observation that there is homology between the sporadic and inherited disease, involving OS, iron dysregulation, and a defect in the ubiquitin-proteasome system (UPS). However, to date, no large-scale gene expression profile has been performed with any of the familial cases of PD, which could shed light on the cross talk of genes participating in the cascade of neurodegeneration.

CONCLUSION: ALL ROADS LEAD TO ROME

In spite of the vast information regarding the pathology and etiology of PD, it is still premature to assert what is the primary event(s) that triggers the development of PD in sporadic and familial forms. Our large-scale analysis of gene expression profiles of sporadic PD SNpc has shown for the first time a pattern of homology with the genetic cases involving mutated genes. One of the most significant linkages between them is the reduction in the levels of selective components of the UPS, together with a progressive dysregulation of extracellular matrix/cytoskeleton components, concurrent with a state of OS and inflammation (FIG. 3). The gene-gene interaction and the pathogenic molecular mechanisms by which the mutated genes cause PD are not known. Nevertheless, it can be assumed that the molecular interactions and final pathway must be common to both sporadic and familial disease (genetic). Thus, "all roads lead to Rome" (FIG. 4), namely, a convergence of mechanisms involved in DA neuron death in both forms of PD. The cascade of gene events that we have identified in the sporadic disease may act independently or cooperatively during the course of the disease, leading eventually to the demise of dopaminergic neurons. Thus, subtle alterations in the kinetics of the different affected proteins may have, during the decades, a cumulative effect underlying the slowly progressive neurodegeneration of the DA-containing neurons in PD. Effective therapies will probably require the simultaneous modulation of several components of the UPS and mitochondria, as well as intervention at the level of iron chelation and molecular chaperone induction, employing polypharmacology or recently developed multifunctional neuroprotective drugs (for review, see ref. 87).

REFERENCES

1. YOUDIM, M.B., D. BEN-SHACHAR & P. RIEDERER. 1993. The possible role of iron in the etiopathology of Parkinson's disease. Mov. Disord. **8:** 1–12.
2. RIEDERER, P. *et al.* 1989. Transition metals, ferritin, glutathione, and ascorbic acid in parkinsonian brains. J. Neurochem. **52:** 515–520.
3. GOTZ, M.E. *et al.* 1994. Oxidative stress: free radical production in neural degeneration. Pharmacol. Ther. **63:** 37–122.
4. YOUDIM, M.B.H. & P. RIEDERER. 1997. Understanding Parkinson's disease: the smoking gun is still missing, but growing evidence suggests highly reactive substances called free radicals are central players in this common neurological disorder. Sci. Am. **276:** 52–59.
5. JENNER, P. & C.W. OLANOW. 1996. Oxidative stress and the pathogenesis of Parkinson's disease. Neurology **47:** S161–S170.
6. JELLINGER, K.A. 2003. Neuropathological spectrum of synucleinopathies. Mov. Disord. **18**(suppl. 6)**:** S2–S12.
7. EBADI, M. *et al.* 2001. Ubiquinone (coenzyme q10) and mitochondria in oxidative stress of Parkinson's disease. Biol. Signals Recept. **10:** 224–253.
8. OSTREROVA-GOLTS, N. *et al.* 2000. The A53T alpha-synuclein mutation increases iron-dependent aggregation and toxicity. J. Neurosci. **20:** 6048–6054.
9. TURNBULL, S. *et al.* 2001. α-Synuclein implicated in Parkinson's disease catalyses the formation of hydrogen peroxide *in vitro*. Free Radical Biol. Med. **30:** 1163–1170.
10. FELLETSCHIN, B. *et al.* 2003. Screening for mutations of the ferritin light and heavy genes in Parkinson's disease patients with hyperechogenicity of the substantia nigra. Neurosci. Lett. **352:** 53–56.
11. YOUDIM, M.B.H. & P. RIEDERER. 2004. Iron in the brain, normal and pathological. *In* Encyclopedia of Neuroscience. Elsevier. Amsterdam/New York.
12. ZECCA, L. *et al.* 2004. Iron, brain ageing, and neurodegenerative disorders. Nat. Rev. Neurosci. **5:** 863–873.
13. GRUNBLATT, E., S. MANDEL & M.B.H. YOUDIM. 2000. MPTP and 6-hydroxydopamine-induced neurodegeneration as models for Parkinson's disease: neuroprotective strategies. J. Neurol. **247:** II/95–II/102.
14. DAUER, W. & S. PRZEDBORSKI. 2003. Parkinson's disease: mechanisms and models. Neuron **39:** 889–909.
15. CIECHANOVER, A. & P. BRUNDIN. 2003. The ubiquitin proteasome system in neurodegenerative diseases: sometimes the chicken, sometimes the egg. Neuron **40:** 427–446.
16. DAWSON, T.M. & V.L. DAWSON. 2003. Molecular pathways of neurodegeneration in Parkinson's disease. Science **302:** 819–822.
17. MCNAUGHT, K.S. *et al.* 2002. Selective loss of 20S proteasome alpha-subunits in the substantia nigra pars compacta in Parkinson's disease. Neurosci. Lett. **326:** 155–158.
18. MCNAUGHT, K.S. *et al.* 2003. Altered proteasomal function in sporadic Parkinson's disease. Exp. Neurol. **179:** 38–46.
19. KITADA, T. *et al.* 1998. Mutations in the parkin gene cause autosomal recessive juvenile parkinsonism [see comments]. Nature **392:** 605–608.
20. MURAKAMI, T. *et al.* 2004. Pael-R is accumulated in Lewy bodies of Parkinson's disease. Ann. Neurol. **55:** 439–442.
21. JELLINGER, K. *et al.* 1990. Brain iron and ferritin in Parkinson's and Alzheimer's diseases. J. Neural Transm. Parkinson's Dis. Dementia Sect. **2:** 327–340.
22. TOMPKINS, M.M. & W.D. HILL. 1997. Contribution of somal Lewy bodies to neuronal death. Brain Res. **775:** 24–29.

23. VILA, M. & S. PRZEDBORSKI. 2003. Targeting programmed cell death in neurodegenerative diseases. Nat. Rev. Neurosci. **4:** 365–375.
24. BONIFATI, V. *et al.* 2003. Mutations in the DJ-1 gene associated with autosomal recessive early-onset parkinsonism. Science **299:** 256–259.
25. VALENTE, E.M. *et al.* 2004. Hereditary early-onset Parkinson's disease caused by mutations in PINK1. Science **304:** 1158–1160.
26. PAISAN-RUIZ, C. *et al.* 2004. Cloning of the gene containing mutations that cause PARK8-linked Parkinson's disease. Neuron **44:** 595–600.
27. ZIMPRICH, A. *et al.* 2004. Mutations in LRRK2 cause autosomal-dominant parkinsonism with pleomorphic pathology. Neuron **44:** 601–607.
28. GRUNBLATT, E. *et al.* 2004. Gene expression profiling of parkinsonian substantia nigra pars compacta; alterations in ubiquitin-proteasome, heat shock protein, iron and oxidative stress regulated proteins, cell adhesion/cellular matrix, and vesicle trafficking genes. J. Neural Transm. **111:** 1543–1573.
29. DENNIS, G., JR. *et al.* 2003. DAVID: database for annotation, visualization, and integrated discovery. Genome Biol. **4:** P3.
30. KAMURA, T. *et al.* 1999. Rbx1, a component of the VHL tumor suppressor complex and SCF ubiquitin ligase. Science **284:** 657–661.
31. SEMPLE, C.A. 2003. The comparative proteomics of ubiquitination in mouse. Genome Res. **13:** 1389–1394.
32. LIANI, E. *et al.* 2004. Ubiquitylation of synphilin-1 and alpha-synuclein by SIAH and its presence in cellular inclusions and Lewy bodies imply a role in Parkinson's disease. Proc. Natl. Acad. Sci. USA **101:** 5500–5505.
33. ZHANG, J. & D.R. GOODLETT. 2004. Proteomic approach to studying Parkinson's disease. Mol. Neurobiol. **29:** 271–288.
34. MEREDITH, G.E., G.M. HALLIDAY & S. TOTTERDELL. 2004. A critical review of the development and importance of proteinaceous aggregates in animal models of Parkinson's disease: new insights into Lewy body formation. Parkinsonism Relat. Disord. **10:** 191–202.
35. STAROPOLI, J.F. *et al.* 2003. Parkin is a component of an SCF-like ubiquitin ligase complex and protects postmitotic neurons from kainate excitotoxicity. Neuron **37:** 735–749.
36. DEV, K.K. *et al.* 2003. Part I: parkin-associated proteins and Parkinson's disease. Neuropharmacology **45:** 1–13.
37. VOGES, D., P. ZWICKL & W. BAUMEISTER. 1999. The 26S proteasome: a molecular machine designed for controlled proteolysis. Annu. Rev. Biochem. **68:** 1015–1068.
38. COUX, O., K. TANAKA & A.L. GOLDBERG. 1996. Structure and functions of the 20S and 26S proteasomes. Annu. Rev. Biochem. **65:** 801–847.
39. GLICKMAN, M.H. & A. CIECHANOVER. 2002. The ubiquitin-proteasome proteolytic pathway: destruction for the sake of construction. Physiol. Rev. **82:** 373–428.
40. GLICKMAN, M.H. *et al.* 1998. A subcomplex of the proteasome regulatory particle required for ubiquitin-conjugate degradation and related to the COP9-signalosome and eIF3. Cell **94:** 615–623.
41. STRICKLAND, E. *et al.* 2000. Recognition of misfolding proteins by PA700, the regulatory subcomplex of the 26S proteasome. J. Biol. Chem. **275:** 5565–5572.
42. ADAMS, J. 2003. The proteasome: structure, function, and role in the cell. Cancer Treat. Rev. **29**(suppl. 1)**:** 3–9.
43. GHEE, M., A. FOURNIER & J. MALLET. 2000. Rat alpha-synuclein interacts with Tat binding protein 1, a component of the 26S proteasomal complex. J. Neurochem. **75:** 2221–2224.
44. SNYDER, H. *et al.* 2003. Aggregated and monomeric alpha-synuclein bind to the S6′ proteasomal protein and inhibit proteasomal function. J. Biol. Chem. **278:** 11753–11759.
45. MARX, F.P. *et al.* 2004. Parkinson's disease associated mutant synphilin-1 mediates proteasomal inhibition and interacts with regulatory proteasomal protein S6. Mov. Disord. **19:** S83.
46. RIBEIRO, C.S. *et al.* 2002. Synphilin-1 is developmentally localized to synaptic terminals, and its association with synaptic vesicles is modulated by alpha-synuclein. J. Biol. Chem. **277:** 23927–23933.
47. WAKABAYASHI, K. *et al.* 2000. Synphilin-1 is present in Lewy bodies in Parkinson's disease. Ann. Neurol. **47:** 521–523.

48. COHLBERG, J.A. *et al.* 2002. Heparin and other glycosaminoglycans stimulate the formation of amyloid fibrils from alpha-synuclein *in vitro*. Biochemistry **41:** 1502–1511.
49. GORDON, C. *et al.* 1993. Defective mitosis due to a mutation in the gene for a fission yeast 26S protease subunit. Nature **366:** 355–357.
50. GHISLAIN, M., A. UDVARDY & C. MANN. 1993. *S. cerevisiae* 26S protease mutants arrest cell division in G2/metaphase. Nature **366:** 358–362.
51. COPANI, A. *et al.* 2001. Activation of cell-cycle-associated proteins in neuronal death: a mandatory or dispensable path? Trends Neurosci. **24:** 25–31.
52. PADMANABHAN, J. *et al.* 1999. Role of cell cycle regulatory proteins in cerebellar granule neuron apoptosis. J. Neurosci. **19:** 8747–8756.
53. GRUNBLATT, E. *et al.* 2001. Gene expression analysis in *N*-methyl-4-phenyl-1,2,3,6-tetrahydropyridine mice model of Parkinson's disease using cDNA microarray: effect of *R*-apomorphine. J. Neurochem. **78:** 1–12.
54. VERDAGUER, E. *et al.* 2002. Kainic acid–induced apoptosis in cerebellar granule neurons: an attempt at cell cycle re-entry. Neuroreport **13:** 413–416.
55. MUCHOWSKI, P.J. & J.L. WACKER. 2005. Modulation of neurodegeneration by molecular chaperones. Nat. Rev. Neurosci. **6:** 11–22.
56. ZINSMAIER, K.E. & P. BRONK. 2001. Molecular chaperones and the regulation of neurotransmitter exocytosis. Biochem. Pharmacol. **62:** 1–11.
57. KLUCKEN, J. *et al.* 2004. Hsp70 reduces α-synuclein aggregation and toxicity. J. Biol. Chem. **279:** 25497–25502.
58. AULUCK, P.K. *et al.* 2002. Chaperone suppression of alpha-synuclein toxicity in a *Drosophila* model for Parkinson's disease. Science **295:** 865–868.
59. BONINI, N.M. 2002. Chaperoning brain degeneration. Proc. Natl. Acad. Sci. USA **99:** 16407–16411.
60. WU, Y.R. *et al.* 2004. Analysis of heat-shock protein 70 gene polymorphisms and the risk of Parkinson's disease. Hum. Genet. **114:** 236–241.
61. MURATA, S., T. CHIBA & K. TANAKA. 2003. CHIP: a quality-control E3 ligase collaborating with molecular chaperones. Int. J. Biochem. Cell Biol. **35:** 572–578.
62. SHERMAN, M.Y. & A.L. GOLDBERG. 2001. Cellular defenses against unfolded proteins: a cell biologist thinks about neurodegenerative diseases. Neuron **29:** 15–32.
63. STENOIEN, D.L. *et al.* 1999. Polyglutamine-expanded androgen receptors form aggregates that sequester heat shock proteins, proteasome components, and SRC-1, and are suppressed by the HDJ-2 chaperone. Hum. Mol. Genet. **8:** 731–741.
64. DE FERRARI, G.V. & N.C. INESTROSA. 2000. Wnt signaling function in Alzheimer's disease. Brain Res. Brain Res. Rev. **33:** 1–12.
65. EPSTEIN, A.C. *et al.* 2001. *C. elegans* EGL-9 and mammalian homologs define a family of dioxygenases that regulate HIF by prolyl hydroxylation. Cell **107:** 43–54.
66. LEE, J.W. *et al.* 2004. Hypoxia-inducible factor (HIF-1) alpha: its protein stability and biological functions. Exp. Mol. Med. **29**(36)**:** 1–12.
67. HANSON, E.S., M.L. RAWLINS & E.A. LEIBOLD. 2003. Oxygen and iron regulation of iron regulatory protein 2. J. Biol. Chem. **278:** 40337–40342.
68. WANG, J. *et al.* 2004. Iron-mediated degradation of IRP2, an unexpected pathway involving a 2-oxoglutarate-dependent oxygenase activity. Mol. Cell. Biol. **24:** 954–965.
69. PONKA, P. 2004. Hereditary causes of disturbed iron homeostasis in the central nervous system. Ann. N.Y. Acad. Sci. **1012:** 267–281.
70. MEYRON-HOLTZ, E.G. *et al.* 2004. Genetic ablations of iron regulatory proteins 1 and 2 reveal why iron regulatory protein 2 dominates iron homeostasis. EMBO J. **23:** 386–395.
71. LAVAUTE, T. *et al.* 2001. Targeted deletion of the gene encoding iron regulatory protein-2 causes misregulation of iron metabolism and neurodegenerative disease in mice. Nat. Genet. **27:** 209–214.
72. MINCHENKO, O., I. OPENTANOVA & J. CARO. 2003. Hypoxic regulation of the 6-phosphofructo-2-kinase/fructose-2,6-bisphosphatase gene family (PFKFB-1–4) expression *in vivo*. FEBS Lett. **554:** 264–270.
73. BERDING, G. *et al.* 2001. Resting regional cerebral glucose metabolism in advanced Parkinson's disease studied in the off and on conditions with [(18)F]FDG-PET. Mov. Disord. **16:** 1014–1022.

74. HARRINGTON, K.A. *et al.* 1996. Dopamine transporter (Dat) and synaptic vesicle amine transporter (VMAT2) gene expression in the substantia nigra of control and Parkinson's disease. Brain Res. Mol. Brain Res. **36:** 157–162.
75. BROOKS, D.J. 2003. Imaging end points for monitoring neuroprotection in Parkinson's disease. Ann. Neurol. **53**(suppl. 3)**:** S110–S118; discussion, pp. S118–S119.
76. OUIMET, C.C., H.C. HEMMINGS, JR. & P. GREENGARD. 1989. ARPP-21, a cyclic AMP–regulated phosphoprotein enriched in dopamine-innervated brain regions. II. Immunocytochemical localization in rat brain. J. Neurosci. **9:** 865–875.
77. TSOU, K., J.A. GIRAULT & P. GREENGARD. 1993. Dopamine D1 agonist SKF 38393 increases the state of phosphorylation of ARPP-21 in substantia nigra. J. Neurochem. **60:** 1043–1046.
78. GALTER, D. *et al.* 2003. ALDH1 mRNA: presence in human dopamine neurons and decreases in substantia nigra in Parkinson's disease and in the ventral tegmental area in schizophrenia. Neurobiol. Dis. **14:** 637–647.
79. GRIMM, J. *et al.* 2004. Molecular basis for catecholaminergic neuron diversity. Proc. Natl. Acad. Sci. USA **101:** 13891–13896.
80. AGID, Y., F. JAVOY & M.B.H. YOUDIM. 1973. Monoamine oxidase and aldehyde dehydrogenase activity in the striatum of rats after 6-hydroxydopamine lesion of the nigrostriatal pathway. Br. J. Pharmacol. **48:** 175–178.
81. DUNCAN, R.J. *et al.* 1972. Aldehyde dehydrogenase and monoamine oxidase in the striatum of cats with nigrostriatal lesions. J. Neurochem. **19:** 2007–2010.
82. COLLINS, G.G. *et al.* 1970. Multiple forms of human brain mitochondrial monoamine oxidase. Nature **225:** 817–820.
83. O'CARROLL, A.M. *et al.* 1983. The deamination of dopamine by human brain monoamine oxidase: specificity for the two enzyme forms in seven brain regions. Naunyn-Schmiedeberg's Arch. Pharmacol. **322:** 198–202.
84. MARDH, G. & B.L. VALLEE. 1986. Human class I alcohol dehydrogenases catalyze the interconversion of alcohols and aldehydes in the metabolism of dopamine. Biochemistry **25:** 7279–7282.
85. HJELLE, J.J. & D.R. PETERSEN. 1983. Hepatic aldehyde dehydrogenases and lipid peroxidation. Pharmacol. Biochem. Behav. **18**(suppl. 1)**:** 155–160.
86. BUERVENICH, S. *et al.* 2005. A rare truncating mutation in ADH1C (G78Stop) shows significant association with Parkinson disease in a large international sample. Arch. Neurol. **62:** 74–78.
87. YOUDIM, M.B. & J.J. BUCCAFUSCO. 2005. Multi-functional drugs for various CNS targets in the treatment of neurodegenerative disorders. Trends Pharmacol. Sci. **26:** 27–35.
88. IMAI, Y. *et al.* 2002. CHIP is associated with parkin, a gene responsible for familial Parkinson's disease, and enhances its ubiquitin ligase activity. Mol. Cell **10:** 55–67.
89. NOUREDDINE, M.A. *et al.* 2005. Genomic convergence to identify candidate genes for Parkinson disease: SAGE analysis of the substantia nigra. Mov. Disord. In press. [Epub ahead of print: 17 June 2005.]
90. ZHANG, Y. *et al.* 2005. Transcriptional analysis of multiple brain regions in Parkinson's disease supports the involvement of specific protein processing, energy metabolism, and signaling pathways, and suggests novel disease mechanisms. Am. J. Med. Genet. Neuropsychiatr. Genet. **B137**(1)**:** 5–16.
91. HAUSER, M.A. *et al.* 2005. Expression profiling of substantia nigra in Parkinson disease, progressive supranuclear palsy, and frontotemporal dementia with parkinsonism. Arch. Neurol. **62**(6)**:** 917–921.

Neuronal Growth-Promoting and Inhibitory Cues in Neuroprotection and Neuroregeneration

STEPHEN D. SKAPER

Department of Neuro Cell Sciences, Neurology and GI Centre of Excellence for Drug Discovery, GlaxoSmithKline Research and Development Limited, Harlow, United Kingdom

ABSTRACT: During development of the nervous system, neurons extend axons over considerable distances in a highly stereospecific fashion in order to innervate their targets in an appropriate manner. This involves the recognition, by the axonal growth cone, of guidance cues that determine the pathway taken by the axons. These guidance cues can act to promote and/or repel growth cone advance. The directed growth of axons is partly governed by cell adhesion molecules (CAMs) on the neuronal growth cone that bind to CAMs on the surface of other axons or nonneuronal cells. *In vitro* assays have established the importance of the CAMs (NCAM, N-cadherin, and L1) in promoting axonal growth over cells. Compelling evidence implicates the fibroblast growth factor receptor tyrosine kinase as the primary signal transduction molecule in the CAM pathway. CAMs are important constituents of synapses, and they appear to play important and diverse roles in regulating synaptic plasticity associated with learning and memory. Synthetic NCAM peptide mimetics corresponding to the binding site of NCAM for the fibroblast growth factor receptor promote synaptogenesis, enhance presynaptic function, and facilitate memory consolidation. Dimeric versions of functional binding motifs of N-cadherin behave as N-cadherin agonists, promoting both neuritogenesis and neuronal cell survival. Negative extracellular signals that physically direct neurite growth have also been described. The latter include the myelin inhibitory proteins, Nogo, myelin-associated glycoprotein, and oligodendrocyte-myelin glycoprotein. Potentiation of outgrowth-promoting signals, together with antagonism of myelin proteins or their convergent receptor, NgR, and its second messenger pathways, may provide new opportunities in the rational design of treatments for acute brain injury and neurodegenerative disorders.

KEYWORDS: cell adhesion molecules; fibroblast growth factor receptor; neuroprotection; neuroregeneration; myelin; Nogo; Rho kinase

Address for correspondence: Stephen D. Skaper, Department of Neuro Cell Sciences, Neurology and GI Centre of Excellence for Drug Discovery, GlaxoSmithKline Research and Development Limited, New Frontiers Science Park, Third Avenue, Harlow, Essex CM19 5AW, United Kingdom. Voice: +44-(0)1279-622350; fax: +44-(0)1279-622660.
stephen_d_skaper@gsk.com

Ann. N.Y. Acad. Sci. 1053: 376–385 (2005). © 2005 New York Academy of Sciences.
doi: 10.1196/annals.1344.032

INTRODUCTION

Nervous system development evolves from the well-orchestrated processes of neural induction, cell proliferation, differentiation, cell migration, survival, and synapse formation.[1,2] The directed growth of axons is fundamental to synapse formation. Receptors for guidance molecules are present on growth cones and their filopodia, and interactions with cognate ligands could result in promotion, inhibition, attraction, or repulsion of the growth cone. A broad spectrum of putative growth-promoting and/or guidance molecules has been identified to date. These include neurotrophic factors,[3,4] chemoattractants such as netrin 1 and 2,[5] chemorepellents from the collapsin/semaphorin family,[6–8] and cell adhesion molecules (CAMs).[2,9] The importance of the last class of molecules is evidenced by the severe neurological deficits found in humans with mutations in the L1 gene, which can include a complete absence of corticospinal tracts.[10]

Growth inhibitory molecules present in the central nervous system (CNS) myelin contribute, at least in part, to the inability of mammalian CNS axons to regenerate upon injury.[11] In recent years, some molecular determinants of axonal regeneration and plasticity in the adult brain have been defined.[12] Three proteins, Nogo-A,[13–15] myelin-associated glycoprotein (MAG),[16,17] and oligodendrocyte-myelin glyco-

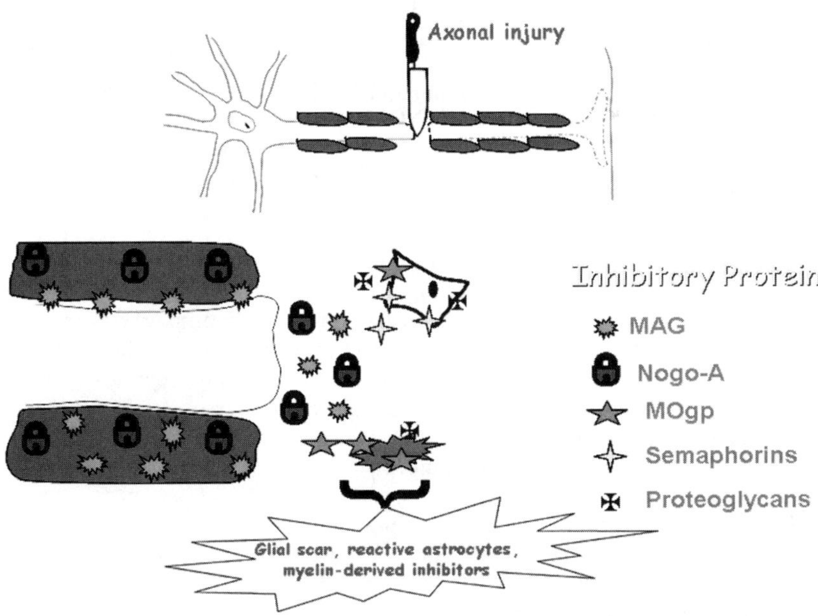

FIGURE 1. Strategies for CNS regeneration. Mechanical injury or traumatic injury, or chronic neurodegenerative disease, can result in neurons being “disconnected” from their innervation fields, leading to a loss of critical tissue-derived trophic support. Regeneration may be promoted by replacement of neurotrophic factors, by stimulation of axonal outgrowth and/or cell survival with adhesion molecules, and by agents capable of overriding the outgrowth inhibitory environment.

protein (OMgp),[18] appear to be responsible for this inhibition of axonal growth. This myelin inhibitory biology leads to the hypothesis that modulation of the interactions of these myelin proteins with their axonal receptor(s) would overcome the inhibitory effects of CNS myelin and promote axon regeneration, leading to improved functional recovery after CNS injury (see FIG. 1). Much recent work has focused upon the identification and characterization of signal transduction pathways for both CAMs and myelin-associated inhibitors. This paper briefly summarizes current knowledge on this topic.

CAMs, NEURONAL PLASTICITY, AND NEUROPROTECTION

Cell-cell interactions mediated by CAMs are fundamental to numerous developmental processes. In the nervous system, the ability of neurons to extend axons and innervate their targets in an appropriate manner is governed to a large extent by the binding of CAMs on the surface of other axons or nonneuronal cells.[19,20] The neuronal receptors important for general cell contact–dependent axonal growth are the β1-integrins, which recognize extracellular matrix molecules; and, in mammals, three CAMs, namely, the neural cell adhesion molecule (NCAM), N-cadherin, and L1, promote axonal growth during development.[2]

N-Cadherin is a member of the classical cadherin family of transmembrane glycoproteins that mediate cellular recognition via homophilic (binding with other N-cadherin molecules on neighboring cells) interaction.[21] In the nervous system, N-cadherin function has been implicated in cell migration,[22] axonal growth and guidance,[23] and synapse formation and synaptic plasticity.[24,25] In addition to homophilic binding, cadherins have been shown to interact with many adaptor or signaling molecules, including the fibroblast growth factor receptor (FGFR). Neurite outgrowth stimulated by N-cadherin is inhibited by a variety of agents that block FGFR function in neurons.[26–28] Soluble forms of some adhesion molecules,[29] including N-cadherin,[30] are effective also in promoting axonal growth. The homophilic binding site resides in extracellular domain 1 (ECD1),[31] and peptide mimetics of two linear sequences from ECD1 (HAVDI and INPISGQ) function as specific N-cadherin antagonists.[32,33] This information was then used to design cyclic peptides containing a tandem repeat of the individual motifs, which function as N-cadherin agonists and stimulate neurite outgrowth.[34] A recent study has shown that a dimeric version (SW4 peptide) of a short N-cadherin binding motif (HAVDI) is capable of promoting the survival of several populations of CNS neurons, under distinct paradigms of injury, in an FGFR-dependent manner.[35] An example of this is illustrated in FIGURE 2 for hippocampal neurons subjected to glutamate-induced excitotoxicity. The neuroprotective effects of SW4 displayed a concentration-dependence similar to those inducing neuritogenesis.[34] The responses to the dimeric agonist peptide were inhibited by a monomeric version of the same motif (itself a highly specific N-cadherin antagonist[32]) and by a specific FGFR antagonist. These data suggest that the dimeric agonist peptide functions by binding to and clustering N-cadherin in neurons, and thereby activating an N-cadherin/FGFR signaling cascade.[35] The neural CAMs, L1 and CHL1,[36] and the synthetic NCAM peptide ligand, C3d,[37] have been reported to display survival-promoting effects (albeit modest) on cultured CNS neurons. The

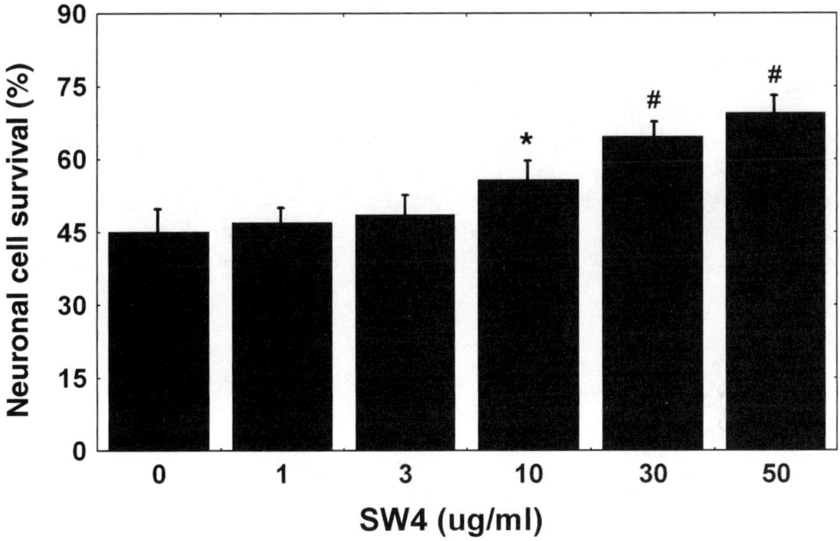

FIGURE 2. The dimeric HAVDI peptide (SW4) attenuates glutamate excitotoxicity to hippocampal neurons *in vitro*. Cells at 8 days in culture (>95% neuronal[35]) were incubated with the SW4 peptide for 48 h, followed by challenge with 50 μM glutamate for 24 h. Data are means ± SD (3 experiments) expressed relative to no glutamate as control (100%). Under these conditions, survival with 25 ng/mL FGF-2 was 82.2±1.5%, consistent with earlier reports for this model.[74] $^{*}P < 0.05$ or $^{\#}P < 0.01$ vs. glutamate only. [Reprinted from fig. 3 of ref. 35, copyright 2004, with permission from Elsevier.]

neurotropic and neurotrophic effects of CAMs strengthen the emerging role for adhesion molecules in synaptic plasticity,[38,39] as discussed below.

CAMs are important constituents of synapses, with well-recognized roles in building and maintaining synaptic structure during brain development. Growing evidence indicates that CAMs play important and diverse roles in regulating synaptic plasticity associated with learning and memory.[40,41] The role of NCAM in cognitive processes is demonstrated by studies in which interference with NCAM function through the administration of antibodies or gene inactivation has resulted in impaired long-term potentiation[42,43] and learning and memory deficits.[44,45] As with N-cadherin, synthetic NCAM peptide mimetics have now become available.[46] After homophilic binding, NCAM promotes neurite outgrowth through mechanisms involving interaction with the FGFR.[47,48] The recently identified FG loop (FGL) peptide, a 15-amino-acid sequence corresponding to the binding site of NCAM for the FGFR1, has been shown to bind to and activate FGFR1 and to stimulate neurite outgrowth.[48] Intracerebroventricular administration of the NCAM mimetic FGL peptide increases memory strength in rats and enhances presynaptic function in primary hippocampal neurons.[49] These results provide the first evidence for a memory-facilitating effect resulting from a treatment that mimics NCAM function.

GROWTH INHIBITORY MOLECULES

In contrast to fish, amphibia, and the mammalian peripheral nerves and developing central nerves, adult central mammalian neurons do not regrow functional axons after damage. It is not the absence of growth-promoting molecules in the CNS, but rather the presence of axonal outgrowth inhibitors in CNS astroglial "scars"[50] and CNS myelin[51,52] that suppresses the regrowth of damaged axons. In particular, two components present in CNS myelin have been characterized as potent inhibitors of axonal growth: MAG[16,17] and Nogo-A, the largest transcript of the recently identified *nogo* gene (formerly called NI-220).[13–15] Other inhibitors include chondroitin

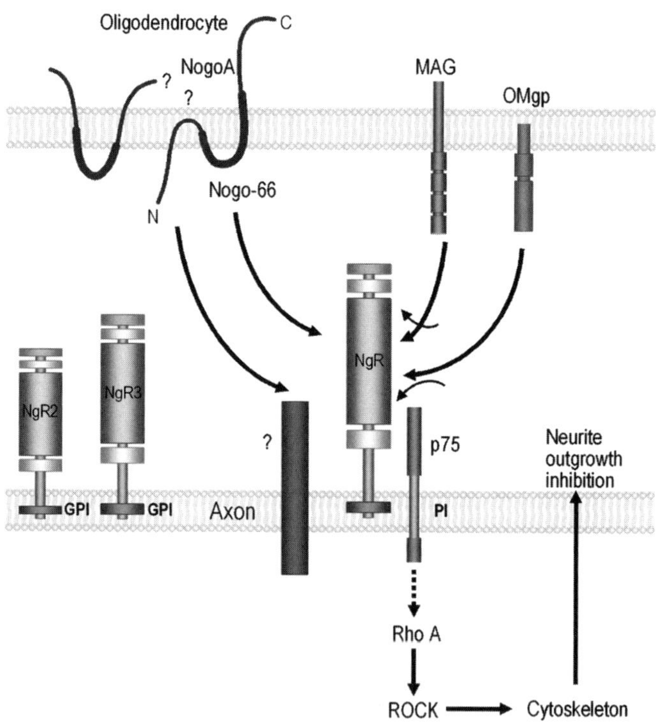

FIGURE 3. The Nogo receptor and inhibition of axonal regeneration. The leucine-rich repeat domains of the Nogo receptor (NgR) are necessary for interaction with Nogo-66, MAG, and OMgp. NgR does not transduce signals directly, but utilizes coreceptor molecules, for example, p75 or others. Coreceptor activation, in turn, activates the Rho and ROCK pathway to modulate the cytoskeleton and neurite growth. While structurally similar to NgR1, NgR2 and NgR3 display essentially no binding to known myelin-derived NgR ligands. GPI, glycosylphosphatidylinositol; ROCK, Rho-associated kinase. [Reproduced from fig. 2 of ref. 60 (www.nature.com/reviews), copyright 2003, with permission from Macmillan Magazines Limited.]

sulfate proteoglycans[53] and OMgp.[18] Nogo is a member of the Reticulon family and occurs in three forms, Nogo-A, -B, and -C, which are generated from alternate splicing.[13–15] Nogo-A, -B, and -C all contain a 66-amino-acid extracellular domain (Nogo-66) that alone can inhibit neurite outgrowth and induce growth cone collapse.[13–15] MAG is a type I membrane protein composed of 5 extracellular immunoglobulin (Ig)–like domains,[16,17] whereas OMgp is a glycosylphosphatidylinositol-anchored protein.[18] Remarkably, a single neuronal protein, the Nogo-66 receptor (NgR), binds Nogo, MAG, and OMgp.[54–57] The p75 low-affinity neurotrophin receptor protein has been implicated in transducing a myelin/NgR signal to the axonal interior[58,59] (see FIG. 3).

The presence of myelin-derived inhibitors suggests that blocking their action might allow the intrinsic growth potential of CNS axons to be unmasked.[60] Indeed, neutralizing Nogo-A with IN-1 antibody induced CNS axon regeneration and improved recovery after various lesions.[61,62] Targeting the axonal NgR with a competitive antagonist compound has the potential to block the action of the three known myelin inhibitors. Both intrathecal[63] and delayed systemic application[64] of NEP1–40 (Nogo extracellular peptide, residues 1–40) produced significant axonal regrowth after spinal cord hemitransection injury, as well as enhanced locomotor recovery.[64] However, these reagents only target a single myelin protein, Nogo, which may not be sufficient to facilitate maximal CNS axonal regeneration because other inhibitors such as MAG and OMgp are present in the CNS myelin environment. In rats with middle cerebral artery occlusion, both the recovery of motor skills and corticofugal axonal plasticity are promoted by intracerebroventricular administration of a function-blocking NgR fragment, sNgR310-Fc [an Ig-fusion protein containing a soluble fragment of NgR encompassing the ligand binding domain (sNgR310)].[65] Stroke lesion size was not significantly reduced in the sNgR310-Fc protein–treated group,[65] suggesting that reduction of NgR function after stroke allows increased anatomical plasticity and improved motor performance that are not attributable to neuroprotection. Comparable results were obtained in $ngr^{-/-}$ mice with photothrombotic cortical lesion.[65] A newly described neutralizing anti-Nogo-66 receptor monoclonal antibody 7E11 was reported to be a more potent inhibitor than sNgR310-Fc in *in vitro* competition binding assays and in a neurite outgrowth assay against CNS myelin.[66] Further experiments in relevant animal models may prove the relevance of anti-NgR antibodies in promoting CNS axonal regeneration.

The signaling mechanisms responsible for the transduction of the inhibitory properties of Nogo-A and MAG domains are not well understood. Recent evidence supports the notion that cytoskeletal components required for proper axonal pathfinding and the formation of axons and dendrites are differentially regulated by members of the Rho family, including RhoA, Rac1, and Cdc42.[67] Rho proteins serve as a molecular switch by cycling between an inactive GDP-bound state and an active GTP-bound state. The most important effector of RhoA in the growth cone is probably the serine-threonine kinase Rho-kinase ROCK.[68] Data indicate that MAG activates RhoA by increasing the proportion of the protein bound to GTP;[69] Nogo-66 and myelin utilize this same signaling pathway (see FIG. 3).[70,71] Pharmacological studies *in vitro* and *in vivo* indicate that ROCK plays a prime role in mediating myelin-induced inhibition via NgR[71,72] and that Rho pathway inactivation can promote spinal cord repair[72] and enhance axonal regeneration after corticospinal tract lesions in the adult rat.[70]

CONCLUDING REMARKS

Information is encoded in the CNS through networks of neurons that are functionally connected by synapses. CAMs have well-recognized roles in building and maintaining synaptic structure during brain development. Growing evidence indicates that CAMs also play important and diverse roles in regulating synaptic plasticity and learning and memory. It is now clear that NCAM, N-cadherin, and L1 stimulate neurite outgrowth by activating the FGFR in neurons. Intriguing new data suggest that CAMs may promote also neuronal cell survival, perhaps by an FGFR signaling cascade. Synthetic CAM peptide agonists may represent a starting point for the development of nonpeptide mimetics with the potential as therapeutic agents promoting cell survival and regeneration. While the developing CNS is highly plastic, the adult brain and spinal cord have little innate capacity for repair. A growing body of knowledge now points to the myelin inhibitory protein Nogo and other myelin molecules such as MAG as being key players underlying this lack of regenerative ability. Convergence of these myelin-associated components on the NgR, and identification of the associated intracellular second messengers, provides an opportunity to develop rational interventions to promote CNS axon regeneration after injury. The NgR provides an attractive therapeutic target because of its essential role, high-affinity interactions, and neural specificity. There is also interest and demonstrated efficacy for blockade of Rho and ROCK; however, as these signaling molecules are present in all cell types of the body, specificity is a concern. Neuroprotective effects of targeting the NgR pathway have not been reported, although antibodies to MAG are neuroprotective in brain ischemia and prevent glutamate-induced oligodendrocyte death.[73] Understanding of how signals from extracellular factors associated with myelin and the injury site are integrated with outgrowth-promoting signals and neurotrophic factors to regulate axonal elongation should further facilitate the development of interventions to improve the outcome of both acute CNS injury and chronic neurodegenerative disorders.

REFERENCES

1. Tessier-Lavigne, M. & C.S. Goodman. 1996. The molecular biology of axonal guidance. Science **274:** 1123–1133.
2. Walsh, F.S. & P. Doherty. 1997. Neural cell adhesion molecules of the immunoglobulin superfamily: role in axonal growth and guidance. Annu. Rev. Cell. Dev. Biol. **13:** 425–456.
3. Ip, N.Y. & G.D. Yancopoulos. 1996. The neurotrophins and CNTF: two families of collaborative neurotrophic factors. Annu. Rev. Neurosci. **19:** 491–515.
4. Skaper, S.D. & F.S. Walsh. 1998. Neurotrophic molecules: strategies for designing effective therapeutic molecules in neurodegeneration. Mol. Cell. Neurosci. **12:** 179–193.
5. Serefini, T., T.E. Kennedy, M.J. Galko *et al.* 1994. The netrins define a family of axon outgrowth-promoting proteins homologous to *C. elegans* UNC-6. Cell **78:** 409–424.
6. Mueller, B.K. 1999. Growth cone guidance: first steps toward a deeper understanding. Annu. Rev. Neurosci. **22:** 351–388.
7. Fournier, A.E. & S.M. Strittmatter. 2001. Repulsive factors and axon regeneration in the CNS. Curr. Opin. Neurobiol. **11:** 89–94.
8. Kolodkin, A.L. 1996. Semaphorins: mediators of repulsive growth cone guidance. Trends Cell Biol. **6:** 15–22.
9. Goodman, C.S. 1996. Mechanisms and molecules that control growth cone guidance. Annu. Rev. Neurosci. **19:** 341–377.

10. KENWRICK, S., A. WATKINS & E. DE ANGELIS. 2000. Neural cell recognition molecule L1: relating biological complexity to human disease mutations. Hum. Mol. Genet. **9:** 879–886.
11. CAJAL, R.S. 1928. Degeneration and Regeneration of the Nervous System. Hafner. New York.
12. MCGEE, A.W. & S.M. STRITTMATTER. 2003. The Nogo-66 receptor: focusing myelin inhibition of axon regeneration. Trends Neurosci. **26:** 193–198.
13. CHEN, M.S., A.B. HUBER, M.E. VAN DER HAAR *et al.* 2000. Nogo-A is a myelin-associated neurite outgrowth inhibitor and an antigen for monoclonal antibody IN-1. Nature **403:** 434–439.
14. GRANDPRE, T., F. NAKAMURA, T. VARTANIAN *et al.* 2000. Identification of the Nogo inhibitor of axon regeneration as a Reticulon protein. Nature **403:** 439–444.
15. PRINJHA, R., S.E. MOORE, M. VINSON *et al.* 2000. Inhibitor of neurite outgrowth in humans. Nature **403:** 383–384.
16. MCKERRACHER, L., S. DAVID, D.L. JACKSON *et al.* 1994. Identification of myelin-associated glycoprotein as a major myelin-derived inhibitor of neurite outgrowth. Neuron **13:** 805–811.
17. MUKHOPADHYAY, G., P. DOHERTY, F.S. WALSH *et al.* 1994. A novel role for myelin-associated glycoprotein as an inhibitor of axonal regeneration. Neuron **13:** 757–767.
18. WANG, K.C., V. KOPRIVICA, J.A. KIM *et al.* 2002. Oligodendrocyte-myelin glycoprotein is a Nogo receptor ligand that inhibits neurite outgrowth. Nature **417:** 941–944.
19. DODD, J. & J.M. JESSELL. 1988. Axon guidance and the patterning of neuronal projections in vertebrates. Science **242:** 692–699.
20. GOODMAN, C.S. & C.J. SHATZ. 1993. Developmental mechanisms that generate precise patterns of neuronal connectivity. Cell/Neuron **72**(suppl. 10)**:** 77–98.
21. TAKEICHI, M. 1995. Morphogenetic role of classic cadherins. Curr. Opin. Cell Biol. **7:** 619–627.
22. BARAMI, K., B. KIRSCHENBAUM, V. LEMMON *et al.* 1994. N-Cadherin and Ng-CAM/8D9 are involved serially in the migration of newly generated neurons into the adult songbird brain. Neuron **13:** 567–582.
23. MATSUNAGA, M., K. HATTA, A. NAGAFUCHI *et al.* 1988. Guidance of optic nerve fibers by N-cadherin adhesion molecules. Nature **334:** 62–64.
24. INOUE, A. & J.R. SANES. 1997. Lamina-specific connectivity in the brain: regulation by N-cadherin, neurotrophins, and glycoproteins. Science **276:** 1428–1431.
25. BOZDAGI, O., W. SHAN, H. TANAKA *et al.* 2000. Increasing numbers of synaptic puncta during late-phase LTP: N-cadherin is synthesized, recruited to synaptic sites, and required for potentiation. Neuron **28:** 245–259.
26. SAFFELL, J.L., E.J. WILLIAMS, I.J. MASON *et al.* 1997. Expression of a dominant negative FGF receptor inhibits axonal growth and FGF receptor phosphorylation stimulated by CAMs. Neuron **18:** 231–242.
27. WILLIAMS, E-J., J. FURNESS, F.S. WALSH *et al.* 1994. Activation of the FGF receptor underlies neurite outgrowth stimulated by L1, N-CAM, and N-cadherin. Neuron **13:** 583–594.
28. WILLIAMS, E-J., G. WILLAMS, F.V. HOWELL *et al.* 2001. Identification of an N-cadherin motif that can interact with the fibroblast growth factor receptor and is required for axonal growth. J. Biol. Chem. **276:** 43879–43886.
29. DOHERTY, P., E. WILLIAMS & F.S. WALSH. 1995. A soluble form of the L1 glycoprotein stimulated neurite outgrowth. Neuron **14:** 57–66.
30. UTTON, M.A., B. EICKHOLT, F.V. HOWELL *et al.* 2001. Soluble N-cadherin stimulates fibroblast growth factor receptor dependent neurite outgrowth and N-cadherin and the fibroblast growth factor receptor co-cluster in cells. J. Neurochem. **76:** 1421–1430.
31. KOCH, A.W., D. BOZIC, O. PERTZ *et al.* 1999. Homophilic adhesion by cadherins. Curr. Opin. Struct. Biol. **9:** 275–281.
32. WILLIAMS, E., G. WILLIAMS, B.J. GOUR *et al.* 2000. A novel family of cyclic peptide antagonists suggests that N-cadherin specificity is determined by amino acids that flank the HAV motif. J. Biol. Chem. **275:** 4007–4012.
33. WILLIAMS, E.J., G. WILLIAMS, B. GOUR *et al.* 2000. INP, a novel N-cadherin antagonist targeted to the amino acids that flank the HAV motif. Mol. Cell. Neurosci. **15:** 456–464.

34. Williams, G., E-J. Williams & P. Doherty. 2002. Dimeric versions of two short N-cadherin binding motifs (HAVDI and INPISG) function as N-cadherin agonists. J. Biol. Chem. **277:** 4361–4367.
35. Skaper, S.D., L. Facci, G. Williams *et al.* 2004. A dimeric version of the short N-cadherin binding motif HAVDI promotes neuronal cell survival by activating an N-cadherin/fibroblast growth factor receptor signalling cascade. Mol. Cell. Neurosci. **26:** 17–23.
36. Chen, S., N. Mantei, L. Dong *et al.* 1999. Prevention of neuronal cell death by neural cell adhesion molecules L1 and CHL1. J. Neurobiol. **38:** 428–439.
37. Ditlevsen, D.K., L.B. Køhler, M.V. Pedersen *et al.* 2003. The role of phosphatidylinositol 3-kinase in neural cell adhesion molecule–mediated neuronal differentiation and survival. J. Neurochem. **84:** 546–556.
38. Goda, Y. 2002. Cadherins communicate structural plasticity of presynaptic and postsynaptic terminals. Neuron **35:** 1–3.
39. Togashi, H., K. Abe, A. Mizoguchi *et al.* 2002. Cadherin regulates dendritic spine morphogenesis. Neuron **35:** 77–89.
40. Schachner, M. 1997. Neural recognition molecules and synaptic plasticity. Curr. Opin. Cell Biol. **9:** 627–634.
41. Benson, D.L., L.M. Schnapp, L. Shapiro *et al.* 2000. Making memories stick: cell-adhesion molecules in synaptic plasticity. Trends Cell Biol. **10:** 473–482.
42. Luthi, A., J.P. Laurent, A. Figurov *et al.* 1994. Hippocampal long-term potentiation and neural cell adhesion molecules L1 and NCAM. Nature **372:** 777–779.
43. Rønn, L.C.B., E. Bock, D. Linnemann *et al.* 1995. NCAM-antibodies modulate induction of long-term potentiation in rat hippocampal CA1. Brain Res. **677:** 145–151.
44. Doyle, E., P.M. Nolan, R. Bell *et al.* 1992. Intraventricular infusions of anti-neural cell adhesion molecules in discrete posttraining period impair consolidation of a passive avoidance response in the rat. J. Neurochem. **59:** 1570–1573.
45. Cremer, H., R. Lange, A. Christoph *et al.* 1994. Inactivation of the NCAM gene in mice results in size reduction of the olfactory bulb and deficits in spatial learning. Nature **367:** 455–459.
46. Rønn, L.C.B., M. Olsen, S. Ostergaard *et al.* 1999. Identification of a neuritogenic ligand of the neural cell adhesion molecule using a combinatorial library of synthetic peptides. Nat. Biotech. **17:** 1000–1005.
47. Saffell, J.L., F.S. Walsh & P. Doherty. 1994. Expression of NCAM containing VASE in neurons can account for a developmental loss in their neuritic outgrowth response to NCAM in a cellular substratum. J. Cell Biol. **125:** 427–436.
48. Kiselyov, V.V., G. Skladchikova, A.M. Hinsby *et al.* 2003. Structural basis for a direct interaction between FGFR1 and NCAM and evidence for a regulatory role of ATP. Structure **11:** 691–701.
49. Cambon, K., S.M. Hansen, C. Venero *et al.* 2004. A synthetic neural cell adhesion molecule mimetic peptide promotes synaptogenesis, enhances presynaptic function, and facilitates memory consolidation. J. Neurosci. **24:** 4197–4204.
50. Fawcett, J.W. & R.A. Asher. 1999. The glial scar and central nervous system repair. Brain Res. Bull. **49:** 377–391.
51. Schwab, M.E. & H. Thoenen. 1985. Dissociated neurons regenerate into sciatic, but not optic nerve explants irrespective of neurotrophic factors. J. Neurosci. **5:** 2415–2423.
52. Schwab, M.E. & P. Caroni. 1988. Oligodendrocytes and CNS myelin are nonpermissive substrates for neurite growth and fibroblast spreading *in vitro*. J. Neurosci. **8:** 2381–2393.
53. Niederöst, B.P., D.R. Zimmermann, M.E. Schwab *et al.* 1999. Bovine CNS myelin contains neurite growth-inhibitory activity associated with chondroitin sulfate proteoglycans. J. Neurosci. **19:** 8979–8989.
54. Fournier, A.E., T. GrandPre & S.M. Strittmatter. 2001. Identification of a receptor mediating Nogo-66 inhibition of axonal regeneration. Nature **409:** 341–346.
55. Domeniconi, M., Z. Cao, T. Spencer *et al.* 2002. Myelin-associated glycoprotein interacts with the nogo66 receptor to inhibit neurite outgrowth. Neuron **35:** 283–290.
56. Liu, B.P., A. Fournier, T. GrandPre *et al.* 2002. Myelin-associated glycoprotein as a functional ligand for the nogo-66 receptor. Science **297:** 1190–1193.
57. Wang, K.C., V. Koprivica, J.A. Kim *et al.* 2002. Oligodendrocyte-myelin glycoprotein is a Nogo receptor ligand that inhibits neurite outgrowth. Nature **417:** 941–944.

58. WANG, K.C., J.A. KIM, R. SIVASANKARAN *et al.* 2002. p75 interacts with the Nogo receptor as a co-receptor for Nogo, MAG, and OMgp. Nature **420:** 74–78.
59. WONG, S.T., J.R. HENLEY, K.C. KANNING *et al.* 2002. A p75 (NTR) and Nogo receptor complex mediates repulsive signaling by myelin-associated glycoprotein. Nat. Neurosci. **5:** 1302–1308.
60. LEE, D.H.S., S.M. STRITTMATTER & D.W.Y. SAH. 2003. Targeting the Nogo receptor to treat central nervous system injuries. Nat. Rev. Drug Discovery **2:** 872–879.
61. BREGMAN, B.S., E. KUNKEL-BAGDEN, L. SCHNELL *et al.* 1995. Recovery from spinal cord injury mediated by antibodies to neurite growth inhibitors. Nature **378:** 498–501.
62. THALLMAIR, M., G.A. METZ, W.J. Z'GRAGGEN *et al.* 1998. Neurite growth inhibitors restrict plasticity and functional recovery following corticospinal tract lesions. Nat. Neurosci. **1:** 124–131.
63. GRANDPRE, T., S. LI & S.M. STRITTMATTER. 2002. Nogo-66 receptor antagonist peptide promotes axonal regeneration. Nature **417:** 547–551.
64. LI, S. & S.M. STRITTMATTER. 2003. Delayed systemic Nogo-66 receptor antagonist promotes recovery from spinal cord injury. J. Neurosci. **23:** 4219–4227.
65. LEE, J-K., J-E. KIM, M. SIVULA *et al.* 2004. Nogo receptor antagonism promotes stroke recovery by enhancing axonal plasticity. J. Neurosci. **24:** 6209–6217.
66. LI, W., L. WALUS, S.A. RABACCHI *et al.* 2004. A neutralizing anti-Nogo66 receptor monoclonal antibody reverses inhibition of neurite outgrowth by central nervous system myelin. J. Biol. Chem. **279:** 43780–43788.
67. LUO, L. 2000. Rho GTPases in neuronal morphogenesis. Nat. Rev. Neurosci. **1:** 173–180.
68. BITO, H., T. FURUYASHIKI, H. ISHIHARA *et al.* 2000. A critical role for Rho-associated kinase, p160ROCK, in determining axonal outgrowth in mammalian CNS neurons. Neuron **26:** 431–441.
69. YAMASHITA, T., H. HIGUCHI, M. TOHYAMA *et al.* 2002. The p75 receptor transduces the signal from myelin-associated glycoprotein to Rho. J. Cell Biol. **157:** 565–570.
70. FOURNIER, A.E., B.T. TAKIZAWA & S.M. STRITTMATTER. 2003. Rho kinase inhibition enhances axonal regeneration in the injured CNS. J. Neurosci. **23:** 1416–1423.
71. NIEDERÖST, B., T. OERTLE, J. FRITSCHE *et al.* 2002. Nogo-A and myelin-associated glycoprotein mediate neurite growth inhibition by antagonistic regulation of RhoA and Rac1. J. Neurosci. **22:** 10368–10376.
72. DERGHAM, P., B. ELLEZAM, C. ESSAGIAN *et al.* 2002. Rho signalling pathway targeted to promote spinal cord repair. J. Neurosci. **22:** 6570–6577.
73. IRVING, E.A., M. VINSON, C. ROSIN *et al.* 2004. Neuroprotective properties of an anti-MAG monoclonal antibody: a novel approach for the treatment of stroke? J. Cereb. Blood Flow Metab. **25:** 98–107.
74. MATTSON, M.P., M. MURRAIN, P.B. GUTHRIE *et al.* 1989. Fibroblast growth factor and glutamate: opposing roles in the generation and degeneration of hippocampal neuroarchitecture. J. Neurosci. **9:** 3728–3740.

Immune-Modulating Effects of Melatonin, *N*-Acetylserotonin, and *N*-Acetyldopamine

MARY C. PERIANAYAGAM,[a] GREGORY F. OXENKRUG,[b] AND BERTRAND L. JABER[a]

[a]*Division of Nephrology, Department of Medicine,* [b]*Department of Psychiatry, Caritas St. Elizabeth's Medical Center, Tufts University School of Medicine, Boston, Massachusetts, USA*

ABSTRACT: Melatonin and *N*-acetylserotonin (NAS) have antioxidant properties. In the present study, we examined whether melatonin, NAS, and *N*-acetyldopamine (NAD) have a modulatory effect on tumor necrosis factor-α (TNF-α) synthesis and superoxide production. Differentiated THP-1-derived human monocytes were coincubated with *Escherichia coli* lipopolysaccharide (LPS) and rising concentrations of melatonin, NAS, or NAD. After 24 h, TNF-α was measured in cell supernatants. In addition, the production of superoxide by HL-60-derived human neutrophils upon stimulation with 4-β-phorbol 12-β-myristate 13-α-acetate (PMA) or *N*-formyl methionyl-leucyl-phenylalanine (fMLP) and increasing concentrations of melatonin, NAS, or NAD was determined. Incubation of THP-1-derived monocytes with increasing concentrations of melatonin, NAS, or NAD resulted in a marked decrease in LPS-stimulated TNF-α production, which was dose-dependent and on the order of 96–98%. Incubation of HL-60-derived neutrophils with increasing concentrations of melatonin, NAS, or NAD resulted in a modest decrease in PMA-stimulated superoxide production, which was dose-dependent. At the 100 μM dose, melatonin, NAS, or NAD resulted in a 14±4%, 30±1%, and 29±1% decrease in PMA-stimulated superoxide production, respectively. Coincubation of HL-60 cells with melatonin, NAS, or NAD also resulted in a modest dose-dependent decrease in fMLP-stimulated superoxide production. At the 100 μM dose, melatonin, NAS, or NAD resulted in a 13±1%, 14±1%, and 14±1% decrease in superoxide production, respectively. Our results indicate that the inhibitory effect of melatonin, NAS, or NAD on LPS-induced TNF-α production is robust and dose-dependent. These compounds are equally effective in attenuating the generation of oxidant radicals, although to a lesser degree.

KEYWORDS: lipopolysaccharide (LPS); melatonin; *N*-acetyldopamine (NAD); *N*-acetylserotonin (NAS); tumor necrosis factor-α (TNF-α); superoxide; monocytes; neutrophils

Address for correspondence: Bertrand L. Jaber, M.D., Department of Medicine, Caritas St. Elizabeth's Medical Center, 736 Cambridge Street, Boston, MA 02135. Voice: 617-562-7832; fax: 617-562-7797.
bertrand_jaber@cchcs.org

Ann. N.Y. Acad. Sci. 1053: 386–393 (2005).
doi: 10.1196/annals.1344.033

INTRODUCTION

Gram-negative bacterial sepsis involves the release of bacterial membrane components such as lipopolysaccharide (LPS), which triggers the production of proinflammatory cytokines, including tumor necrosis factor-α (TNF-α) and interleukin-1β, and stimulation of inducible nitric oxide synthase (iNOS), resulting in extensive oxidative stress and tissue injury.[1]

The administration of the pineal secretory products, melatonin or *N*-acetylserotonin (NAS), counteracts the toxic effect of LPS in experimental models of sepsis[2–4] and reduces biomarkers of inflammation and oxidative stress in neonates undergoing surgery.[5] NAS, the immediate precursor and metabolite of melatonin,[6] prevents LPS-induced hypotensive shock[7] and lethality in mice[8] and rats.[4] Melatonin and NAS have also been shown to strongly suppress LPS- and iron-induced lipid peroxidation.[4] In an *in vitro* and *in vivo* mouse model of sepsis, melatonin inhibited LPS-induced TNF-α production.[8] In a rat model of sepsis, NAS reduced circulating TNF-α levels.[9]

In the present study, we evaluated the effect of melatonin, NAS, and *N*-acetyldopamine (NAD) on TNF-α production by THP-1-derived monocytes and explored the effect of these three compounds on superoxide production by HL-60-derived neutrophils.

EXPERIMENTAL METHODS

THP-1 Cell Culture

The human promonocytic THP-1 cell line (American Type Culture Collection, Manassas, VA) was maintained in suspension culture at 0.25×10^6 cells/mL in RPMI-1640 medium supplemented with 2 mM L-glutamine, 10% fetal bovine serum, and 0.05 mM 2-mercaptoethanol in a humidified atmosphere of 5% CO_2 in air at 37°C. Differentiation to monocytes (0.25×10^6 cells/mL) was induced by incubating cells with *trans*-retinoic acid (1 μM), 1,25-dihydroxy-cholecalciferol (0.1 μM), and interferon-γ (0.01 mg/L) (Sigma, St. Louis, MO). After 3 days, cells were detached using trypsin-EDTA and washed in PBS, and 1×10^6 cells were used for each experimental condition.

Cytokine Production by THP-1-Derived Monocytes

Differentiated THP-1 cells were coincubated with 10 ng/mL of purified LPS from *Escherichia coli* (Sigma) and increasing concentrations (0–400 μM) of melatonin, NAS, or NAD (Sigma) in RPMI-1640 cell culture medium at 37°C in a humidified atmosphere supplemented with 5% CO_2. After 24-h incubation, cell supernatants were harvested, and TNF-α was measured by a sandwich enzyme-linked immunosorbent assay (ELISA), according to the manufacturer's instructions (Quantikine®, R&D Systems, Minneapolis, MN). The lower limit of detection for TNF-α was 1.6 pg/mL. The average intra-assay coefficient of variation for TNF-α was 5%.

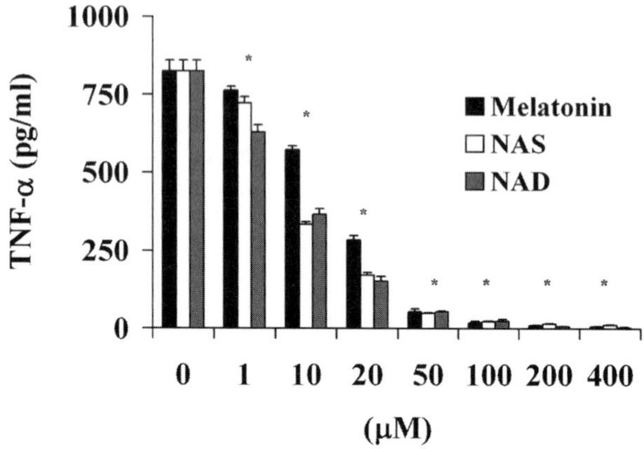

FIGURE 1. Effect of melatonin, NAS, or NAD on LPS-stimulated TNF-α production. Differentiated THP-1 cells were coincubated with LPS (10 ng/mL) and increasing concentrations of melatonin, NAS, or NAD (0–400 μM) for 24 h. Cell supernatants were assayed for TNF-α by ELISA. $*P = 0.03$ vs. control. Data are presented as mean ± SEM ($N = 6$).

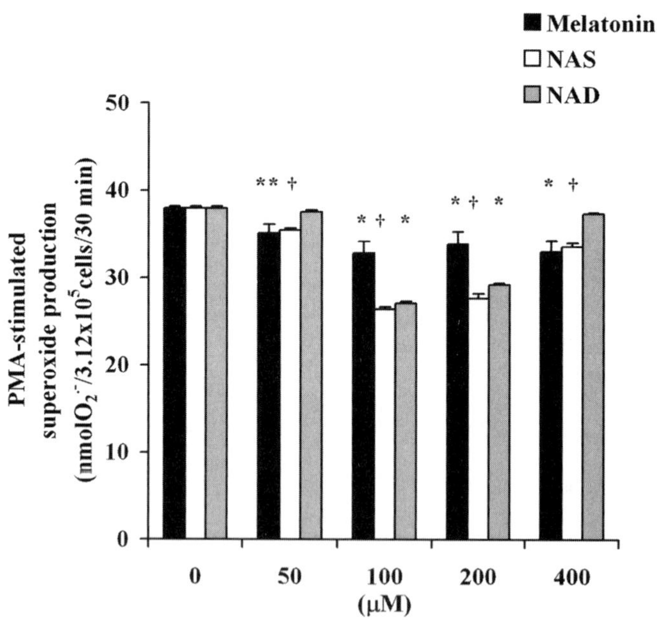

FIGURE 2. Effect of melatonin, NAS, or NAD on superoxide production by PMA-stimulated HL-60-derived neutrophils. Differentiated HL-60 cells were stimulated with PMA in the presence or absence of increasing concentrations of melatonin, NAS, or NAD (0–400 μM), superoxide dismutase, and ferri-cytochrome C for 30 min. The production of superoxide ($O_2^{\bullet -}$) by differentiated neutrophils was determined by measuring the capacity of cells to reduce ferri- to ferro-cytochrome C. $*P = 0.03$ vs. control; $**P = 0.05$ vs. control; $^{\dagger}P = 0.03$ vs. control. Data are presented as mean ± SEM ($N = 6$).

HL-60 Cell Culture

The human promyelocytic leukemia HL-60 cell line (American Type Culture Collection) was maintained in suspension culture at 0.3×10^6 cells/mL in Iscove's modified Dulbecco's medium supplemented with 2 mM L-glutamine and 20% fetal bovine serum in a humidified atmosphere of 5% CO_2 in air at 37°C. HL-60 cells were differentiated into neutrophils by the addition of 1.25% DMSO to the culture medium at 37°C in a 5% CO_2 incubator. After 5 days, cells were washed in PBS, and 1×10^6 cells were used for each experimental condition.

Superoxide Production by HL-60-Derived Neutrophils

The production of superoxide ($O_2^{\bullet-}$) by differentiated neutrophils was determined by measuring the capacity of cells to reduce ferri- to ferro-cytochrome C. In brief, cells were coincubated with increasing concentrations (0–400 μM) of melatonin, NAS, or NAD in the presence of ferri-cytochrome C (Sigma, 12.3 mg/mL), 4-β-phorbol 12-β-myristate 13-α-acetate (PMA; Sigma, 10 nM), or *N*-formyl methionyl-leucyl-phenylalanine (fMLP; Sigma, 10 μM), with or without superoxide dismutase (SOD; Sigma, 1 mg/mL). After 30-min incubation at 37°C, tubes were placed on ice and centrifuged at 14,000 rpm for 1 min. The amount of $O_2^{\bullet-}$ produced was quantified by measuring the change in spectrophotometric absorbance of the cell-free supernatant at dual wavelength (550-nm test filter with a reference wavelength of 570 nm), by using a microplate reader (MRX II; Dynatech Laboratories, Chantilly, VA). The results are expressed as nanomoles of $O_2^{\bullet-}$ produced/3.12×10^5 cells per 30 min.

Statistical Analysis

Statistical analysis was performed using the Statistical Package for Social Sciences version 10.0 (SPSS, Chicago, IL). Comparisons between groups were made by ranked nonparametric Kruskal-Wallis analysis of variance (ANOVA) or Friedman test, and two-tailed Mann-Whitney test (unpaired and paired) for continuous variables. Results are expressed as means ± standard error of the mean (SEM). Differences were considered statistically significant at $P < 0.05$.

RESULTS

Effect of Melatonin, NAS, or NAD on LPS-Stimulated TNF-α Production

Incubation of THP-1-derived monocytes with increasing concentrations of melatonin, NAS, or NAD resulted in a marked decrease in LPS-stimulated TNF-α production, which was dose-dependent. Indeed, as shown in FIGURE 1, compared with control conditions, melatonin, NAS, or NAD significantly inhibited TNF-α production by 96–98% ($P = 0.03$).

Effect of Melatonin, NAS, or NAD on PMA-Stimulated Superoxide Production

Incubation of HL-60-derived neutrophils with increasing concentrations of melatonin, NAS, or NAD resulted in a modest decrease in PMA-stimulated superoxide production, which was dose-dependent. Indeed, as shown in FIGURE 2, compared with PMA-stimulated conditions, cells treated with PMA and melatonin at 50, 100, 200, and 400 μM resulted in a 7±3% (P = 0.05), 14±4% (P = 0.03), 11±4% (P = 0.03), and 13±3% (P = 0.03) decrease in superoxide production, respectively.

Similarly, compared with PMA-stimulated conditions, cells treated with PMA and NAS at 50, 100, 200, and 400 μM resulted in a 6±1% (P = 0.03), 30±1% (P = 0.03), 27±2% (P = 0.03), and 11±1% (P = 0.03) decrease in superoxide production, respectively. Of note, compared with 100 μM NAS, 400 μM NAS resulted in a lower degree of suppression of superoxide production.

Finally, compared with PMA-stimulated conditions, cells treated with PMA and NAD at 100 and 200 μM resulted in a significant 29±1% (P = 0.03) and 23±1% (P = 0.03) decrease in superoxide production, respectively, whereas the doses of 50 and 400 μM had no impact (FIG. 2).

The maximum inhibition of superoxide production was observed with 100 μM melatonin, NAS, or NAD. However, at the 100 μM dose, NAS as well as NAD displayed a more potent inhibitory effect on superoxide production compared with melatonin.

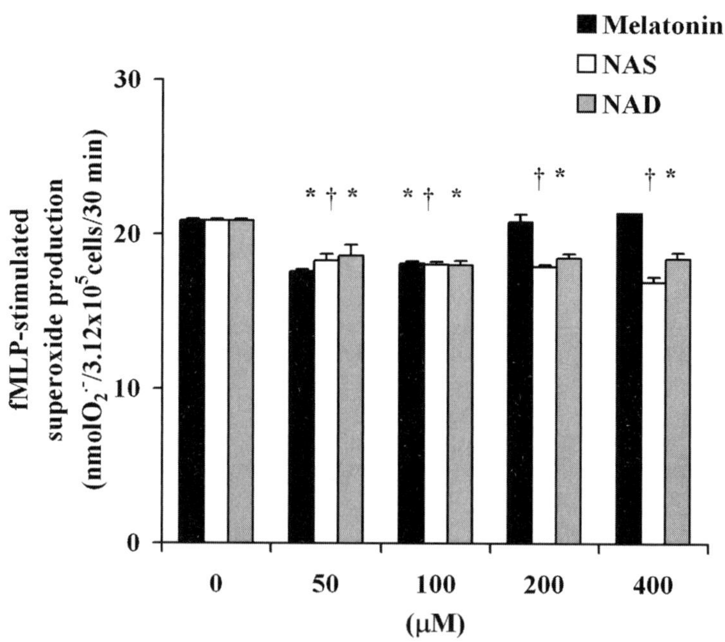

FIGURE 3. Effect of melatonin, NAS, or NAD on superoxide production by fMLP-stimulated HL-60-derived neutrophils. Differentiated HL-60 cells were stimulated with fMLP in the presence or absence of increasing concentrations of melatonin, NAS, or NAD (0–400 μM), superoxide dismutase, and ferri-cytochrome C for 30 min. The production of superoxide ($O_2^{\bullet -}$) by differentiated neutrophils was determined by measuring the capacity of cells to reduce ferri- to ferro-cytochrome C. *P = 0.03 vs. control; †P = 0.03 vs. control. Data are presented as mean ± SEM (N = 6).

Effect of Melatonin, NAS, or NAD on fMLP-Stimulated Superoxide Production

Incubation of HL-60-derived neutrophils with increasing concentrations of melatonin, NAS, or NAD resulted in a modest decrease in fMLP-stimulated superoxide production, which was dose-dependent. Indeed, as shown in FIGURE 3, compared with fMLP-stimulated conditions, cells treated with fMLP and melatonin at 50 and 100 μM resulted in a 16±1% ($P = 0.03$) and 13±1% ($P = 0.03$) decrease in superoxide production, respectively. The 200 and 400 μM doses of melatonin did not confer any additional inhibitory effect.

Similarly, compared with fMLP-stimulated conditions, fMLP and NAS–treated cells at 50, 100, 200, and 400 μM resulted in a 13±2% ($P = 0.03$), 14±1% ($P = 0.03$), 14±1% ($P = 0.03$), and 19±2% ($P = 0.03$) decrease in superoxide production, respectively (FIG. 3).

Finally, compared with fMLP-stimulated conditions, cells treated with fMLP and NAD at 50, 100, 200, and 400 μM resulted in a 11±3% ($P = 0.03$), 14±1% ($P = 0.03$), 11±2% ($P = 0.03$), and 12±2% ($P = 0.03$) decrease in superoxide production, respectively (FIG. 3).

Of note, in response to the 200 and 400 μM doses of melatonin, fMLP-stimulated cells produced more superoxide compared with the 50 and 100 μM doses. It appears that higher concentrations of melatonin are pro-oxidant, favoring superoxide anion production by HL-60-derived neutrophils.

DISCUSSION

In the present study, we demonstrated that melatonin, NAS, or NAD suppresses LPS-stimulated TNF-α synthesis by monocytic cells in a dose-dependent manner. Low-dose NAD was more potent in blocking TNF-α production compared with melatonin and NAS. In addition, melatonin, NAS, or NAD attenuated PMA- and fMLP-stimulated superoxide production in HL-60-differentiated neutrophils.

Melatonin, in addition to its hormonal function, has antioxidant activity and is protective in many *in vivo* and *in vitro* models of oxidative damage.[10] Melatonin has been shown to inhibit low-density lipoprotein oxidation,[11] and protect against experimental pulmonary damage,[12] stroke,[13] LPS-induced hepatotoxicity,[14] ethanol-induced gastroduodenal injury,[15] and viral encephalitis.[16] Our data support previous findings of the protective effect of melatonin on LPS-induced TNF-α production.

The effect of NAS on LPS-induced TNF-α production is controversial. In animal models of sepsis, NAS has been shown to attenuate the increase in plasma TNF-α levels caused by LPS.[8,9] However, *in vitro* studies have failed to demonstrate a direct effect of NAS on LPS-stimulated TNF-α production in human monocytes.[8] Our data confirm that NAS attenuates LPS-induced TNF-α production. Our study is the first to demonstrate the protective effect of NAD on LPS-induced TNF-α production.

The melatonin and NAS protective effect against LPS-stimulated TNF-α production may be mediated through inhibition of nitric oxide (NO) production. Nitric oxide is a potent endogenous vasodilator produced from L-arginine by NO synthase (NOS). Three different isoforms of NOS have been isolated, cloned, sequenced, and expressed. Under physiological conditions, the vascular endothelium expresses constitutive eNOS to release NO, which regulates blood vessels and blood pressure. Upon cytokine and LPS stimulation, an inducible form of NOS (iNOS) is expressed and produces NO, which activates macrophages. Originally, iNOS was purified and cloned from an immunoactivated macrophage cell line, whereas neuronal NOS (nNOS) was originally purified and cloned from neuronal tissues. However, nNOS is more widely distributed, with an important level of expression in skeletal muscle. NOS requires tetrahydrobiopterin (BH4) as an essential cofactor.[17] Biosynthesis of BH4 occurs from guanosine triphosphate (GTP), through the cooperation of GTP cyclohydrolase I (GTPCH), 6-pyruvoyltetrahydropterin synthase, and sepiapterin reductase (SPR).

Previous work has shown that LPS-induced oxidant stress is mediated in part by an increase in NOS activity and NO generation.[7] Melatonin, NAS, and NAD strongly suppress LPS- and iron-induced lipid peroxidation[4] (also see Oxenkrug and Requintina, this volume). Since melatonin has been shown to downregulate the expression of iNOS,[18] this hypothesis lends itself to the protective effect of the other two compounds. In addition to SPR, GTPCH activity is required for the biosynthesis of BH4. Since TNF-α is known to increase GTPCH activity,[19] inhibition of TNF-α synthesis by melatonin, NAS, or NAD also contributes to the reduction in NO generation.

Finally, in our study, all three compounds were more potent in attenuating superoxide production by a receptor-independent stimulus (PMA) compared with a receptor-mediated stimulus (fMLP). It is noteworthy that the antioxidant effects of melatonin and NAS have recently been shown to be melatonin receptor–independent (see Requintina and Oxenkrug, this volume).

In conclusion, melatonin, NAS, or NAD attenuates LPS-stimulated TNF-α production, as well as PMA- and fMLP-stimulated superoxide production. Further studies are required to determine the role of melatonin, NAS, or NAD in iNOS expression.

REFERENCES

1. Faure, E., L. Thomas, H. Xu *et al.* 2001. Bacterial lipopolysaccharide and IFN-gamma induce Toll-like receptor 2 and Toll-like receptor 4 expression in human endothelial cells: role of NF-kappaB activation. J. Immunol. **166:** 2018–2024.
2. Sewerynek, E., D. Melchiorri, L. Chen & R.J. Reiter. 1995. Melatonin reduces both basal and bacterial lipopolysaccharide-induced lipid peroxidation *in vitro*. Free Radical Biol. Med. **19:** 903–909.
3. Maestroni, G.J. 1996. Melatonin as a therapeutic agent in experimental endotoxic shock. J. Pineal Res. **20:** 84–89.
4. Requintina, P.J. & G.F. Oxenkrug. 2003. Differential effects of lipopolysaccharide on lipid peroxidation in F344N, SHR rats and BALB/c mice, and protection of melatonin and NAS against its toxicity. Ann. N.Y. Acad. Sci. **993:** 325–333.
5. Gitto, E., C. Romeo, R.J. Reiter *et al.* 2004. Melatonin reduces oxidative stress in surgical neonates. J. Pediatr. Surg. **39:** 184–189.
6. Young, I.M., R.M. Leone, P. Francis *et al.* 1985. Melatonin is metabolized to *N*-acetyl serotonin and 6-hydroxymelatonin in man. J. Clin. Endocrinol. Metab. **60:** 114–119.
7. Klemm, P., J. Ostrowski, T. Morath *et al.* 1993. *N*-Acetylserotonin prevents the hypotension induced by bacterial lipopolysaccharides in the rat. Eur. J. Pharmacol. **250:** R9–R10.
8. Sacco, S., L. Aquilini, P. Ghezzi *et al.* 1998. Mechanism of the inhibitory effect of melatonin on tumor necrosis factor production *in vivo* and *in vitro*. Eur. J. Pharmacol. **343:** 249–255.

9. Klemm, P., M. Hecker, H. Stockhausen *et al.* 1995. Inhibition by *N*-acetyl-5-hydroxytryptamine of nitric oxide synthase expression in cultured cells and in the anaesthetized rat. Br. J. Pharmacol. **115:** 1175–1181.
10. Reiter, R.J., L. Tang, J.J. Garcia & A. Munoz-Hoyos. 1997. Pharmacological action of melatonin in oxygen radical pathophysiology. Life Sci. **60:** 2255–2271.
11. Pieri, C., M. Marra, R. Gaspar & S. Damjanovich. 1996. Melatonin protects LDL from oxidation, but does not prevent the apolipoprotein derivatization. Biochem. Biophys. Res. Commun. **222:** 256–260.
12. Melchiorri, D., R.J. Reiter, A.M. Attia *et al.* 1995. Potent protective effect of melatonin on *in vivo* paraquat-induced oxidative damage in rats. Life Sci. **56:** 83–89.
13. Manev, H., C.M. Cagnoli, A. Kharlamov *et al.* 1995. *In vitro* and *in vivo* neuroprotection with melatonin against the toxicity of singlet oxygens. Soc. Neurosci. Abstr. **21:** 1518.
14. Sewerynek, E., D. Melchiorri, R.J. Reiter *et al.* 1995. Lipopolysaccharide-induced hepatotoxicity is inhibited by the antioxidant melatonin. Eur. J. Pharmacol. **293:** 327–334.
15. Melchiorri, D., E. Sewerynek, R.J. Reiter *et al.* 1997. Suppressive effect of melatonin administration on ethanol-induced gastroduodenal injury in rats *in vivo*. Br. J. Pharmacol. **121:** 264–270.
16. Ben-Nathan, D., G.J. Maestroni, S. Lustig & A. Conti, 1995. Protective effects of melatonin in mice infected with encephalitis viruses. Arch. Virol. **140:** 223–230.
17. Thony, B., G. Auerbach & N. Blau. 2000. Tetrahydrobiopterin biosynthesis, regeneration, and functions. Biochem. J. **347**(part 1)**:** 1–16.
18. Dong, W.G., Q. Mei, J.P. Yu *et al.* 2003. Effects of melatonin on the expression of iNOS and COX-2 in rat models of colitis. World J. Gastroenterol. **9**(6)**:** 1307–1311.
19. Werner, E.R., G. Werner-Felmayer, D. Fuchs *et al.* 1991. Impact of tumour necrosis factor-alpha and interferon-gamma on tetrahydrobiopterin synthesis in murine fibroblasts and macrophages. Biochem. J. **280**(part 3)**:** 709–714.

N-Acetyldopamine Inhibits Rat Brain Lipid Peroxidation Induced by Lipopolysaccharide

GREGORY F. OXENKRUG AND PURA J. REQUINTINA

Melatonin Clinic and Pineal Research Laboratory, Department of Psychiatry, Caritas St. Elizabeth's Medical Center/Tufts University School of Medicine, Boston, Massachusetts, USA

ABSTRACT: The effects of *N*-acetyldopamine, a sepiapterin reductase inhibitor, on lipopolysaccharide-induced lipid peroxidation were examined in rat brain homogenates *in vitro*. Lipid peroxidation in the form of malondialdehyde (MDA) was evaluated by the measurement of thiobarbituric acid (TBA) reactive substances. *N*-Acetyldopamine inhibited the formation of MDA in a concentration-dependent manner. The effect was similar to that of *N*-acetyl-serotonin, but stronger than that of the endogenous antioxidant agent, melatonin. Possible clinical applications of *N*-acetyldopamine and its derivatives are discussed.

KEYWORDS: *N*-acetyldopamine; *N*-acetylserotonin; sepsis; lipid peroxidation; lipopolysaccharide; malondialdehyde; brain; sepiapterin reductase

INTRODUCTION

Septic shock represents a major cause of death in intensive care units. Septic shock is characterized by hypotension, hyporeactivity to vasoconstrictor agents, inadequate tissue perfusion, vascular damage, and disseminated intravascular coagulation leading to multiple organ failure and death. Septic shock is also considered as a systematic inflammatory response caused not only by gram-negative and gram-positive bacteria, but also by noninfectious disorders such as ischemia and trauma.[1,2] Pathogenic mechanisms of septic shock involve the release of bacterial membrane component lipopolysaccharide (LPS). LPS triggers the production of the inflammatory cytokines such as tumor necrosis factor-α (TNF-α)[3] and enhances the activities of enzymes (including sepiapterin reductase) involved in the *de novo* synthesis of tetrahydrobiopterin (BH_4),[4,5] the requisite cofactor for nitric oxide synthase (NOS).[6] This could lead to the increase of inducible nitric oxide synthase (iNOS) and excessive formation of reactive oxygen species,[3] and consequently extensive oxidative damage. Melatonin, the pineal hormone, counteracted LPS toxicity in laboratory animals[7–9] and prevented lethality in patients suffering from septic shock.[10] *N*-Acetylserotonin (NAS), the immediate precursor and metabolite[11] of melatonin, protected against

Address for correspondence: Dr. Gregory Oxenkrug, Melatonin Clinic and Pineal Research Laboratory, Department of Psychiatry, Caritas St. Elizabeth's Medical Center, Boston, MA 02135. Voice: 617-636-0219; fax: 617-636-8442.
goxenkrug@tufts-nemc.org

Ann. N.Y. Acad. Sci. 1053: 394–399 (2005).
doi: 10.1196/annals.1344.034

LPS-induced hypotensive shock in rats[12] and lethal effect in mice.[9,13] The protective effect of NAS against LPS toxicity was attributed to its ability to inhibit sepiapterin reductase (SPR).[14] This study aimed to evaluate the effect of another SPR inhibitor, *N*-acetyldopamine (NADA), on LPS-induced oxidative damage in the *in vitro* model. The effect of NADA on lipid peroxidation was compared to NAS and melatonin, a powerful endogenous antioxidant.[15]

MATERIALS AND METHODS

NADA, melatonin, 2-thiobarbituric acid (TBA), and LPS (*Escherichia coli* 0127:B8) were purchased from Sigma Chemical (St. Louis, MO).

The formation of thiobarbituric substances (TBARS) was used as an index of induced oxidative damage to lipid membranes. Lipid peroxidation was induced by LPS (400 μg/mL). TBARS was measured as described elsewhere.[9] Briefly, brain tissues from untreated F344N rats were homogenized in 20 mM Tris buffer using a Tissue Tearor™ (Biospec Products, Inc.) at a ratio of 1:5 (w/v). After centrifugation, 200 μL of homogenate was then incubated for 1 h at 37°C in Tris buffer (control), Tris buffer + LPS, NADA + LPS, NAS + LPS, melatonin + LPS, or NADA + NAS + LPS (for concentrations of NADA, melatonin, and NAS, see RESULTS). TBARS was assayed by the addition of 250 μL of 1% TBA and 250 μL of 1 N HCl and incubated at 80°C in water bath for 20 min. After cooling in ice, 200 μL of acetonitrile was added and reaction mixtures were centrifuged at 10,000 rpm for 5 min. The absorbance of the organic mixture was measured at 535 nm. The concentration of malondialdehyde (MDA) in the tissue was calculated by using a standard curve prepared from the MDA standard, 1,1,3,3-tetramethoxypropane, obtained from Oxis Health Products (Portland, OR). Each sample was done in duplicate. The results were expressed as μmol MDA/mg protein and are means ± SD. Data were statistically treated by one-way ANOVA followed by individual mean comparisons using Student's *t* test.

Protein content was determined using the Lowry method using a protein kit obtained from Sigma Chemical (St. Louis, MO).

RESULTS

LPS induced a 9-fold increase of MDA levels in brain tissue. NADA inhibited LPS-induced formation of MDA in a dose-dependent manner starting from a concentration of 50 μM and reaching complete inhibition at 200 μM (FIG. 1). The effect of NAS on LPS-induced lipid peroxidation was similar to that of NADA (FIG. 2). Melatonin reached statistically significant inhibition of LPS-induced lipid peroxidation at a concentration of 800 μM (FIG. 3). Combination of NADA and NAS exerted additive effects (FIG. 4).

DISCUSSION

To the best of our knowledge, this is the first observation of the inhibiting effect of NADA on LPS-induced lipid peroxidation. The effect of NAS was similar to that

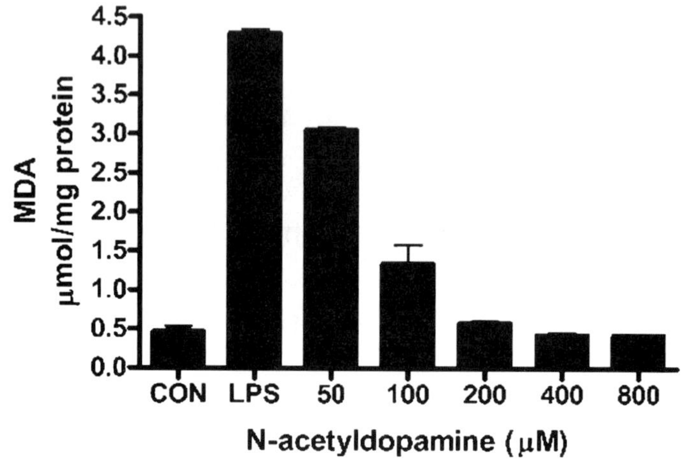

FIGURE 1. The effect of different concentrations of *N*-acetyldopamine on the level of lipid peroxidation induced by lipopolysaccharide (LPS) in rat brain tissues. Terms: MDA, malondialdehyde; CON, control (no LPS added); LPS, only lipopolysaccharide (400 μM) was added. All other groups: LPS + different concentrations of *N*-acetyldopamine. Results expressed as mean ± SD ($n = 6$). MDA level of the LPS group was higher than that in any other group ($P < 0.001$).

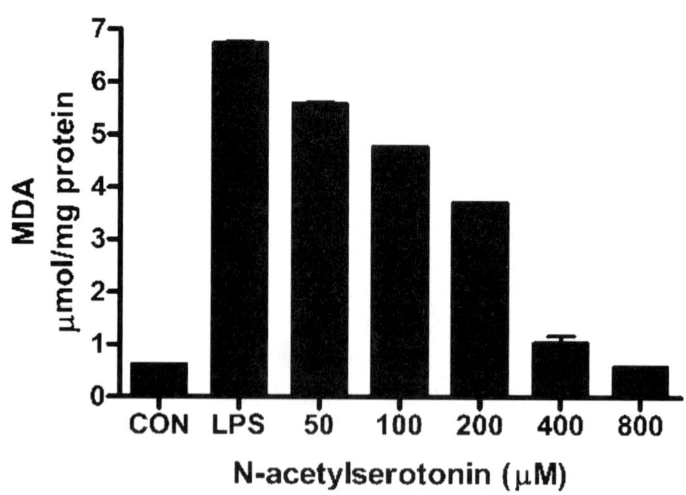

FIGURE 2. The effect of different concentrations of *N*-acetylserotonin on the level of lipid peroxidation induced by lipopolysaccharide (LPS) in rat brain tissues. Terms: MDA, malondialdehyde; CON, control (no LPS added); LPS, only lipopolysaccharide (400 μM) was added. All other groups: LPS + different concentrations of *N*-acetylserotonin. Results expressed as mean ± SD ($n = 6$). MDA level of the LPS group was higher than that in any other group ($P < 0.001$).

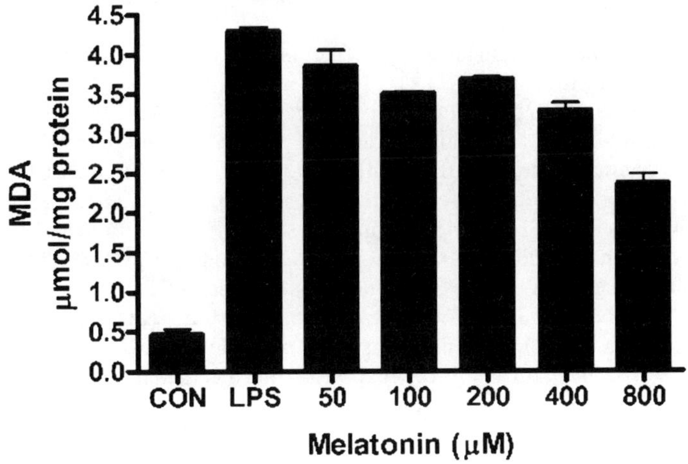

FIGURE 3. The effect of different concentrations of melatonin on the level of lipid peroxidation induced by lipopolysaccharide (LPS) in rat brain tissues. Terms: MDA, malondialdehyde; CON, control (no LPS added); LPS, only lipopolysaccharide (400 μM) was added. All other groups: LPS + different concentrations of melatonin. Results expressed as mean ± SD ($n = 6$). MDA level of the LPS + melatonin (800 μM) group was significantly different from that of any other group ($P < 0.001$).

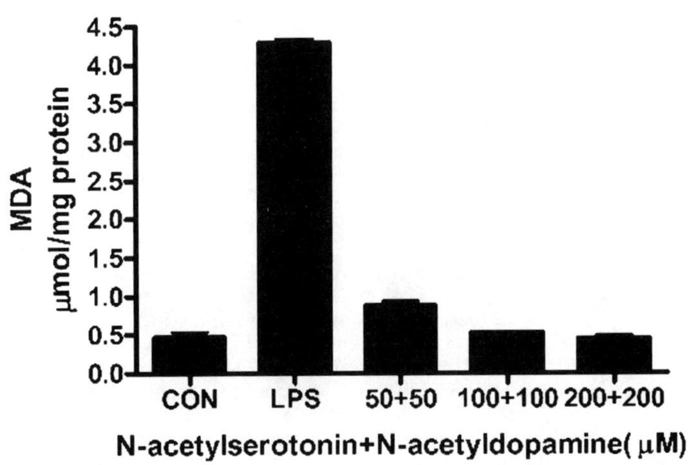

FIGURE 4. The effect of combination of NAS and NADA on the level of lipid peroxidation induced by lipopolysaccharide (LPS) in rat brain tissues. Terms: MDA, malondialdehyde; CON, control (no LPS added); LPS, only lipopolysaccharide (400 μM) was added. All other groups: LPS + NAS and NADA. Results expressed as mean ± SD ($n = 6$). MDA level of the LPS-only group was significantly different from that of any other group ($P < 0.001$).

of NADA, and the inhibiting effects of both NADA and NAS were much stronger than that of melatonin. The effect of melatonin was in the same range as described in the literature.[7] The mechanism of this effect is not clear. It is noteworthy that K_i values for SPR inhibition by NADA and NAS are very close (0.12 and 0.17 μM, respectively), while the K_i for melatonin is much higher (25 μM).[16,17] Since we have observed the similar pattern for inhibition of LPS-induced lipid peroxidation in rat brain tissues, one might suggest that inhibition of SPR might be one of the factors responsible for the protective effect of tested compounds against LPS. Therefore, NADA derivatives with SPR-inhibiting qualities, that is, *N*-chloroacetyldopamine, *N*-acetyl-*m*-tyramine,[17] and *N*-acetyl-3-*O*-methyldopamine (NAMDA),[18] might also provide protection against LPS toxicity. Indeed, blockade of BH_4 using NAMDA has been shown to be beneficial in protecting neurons after transient forebrain ischemia in rats.[18] However, some iNOS inhibitors were not able to prevent the hepatotoxic effects of LPS.[19] Thus, further investigation of the mechanisms of the protective effect of NADA against LPS is warranted.

NADA plays an important role in insect physiology.[20] Although it has been also discovered in human liver,[21] kidney, and urine,[22] and it is being synthesized in human platelets,[23] its role in mammal physiology is not clear. Studies to evaluate the effect of NADA *in vivo* are scarce. It was previously reported that NADA showed significant antitumor activity in experimental L1210 and P388 leukemias in mice.[24] Possible clinical application of NADA, besides the treatment of septic shock and systemic inflammatory response syndrome, might be for some other conditions associated with oxidative damage such as carcinogenesis, mutation, degenerative disorders (Parkinson's and Alzheimer's disorders), toxic effects of chemotherapy and radiation therapy, demyelination disorders (multiple sclerosis),[25] severe burns,[26] and psychoses,[27] and as an antiaging intervention.[28,29]

REFERENCES

1. TRACEY, K.J. & A. CERAMI. 1994. Tumor necrosis factor: a pleiotropic cytokine and therapeutic target. Annu. Rev. Med. **45:** 491–503.
2. REYNOLDS, F.D., R. DAUCHY, D. BLASK *et al.* 2003. The pineal gland hormone melatonin improves survival in a rat model of sepsis shock induced by zymosan A. Surgery **134:** 474–479.
3. FAURE, E., L. THOMAS, H. XU *et al.* 2001. Bacterial lipopolysaccharide and IFN-gamma induce Toll-like receptor 2 and Toll-like receptor 4 expression in human endothelial cells: role of NF-kappaB activation. J. Immunol. **166:** 2018–2024.
4. MORI, K., A. NAKASHIMA, T. NAGATSU & A. OTA. 1997. Effect of lipopolysaccharide on the gene expression of the enzymes involved in tetrahydrobiopterin *de novo* biosynthesis in murine neuroblastoma cell line N1E-115. Neurosci. Lett. **238:** 21–24.
5. FUJIWARA, K., K. MORI *et al.* 2004 Tetrahydrobiopterin biosynthesis in white and brown adipose tissues is enhanced following intraperitoneal administration of bacterial lipopolysaccharide. Biochim. Biophys. Acta Gen. Subj. **1670:** 181–198.
6. THONY, B., G. AUERBACH & N. BLAU. 2000. Tetrahydrobiopterin biosynthesis, regeneration, and functions. Biochem. J. **347:** 1–16.
7. SEWERYNEK, E., D. MELCHIORRI, L. CHEN & R.J. REITER. 1995. Melatonin reduces both basal and bacterial lipopolysaccharide-induced lipid peroxidation *in vitro*. Free Radical Biol. Med. **19:** 903–909.
8. MAESTRONI, G.J.M. 1996. Melatonin as a therapeutic agent in experimental endotoxic shock. J. Pineal Res. **20:** 84–89.

9. REQUINTINA, P.J. & G.F. OXENKRUG. 2003. Differential effects of lipopolysaccharide on lipid peroxidation in F344N, SHR rats and BALB/c mice, and protection of melatonin and NAS against its toxicity. Ann. N.Y. Acad. Sci. **993:** 325–333.
10. GITTO, E., C. ROMEO, R.J. REITER *et al.* 2004. Melatonin reduces oxidative stress in surgical neonates. J. Pediatr. Surg. **39:** 184–189.
11. YOUNG, I.M., R.M. LEONE, P. FRANCIS *et al.* 1985. Melatonin is metabolized to *N*-acetyl serotonin and 6-hydroxymelatonin in man. J. Clin. Endocrinol. Metab. **60:** 114–119.
12. KLEMM, P., J. OSTROWSKI, T. MORATH *et al.* 1993. *N*-Acetylserotonin prevents the hypotension induced by bacterial lipopolysaccharides in the rat. Eur. J. Pharmacol. **250:** R9–R10.
13. SACCO, S., L. AQUILINI, P. GHEZZI *et al.* 1998. Mechanism of the inhibitory effect of melatonin on tumor necrosis factor production *in vivo* and *in vitro*. Eur. J. Pharmacol. **343:** 249–255.
14. KLEMM, P., M. HECKER, H. STOCKHAUSEN *et al.* 1995. Inhibition by *N*-acetyl-5-hydroxy-tryptamine of nitric oxide synthase expression in cultured cells and in the anaesthetized rat. Br. J. Pharmacol. **115:** 1175–1181.
15. REITER, R.J., D.X. TAN & S. BURKHARDT. 2002. Reactive oxygen and nitrogen species and cellular and organismal decline: amelioration with melatonin. Mech. Ageing Dev. **123:** 1007–1019.
16. KATOH, S., T. SUEOKA, & S. YAMADA. 1982. Direct inhibition of brain sepiapterine reductase by catecholamine and indoleamine. Biochem. Biophys. Res. Commun. **105:** 75–81.
17. SMITH, G.K., D.S. DUCH, M.P. EDELSTEIN & E.C. BIGHAM. 1992. New inhibitors of sepiapterine reductase: lack of an effect of intracellular tetrahydrobiopterin depletion upon *in vitro* proliferation of two human cell lines. J. Biol. Chem. **267:** 5599–5607.
18. CHO, S., B.T. VOLPE *et al.* 1999. Blockade of tetrahydrobiopterin synthesis protects neurons after transient forebrain ischemia in rat: a novel role for the cofactor. J. Neurosci. **19:** 878–889.
19. SAKAGUCHI, S., S. FURISAWA, K. YOKOTA *et al.* 2000. Effect of nitric oxide synthase inhibitors on lipid peroxide formation in liver caused by endotoxin challenge. Pharmacol. Toxicol. **86:** 162–168.
20. SASAKI, K. & T. NAGAO. 2001. Distribution and levels of dopamine and its metabolites in brains of reproductive workers in honeybees. J. Insect Physiol. **47:** 1205–1216.
21. KHOO, B.Y., K.H. SIT & K.P. WONG. 1990. Sulphate conjugation in human liver: direct measurement of *N*-acetyldopamine-sulphate. Biochem. Pharmacol. **40:** 1021–1026.
22. ELCHISAK, M.A. & E.A. HAUSNER. 1984. Demonstration of *N*-acetyldopamine in human kidney and urine. Life Sci. **35:** 2561–2569.
23. KHOO, B.Y., K.H. SIT & K.P. WONG. 1988. The human platelet as an independent unit for sulfate conjugation. Life Sci. **42:** 1165–1171.
24. WICK, M.M. & A. MUI. 1981. Synthesis and biologic evaluation of the dopamine analog *N*-acetyldopamine in experimental leukemia in mice. J. Natl. Cancer Inst. **66:** 351–354.
25. KOHEN, R. & A. NYSKA. 2002. Oxidation of biological systems: oxidative stress phenomena, antioxidants, redox reactions, and methods for their quantification. Toxicol. Pathol. **30:** 620–650.
26. DAVIS, K.A., J.M. SANTANIELLO, L.K. HE *et al.* 2004. Burn injury and pulmonary sepsis: development of a clinically relevant model. J. Trauma **56:** 272–278.
27. ROSENBERGER, T.A., N.E. VILLACRESES, J.T. HOVDA *et al.* 2004. Rat brain arachidonic acid metabolism is increased by a 6-day intracerebral ventricular infusion of bacterial lipopolysaccharide. J. Neurochem. **88:** 1168–1178.
28. OXENKRUG, G.F. 2003. Anti-aging effect of (–)deprenyl and inhibition of lipid peroxidation by *N*-acetylserotonin and mating. *In* Monoamine Oxidase Inhibitors and Their Role in Neurotransmission (Drug Development), pp. 307–317. Medicina. Budapest.
29. OXENKRUG, G., P.J. REQUINTINA & S. BACHURIN. 2001. Antioxidant and antiaging activity of *N*-acetylserotonin and melatonin in the *in vivo* models. Ann. N.Y. Acad. Sci. **939:** 190–199.

The *In Vitro* Effect of Estradiol and Testosterone on Iron-Induced Lipid Peroxidation in Rat Brain and Kidney Tissues

PURA J. REQUINTINA AND GREGORY F. OXENKRUG

Melatonin Clinic and Pineal Research Laboratory, Department of Psychiatry, Tufts University School of Medicine, Boston, Massachusetts, USA

ABSTRACT: The effects of estradiol and testosterone on iron-induced lipid peroxidation were compared in rat brain and kidney homogenates *in vitro*. Lipid peroxidation in the form of malondialdehyde (MDA) was evaluated by the measurement of thiobarbituric acid (TBA) reactive substances. Estradiol inhibited lipid peroxidation in both tissues studied in a dose-dependent manner. The effect was five times stronger in brain than in kidney. Testosterone did not affect lipid peroxidation in either tissue. Estradiol-induced inhibition of brain lipid peroxidation might contribute to the neuroprotective effect of estrogens.

KEYWORDS: estradiol; testosterone; brain; kidney; lipid peroxidation

INTRODUCTION

Beyond the key role in reproductive and cognitive functions, estrogens have been shown to protect against neurodegeneration associated with acute and chronic injuries of the adult brain. Estrogens were reported to inhibit lipid peroxidation in brain tissues.[1,2] However, some data suggested an *in vivo* pro-oxidant effect of estrogens in estrogen-induced kidney carcinogenesis in hamsters.[3] The data on the antioxidant effect of testosterone have also been controversial. While some researchers reported increased lipid peroxidation in rabbit testes after chronic testosterone treatment,[4] and in aorta walls of rats in *in vivo* and *in vitro* experiments,[5] there have also been data indicating the protective effect of testosterone against oxidative alcohol- and paracetamol-induced liver damage.[6] Since the effect of estrogens on lipid peroxidation appeared to be organ-specific, the present study aimed to compare the effects of estradiol and testosterone on iron-induced lipid peroxidation in rat central (brain) and peripheral (kidney) tissues *in vitro*.

Address for correspondence: Dr. Pura J. Requintina, Melatonin Clinic and Pineal Research Laboratory, Department of Psychiatry, Caritas St. Elizabeth's Medical Center, Boston, MA 02135. Voice: 617-789-3374; fax: 617-789-2066.
requintina@cox.net

Ann. N.Y. Acad. Sci. 1053: 400–404 (2005).
doi: 10.1196/annals.1344.035

MATERIALS AND METHODS

Brain and kidney tissues were collected from Fischer 344N male rats, 100–150 g body weight, obtained from Charles River (Wilmington, MA). The tissues were frozen in dry ice and kept at −70°C until analyses.

Estradiol, testosterone, Tris, 2-thiobarbituric acid (TBA), $FeCl_2$, ascorbic acid, and acetonitrile were purchased from Sigma Chemical (St. Louis, MO). The formation of thiobarbituric substances (TBARS) was used as an index of induced oxidative damage to lipid membranes. TBARS was measured as described elsewhere.[7] Briefly, tissues (brain and kidney) from untreated F344N rats were homogenized in 20 mM Tris buffer using a Tissue Tearor™ (Biospec Products, Inc.) at a ratio of 1:5 (w/v). After centrifugation, 200 μL of homogenate was then incubated for 1 h at 37°C in Tris buffer (control) or with estradiol or testosterone added (10–800 μM). Iron-induced peroxidation was induced by adding 25 μL of 1 mM $FeCl_2$ and 25 μL of 1 mM ascorbic acid to 200 mL of tissue homogenate. TBARS was assayed by the addition of 250 μL of 1% TBA and 250 μL of 1 N HCl followed by incubation in an 80°C water bath for 20 min. After cooling in ice, 200 μL of acetonitrile was added and reaction mixtures were centrifuged at 10,000 rpm for 5 min. The absorbance of the organic mixture was measured at 535 nm. The concentration of malondialdehyde (MDA) in the tissue was calculated by using a standard curve prepared from the MDA standard, 1,1,3,3-tetramethoxypropane, obtained from Oxis Health Products (Portland, OR). Protein content was determined by the Lowry method using a protein kit obtained from Sigma Chemical (St. Louis, MO). Each sample was done in duplicate. Results were expressed as μmol MDA/mg protein and are mean ± SD. Data were statistically evaluated by one-way ANOVA followed by individual mean comparisons using Student's *t* test.

RESULTS

Estradiol suppressed lipid peroxidation in both brain and kidney tissues in a dose-dependent manner. However, the effect was more pronounced in brain than in kidney. The effective starting concentration of estradiol in brain (FIG. 1) was 10 μM, while in kidney it was 50 μM (FIG. 2).

Testosterone did not affect lipid peroxidation in both tissues (FIG. 3).

DISCUSSION

Our results indicated that estradiol was much more effective against lipid peroxidation in brain than in kidney tissue, while testosterone was not effective in either tissue studied. Our data are in good agreement with the previously reported observation of 70% inhibition of lipid peroxidation in brain by 10 μM estradiol.[1] Several studies have reported on the neuroprotective effect of estrogen. Estrogen treatment attenuates the molecular signals of apoptosis in ethanol-withdrawn rats, thereby decreasing the associated behavioral deficits.[8] Estrogen was also neuroprotective against middle cerebral artery occlusion–induced cell death in adult rats,[9] and it reduced brain injury in neonatal rats.[10]

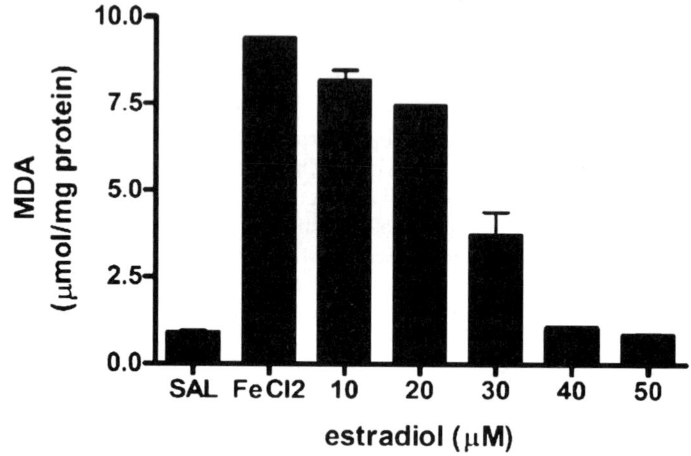

FIGURE 1. The effect of different concentrations of estradiol on lipid peroxidation induced by $FeCl_2$ in rat brain tissues. Terms: MDA, malondialdehyde; SAL, saline control (no $FeCl_2$ added); $FeCl_2$, only $FeCl_2$ was added. All other groups: $FeCl_2$ + different concentrations of estrogen. Results expressed as mean ± SD ($n = 6$). MDA level of the $FeCl_2$ group was higher than in any other group ($P < 0.001$).

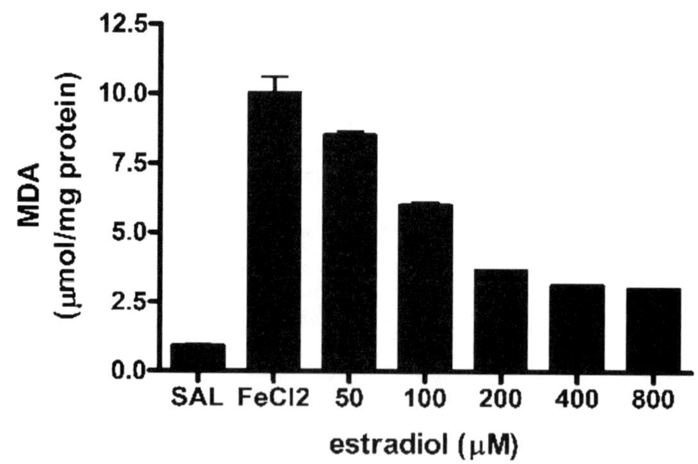

FIGURE 2. The effect of different concentrations of estradiol on lipid peroxidation induced by $FeCl_2$ in rat kidney tissues. Terms: MDA, malondialdehyde; SAL, saline control (no $FeCl_2$ added); $FeCl_2$, only $FeCl_2$ was added. All other groups: $FeCl_2$ + different concentrations of estrogen. Results expressed as mean ± SD ($n = 6$). MDA level of the $FeCl_2$ group was higher than in any other group ($P < 0.001$).

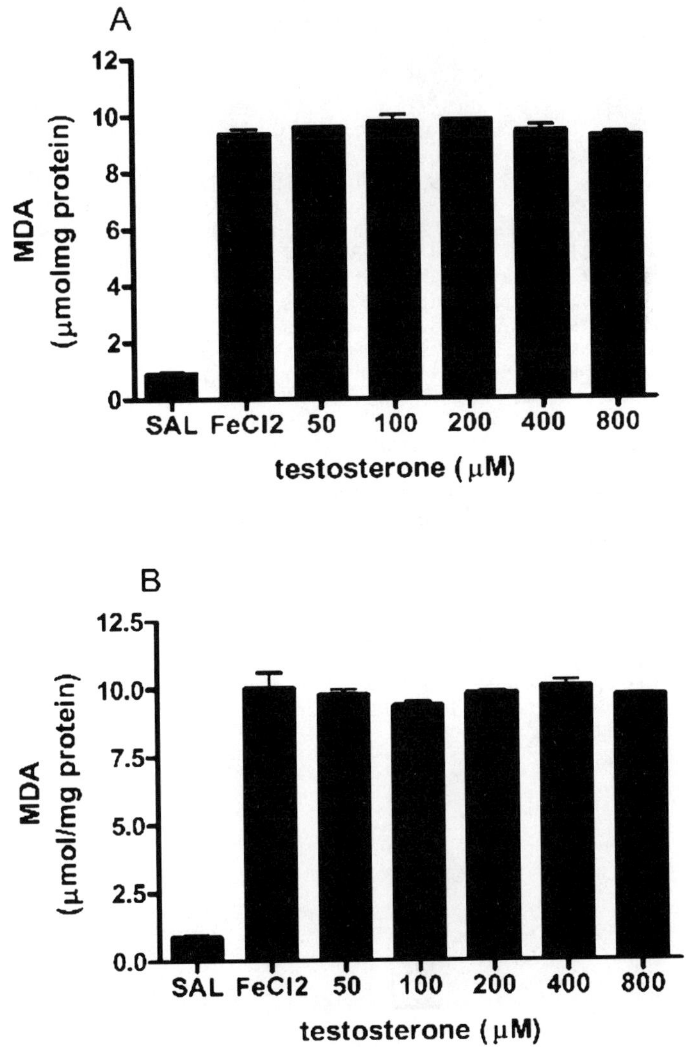

FIGURE 3. The effect of different concentrations of testosterone on lipid peroxidation induced by $FeCl_2$ in rat **(A)** brain and **(B)** kidney tissues. Terms: MDA, malondialdehyde; SAL, saline control (no $FeCl_2$ added); $FeCl_2$, only $FeCl_2$ was added. All other groups: $FeCl_2$ + different concentrations of testosterone. Results expressed as mean ± SD ($n = 6$). No significant difference between the MDA level of the $FeCl_2$ group and any other group.

The present study, showing the pronounced effectiveness of estradiol in inhibiting brain lipid peroxidation, adds to the growing body of evidence indicating that this capability might contribute to the neuroprotective effect of estrogens. Since most studies were done in the *in vitro* model, more *in vivo* studies should be performed to elucidate the effect of estrogens (and testosterone) on lipid peroxidation. These studies are important in considering whether hormone replacement therapy is beneficial for postmenopausal women.

REFERENCES

1. Vedder, H., N. Anthes, G. Stumm *et al.* 1999. Estrogen hormones reduce lipid peroxidation in cells and tissues of the central nervous system. J. Neurochem. **72:** 2531–2538.
2. Jung, M.E., M. Rewal *et al.* 2004. Estrogen protects against lipid peroxidation in ethanol-withdrawn rats. Pharmacol. Biochem. Behav. **79:** 573–586.
3. Wang, M.Y. & J.G. Liehr. 1995. Induction by estrogens of lipid peroxidation and lipid peroxide–derived malonaldehyde-DNA adducts in male Syrian hamsters: role of lipid peroxidation in estrogen-induced kidney carcinogenesis. Carcinogenesis **16:** 1941–1945.
4. Aydilek, N., M. Aksakal & A.Z. Karakilcik. 2004. Effects of testosterone and vitamin E on the antioxidant system in rabbit testis. Andrologia **36:** 277–281.
5. Karachentsev, A.N. & I.A. Mel'chenko. 1997. Effect of sex hormones on lipid peroxidation in the rat aorta. Eksp. Klin. Farmakol. **60:** 13–16. [In Russian.]
6. Jaya, D.S., J. Augstine & V.P. Menon. 1995. Protective effect of testosterone against alcohol and paracetamol induced hepatotoxicity in rats. Indian J. Exp. Biol. **33:** 194–200.
7. Kohen, R. & A. Nyska. 2002. Oxidation of biological systems: oxidative stress phenomena, antioxidants, redox reactions, and methods of their quantifications. Toxicol. Pathol. **30:** 620–650.
8. Jung, M.E., M.B. Gatch & J.W. Simpkins. 2005. Estrogen neuroprotection against the neurotoxic effects of ethanol withdrawal: potential mechanisms. Exp. Biol. Med. **230:** 8–22.
9. Rau, S.W., D.B. Dubal *et al.* 2003. Estradiol attenuates programmed cell death after stroke-like injury. J. Neurosci. **23:** 11420–11426.
10. Feng, Y., J.D. Fratkins & M.H. LeBlanc. 2005. Estrogen attenuates hypoxic-ischemic brain injury in neonatal rats. Eur. J. Pharmacol. **507:** 77–86.

Questions and Answers

Session VIII: Mechanisms of Neuroprotection (2)

QUESTIONS FOR STEPHEN SKAPER

From Chia-Yi Kuan

What is the dose response of the dimeric N-cadherin binding motif peptide in stimulating neurite outgrowth? Could it be possible that this peptide at low dose serves as a bridge to stimulate neurite outgrowth, whereas at high dose it may saturate all potential binding sites and block neurite outgrowth?

ANSWER: The neuroprotective effect of the N-cadherin dimeric peptide agonist is observed over a concentration range that is similar to that inducing neuritogenesis. Even higher concentrations (>30 μg/mL) of the HAVDI agonist peptide may cause a modest reduction in the level of neurite outgrowth, which could be due to saturation of binding sites, although such inhibition was not seen for neuronal cell survival. While a saturation effect for neurite outgrowth cannot be excluded, this is not possible to address for technical reasons.

From Philip Lazarovici

The only model that you favor for the N-CAM active domain synthetic peptide neurite outgrowth/survival effect is by coupling to FGF receptors. Can you indicate the evidence for this?

ANSWER: Four lines of evidence suggest that an interaction with N-cadherin is required for the neurite outgrowth response stimulated by the dimeric HAVDI peptide. First, the response to peptide is inhibited by monomeric mimetics of the corresponding motif, and these have previously been established to function as specific N-cadherin antagonists. Second, the recombinant extracellular domain 1 (ECD1) protein of N-cadherin inhibits the agonist peptide responses, suggesting that they share a common cellular binding site. Given the molar ratio of the peptides to the soluble ECD1 protein (~300:1), we can conclude that ECD1 competes for peptide binding to a cellular site as opposed to acting as a soluble sink for the peptides in solution. Third, the neurite outgrowth response to agonist peptide is inhibited by a monovalent F(ab′) fraction of an antiserum that reacts specifically with a small motif in ECD4 of N-cadherin. This reagent inhibits the neurite outgrowth response stimulated by native N-cadherin in the absence of any effect on neurite outgrowth stimulated by a range of other molecules. Fourth, neurite outgrowth stimulated by native N-cadherin requires FGF receptor function in the neuron. We have shown that a highly specific FGF receptor antagonist (PD173074) inhibits the agonist peptide responses. Likewise, the neuroprotective effects of the peptide agonist were inhibited by a monomeric version of the same motif and by PD173074, and were not mimicked by the linear peptide.

Ann. N.Y. Acad. Sci. 1053: 405–406 (2005). © 2005 New York Academy of Sciences.
doi: 10.1196/annals.1344.067

QUESTION FOR SILVIA MANDEL AND ORLY WEINREB

From Syed Ali

In your last slide, you summarized the whole cascade in which you suggest that nitric oxide/peroxynitrite and superoxide are responsible for dopaminergic neurotoxicity. What if you used a powerful antioxidant that can block the generation of ON/ONOO/O? Can it be used as a neuroprotective agent instead of targeting specific genes along the pathway as shown by Orly Weinreb? Are 1.5-fold changes large enough to produce Parkinson's disease (PD) or dopaminergic neurotoxicity?

ANSWER: So far, only vitamin E has been examined clinically in studies in PD as an antioxidant. The results have been negative. It is possible that a powerful antioxidant would be neuroprotective. However, our gene expression studies in the MPTP model of PD and substantia nigra of PD brains have shown a cascade of events in the neurodegenerative process, indicating that a single neuroprotective drug may not be sufficient to induce neuroprotection. The 1.5 threshold was set initially to filter as many nonspecific gene changes as possible, but the results were further analyzed based on the biologic processes and molecular pathways that the genes take part in. The most relevant gene alterations are being currently corroborated by immunohistochemistry.

QUESTION FOR ORLY WEINRAB

From Philip Lazarovici

I would like to caution you regarding rasagiline's upregulation effect on the "PKC isoform" gene, which may be interpreted as a tumor formation effect? This aspect requires special attention!

ANSWER: Increased expressions of PKCα and ε have consistently been shown to have a protective effect, while those of PKCδ and γ induce cell death. In our hands, rasagiline upregulates PKCα and ε and downregulates γ *in vitro*, where rasagiline protects PC12 cells from death induced by serum withdrawal. We have not observed any tumor formation in chronic studies with rasagiline in cell culture and *in vivo* studies with mice or rats. We believe that the activation of PKC may be one reason why rasagiline has a neurorescue activity when given chronically after lessening of the dopamine neurons by MPTP in mice (Sagi *et al.*, submitted), and neuroprotective activity in PC12 cells, where PKC inhibitor prevents its neuroprotective activity (Weiner *et al.*, 2004).

Neuroprotective Effects of Neurotrophins and Melanocortins in Spinal Cord Injury

An Experimental Study in the Rat Using Pharmacological and Morphological Approaches

HARI SHANKER SHARMA

Laboratory of Cerebrovascular Research, Department of Surgical Sciences, Anesthesiology, and Intensive Care Medicine, University Hospital, Uppsala University, SE-75185 Uppsala, Sweden

ABSTRACT: Spinal cord injury (SCI) induces lifetime disability, and no suitable therapy is available to treat victims or to minimze their sufferings. Recently, neurotrophins and compounds acting at melanocortin receptors have been been identified as potential neuroprotective agents. In this investigation, the neuroprotective effects of neurotrophins and melanocortins on the pathophysiology of SCI were examined in a rat model. The SCI was produced by making a longitudinal incision into the right dorsal horn of the T10–11 segments under equithesin anesthesia. In separate groups, neurotrophins [BDNF or IGF-1 (0.1–1 μg/10 μL in saline)] or melanocortins (ME10092, ME10354, ME10393, ME10431, and ME10501, having affinities to melanocortin receptors; 1–10 μg in saline) were applied topically over the traumatized cord segment within 5–10 min after SCI and the rats were allowed to survive for 5 h. A focal SCI resulted in widespread disruption of the blood–spinal cord barrier (BSCB) to Evans blue albumin (EBA), $^{[131]}$iodine, or lanthanum tracers and exhibited profound edema formation and cell or tissue destruction. Topical application of BDNF, IGF-1, or ME10501 (having high affinity to melanocortin-4 receptor, MCR-4) in high quantity markedly attenuated BSCB disruption, edema formation, and nerve cell, glial cell, and axonal injuries. On the other hand, low doses of neurotrophins or melanocortins were not effective in attenuating pathophysiology of SCI. These observations suggest that neurotrophins (BDNF and IGF-1) and melanocortins (with high affinity to MCR-4) are capable of inducing neuroprotection if applied shortly after trauma in high doses. Taken together, the results indicate that neurotrophins and melanocortins participate in the pathophysiology of spinal cord cell and tissue injury following trauma.

KEYWORDS: spinal cord injury; melanocortins; brain-derived neurotrophic factor; insulin-like growth factor-1; blood–spinal cord barrier; neuroprotection

Address for correspondence: Hari Shanker Sharma, Dr. Med. Sci., Laboratory of Cerebrovascular Research, Department of Surgical Sciences, Anesthesiology, and Intensive Care Medicine, University Hospital, Uppsala University, SE-75185 Uppsala, Sweden. Voice: +46-18-611-9208; fax: +46-18-55-93-57.
sharma@surgsci.uu.se

Ann. N.Y. Acad. Sci. 1053: 407–421 (2005).
doi: 10.1196/annals.1344.036

INTRODUCTION

Spinal cord injury (SCI) is a serious clinical problem that imposes huge responsibility and costs on society.[1–3] The prevalence of SCI is about 30 to 50 cases per million population per year in the United States, which is quite comparable to Europe and other continents.[1] Most cases of SCI are due to motor vehicle accidents, followed by falls, penetrating injuries like gunshots or knife wounds, and sports injuries.[1,2] The symptoms of SCI include quadruplegia causing paralysis of the upper and lower extremities, followed by paraplegia involving only the lower extremity.[3] About half of the patients with cord trauma have complete injuries without any signs of voluntary motor or sensory perception below the level of the lesion.[1,3] The victims of cord trauma are mainly young men in their early 20s to 30s.[2] Thus, efforts should be made to improve the quality of life of the young victims and to reduce the clinical burden in society. To date, no suitable therapy for the victims of SCI is available. Hence, new therapeutic strategies with the possibility of regeneration of the lesioned spinal cord axons are needed to improve the quality of life of patients with SCI.

The term "neuroprotection" is commonly used to denote rescue of nerve cells.[4] However, in the central nervous system (CNS), the nonneural cells, that is, glial cells and endothelial cells, are equally important for brain function and actively participate in the secondary injury process.[5] The number of nonneural cells far exceeds the number of neural cells in the CNS. Thus, the involvement of glial cells and endothelial cells in the secondary injury process following SCI requires further attention.

One of the early consequences of SCI includes alterations in the fluid microenvironment, caused by breakdown of the blood–spinal cord barrier (BSCB) permeability.[1,3] The BSCB resides within the endothelial cells of the microvessels of the spinal cord that are connected with tight junctions (FIG. 1A, a). The spinal cord microvessels are surrounded by astrocytic end feet that cover more than 85% of their surface (FIG. 1A, a). In normal conditions, the BSCB strictly regulates the spinal cord fluid microenvironment.[1,3,5] However, following SCI, a breakdown of the BSCB will allow entry of serum proteins into the spinal cord fluid microenvironment, leading to vasogenic edema formation and cell injury.[1–3] Several neurochemical mediators and injury-related factors participating in the secondary injury cascade are involved in BSCB disturbances and play important roles in long-term cell and tissue injury.[5,6] Thus, efforts should be made to attenuate BSCB dysfunction and the secondary injury cascades to reduce cell injury and to minimize functional disability.

Another approach to enhance functional recovery after SCI is to promote neuroregeneration (cf. refs. 1, 3, and 7). One way to enhance spinal cord regeneration is to use neurotrophins and related compounds.[1,2,7,8] Neurotrophins are a family of growth factors consisting of nerve growth factor (NGF), brain-derived neurotrophic factor (BDNF), insulin-like growth factor (IGF), neurotrophin-3 (NT-3), and neurotrophin-4/5 (NT-4/5).[3,7,8] The other growth factors include glial-derived neurotrophic factor (GDNF), ciliary neurotrophic factor (CNTF), and transforming growth factor-β (TGF-β).[1,3,4,8,9] Exogenous administration of NT-3, NGF, and BDNF increases axonal sprouting following bilateral transection in the spinal cord of adult rats, indicating that neurotrophins influence regeneration of the lesioned neurons in the spinal cord.[1,3,7,8] Most of these studies largely deal with regeneration of axons within the spinal cord. Thus, the influence of neurotrophins on restoration of sensory and motor function as well as structural changes in the spinal cord requires further investigation.

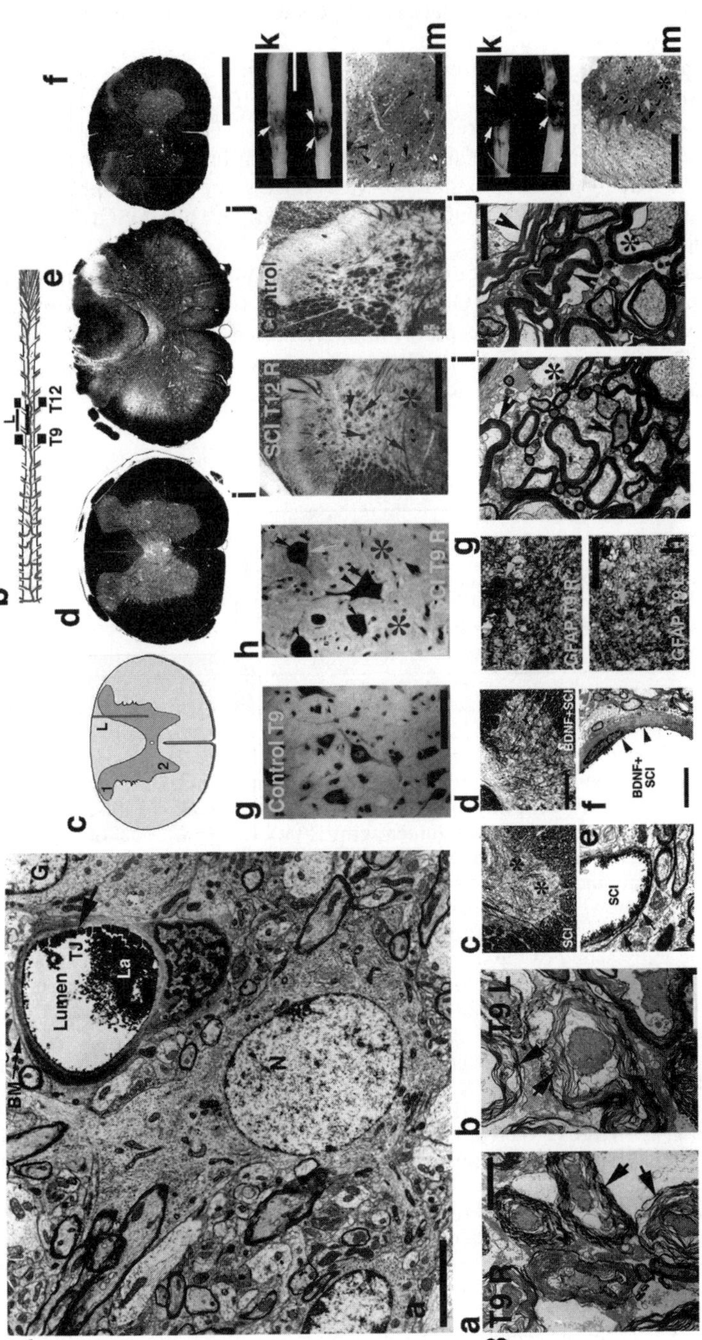

FIGURE 1. *See following page for legend.*

Apart from neurotrophins, melanocortin peptides such as α-melanocyte stimulating hormone (α-MSH) and adrenocorticotropin (ACTH) or its fragments exert trophic effects and influence functional recovery following peripheral nerve lesion and cortical brain damage through receptor-mediated effects.[10,11] Several melanocortin receptors, for example, MSH receptor (MC1-R), ACTH receptor (MC2-R), MC3-R, MC4-R, and MC5-R, have been identified in the rat brain and spinal cord.[12] These multiple melanocortin receptors and α-MSH have some neurotrophic and/or neuroprotective effects in brain damage.[10,11] However, their role in SCI-induced cell and tissue injuries is still unclear.

To understand the role of neurotrophins and melanocortins in the pathophysiology of SCI, the effects of BDNF, IGF-1, and melanocortins (having varying affinity and selectivity to melanocortin receptors) were examined in the present investigation on trauma-induced alterations in BSCB permeability, edema formation, and cell or tissue injuries in a rat model.

FIGURE 1. [A] (a) Low-power electron micrograph of the rat spinal cord showing structure of the blood–spinal cord barrier (BSCB). The endothelial cells are connected with tight junctions (TJ, *arrow*) and are surrounded by a thick basement membrane (BM). The glial cells (G) and the astrocytic processes around the microvessel are apparent. A nerve cell (N) in close proximity with the endothelial cell is clearly seen. The electron dense tracer lanthanum (La) is confined into the lumen (bar: 1 μm). **(b)** New model of spinal cord injury (SCI) that comprises a focal incision (L) into the right dorsal horn of the T10–11 segments. Tissue pieces from the adjacent T9 and T12 are taken for investigation. **(c)** Cross section of the spinal cord shows that the deepest part of the lesion (L) is limited to Rexed's laminae VII and VIII, leaving white matters largely intact. Arabic numerals represent the areas used for electron microscopy of the dorsal horn (bars: 5 μm, b; 2 μm, c). **(d–f)** Toluidine blue–stained, 1-μm-thick, Epon-embedded spinal cord sections from the T9 segment of a control (d), 5-h spinal cord injured (e), and BDNF-treated injured (f) rat. Paraffin-embedded, 3-μm-thick sections stained with Nissl **(g, h)**, myelin basic protein (MBP) **(i, j)**, or hematoxylin and eosin **(m)**. SCI induced marked nerve cell damage **(h)** and loss of MBP immunostaining **(i)** compared to respective controls **(g, j)**. Treatment with ME10501 reduced gross pathological changes in the cord after 5-h SCI **(k)** and cell changes in the ventral horn of the T9 segment (m). Bars: (g, h) 30 μm; (i, j) 90 μm; (k) 3 μm; (m) 150 μm. **[B] (a, b)** Ultrastructural changes in myelin in the ipsi- (a) and contralateral (b) spinal cord following 5-h SCI. BDNF **(i)** or IGF-1 **(j)** considerably attenuated SCI-induced myelin damage. Extravasation of lanthanum across the BSCB **(e)** is prevented by BDNF treatment **(f)**. MBP immunostaining and axonal damage are also considerably reduced by BDNF **(d)** compared to untreated SCI **(c)**. Activation of astrocytes as seen using glial fibrillary acidic protein (GFAP) immunoreactivity is most pronounced in the ipsilateral side **(g)** compared to the contralateral half **(h)** of the T9 spinal cord segment after 5-h SCI. At this time, pathology of the spinal cord shows visual swelling, hemorrhage, and edema **(k)**, as well as damage to motoneurons **(m)**. Bars: (a, b) 1 μm; (c, d) 100 μm; (e, f) 2 μm; (g, h) 60 μm; (i, j) 1.5 μm; (k) 3 μm; (m) 150 μm. [Data modified after various sources: refs. 1, 2, 6, 16, 17, 19, 21, and 22.]

TABLE 1. A comparison of facts between clinical and experimental SCI

Clinical SCI	Experimental SCI
(1) Multifactorial: flexion, extension, rotation, compression, concussion, contusion, laceration	Simple: weight-drop, incision,[a] compression, transection, hemisection, electrolytic lesion
(2) Complex forces are active at the time of injury	Only one injury factor is present
(3) Closed vertebral system injury	Open vertebral system injury after laminectomy
(4) Usually anterior compression	Mainly posterior compression
(5) Mainly occurs during conscious state	Produced under anesthesia
(6) Unlimited or uncontrolled time interval between injury and firsthand hospital examination	Carefully controlled time schedule
(7) No two SCI cases are similar	Identical SCI can be produced

NOTE: Compiled from various sources (for review, see refs. 1, 2, 6, and 8). For details, see text.
[a]From author's own investigation.

MATERIALS AND METHODS

Animals

Experiments were carried out on 145 male Wistar rats (200–250 g body weight; age: 15–18 weeks) under equithesin anesthesia (3 mL/kg, ip) and according to the guidelines of the National Institutes of Health (NIH) and the Local Committee of Care for Experimental Animals (Uppsala, Sweden).

New Model of SCI

The human cases of SCI are impossible to simulate by any experimental animal model (see TABLE 1).[1,3] Thus, human SCI usually represents an anterior cord compression or damage in conscious state within the closed vertebral system,[8] whereas SCI in animal models is always produced on the posterior side of the cord in anesthetized conditions after laminectomy.[1,3] In addition, human SCI results from several forces of flexion, extension, rotation, and compression at the same time or in combination, whereas only one force is used to induce trauma in animal models.[1,3,8] Fracture of vertebral column or luxation of vertebrae causes concussion, contusion, or laceration of the spinal cord in humans, while these factors are absent in animal models due to laminectomy.[8] Due to the complex nature of human SCI, no two clinical cases are similar.[13]

The existing animal models of SCI comprise weight-drop technique, controlled contusion, and maintained compression (cf. refs. 1 and 3). Studies on SCI-induced repair mechanisms are normally examined following partial to complete transection or hemisection of the cord.[7,8,14,15] However, each method has its own advantages and drawbacks.

We developed an incision model of SCI that has several advantages over the existing animal models. In this model, one segment laminectomy was done on the T10–11 segment to expose the spinal cord. A trauma to the cord was made by making an incision into the right dorsal horn of the T10–11 segments using a scalpel blade.[16,17] The deepest part of the lesion was close to lamina VII–VIII.[16] This experimental condition was approved by the Ethical Committee of Uppsala University (Uppsala, Sweden).

This method of SCI allows reproducible lesions to the axons and fiber tracts of the cord, leaving white matter largely intact (cf. refs. 16–18). The unique advantage of the method is the possibility to study the morphological changes in the ipsi- and contralateral side of the cord in the segments located in the vicinity of the lesion site in the rostral and caudal directions (FIG. 1). The normal animals served as intact controls since previous experiments from the laboratory showed no changes in BSCB permeability, edema formation, and cell injury in the sham group.[1–3]

Treatment with Neurotrophins and Melanocortins

To understand the role of neurotrophins and melanocortins in the pathophysiology of SCI, we examined the effects of BDNF and IGF-1 as well as several low-molecular-weight, nonpeptide compounds with varying affinity and selectivity to the melanocortin receptors on BSCB permeability, edema formation, and cell injury in our rat model.[17,19]

In separate groups of animals, BDNF ($n = 5$) or IGF-I ($n = 5$) (0.1–1 μg in 10 μL phosphate buffer saline) was applied topically at 5, 10, or 30 min after SCI (see FIG. 1). All animals were allowed to survive for 5 h after the SCI.[1,17] Another group of rats were treated with five selected compounds with various affinities to melanocortin receptors (ME10092, ME10354, ME10393, ME10431, or ME10501 in saline). The compounds were applied topically (1, 5, and 10 μg) over the spinal cord for 5 min after SCI, and the rats were allowed to survive for 5 h.[1,19] The untreated traumatized animals were used as controls.

Parameters Measured

BSCB Permeability

BSCB permeability was examined using either Evans blue and/or $^{[131]}$I-sodium in the perifocal T9 and T12 segments.[17,20] The intravascular tracer was washed out by a brief saline rinse through the heart.[20] Tissue pieces from T9, T10–11, and T12 were dissected out, weighed immediately, and counted in a 3-inch-well type gamma counter (energy window: 500–800 keV). After counting the radioactivity, tissue samples were processed for Evans blue measurement using colorimetric techniques.[17,20]

Histopathology of the Spinal Cord

After SCI, the animals were perfused with Somogyi fixative[1,6] and the spinal cord was taken out, photographed for visual swelling, and processed for histological evaluation using standard protocol.[16,17,19] About 3-μm-thick paraffin sections were cut from the T9 and/or T12 segment, stained with hematoxylin and eosin, or Nissl, and examined under a light microscope. Occurrence of sponginess, edema, cell

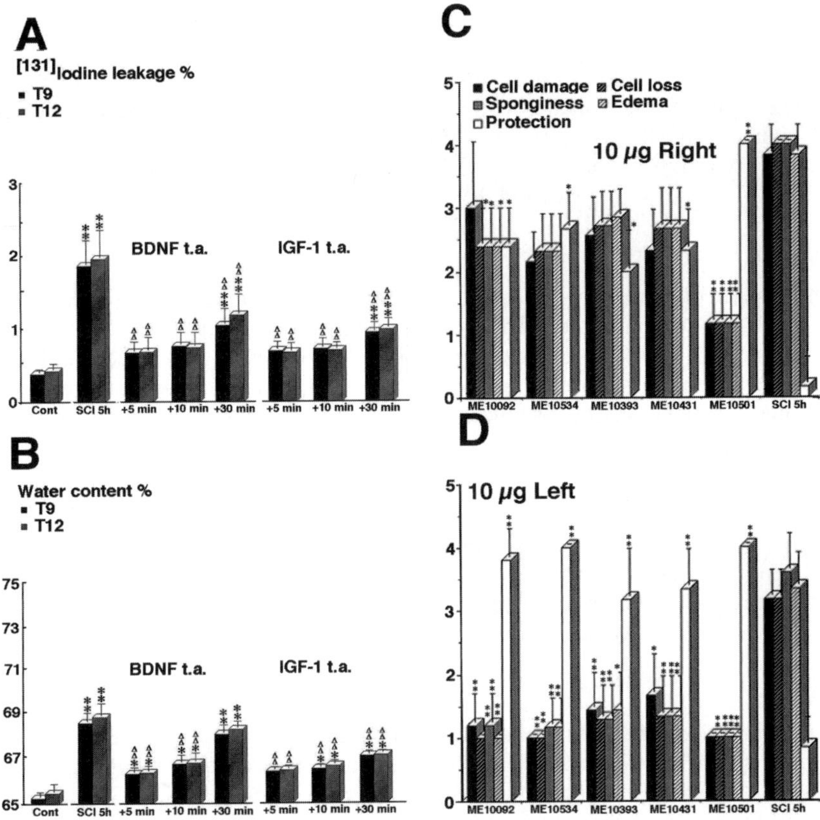

FIGURE 2. Changes in BSCB permeability to radioiodine **(A)** and water content **(B)** following 5-h SCI in T9 and T12 segments and their modifications with BDNF or IGF-1. Semiquantitative analysis of morphological changes following SCI and their modification with five melanocortin compounds in the ipsilateral (*right*) **(C)** or contralateral (*left*) **(D)** T9 segment of the cord. The incision was made on the T10–11 segment of the right dorsal horn (for details, see text). Neurotrophins are able to induce the most pronounced reduction in BSCB permeability and edema formation when applied within 5 to 10 min after SCI (A, B). (C, D) Effect of melanocortins on morphological changes in the T9 segment of the cord after 5-h SCI. The compound ME10501 in high dose (10 μg) was able to induce significant neuroprotection in the ipsilateral side of the cord (C) compared to other compounds. On the other hand, almost all melanocortin compounds in high doses (10 μg) were able to induce considerable neuroprotection in the contralateral side of the cord (D). Values are the mean ± SD of 5–6 rats at each time point. (A, B) $*P < 0.05$, $*P < 0.01$ compared to control (Cont); $^{\Delta\Delta}P < 0.01$ compared to 5-h SCI; ANOVA followed by Dunnett's test from one control group. (C, D) $*P < 0.05$; $**P < 0.01$; chi-square test from 5-h SCI. [Data modified after various sources: refs. 1, 3, 7, and 19.]

injury, cell loss, and/or cell death was examined in a blinded fashion. For each parameter in each individual animal, a rough score of 1 (least) to 4 (maximum) was assigned (FIG. 2) for semiquantitative analysis.[19]

Edema Formation

The spinal cord edema formation was examined by measuring alterations in the cord water content. The spinal cord T9 and T12 segments after SCI were dissected out, weighed immediately, and placed in an oven maintained at 90°C for 72 h to obtain the dry weight of the samples.[16] The water content of the cord was calculated from the differences in the wet and dry weights as described earlier.[20]

Lanthanum Extravasation

The passage of tracer transfer across the BSCB was examined using extravasation of lanthanum.[20] Animals were perfused with fixative containing lanthanum: lanthanum chloride (2.5%).[16,20] Lanthanum is an electron dense tracer seen as black particle within the lumen at the ultrastructural level. Thus, its passage across the endothelial cell can easily be visualized by electron microscopy (for details, see refs. 17 and 20).

Astrocytic Reaction

Activation of astrocytes was examined using glial fibrillary acidic protein (GFAP) immunoreactivity on 3-μm-thick paraffin sections obtained from the T9 or T12 segments using standard protocol.[21] Alterations in perivascular astrocytes were also examined at the ultrastructural level.[1,3,21]

Axonal Damage

The axonal damage was assessed using myelin basic protein (MBP) immunostaining on paraffin-embedded 3-μm-thick sections obtained from the T9 segment of the cord as described earlier.[22] Vesiculation of myelin was examined at the ultrastructural level using standard transmission electron microscopy.[22]

Statistical Analysis of the Data

ANOVA followed by Dunnett's test was applied to evaluate statistical significance of the data obtained for quantitative measurement of BSCB permeability and edema formation. The morphological scores were compared using nonparametric chi-square test.

RESULTS

Effect of Neurotrophins and Melanocortins on Visual Swelling

Five hours of SCI resulted in marked visual swelling, microhemorrhages, and edema around the lesioned site (FIG. 1B, k). Topical application of neurotrophins in high dose (1 μg) (BDNF or IGF-1) considerably attenuated the occurrence of gross visual swelling when applied within 10 min (but not 30 min) after injury without influencing microhemorrhages (results not shown). Topical application of ME10501 given after 5-min injury in high dose (10 μg) resulted in much less edema, distortion of the injured tissue, and microhemorrhages around the lesion site (FIG. 1A, k), whereas only a mild or no effect on visual swelling and spinal cord edema were observed with other melanocortin compounds (ME10092, ME10354, ME10393, or ME1043) (results not shown).

Effect of Neurotrophins and Melanocortins on BSCB Permeability

A focal SCI resulted in profound extravasation of Evans blue and radioiodine (FIG. 2A). Neurotrophins in high doses significantly attenuated BSCB permeability to Evans blue and iodine tracers when administered within 10 min after SCI in high doses (FIG. 2A). The lower dosages of the neurotrophins or their administration after 30-min SCI was not very effective in reducing the BSCB breakdown (results not shown). A marked reduction in extravasation of Evans blue was noted in the spinal cord following trauma in ME10501-treated rats at high dose (TABLE 2). Lower doses of the compound or other melanocortin agents were not effective in reducing Evans blue leakage after SCI (TABLE 2).

Effect of Neurotrophins and Melanocortins on Edema Formation

Profound increase in spinal cord water content occurred in rats subjected to 5-h SCI (FIG. 2B). Topical application of BDNF, IGF-1 (FIG. 2B), and ME10501 (FIGS. 2C and 2D) in high doses within 5 to 10 min significantly attenuated the SCI-induced increase in spinal cord water content in the T9 and T12 segments (FIG. 2, TABLE 2). Lower doses of the compounds or their administration after 30-min SCI did not reduce spinal cord water content significantly (results not shown).

Effect of Neurotrophins and Melanocortins on Morphological Changes

A focal trauma to rat spinal cord induces marked structural changes that can be visualized by light and electron microscopy (FIG. 1). General expansion of the spinal

TABLE 2. Effect of ME10501 on cord water content and BSCB permeability following SCI in rats

Experimental type	n	Spinal cord water %		Evans blue mg %	
		T9	T12	T9	T12
Control	6	65.46 ± 0.22	65.59 ± 0.15	0.28 ± 0.02	0.28 ± 0.03
SCI 5 h	5	68.23 ± 0.31[a]	68.63 ± 0.38[a]	1.15 ± 0.10[a]	1.18 ± 0.15[a]
ME10501 10 μg + SCI	6	66.27 ± 0.46[b,c]	66.09 ± 0.21[b,c]	0.56 ± 0.06[b,c]	0.64 ± 0.08[b,c]
ME10501 5 μg + SCI	6	66.99 ± 0.15[a,c]	66.98 ± 0.31[a,c]	0.76 ± 0.01[a,c]	0.81 ± 0.04[a,c]

NOTE: The compounds were applied topically on the injured spinal cord at 5 min after injury (for details, see text). Values are the mean ± SD; [a]$P < 0.01$, [b]$P < 0.05$, significantly different from control; [c]$P < 0.05$, significantly different from SCI; ANOVA followed by Dunnett's test for multiple group comparison. [Modified after ref. 19.]

cord, sponginess, and edema are quite prominent in untreated injured rats (FIG. 1A, e) compared to controls (FIG. 1A, d). Fine structure of the spinal cord showed profound damage to nerve cells (FIG. 1A, h; FIG. 1B, m), activation of astrocytes (FIG. 1B, g and h), and loss of myelin (FIG. 1A, i) compared to the control group (FIG. 1A, g and j; FIG. 1B, c). The neurotrophins BDNF or IGF-1 in high doses when applied within 10 min after SCI significantly reduced SCI-induced general expansion, edema (FIG. 1A, f), and cell injury (FIG. 1B, d). The spinal cord nerve cells were normal in appearance, and damage to the glial cells or myelin was less pronounced (FIG. 1B, d). This effect of neurotrophins was most pronounced in the contralateral side compared to the ipsilateral half (results not shown).

Topical application of ME10501 (10 μg) at 5 min after injury markedly reduced visual swelling, microhemorrhages, and edema in the spinal cord (FIG. 1A, k). At the light microscopic level, the compound was able to thwart nerve cell damage (FIG. 1A, m) compared to the untreated group (FIG. 1B, k and m). A significant reduction in cell damage, cell loss, and sponginess in the T9 segment of the cord was seen (FIGS. 2C and 2D). This effect of ME10501 is equally pronounced in both right and left sides of the cord (FIGS. 2C and 2D). However, low doses of ME10501 did not exhibit significant neuroprotection (results not shown).

The other melanocortin compounds (ME10092, ME10354, ME10393, and ME10431) at high doses (10 μg) are able to show a moderate degree of neuroprotection in the contralateral cord (FIGS. 2C and 2D). However, these compounds were not effective in reducing cell changes or edema formation in the ipsilateral cord (FIG. 2C) except ME10393, which showed mild neuroprotection at the 5-μg dose in both sides of the cord (results not shown). Low doses of compounds ME10092, ME10354, and ME10393 (1 μg) did not induce any significant neuroprotective effect in the injured side. However, a mild degree of neuroprotection is seen by these compounds in the contralateral cord (results not shown).

Activation of Astrocytes

SCI induced massive upregulation of GFAP in the spinal cord segments. The intensity of GFAP activation was most pronounced in the ipsilateral side (FIG. 1B, g) compared to the contralateral cord (FIG. 1B, h). Application of BDNF or IGF-1 in high doses within 10 min after SCI markedly reduced the activation of GFAP in the spinal cord. This effect was most pronounced in the contralateral side of the cord. Low doses of neurotrophins or their application after 30-min SCI was not effective in reducing GFAP expression in the cord (unpublished observation).

Axonal Injuries

Axonal injuries as seen by myelin damage are frequent in untreated spinal cord–injured animals. Thus, loss of MBP is apparent in spinal cord dorsal and ventral horns (FIG. 1A, j; FIG. 1B, c). At the ultrastructural level, myelin vesiculation is seen in the T9 and T12 segments. The magnitude of myelin injury is most severe in the ipsilateral cord (FIG. 1B, a) compared to the contralateral side (FIG. 1B, b). Treatment with BDNF or IGF-1 in high doses within 10 min after SCI attenuated MBP degradation in the cord and axonal injuries (FIG. 1). At the ultrastructural level, vesiculation of myelin and damage to the axons were considerably reduced in neurotrophin-treated injured animals (FIG. 1). Application of either low doses of BDNF and IGF-1 within 10 min or high doses of the compounds after 30 min was ineffective in reducing MBP degradation and axonal injuries.

Endothelial Cell Membrane Permeability

A focal SCI in rats resulted in extravasation of lanthanum across the endothelial cell (FIG. 1B, e). Lanthanum can be seen within the basement membrane as well as in the endothelial cell cytoplasm (FIG. 1B, e). Topical application of BDNF or IGF-1 when administered in high doses within 10 min after SCI prevented the lanthanum extravasation across the endothelial cells in the spinal cord T9 and T12 segments. In the treated group, lanthanum tracer was mainly confined within the lumen (FIG. 1B, f).

DISCUSSION

The present study shows that topical application of neurotrophins BDNF or IGF-1 and melanocortins with affinity to MCR-4 ME10501 on the traumatized spinal cord induces marked neuroprotective effects. This effect of growth factors and melanocortin compounds appears to be dose-dependent. The most pronounced neuroprotective of these compounds is observed when they are applied over the traumatized cord within 10 min after injury. This indicates that neurotrophins and melanocortins participate in the early consequences of cellular and molecular events during SCI. Thus, in clinical settings, it would be possible to apply neurotrophins or melanocortins at the site of injury to delay or reduce the consequences of spinal cord pathology in trauma victims, a subject that requires additional investigation.

A focal trauma to the cord upregulates nitric oxide synthase (NOS) expression[23] (see also ref. 24, in this volume). Peripheral axotomy induces NOS upregulation in the spinal cord motoneurons.[25] This is significantly reduced with BDNF pretreatment, which is in line with this observation.[26] Activation of NOS results in nitric oxide (NO) production (see ref. 27). NO is a free radical gas and has the capacity to induce membrane disruption and cell injury (see refs. 27 and 28). NO is also associated with neurotoxicity in cells via NMDA receptor activation and influx of Ca^{2+} (see refs. 27 and 28). Previous studies from our laboratory have shown that pretreatment with BDNF or IGF-1 prevented the SCI-induced NOS upregulation around the lesion site.[29,30] This suggests that blockade of NOS expression by neurotrophins could be one of the important mechanisms of neuroprotection in SCI. This assumption gets further support from our previous data that show significant neuroprotection in this model of SCI following blockade of nNOS expression after trauma.[3,7,27]

The melanocortins such as α-MSH and ACTH or its fragments exert trophic effects.[10–13,31] Several melanocortin receptors, for example, MSH receptor (MC1-R), ACTH receptor (MC2-R), MC3-R, MC4-R, and MC5-R, have recently been identified in the brain and spinal cord.[10–13] Local administration of ACTH4–10 and α-MSH after the chemical lesion in nucleus accumbens or in the septal regions accelerates functional recovery in rats.[31] It appears that melanocortins acting through its several receptors can induce similar trophic effects. Since melanocortins are also able to influence NO production (cf. ref. 13), there are reasons to believe that neuroprotection achieved by the compounds having varying affinities to melanocortin receptors are working through NO-mediated pathways. However, further studies using NOS immunohistochemistry in melanocortin-treated injured spinal cords are needed to confirm this hypothesis.

The compound ME10501 appears to be most potent in reducing spinal cord pathophysiology in the present investigation. This compound has very high affinity to MCR-4 receptors. This indicates that the affinity and specificity of compounds to melanocortin receptors are important factors in determining neuroprotection. The strong neuroprotective effects of the MCR-4 agonist ME10501 in SCI further suggest a possible involvement of MC4-R expression in spinal cord pathology that requires additional investigation. MCR-4 is present in the spinal cord and the dorsal root ganglia in rats.[13] An upregulation of spinal melanocortin receptors occurs in a rat model of neuropathic pain that is blocked by drugs influencing MCR-4 (cf. ref. 32). An upregulation of MC4-R mRNA is also seen in the striatum of the non-injured hemisphere following ischemia.[13] These observations suggest that MC4-R is involved in the pathophysiology of CNS injuries, and drugs influencing MCR-4 have new therapeutic potentials in brain or spinal cord trauma. Our studies are thus in close agreement with previous studies showing neurological and functional recovery following SCI or sciatic nerve lesion in rats with α-MSH and related peptides.

Consequences of the BSCB Breakdown in SCI

Topical application of neurotrophins and melanocortins reduced the visual swelling of traumatized cord, indicating that these compounds are able to attenuate edema formation in traumatized cord. Edema formation within the brain or spinal cord following ischemia or trauma is one of the leading causes of cell and tissue injury.[1–3] Accumulation of edema fluid into the extracellular or intracellular compartments within the cord initiates a series of cellular and molecular changes that lead to cell injury and cell death.[5,7,9,13,16,17] Thus, a reduction in edema formation by neurotrophins and melanocortins suggests that these compounds are influencing either the accumulation of edema fluid within the cord microenvironment or attenuating edema-induced cell injury, a feature that requires further investigation. This effect of the compounds appears to be related with their ability to reduce the breakdown of the BSCB to protein tracers, for example, Evans blue albumin and radioiodine. A reduction in BSCB permeability attenuates leakage of plasma proteins and thus likely reduces vasogenic edema formation. This idea gets further support from the data showing a significant reduction in the spinal cord water content in the drug-treated groups (see refs. 1 and 3). Obviously, fewer disturbances in the fluid microenvironment of the spinal cord following trauma will help to reduce cell and tissue injury.

Cell Injury and SCI

The motoneurons and other neuronal populations in the spinal cord are important targets of neurotrophins and melanocortins[1,3] (see refs. 7 and 17). Thus, exogenous supplement of BDNF may induce receptor-mediated effects in the traumatized spinal cord, leading to neuroprotection. Likewise, spinal cord is very rich in IGF, and SCI reduces the IGF content,[7,30] depriving neurons of trophic support and resulting in atrophy or cell death. Exogenous supplement of IGF-1 thus rescues the nerve cells from damage after SCI, resulting in neuroprotection.

Topical application of neurotrophins and melanocortins can gain access within the spinal cord tissue in a short duration. Serotonin or neuronal NOS antisera after their topical application over the spinal cord following injury are able to neutralize their tissue antigens *in vivo* and can prevent the trauma induction of serotonin or neuronal NOS upregulation, respectively, which is in line with this idea.[23,33]

Neurotrophins and melanocortins are able to influence the intracellular cascade following trauma by modifying signal transduction and Ca^{2+} permeability.[1,3,6,17,34,35] Another possibility of neuroprotection caused by neurotrophins and melanocortins is to attenuate the intensity of trauma-induced cellular or oxidative stress (see ref. 17). Less cellular or tissue stress following trauma will result in neuroprotection by reduction in the secondary injury cascades and attenuation in apoptoic and/or necrotic cell deaths, a feature that requires additional investigation.

CONCLUSIONS

In conclusion, the present study provides new experimental evidence regarding involvement of neurotrophins and melanocortins in the early phase of secondary injury cascades following SCI. Exogenous supplement of BDNF or IGF-1 as well as activation of MCR-4 receptors with melanocortins is neuroprotective in SCI. The beneficial effects of these compounds can be observed when they are applied within 10 min after SCI in high concentrations. This would indicate that neurotrophins or melanocortins can be applied on the injury site in trauma victims in clinical situations to thwart or delay the consequences of secondary injury cascades. Reductions in trauma-induced BSCB permeability and edema formation appear to be key events in attenuating cell and tissue injury by these drugs.

ACKNOWLEDGMENTS

This investigation is supported by grants from the Swedish Medical Research Council (2710), Stockholm, Sweden; Melacure Therapeutics, Uppsala, Sweden; Acure Pharma, Uppsala, Sweden; University Grants Commission, New Delhi, India; Medical Research Council, New Delhi, India; and the Alexander von Humboldt Foundation, Bonn, Germany. Critical reading of the manuscript by Anna Skottner and Torbjörn Lundstedt; technical assistance of Inga Hörte, Kärstin Flink, and Katja Deparade; and secretarial assistance of Aruna Sharma are highly appreciated.

REFERENCES

1. SHARMA, H.S. 2005. Pathophysiology of blood–spinal cord barrier in traumatic injury and repair. Curr. Pharm. Des. **11:** 1353–1389.
2. STÅLBERG, E., H.S. SHARMA & Y. OLSSON, Eds. 1998. Spinal Cord Monitoring: Basic Principles, Regeneration, Pathophysiology, and Clinical Aspects. Springer. Wien/New York.
3. SHARMA, H.S. 2004. Pathophysiology of the blood–spinal cord barrier in traumatic injury. *In* The Blood–Spinal Cord and Brain Barriers in Health and Disease, pp. 437–518. Elsevier Academic. San Diego.
4. SHARMA, H.S. 2004. Editorial. Int. J. Neuroprotec. Neuroregen. **1:** 8.
5. SHARMA, H.S. & J. WESTMAN, Eds. 2004. The Blood–Spinal Cord and Brain Barriers in Health and Disease. Elsevier Academic. San Diego.

6. WINKLER, T., H.S. SHARMA, E. STÅLBERG & J. WESTMAN. 1998. Spinal cord bioelectrical activity, edema, and cell injury following a focal trauma to the spinal cord: an experimental study using pharmacological and morphological approach. *In* Spinal Cord Monitoring: Basic Principles, Regeneration, Pathophysiology and Clinical Aspects, pp. 281–348. Springer. Wien/New York.
7. SHARMA, H.S., F. NYBERG, T. GORDH *et al.* 1998. Neurotrophic factors attenuate neuronal nitric oxide synthase upregulation, microvascular permeability disturbances, edema formation, and cell injury in the spinal cord following trauma. *In* Spinal Cord Monitoring: Basic Principles, Regeneration, Pathophysiology and Clinical Aspects, pp. 118–148. Springer. Wien/New York.
8. SCHWAB, M.E. & D. BARTHOLDI. 1996. Degeneration and regeneration of axons in the lesioned spinal cord. Physiol. Rev. **76:** 319–370.
9. BARDE, Y.A. 1994. Neurotrophins: a family of proteins supporting the survival of neurons. Prog. Clin. Biol. Res. **390:** 45–56.
10. VAN DER KRAAN, M., J.B. TATRO, M.L. ENTWISTLE *et al.* 1999. Expression of melanocortin receptors and pro-opiomelanocortin in the rat spinal cord in relation to neurotrophic effects of melanocortins. Mol. Brain Res. **63:** 276–286.
11. VAN DE MEENT, H., F.P. HAMERS, A.J. LANKHORST *et al.* 1997. Beneficial effects of the melanocortin alpha-melanocyte stimulating hormone on clinical and neurophysiological recovery after experimental spinal cord injury. Neurosurgery **40:** 122–130.
12. MOUNTJOY, K.G., L.S. ROBBINS, M.T. MORTRUD & R.D. CONE. 1992. The cloning of a family of genes that encode the melanocortin receptors. Science **257:** 543–546.
13. KAKULAS, B. 2004. Neuropathology: the foundation for new treatments in spinal cord injury. Spinal Cord **42:** 549–563.
14. IANNOTTI, C., Y. PING ZHANG, C.B. SHIELDS *et al.* 2004. A neuroprotective role of glial cell line–derived neurotrophic factor following moderate spinal cord contusion injury. Exp. Neurol. **189:** 317–332.
15. LU, P., H. YANG, L.L. JONES *et al.* 2004. Combinatorial therapy with neurotrophins and cAMP promotes axonal regeneration beyond sites of spinal cord injury. J. Neurosci. **24:** 6402–6409.
16. SHARMA, H.S. & Y. OLSSON. 1990. Edema formation and cellular alterations following spinal cord injury in rat and their modification with *p*-chlorophenylalanine. Acta Neuropathol. (Berlin) **79:** 604–610.
17. SHARMA, H.S. 2003. Neurotrophic factors attenuate microvascular permeability disturbances and axonal injury following trauma to the rat spinal cord. Acta Neurochir. (Wien) Suppl. **86:** 383–388.
18. SHARMA, H.S., T. WINKLER, E. STÅLBERG *et al.* 1991. Evaluation of traumatic spinal cord edema using evoked potentials recorded from the spinal epidural space: an experimental study in the rat. J. Neurol. Sci. **102:** 150–162.
19. SHARMA, H.S., T. LUNDSTEDT, M. FLÄRDH *et al.* 2003. Low molecular weight compounds with affinity to melanocortin receptors exert neuroprotection in spinal cord injury: an experimental study in the rat. Acta Neurochir. (Wien) Suppl. **86:** 399–405.
20. SHARMA, H.S., Y. OLSSON, S. PEARSSON & F. NYBERG. 1995. Trauma induced opening of the blood–spinal cord barrier is reduced by indomethacin, an inhibitor of prostaglandin synthesis: experimental observations in the rat using ^{131}I-sodium, Evans blue, and lanthanum as tracers. Restor. Neurol. Neurosci. **7:** 207–215.
21. SHARMA, H.S., Y. OLSSON & J. CERVÓS-NAVARRO. 1993. *p*-Chlorophenylalanine, a serotonin synthesis inhibitor, reduces the response of glial fibrillary acidic protein induced by trauma to the spinal cord. Acta Neuropathol. (Berlin) **86:** 422–427.
22. SHARMA, H.S., Y. OLSSON & J. CERVÓS-NAVARRO. 1993. Early perifocal cell changes and edema in traumatic injury of the spinal cord are reduced by indomethacin, an inhibitor of prostaglandin synthesis. Acta Neuropathol. (Berlin) **85:** 145–153.
23. SHARMA, H.S., J. WESTMAN, Y. OLSSON & P. ALM. 1996. Involvement of nitric oxide in acute spinal cord injury: an immunohistochemical study using light and electron microscopy in the rat. Neurosci. Res. **24:** 373–384.
24. SHARMA, H.S., R.D. BADGAIYAN, P. ALM *et al.* 2005. Neuroprotective effects of nitric oxide synthase inhibitors in spinal cord injury induced pathophysiology and motor functions: an experimental study in the rat. Ann. N.Y. Acad. Sci. This volume.

25. WU, W. 2000. Response of nitric oxide synthase to neuronal injury. *In* Functional Neuroanatomy of the Nitric Oxide System. Handb. Chem. Neuroanat. Vol. 17, pp. 315–353. Elsevier. Amsterdam/New York.
26. NOVIKOV, L., L. NOVIKOVA & J.O. KELLERTH. 1995. Brain-derived neurotrophic factor promotes survival and blocks nitric oxide synthase expression in adult rat spinal motoneurons after ventral nerve root avulsion. Neurosci. Lett. **200:** 45–48.
27. SHARMA, H.S. & P. ALM. 2004. Role of nitric oxide on the blood-brain and the spinal cord barriers. *In* The Blood–Spinal Cord and Brain Barriers in Health and Disease, pp. 191–230. Elsevier Academic. San Diego.
28. DAWSON, V.L. & T.M. DAWSON. 1996. Nitric oxide neurotoxicity. J. Chem. Neuroanat. **10:** 179–190.
29. SHARMA, H.S., F. NYBERG, J. WESTMAN *et al.* 1998. Brain derived neurotrophic factor and insulin like growth factor-1 attenuate upregulation of nitric oxide synthase and cell injury following trauma to the spinal cord. Amino Acids **14:** 121–130.
30. SHARMA, H.S., F. NYBERG, T. GORDH *et al.* 1997. Topical application of insulin like growth factor-1 reduces edema and upregulation of neuronal nitric oxide synthase following trauma to the rat spinal cord. Acta Neurochir. (Suppl.) **70:** 130–133.
31. WOOLTERINK, G., E. VAN ZANTEN, H. KAMSTEEG *et al.* 1990. Functional recovery after destruction of dopamine systems in the nucleus accumbens of rats. II. Facilitation by the ACTH (4–9) analog ORG 2766. Brain Res. **507:** 101–108.
32. VRINTEN, D.H., C.J. KALKMAN, R.A.H. ADAN & W.H. GISPEN. 2001. Neuropathic pain: a possible role for the melanocortin system? Eur. J. Pharmacol. **429:** 61–69.
33. SHARMA, H.S., J. WESTMAN & F. NYBERG. 1997. Topical application of 5-HT antibodies reduces edema and cell changes following trauma to the rat spinal cord. Acta Neurochir. (Suppl.) **70:** 155–158.
34. PAN, W., A.J. KASTIN & C.G. PICK. 2004. The staircase test in mice after spinal cord injury. Int. J. Neuroprotec. Neuroregen. **1:** 32–37.
35. WINKLER, T., H.S. SHARMA, E. STÅLBERG *et al.* 2003. An L-type calcium channel blocker, nimodipine, influences trauma induced cord conduction and axonal injury in the rat. Acta Neurochir. (Wien) Suppl. **86:** 425–432.

Neuroprotective Effects of Nitric Oxide Synthase Inhibitors in Spinal Cord Injury–Induced Pathophysiology and Motor Functions

An Experimental Study in the Rat

HARI SHANKER SHARMA,[a,b] RAJENDRA D. BADGAIYAN,[b,c] PER ALM,[d] S. MOHANTY,[e] AND LARS WIKLUND[a]

[a]*Department of Surgical Sciences, Anesthesiology, and Intensive Care Medicine, University Hospital, Uppsala University, SE-75185 Uppsala, Sweden*

[b]*Laboratory of Neuroanatomy, Department of Medical Cell Biology, Biomedical Center, Uppsala University, S-75123 Uppsala, Sweden*

[d]*Department of Pathology, University Hospital, Lund University, SE-22185 Lund, Sweden*

[e]*Department of Neurosurgery, Institute of Medical Sciences, Banaras Hindu University, Varanasi 221005, India*

ABSTRACT: The role of nitric oxide (NO) in spinal cord injury (SCI)–induced motor dysfunction, breakdown of the blood–spinal cord barrier (BSCB), edema formation, and cell injury was examined using a pharmacological approach. We used three types of nitric oxide synthase (NOS) inhibitors: a nonselective blocker, L-NAME; an irreversible inhibitor of all isoforms of NOS, L-NMMA; and a long-term competitive inhibitor of neuronal NOS with equal potency to inhibit endothelial NOS, L-NNA. The compounds were administered once daily in separate groups of rats for 7 days. On the 8th day, SCI was performed by making a longitudinal incision into the right dorsal horn of the T10–11 segments, and the rats were allowed to survive 5 h after injury. Long-term treatment with L-NNA attenuated SCI-induced NOS upregulation, BSCB breakdown, edema formation, and cell injury, whereas comparatively less neuroprotection is offered by L-NMMA. The magnitude of neuroprotection is much less evident in injured animals that received L-NAME. Interestingly, SCI-induced motor dysfunction measured according to the Tarlov scale showed close correlation with the magnitude of neuroprotection. Thus, an improvement in motor function was seen in animals pretreated with L-NNA, whereas rats treated with L-NAME or L-NMMA did not show any influence on motor dysfunction after SCI. This observation suggests that inhibition of neuronal NOS is important for neuro-

Address for correspondence: Hari Shanker Sharma, Dr. Med. Sci., Department of Surgical Sciences, Anesthesiology, and Intensive Care Medicine, University Hospital, Uppsala University, SE-75185 Uppsala, Sweden. Voice: +46-18-611-9208; fax: +46-18-55-93-57.
sharma@surgsci.uu.se

[c]Present address: Rajendra D. Badgaiyan, Department of Radiology, Harvard Medical School, Harvard University, William James Hall, 33 Kirkland Street, Cambridge, MA 02138.

Ann. N.Y. Acad. Sci. 1053: 422–434 (2005).
doi: 10.1196/annals.1344.037

protection, and the disturbances in motor function following SCI are associated with the state of spinal cord pathology.

KEYWORDS: spinal cord injury; nitric oxide; nitric oxide synthase; L-NAME; L-NNA; L-NMMA; neuronal NOS; endothelial NOS; blood–spinal cord barrier; edema formation; cell injury; motor dysfunction; spinal cord pathology

INTRODUCTION

The role of nitric oxide (NO) in the pathophysiology of spinal cord injury (SCI), for example, motor dysfunction, disturbances in the blood–spinal cord barrier (BSCB) function, edema formation, and cell injury, are still not well known.[1–3] NO has a very short half-life (less than 5 s) after its synthesis; thus, our knowledge of NO in pathophysiology of central nervous system (CNS) diseases are based on studies using nitric oxide synthase (NOS) expression.[2–4] In several neuropathological conditions, upregulation of NOS occurs in injured neurons, indicating that NO is involved in neurotoxicity.[1,5] NOS is classified into two principal isoforms: (a) constitutive NOS (cNOS), which is further subdivided into neuronal NOS (nNOS, type I) and endothelial NOS (eNOS, type III); and (b) inducible NOS (iNOS, type II), often known as immunologic NOS.[2–5] All these NOS isoforms are expressed in the brain,[4,5] indicating an important regulatory role of NO in CNS function (cf. ref. 1).

Rat spinal cord neurons express nNOS and NOS mRNAs that are concentrated in laminae I–IV and X throughout the spinal cord.[2,5] In the thoracic spinal cord, NOS-positive cells are also located within the dorsal horn, the dorsolateral funiculus, and lateral spinal neurons, and around the central canal region (Rexed lamina X).[6,7] In the spinal cord laminae I–III of the dorsal horn, NOS neurons contain GABA, glycine, and acetylcholine.[8] This suggests that interaction between NO and other neurotransmitters plays an important role in CNS regulation. However, very little is known about the interaction of NOS neurons with microvessels in the spinal cord (cf. refs. 1 and 5). However, it appears that NOS neurons influence spinal cord blood flow (SCBF) and regulate the BSCB function.[5,7]

Increased NOS expression occurs in the dorsal horn (laminae I–III) following spinal cord ischemia or peripheral nerve injury.[9,10] Likewise, spinal cord hemisection or impact injury results in an upregulation of NOS-positive interneurons, especially rostral to lesion.[1,5,7] Previous reports from our laboratory show that a focal incision into the right dorsal horn at the T10–11 segments causes NOS expression around the lesioned site.[11,12] These observations are in line with the idea that focal trauma to the cord induces NOS expression and thus contributes to neurotoxicity in the spinal cord.

Further support for this hypothesis came from the observations that inhibition of neuronal NOS by topical application of nNOS antibodies attenuates BSCB breakdown and edema formation, leading to neuroprotection.[11] Thus, it appears that NOS inhibitors have a potential therapeutic role in the neuroprotective strategies following SCI. In the present investigation, we examine the influence of selective and non-selective NOS inhibitors on SCI-induced BSCB permeability, edema formation, cell injury, and motor disturbances in our rat model.[1,11,13]

MATERIALS AND METHODS

Animals

Experiments were carried out on male Sprague-Dawley rats housed at controlled room temperature, 21 ± 1°C, with a 12-h light and 12-h dark schedule. The rat food and tap water were supplied ad libitum.

Spinal Cord Injury

Under equithesin anesthesia (3 mL/kg, ip), one segment laminectomy was performed at the T10–11 segment. SCI was produced by making a longitudinal incision into the right dorsal horn (about 2 mm deep and 4 mm long).[13] The wound was covered with cotton soaked in saline to prevent a direct exposure of the cord to air. This experimental condition was approved by the Regional Animal Ethics Committee, Uppsala, Sweden. Animals were allowed to survive for 5 h after injury. Equithesin-anesthetized normal rats served as controls.

Functional Paralysis

Functional paralysis of the hind limb was determined using a semiquantitative analysis during open field walking using a modified Tarlov scale.[14,15] These experiments were done according to National Institutes of Health (NIH) Guidelines and Care of Animals and approved by the Animal Care and Experimental Committee of Banaras Hindu University, Varanasi, India. The following score for hind limb function was used: 0 = total paraplegia; 1 = no spontaneous movement, but responds to pinch; 2 = spontaneous movement; 3 = able to support weight, but unable to walk; 4 = walk with gross deficits; 5 = walk with mild deficits; 6 = normal walk.

NOS Immunohistochemistry

The NOS immunohistochemistry was examined on Vibratome sections (40 μm thick) for nNOS and iNOS using polyclonal antibodies according to commercial protocol.[16]

BSCB Permeability

The BSCB permeability was examined using Evans blue and radiolabeled iodine ($^{[131]}$iodine) or peptide ($^{[125]}$Met-Enk-Arg-Phe, MEAP) as described earlier.[11] The radiolabeled tracers were administered at 5 min before sacrifice. The intravascular tracers were washed out by transcardiac perfusion with 0.9% saline at room temperature.[11,17] The tissue pieces from T9, T10–11, and T12 were dissected out and counted for radioactivity. The radioactivity in the whole blood sample obtained from cardiac puncture immediately before perfusion was also determined (cf. ref. 11). Extravasation of radiotracer in tissue was expressed as percentage of whole blood radioactivity.[1,12–14]

Spinal Cord Edema Formation

The water content of the spinal cord was determined to evaluate spinal cord edema formation.[11–13] For this purpose, after counting the radioactivity, the tissue samples were placed in an oven at 90°C to obtain their dry weight. The water content was calculated from the difference between dry and wet weights of the samples.[13]

Spinal Cord Cell Injury

Cell changes, sponginess, and edema were also examined in paraffin-embedded, 3-µm-thick sections stained with hematoxylin and eosin (H & E) or Nissl using light microscopy.[12–14] Ultrastructural changes in endothelial cells, nerve cells, glial cells, and myelin were examined using electron microscopy.[1,12,18] The passage of tracer across the BSCB was examined using lanthanum at the ultrastructural level.[18,19] For this purpose, animals were perfused with fixative (4% buffered paraformaldehyde) containing 2.5% lanthanum chloride (Sigma) immediately after washout with 0.9% saline.[19] Tissue pieces from the T9 to T12 were processed for standard transmission electron microscopy.[19,20]

Treatment with NOS Inhibitors

We used three different kinds of NOS inhibitors in this investigation:[1,11] a non-selective blocker of NOS, L-NAME;[21] an irreversible inhibitor of all isoforms of NOS, L-NMMA;[22] and a long-term competitive inhibitor of nNOS with equal potency to inhibit eNOS, L-NNA.[23] These were administered separately in different groups of animals once daily for 7 days (TABLE 1). On the day of experiments, one dose of the drug was administered at 30 min before SCI (TABLE 1). In a separate group of animals, L-NAME was also applied (100 µg/mL in phosphate-buffered saline) topically over the traumatized cord for 10 s or administered intravenously (25 µg/kg/min for 15 min) at 2 min after SCI (TABLE 1) (cf. refs. 1 and 11).

TABLE 1. Pharmacological manipulation with NOS inhibitors in SCI

Drug prototype (Tocris, U.K.)	Dose/route (mg/kg)	Schedule, no. of injections	Principal function
L-NAME hydrochloride	30 mg, ip	1 daily, 7 days; 30 min before SCI	Nonselective NOS inhibitor
L-NAME	25 µg/kg/min for 15 min, iv	2 min after SCI, continuous infusion	
L-NAME	2 µg in 20 µL in 20 s	2 min after SCI, topical application	
L-NMMA	35 mg, ip	1 daily, 7 days; 30 min before SCI	Competitive, irreversible inhibitor of all 3 isoforms
L-NNA	20 mg, ip	1 daily, 7 days; 30 min before SCI	NOS inhibitor (nNOS = eNOS >> iNOS)

NOTE: Data compiled from various sources. Terms: L-NAME, N^G-nitro-L-arginine methyl ester; L-NMMA, N^G-monomethyl-L-arginine acetate; L-NNA, N^G-nitro-L-arginine; NOS, nitric oxide synthase. See refs. 1 and 11.

Statistical Analysis

Student's unpaired *t* test was applied to evaluate statistical significance of the quantitative data obtained. Chi-square test was applied to evaluate semiquantitative data. A P value of less than 0.05 was considered significant.

RESULTS

Functional Paralysis

Untreated traumatized rats showed functional paralysis of the ipsilateral hind limb at 5 h after SCI (TABLE 2).[14] Pretreatment with L-NNA significantly improved motor functions; however, only a mild improvement in hind limb paralysis was observed with L-NMMA (TABLE 2). On the other hand, pretreatment or postinjury treatment with L-NAME did not influence trauma-induced functional paralysis (TABLE 2).

Spinal Cord Pathology

Untreated traumatized rats showed extensive visual swelling of the spinal cord, microhemorrhages, and edema around the lesion site (FIG. 1). Pretreatment with long-term L-NAME or its acute administration either topically or intravenously did not reduce SCI-induced cord pathology (FIG. 1). However, long-term treatment with L-NNA markedly attenuated visual swelling, hemorrhages, and edematous expansion of the cord. Reduction in visual swelling and edematous expansion was only mildly reduced by L-NMAA (TABLE 2).

NOS Immunostaining

SCI induced a marked upregulation of nNOS and iNOS in T9 and T12 segments that is mainly confined to the injured cells located in the edematous regions of the spinal cord (FIG. 1). Pretreatment with NOS inhibitors attenuated nNOS and iNOS upregulation in the cord. However, this effect was most pronounced in animals that received selective NOS inhibitors compared to the nonselective L-NAME (TABLE 2). The most marked reduction in nNOS upregulation was seen in the L-NNA-treated group (TABLE 2). The compound L-NMMA slightly—but significantly—reduced the upregulation of iNOS in the injured segment (TABLE 2).

Long-term treatment or postinjury administration of L-NAME either given locally or systemically did not prevent SCI-induced NOS expression (FIG. 1, TABLE 2). However, a slight reduction in the magnitude and intensity of nNOS upregulation was seen near the lesion site (FIG. 1).

BSCB Permeability and Edema Formation

Extravasation of Evans blue and $^{[131]}$iodine tracer was observed at 5 h in the spinal cord T9 and T12 segments showing marked visual swelling and expansion of the cord (TABLE 2).[19] Measurement of the spinal cord water content revealed more than 14% and 16% increases in volume swelling in the T9 and T12 segments, respectively (TABLE 2).[11] The permeability of radiolabeled peptide MEAP in normal ani-

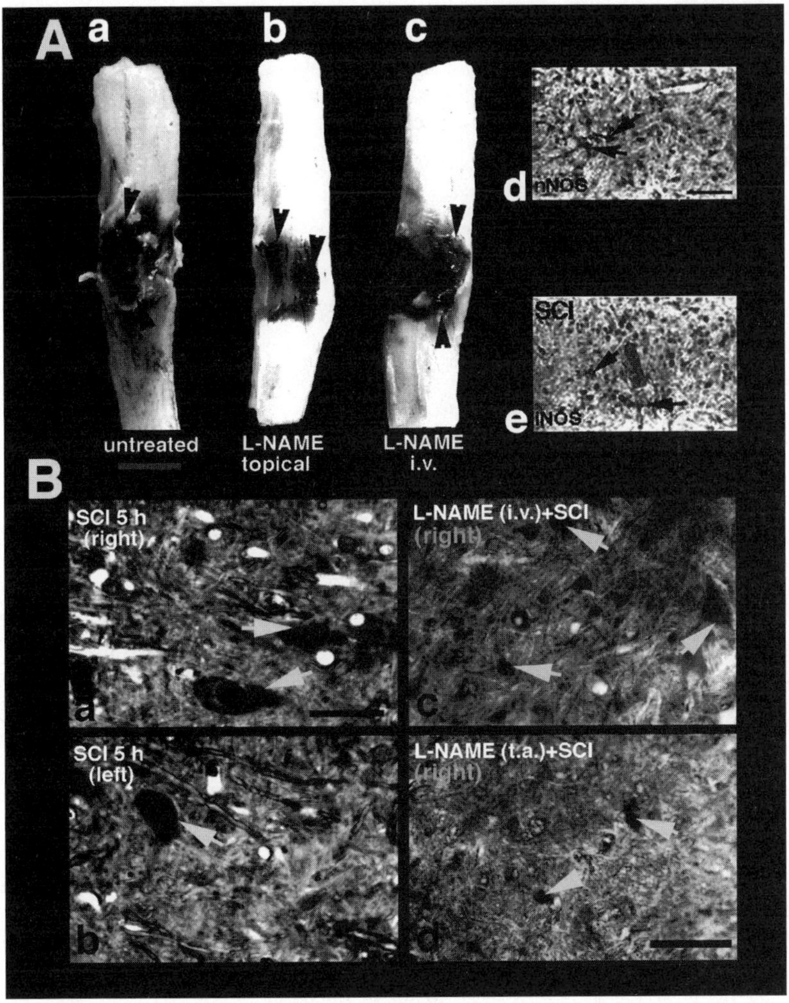

FIGURE 1. **[A]** Gross pathological changes in the spinal cord following 5 h after injury **(a)** and their modification with a nonspecific nitric oxide synthase (NOS) inhibitor drug L-NAME given topically **(b)** or systemically **(c)**. SCI was made by an incision into the right dorsal horn of the T10–11 segments. Untreated injured spinal cord exhibits profound visual swelling and hemorrhages around the lesion site (A, a; *arrowheads*). Treatment with L-NAME did not reduce visual swelling, hemorrhage, or expansion of the spinal cord at 5-h SCI (b, c). **(d, e)** Profound upregulation of nNOS (d) and iNOS (e) in the spinal cord (*arrowheads*) following 5-h SCI is mainly apparent in the distorted cells located in the edematous region. **[B]** Neuronal NOS expression in the untreated injured cord in the T9 segment (*right*, **a**, ipsilateral; *left*, **b**, contralateral side) following 5-h SCI and its modification with intravenous **(c)** or topical application **(d)** of L-NAME. Pronounced upregulation of NOS-positive neurons (brown reaction product, *arrows*) in the ipsilateral and contralateral side of the T9 segment is apparent (a, b). Neither topical nor intravenous administration of L-NAME is able to reduce NOS upregulation following SCI (c, d). Bars: [A] (a, c) 3 mm; (d, e) 100 μm; [B] (a, b) 25 μm; (c, d) 50 μm. [Data modified from refs. 1, 11, and 16.]

TABLE 2. Effect of NOS inhibitors on SCI-induced pathophysiology in the T9 segment

Type of experiment	n	Hind limb (R) function: Tarlov scale	BSCB permeability			Spinal cord edema		NOS immunostaining		Cell injury	
			$^{[131]}$Iodine (%)	$^{[125]}$MEAP (%)	Lanthanum exudation	Cord width (mm)	Water content (%)	nNOS	iNOS	Nerve cell	Myelin
Control	6	6 ± 0	0.24 ± 0.08	0.34 ± 0.10	Nil	3 ± 0.5	66.34 ± 0.23	1 ± 1	0	Nil	Nil
5-h SCI	8	2 ± 1^{a}	1.56 ± 0.12^{b}	1.67 ± 0.11^{b}	++++	5 ± 0.5^{b}	69.54 ± 0.18^{b}	28 ± 6^{a}	12 ± 2^{a}	++++	++++
L-NAME, ip	6	2 ± 2^{a}	1.16 ± 0.18^{b}	1.06 ± 0.14^{b}	++++	5 ± 1^{b}	69.23 ± 0.08^{b}	22 ± 4^{a}	10 ± 6^{a}	++++	++++
L-NAME, iv	8	2 ± 1^{a}	1.78 ± 0.23^{b}	1.87 ± 0.33^{b}	++++	6 ± 2^{b}	69.76 ± 0.32^{b}	24 ± 8^{a}	11 ± 7^{a}	++++	++++
L-NAME, ta	6	2 ± 2^{a}	1.58 ± 0.12^{b}	1.89 ± 0.18^{b}	++++	6 ± 3^{b}	69.69 ± 0.23^{b}	22 ± 6^{a}	12 ± 4^{a}	++++	++++
L-NMMA, ip	8	$4 \pm 1^{a,b}$	$1.03 \pm 0.08^{b,c}$	$1.08 \pm 0.06^{b,c}$	+++	5 ± 2^{b}	$68.87 \pm 0.11^{b,c}$	18 ± 6^{a}	$8 \pm 4^{a,c}$	+++	+++
L-NNA, ip	6	5 ± 2^{c}	$0.89 \pm 0.12^{b,c}$	$0.92 \pm 0.06^{b,c}$	++	4 ± 1^{c}	$67.56 \pm 0.12^{b,c}$	$8 \pm 4^{a,c}$	$8 \pm 6^{a,c}$	++	++

NOTE: Values are mean ± SD. Tarlov scale (R = right hind limb): 0 = total paraplegia; 1 = no spontaneous movement, but responds to pinch; 2 = spontaneous movement; 3 = able to support weight, but unable to walk; 4 = walk with gross deficits; 5 = walk with mild deficits; 6 = normal walk; nil = absent; ++++ = extensive; +++ = moderate; ++ = mild; $^{a}P < 0.01$, chi-square test (semiquantitative analyses) compared to control; $^{b}P < 0.01$, Student's unpaired t test compared to control; $^{c}P < 0.05$ compared to 5-h SCI. For details, see text.

mals was quite comparable to that of $^{[131]}$iodine (TABLE 2).[1] However, the increased permeability of MEAP in spinal cord segments after SCI is far greater than that of iodine (TABLE 2).[11] The compound L-NNA was also able to attenuate lanthanum extravasation across the spinal cord microvessel following SCI, a feature not seen in rats treated with L-NAME. A slight reduction in lanthanum extravasation was observed in animals pretreated with L-NMMA (TABLE 2).

Long-term treatment with L-NNA significantly attenuated SCI-induced BSCB breakdown and edema formation at 5 h after SCI (TABLE 2). Comparatively less reduction in BSCB breakdown or edema formation was seen with L-NMMA pretreatment (TABLE 2). The magnitude of BSCB breakdown, edema formation, or spinal cord expansion in L-NAME-pretreated injured animals was very similar to that of untreated traumatized rats (TABLE 2). Postinjury treatment with L-NAME did not reduce the spinal cord width, edema formation, or volume swelling (TABLE 2). Extravasation of Evans blue, $^{[131]}$iodine, or MEAP in the cord was very similar to that of untreated traumatized rats (TABLE 2).

Spinal Cord Cell Injury

A focal SCI induced profound nerve cell, glial cell, endothelial cell, and myelin injury (TABLE 2).[17] Long-term pretreatment or acute postinjury administration of L-NAME did not reduce the magnitude or severity of dark and distorted neurons, membrane damage, edema, and sponginess (results not shown). However, long-term pretreatment with selective NOS inhibitors markedly attenuated SCI-induced cell injury. This effect was most pronounced in traumatized animals that received L-NNA (TABLE 2).

At the ultrastructural level, membrane damage, myelin vesiculation, and extravasation of lanthanum across the endothelial cells were much less evident in L-NNA-treated injured rats. On the other hand, the influence of L-NMAA was much less pronounced. The L-NAME either given as pre- or postinjury treatment was ineffective in reducing spinal cord cell and tissue injury (results not shown).

DISCUSSION

The salient new findings of this study suggest that selective long-term inhibitors of nNOS are able to induce neuroprotection in SCI. This is evident from the fact that long-term treatment with L-NNA significantly attenuated SCI-induced NOS upregulation, BSCB breakdown, edema formation, and cell injury. This observation is in line with the idea that inhibition of nNOS is important for neuroprotection. On the other hand, comparatively less neuroprotection offered by L-NMMA suggests that blockade of all the isoforms of NOS in SCI is not beneficial. The magnitude of neuroprotection is much less in injured animals that received the nonselective inhibitor of NOS, L-NAME. Since L-NAME is able to inhibit eNOS as well, it appears that blockade of eNOS in SCI induces adverse cell reaction.

Our basic aim of this investigation is to find out if upregulation of NOS is involved in the pathophysiology of the spinal cord following trauma. To achieve this goal, we used long-term treatment with several NOS inhibitors. Previously, we used chronic L-NAME treatment and examined NOS immunohistochemistry in the spinal cord following peripheral nerve lesion (see refs. 1 and 20). Our results show that chronic L-NAME treatment did not abolish NOS expression in the cord. However, chronic treatment with L-NAME significantly attenuated neurodegenerative changes in the spinal cord following spinal nerve lesion. This observation suggests that NOS upregulation is somehow related with the neurodegeneration and supports the idea that NOS inhibitors could induce neuroprotection depending on their ability to inhibit NOS expression. To further confirm this hypothesis, in a selective group of rats, L-NAME was applied topically or intravenously at 2 min after SCI. The results of this investigation clearly demonstrated that this dose of L-NAME was not able to attenuate NOS expression nor the pathological changes in the spinal cord. Taken together, these observations strongly support the involvement of NO in the pathophysiology of SCI. However, further studies are needed to find out suitable therapeutic strategies in clinical condition to inhibit NOS expression after SCI. This is a subject that is currently being investigated in our laboratory.

The other important finding from this study shows that the intensity of SCI-induced motor dysfunction is closely associated with the magnitude of trauma-induced spinal cord edema and cell injury. An improvement in the right hind limb function measured using the Tarlov scale closely corresponds to the magnitude of neuroprotection offered by NOS inhibitor compounds and is in line with this idea. Thus, an improvement in motor function was seen in animals pretreated with L-NNA, whereas rats treated with L-NAME or L-NMMA did not show much improvement in motor function after SCI.

The SCI-induced motor impairment improves over time even without any treatment.[20] Thus, it would be interesting to compare long-term motor dysfunction in untreated traumatized rats with animals pretreated with selective NOS inhibitors. However, due to limitation of our experimental protocol, we could not assess motor function beyond 5 h after SCI. Nevertheless, our investigations showed that prior inhibition of NOS was able to improve motor disturbances in the present investigation as early as 5 h after SCI. This suggests that NOS inhibitors may have some role in motor dysfunction after SCI. Further posttrauma treatment of NOS inhibitors on motor dysfunction will clarify this point.

These observations suggest that disturbances in motor function are associated with the state of spinal cord pathology following trauma.[24,25] Furthermore, our observations indicate that NOS upregulation is associated with spinal cord pathology and thus motor dysfunction, not reported earlier.

In the present investigation, a focal SCI induced an upregulation of nNOS and iNOS in the traumatized as well as adjacent noninjured spinal cord segments. Expression of iNOS is confined mostly to the injured segment, whereas distribution of nNOS is more widespread in the cord following SCI. The nNOS expression was normally seen in the edematous regions of the spinal cord containing damaged nerve cells. This indicates that upregulation of nNOS is injurious to cord, and iNOS upregulation is associated with intense cell injury. A prolonged and sustained release of NO from the iNOS supports this idea.[26] Expression of nNOS in remote regions suggests that the spread of injury factors or edema fluid in the adjacent segments of the spinal cord probably triggers the upregulation of nNOS. Since normal spinal cord segments did not express nNOS, it may be that cells expressing nNOS activity are more vulnerable to SCI-induced cell death.[1,3–5]

There are reasons to believe that production of NO following activation of NOS is contributing to membrane disruption, edema formation, and breakdown of the BSCB permeability in SCI. Breakdown of the BSCB is largely responsible for edema formation in the spinal cord.[13,14,17,18] Direct damage to the endothelial cell membrane is likely to allow accumulation of water in the spinal cord extra- and intracellular compartments, leading to vacuolation, swelling, and/or cell death.[17–20] Measurement of spinal cord water content alone is not sufficient enough to determine accumulation of water in the extra- or intracellular compartments.[16,18] Ultrastructural studies, however, support the idea that water accumulation can occur in both the extra- and intracellular compartments in this model after SCI.[20,26,27]

A direct membrane disruption responsible for BSCB breakdown in SCI is further supported with the finding of lanthanum infiltration into the endothelial cell cytoplasm.[17,18] Damage to the endothelial cell membrane following SCI appears to be mediated through NO toxicity.[1,11] This is supported by the fact that pretreatment with L-NNA that inhibited nNOS upregulation significantly attenuated BSCB disruption. In contrast, the other NOS inhibitors that failed to reduce nNOS effectively did not prevent BSCB disruption.

Several lines of evidence suggest that upregulation of nNOS is associated with increased NO production that is responsible for CNS toxicity in various injury models.[1–3,5,12,16,18,20] The fact that nNOS null mice are quite resistant to ischemia-induced cell damage in the brain is line with this hypothesis (cf. ref. 5). Further support regarding the involvement of nNOS in the pathophysiology of SCI came from our observations that topical application of antibody raised against nNOS is capable of attenuating edema formation, BSCB disruption, and cell injury.[1,11,18,20] This beneficial effect of the antiserum is related to its ability to inhibit nNOS upregulation.[11,12] This indicates that NOS inhibitors are neuroprotective in nature. However, NOS inhibitors in ischemia, stroke, or infarction provide contradictory results, making the hypothesis that NO is involved in cell injury and cell death a bit controversial.[1,26,28] There are indications that blockade of eNOS aggravates ischemic injury, whereas blockade of nNOS in pathological conditions is beneficial for cell survival (cf. refs. 3 and 28). Thus, inhibition of selective NOS is important for cell injury or survival.

The mechanisms by which CNS injuries induce NOS upregulation are still speculative. It appears that profound cellular stress, release of neurochemicals, lipid peroxidation, and generation of free radicals may play important roles in NO production.[11,18,20] Generation of free radicals triggers the opening of cation-permeable channels, resulting in an increased accumulation of intracellular Ca^{2+} in the brain microenvironment.[29–32] The intracellular Ca^{2+} then binds to calmodulin, a cofactor of NOS, and stimulates NOS activity.[4,28,33] Overproduction of NO contributes to neurotoxicity through generation of oxidant compounds such as peroxynitrite and superoxide anion.[34–36] Neuroprotection offered by superoxide dismutase in cell culture studies following glutamate or other NO donors supports this idea.[28]

Alternatively, damage to DNA by the NO- and $ONOO^-$-induced activation of nuclear enzyme poly(ADP-ribose) synthetase (PARS) is quite likely.[28,37–39] Activation of PARS causes cell death by rapid depletion of cell energy. Ability of PARS inhibitors to protect cortical cell cultures following glutamate and NO neurotoxicity supports this hypothesis.[40]

In the present investigation, L-NNA effectively inhibited nNOS and was thus able to induce neuroprotection. The compound L-NAME neither blocked NOS upregulation effectively nor induced neuroprotection. It may be that application of L-NAME topically or systemically is not sufficiently adequate to inhibit NOS effectively.[1,11,28] Furthermore, blockade of eNOS expression by L-NAME may also induce adverse cellular reactions.[28]

CONCLUSIONS

Taken together, our results clearly demonstrate that blockade of NOS expression with selective NOS inhibitors is instrumental in attenuating SCI-induced BSCB disturbances, edema formation, cell reactions, and improved motor functions. However, to explore the potential role of NOS inhibitors in the clinical situation, further studies using postinjury treatments with these drugs are needed. It remains to be seen whether NOS inhibitors given at various intervals after SCI are still able to improve motor functions and/or spinal cord cell injury, a feature currently being investigated in our laboratory.

ACKNOWLEDGMENTS

The research described in this review is supported by grants from the Swedish Medical Research Council, No. 2710 (to H. S. Sharma and L. Wiklund) and No. 11205 (to P. Alm and H. S. Sharma); the Alexander von Humboldt Foundation, Bonn, Germany (to H. S. Sharma); University Grants Commission, New Delhi, India (to H. S. Sharma); the Indian Council of Medical Research, New Delhi, India (to H. S. Sharma); Astra-Zeneca, Mölndal, Sweden (to H. S. Sharma); and IPSEN-Medical, Paris, France (to H. S. Sharma). The technical assistance of Kärstin Flink, Kerstin Rystedt, Inga Hörte, and Margareta Butler, and the secretarial assistance of Aruna Sharma are highly appreciated. The computer assistance of Suraj Sharma is acknowledged with thanks.

REFERENCES

1. Sharma, H.S. & P. Alm. 2004. Role of nitric oxide on the blood-brain and the spinal cord barriers. *In* The Blood–Spinal Cord and Brain Barriers in Health and Disease, pp. 191–230. Elsevier Academic Press. San Diego.
2. Bredt, D.S. 1995. Molecular characterization of nitric oxide synthase. *In* Nitric Oxide Synthase in the Nervous System, pp. 1–19. Academic Press. Boston/New York.
3. Dawson, T.M., J. Zhang, V.L. Dawson & S.H. Snyder. 1994. Nitric oxide: cellular regulation and neuronal injury. Prog. Brain Res. **103:** 365–369.
4. Dawson, T.M. & S.H. Snyder. 1994. Gases as biological messenger: nitric oxide and carbon monoxide in the brain. J. Neurosci. **14:** 5147–5159.
5. Wu, W. 2000. Response of nitric oxide synthase to neuronal injury. *In* Functional Neuroanatomy of the Nitric Oxide System. Handb. Chem Neuroanat. Vol. 17, pp. 315–353. Elsevier. Amsterdam/New York.
6. Vogel, M., G. Luck, S. Bachmann & D. Blottner. 1997. NOS type-1 mRNA expression and protein localization in spinal autonomic neurons. NeuroReport **8:** 3389–3393.
7. Vincent, S.R. 1994. Nitric oxide: a radical neurotransmitter in the central nervous system. Prog. Neurobiol. **42:** 129–160.

8. SPIKE, R.C., A.J. TODD & H.M. JOHNSTON. 1993. Coexistence of NADPH-diaphorase with GABA, glycine, and acetylcholine in rat spinal cord. J. Comp. Neurol. **335:** 320–333.
9. MARSALA, J., D. KLUCHOVA & M. MARSALA. 1997. Spinal cord gray matter layers rich in NADPH-diaphorase-positive neurons are refractory to ischemia-reperfusion-induced injury: a histochemical and silver impregnation study in rabbit. Exp. Neurol. **143:** 165–179.
10. HAMA, A.T. & J. SAGEN. 1994. Induction of spinal NADPH-diaphorase by nerve injury is attenuated by adrenal medullary transplants. Brain Res. **640:** 345–351.
11. SHARMA, H.S., J. WESTMAN, Y. OLSSON & P. ALM. 1996. Involvement of nitric oxide in acute spinal cord injury: an immunohistochemical study using light and electron microscopy in the rat. Neurosci. Res. **24:** 373–384.
12. SHARMA, H.S., F. NYBERG, T. GORDH *et al.* 1998. Neurotrophic factors attenuate neuronal nitric oxide synthase upregulation, microvascular permeability disturbances, edema formation, and cell injury in the spinal cord following trauma. *In* Spinal Cord Monitoring: Basic Principles, Regeneration, Pathophysiology, and Clinical Aspects, pp. 118–148. Springer. Wien/New York.
13. SHARMA, H.S. & Y. OLSSON. 1990. Edema formation and cellular alterations following spinal cord injury in rat and their modification with *p*-chlorophenylalanine. Acta Neuropathol. (Berlin) **79:** 604–610.
14. SHARMA, H.S., T. GORDH, S. MOHANTY & P-O. SJÖQUIST. 2005. Spinal cord injury induced heat shock protein expression is reduced by an antioxidant compound H-290/51: an experimental study using light and electron microscopy in the rat. J. Neural Transm. In press.
15. KAMENCIC, H., R.W. GRIEBEL, A.W. LYON *et al.* 2001. Promoting glutathione synthesis after spinal cord trauma decreases secondary damage and promotes retention of function. FASEB J. **15:** 243–250.
16. SHARMA, H.S., P-O. SJÖQUIST & P. ALM. 2003. A new antioxidant compound H-290/51 attenuates spinal cord injury induced expression of constitutive and inducible isoforms of nitric oxide synthase and edema formation in the rat. Acta Neurochir. (Wien) Suppl. **86:** 415–420.
17. SHARMA, H.S. 2005. Neuroprotective effects of neurotrophins and melanocortins in spinal cord injury: an experimental study in the rat using pharmacological and morphological approaches. Ann. N.Y. Acad. Sci. This volume.
18. SHARMA, H.S. 2005. Pathophysiology of blood–spinal cord barrier in traumatic injury and repair. Curr. Pharm. Des. **11:** 1353–1389.
19. SHARMA, H.S., Y. OLSSON, S. PEARSSON & F. NYBERG. 1995. Trauma induced opening of the blood–spinal cord barrier is reduced by indomethacin, an inhibitor of prostaglandin synthesis: experimental observations in the rat using ^{131}I-sodium, Evans blue, and lanthanum as tracers. Restor. Neurol. Neurosci. **7:** 207–215.
20. SHARMA, H.S. 2004. Pathophysiology of the blood–spinal cord barrier in traumatic injury. *In* The Blood–Spinal Cord and Brain Barriers in Health and Disease, pp. 437–518. Elsevier Academic Press. San Diego.
21. MOORE, P.K. & R.L. HANDY. 1997. Selective inhibitors of neuronal nitric oxide synthase—is no NOS really good NOS for the nervous system? Trends Pharmacol. Sci. **18:** 204–11.
22. REIF, D.W. & S.A. MCCREEDY. 1995. *N*-Nitro-L-arginine and *N*-monomethyl-L-arginine exhibit a different pattern of inactivation toward the three nitric oxide synthases. Arch. Biochem. Biophys. **320:** 170–176.
23. DWYER, M.A., D.S. BREDT & S.H. SNYDER. 1991. Nitric oxide synthase: irreversible inhibition by L-NG-nitroarginine in brain *in vitro* and *in vivo*. Biochem. Biophys. Res. Commun. **176:** 1136–1141.
24. PAN, W.A., J. KASTIN & C.G. PICK. 2004. The staircase test in mice after spinal cord injury. Int. J. Neuroprotec. Neuroregen. **1:** 32–37.
25. SHARMA, H.S. 2004. Editorial. Int. J. Neuroprotec. Neuroregen. **1:** 8.
26. SHARMA, H.S., P. ALM & J. WESTMAN. 1998. Nitric oxide and carbon monoxide in the pathophysiology of brain functions in heat stress. Prog. Brain Res. **115:** 297–333.

27. GORDH, T., H.S. SHARMA, P. ALM & J. WESTMAN 1998. Spinal nerve lesion induces upregulation of neuronal nitric oxide synthase in the spinal cord. Amino Acids **14:** 105–112.
28. DAWSON, V.L. & T.M. DAWSON. 1996. Nitric oxide neurotoxicity. J. Chem. Neuroanat. **10:** 179–190.
29. CHO, H.J., Q.W. XIE, J. CALAYCAY *et al.* 1992. Calmodulin is a subunit of a nitric oxide synthase from macrophages. J. Exp. Med. **176:** 599–604.
30. DARLEY-USMAR, V.M., N. HOGG, V.J. O'LEARY *et al.* 1992. The simultaneous generation of superoxide and nitric oxide can initiate lipid peroxidation in human low density lipoprotein. Free Radical Commun. **17:** 9–20.
31. HIRSCH, J., J. LEIPZIGER, U. FROBE & E. SCHLATTER. 1993. Regulation and possible physiological role of the Ca(2+)-dependent K+ channel of cortical collecting ducts of the rat. Pflüg. Arch. **422:** 492–498.
32. KURENNY, D.E., L.L. MOROZ, R.W. TURNER *et al.* 1994. Modulation of ion channels in rod photoreceptors by nitric oxide. Neuron **13:** 315–324.
33. KOCH, K.W., H.G. LAMBRECHT, M. HABERECHT *et al.* 1994. Functional coupling of a Ca^{2+}/calmodulin-dependent nitric oxide synthase and a soluble guanylyl cyclase in vertebrate photoreceptor cells. EMBO J. **13:** 3312–3320.
34. OURY, T.D., V-S. HO, C.A. PIANTADOSI & J.D. CRAPO. 1992. Extracellular superoxide dismutase, nitric oxide, and central nervous system O_2 toxicity. Proc. Natl. Acad. Sci. USA **89:** 9715–9719.
35. LIPTON, S.A., D.J. SINGEL & J.S. STAMLER. 1994. Neuroprotective and neurodestructive effects of nitric oxide and redox congeners. Ann. N.Y. Acad. Sci. **738:** 382–387.
36. STAMLER, J.S. 1994. Redox signalling: nitrosylation and related target interactions of nitric oxide. Cell **78:** 931–936.
37. LAUTIER, D., J. LAGUEUX, J. THIBODEAU *et al.* 1993. Molecular and biochemical features of poly (ADP-ribose) metabolism. Mol. Cell. Biochem. **122:** 171–193.
38. BECKMAN, J.S. 1994. The double-edged role of nitric oxide in brain function and superoxide-mediated injury. J. Dev. Physiol. **15:** 53–59.
39. BOLANOS, J.P., S.J.R. HEALES, J.M. LAND & J.B. CLARK. 1995. Effect of peroxynitrite on the mitochondrial respiratory chain: differential susceptibility of neurones and astrocytes in primary culture. J. Neurochem. **64:** 1965–1972.
40. ZHANG, Z.G., M. CHOPP, S. GAUTAM *et al.* 1994. Upregulation of neuronal nitric oxide synthase and mRNA, and selective sparing of nitric oxide synthase–containing neurons after focal cerebral ischemia in rat. Brain Res. **654:** 85–95.

Acrylamide Stimulates Glutamine Uptake in Fischer 344 Rat Astrocytes by a Mechanism Involving Upregulation of the Amino Acid Transport System N

QI WU,[a] MARTA SIDORYK,[b] LYSETTE MUTKUS,[a] MAGDALENA ZIELIŃSKA,[b] JAN ALBRECHT,[b] AND MICHAEL ASCHNER[a,c]

[a]*Department of Physiology and Pharmacology, Wake Forest University School of Medicine, Winston-Salem, North Carolina, USA*

[b]*Department of Neurotoxicology, Medical Research Center, Polish Academy of Sciences, Warsaw, Poland*

[c]*Department of Pediatrics and Pharmacology, and the Kennedy Center, Vanderbilt University Medical Center, Nashville, Tennessee, USA*

ABSTRACT: High demand of neoplastic tissues for glutamine (Gln) is met by its active transport across cell membranes. Chronic treatment with acrylamide in rodents is associated with an increased incidence of neoplasms, including astrocytomas. In this study, 24-h acrylamide treatment significantly increased the initial rate of L-[G-^{3}H]glutamine uptake in astrocyte cultures derived from the acrylamide-sensitive Fischer 344 rat, and this effect could be fully inhibited by histidine, a model substrate for the amino acid transport system N. RT-PCR analysis revealed that acrylamide treatment caused a significant increase in the astrocytic expression of the mRNA coding for the major system N protein, SNAT3, which is specifically overexpressed in malignant gliomas *in situ*. The acrylamide-induced upregulation of astrocytic Gln transport via system N is likely to affect Gln homeostasis in these cells and may be causally related to the increased astrocytoma incidence observed in Fischer 344 rats.

KEYWORDS: acrylamide; amino acid transport system N; astrocyte; Fischer 344 rat; glutamine (Gln)

INTRODUCTION

Acrylamide (2-propenamide) is commonly used as a polymer in flocculants for drinking and waste water purification, for thickening of agricultural sprays, in polyacrylamide gel chromatography electrophoresis and soil stabilization, and in the paper and pulp industries.[22] Recent studies have also demonstrated human exposure

Address for correspondence: Michael Aschner, Ph.D., Department of Pediatrics, B-3307 Medical Center North, Vanderbilt University School of Medicine, Nashville, TN 37232-2495. Voice: 615-322-8024; fax: 615-322-6541.
michael.aschner@vanderbilt.edu

Ann. N.Y. Acad. Sci. 1053: 435–443 (2005).
doi: 10.1196/annals.1344.038

to acrylamide from processed foods.[31,38,44] The acrylamide monomer is a well-characterized neurotoxicant, and excessive exposure is purported to lead to both peripheral and central neuropathy,[7,13,39] effects that are potentially mediated via changes in neurofilament structure and distribution.[11,16]

Recent studies from our laboratory suggest that acute exposure to acrylamide causes significant changes in the expression of glutamine synthetase [the astrocyte-specific enzyme that catalyzes glutamine (Gln) formation from glutamate (Glu)] and the glutamate/aspartate transporter (GLAST), thus potentially altering Glu homeostasis.[3] Acute acrylamide treatment also promoted astrocytic proliferation.[4] Chromosomal aberrations, increased sister chromatid exchanges, unscheduled DNA synthesis, and induction of DNA fragments[6,21,36,40,41] have also been associated with exposure to acrylamide. In rats, chronic exposure to acrylamide via drinking water (0.01, 0.1, 0.5, or 2.0 mg acrylamide/kg body wt/day for 2 years) is associated with neoplasia of the thyroid, adrenal medulla, testicular mesothelium, and mammary glands.[17,20] In addition, male rats receiving 2.0 mg acrylamide/kg/day had increased incidence of astrocytomas.[20] The mechanism(s) involved in the induction of tumors by acrylamide is not understood.

Gln is a key factor in the growth and metabolism of neoplastic tissue.[1,12,28,32,42] In CNS-derived tumors and tumor cell lines, Gln is predominantly metabolized to glutathione (GSH)[29,34] and Glu.[30] Whereas GSH accounts for tumor chemoresistance[26] and radioresistance,[18,25] the accumulation of Glu in the extracellular space contributes to excitotoxicity via overactivation of neuronal *N*-methyl D-aspartate (NMDA) receptors[32,33] and increased cell death.

Because Gln synthesis in most neoplastic tissues is too low to meet the cellular demand for this amino acid, Gln uptake is widely recognized as rate-limiting for Gln utilization.[12,42,43] In mammalian tissues, Gln is transported by a plethora of amino acid permeases that are classified by their substrate specificity.[8] Of the different Gln transport systems operating in the CNS, system N is the one that exhibits the highest specificity for Gln. SN1, recently renamed as SNAT3 (for the updated nomenclature, see ref. 23), is the dominating N system transporting protein that, within the CNS, is located almost exclusively in astrocytes.[10] Increased expression of SNAT3 appears to be a specific feature of highly malignant human gliomas *in situ*.[37]

Given the observation that acrylamide has produced malignant gliomas,[20] the present study was undertaken to examine the effect of acrylamide on astrocytic Gln transport and transporter mRNA expression. We focused on the effect of acrylamide on the N-system-mediated uptake, analyzing the uptake in the presence or absence of histidine, a model system N substrate and thus inhibitor of N-system-mediated Gln uptake. SNAT3 mRNA expression was also analyzed using the RT-PCR technique.

METHODS

Materials

L-[G-^{3}H]Glutamine (specific activity: 37 MBq/mL, 1 mCi/mL) was purchased from Amersham Biosciences (Arlington Heights, IL). Minimal essential medium (MEM) with Earle's salts, Dulbecco's modified medium with Earle's salts, Ham's F-12 nutrient mixture, neurobasal medium, B-27 supplement, heat-inactivated horse serum, fetal bovine serum, L-glutamine, penicillin, streptomycin, Fungizone, β-mercaptoethanol, and dispase were all purchased from Life Technologies (Gaithersburg, MD). Threonine, histidine, and methylaminoisobutyric (MeAIB) were purchased from Sigma Chemical (St. Louis, MO). All other reagents were purchased from either Sigma Chemical or Fisher Scientific (Pittsburgh, PA) and were of cell culture quality or higher.

Astrocyte Cell Cultures

Primary cultures of astrocytes from cerebral cortices of newborn (1-day-old) Fischer 344 rats were established as previously detailed.[2] Briefly, subsequent to removal of the meninges, the cerebral cortices were digested with bacterial neutral protease (dispase) and astrocytes recovered by repeated aspiration of dissociated cells. Twenty-four hours subsequent to initial plating of cells in poly-D-lysine-coated Corning 35-mm dishes, the media were changed to preserve the adhering astrocytes and remove neurons and oligodendrocytes. The cultures were kept at 37°C in a 5% CO_2/95% air incubator for 4–5 weeks in MEM with Earle's salts supplemented with 10% heat-inactivated horse serum, 100 U/mL penicillin, 100 μg/mL streptomycin, and 0.25 μg/mL Fungizone. The media were changed twice per week. These monolayer, surface-adhering cultures were >95% positive for the astrocytic marker, glial fibrillary acidic protein (GFAP).

Glutamine Uptake Studies

Astrocytic cultures were grown in supplemented MEM medium (see above) in 6-well plates. After reaching confluency at 3 weeks in culture, the cells were treated for 24 h with ±0.1 or 1.0 mM acrylamide. This was followed by three washes with 2 mL of a HEPES-buffered solution containing 122 mM NaCl, 3.3 mM KCl, 0.4 mM $MgSO_4$, 1.3 mM $CaCl_2$, 1.2 mM KH_2PO_4, 25 mM HEPES, and 10 mM D-(+)-glucose. The buffer was adjusted to a pH of 7.4 by the addition of 10 N NaOH. Subsequently, the astrocytes were incubated for 5 min in a warmed HEPES-buffered solution containing the radiotracer L-[G-^{3}H]Gln (Amersham, Arlington Heights, IL) at 1 μCi/mL in the presence of unlabeled L-Gln at 50 μM. For competition experiments, histidine was added at 50-fold excess of the total Gln concentration, together with L-[G-^{3}H]Gln. Uptake of Gln was terminated by rapidly removing the radioactive buffer and immediately washing the wells three times with 2 mL of ice-cold mannitol buffer (pH 7.4) with the following composition: 290 mM mannitol, 10 mM Tris-nitrate, and 0.5 mM $Ca(NO_3)_2$. Cells were solubilized in 2 mL of 1 N NaOH for determinations of radioactivity and protein content. An aliquot of 750 μL of sample was neutralized in 75 μL of 10 N HCl, and radioactivity was determined by liquid scintillation spectroscopy. Protein content was determined using a 25 μL aliquot of the sample neutralized in 1 N HCl and quantified using a bicinchoninic acid assay (BCA) protein assay reagent kit (Pierce, Rockford, IL). All levels of radioactivity were corrected for protein levels and calculated as DPM/μg protein.

RT-PCR Analysis

RT-PCR was performed essentially as described by Sidoryk *et al.*[37] Total RNA was isolated using the TRIzol Reagent (Life Technologies), and total RNA (5 μg) was reverse-transcribed with the Superscript II and oligo $(dT)_{12–18}$ primers (Gibco/BRL, now Invitrogen, Rockville, MD). Each cDNA sample (2 μL) was then amplified by PCR using 5′-aggtggacccatttgatgtg and 5′-gtcccagagacccagtcagt glutamine transporter SN1 (SNAT3) primers. GAPDH served as a constitutive marker, using the primers 5′-tgaaggtcggagtcaacggatttgg-3′ and 5′-catgtaggcatgaggtccaccac-3′.[35,37] The primers were obtained from TIB Biomol (Poznañ, Poland). Following 30 cycles of amplification (previously described[14]), the PCR products were resolved on 1.2% agarose gels in an ethidium bromide–containing buffer with 418-bp SNAT3 run as standard. The bands were recorded using the Nucleovision system (Nucleotech, San Carlos, CA), and densitometric analysis was carried out using the GelExpert 4.0 program. For sequence analysis, the bands were extracted from the agarose with a DNA cleanup kit (Akor Laboratories, Titusville, NJ). Reactions were run on a Perkin-Elmer ABI type 383 sequencer.

Statistical Analysis

All experiments were conducted with a minimum of three replicates. The data were analyzed with GraphPad InStat version 3.02 for Windows (GraphPad Software, San Diego, CA). One-way analysis of variance was used to test for effects of acrylamide on the neutral amino acid transporter ASCT2 and SNAT3 mRNA expression, as well as cell Gln uptake under the various experimental conditions. Newman-Keuls post-hoc test was used to evaluate mean differences. The alpha level for the analyses was $P < 0.05$.

RESULTS

FIGURE 1 illustrates the effect of acrylamide on Gln uptake in Fischer 344 astrocytes. Following 24-h treatment with 0.1 or 1.0 mM acrylamide, we assessed the initial rate (5 min) of L-[G-^{3}H]Gln uptake in the presence or absence of a 50-fold excess of the model N system substrate, histidine. [G-^{3}H]Gln uptake in astrocytes was concentration-dependently increased by 0.1 and 1.0 mM acrylamide (120±8.0% and 141±2.0%, respectively; mean ± SEM), and this effect was statistically significant in the presence of 1.0 mM acrylamide ($P < 0.05$). When present with L-[G-^{3}H]Gln for the 5-min uptake period, histidine led to a significant decrease in Gln uptake by astrocytes (***$P < 0.001$ vs. control). The presence of histidine for the 5-min L-[G-^{3}H]Gln uptake period was also effective in decreasing the stimulatory effect of both 0.1 and 1.0 mM acrylamide, to the extent that astrocytic L-[G-^{3}H]Gln uptake was indistinguishable from cells treated with histidine alone (*$P < 0.05$ and **$P < 0.01$ for 0.1 mM acrylamide + histidine and 1.0 mM acrylamide + histidine, respectively, vs. control, and indistinguishable from histidine alone).

FIGURE 2 depicts the effect of 6-h acrylamide treatment on the expression of SNAT3 in neonatal rat (Fischer 344) astrocyte cultures. The ratio of SNAT3 to GAPDH (a constitutive marker) was 0.23 ± 0.02 (mean ± SD) in untreated astrocytes, and it significantly (*$P < 0.05$) increased in the presence of 0.1 and 1.0 mM acrylamide (0.92 ± 0.10 and 0.75 ± 0.12, respectively; for a representative electrophoretic separation, see FIG. 3).

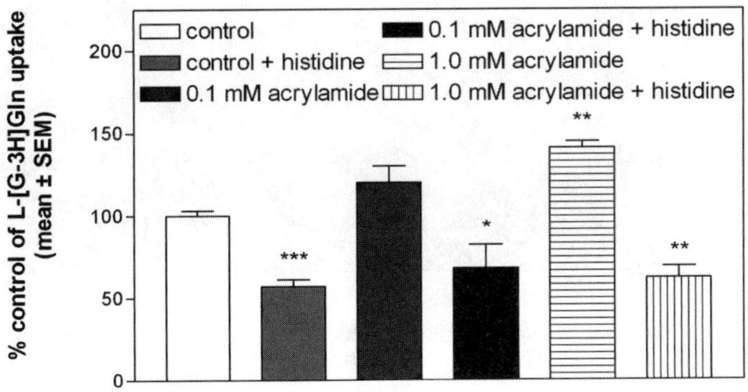

FIGURE 1. Initial rates (5 min) of L-[G-^{3}H]Gln uptake (final concentration: 50 μM) in control and acrylamide (0.1 or 1.0 mM for 24 h)–treated astrocytes in the presence and absence of histidine (100 μM), a model substrate for the N transport system. Data are expressed as mean ± SEM; *$P < 0.05$, **$P < 0.01$, ***$P < 0.001$; $n = 3$.

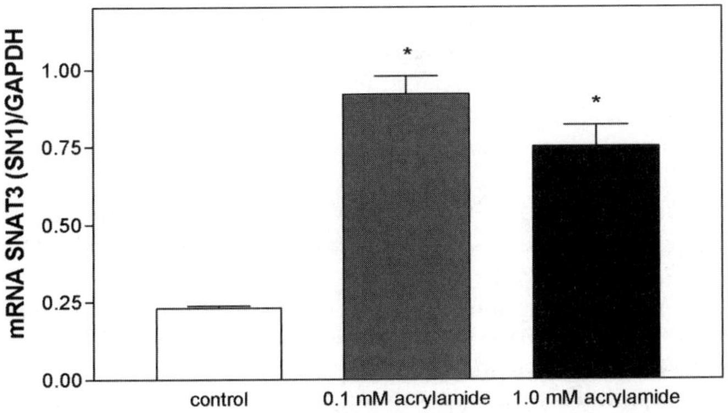

FIGURE 2. The effect of 6-h acrylamide treatment on the expression of SNAT3 mRNA in neonatal rat (Fischer 344) astrocyte cultures is depicted as the relative mRNA ratio of SNAT3 to GAPDH (a constitutive marker). Data are expressed as mean ± SD; *$P < 0.05$; $n = 3$.

FIGURE 3. Representative agarose gel electrophoresis of the PCR products. The sizes of SNAT3 mRNA and GAPDH mRNA are ~500 kb and ~1000 kb, respectively.

DISCUSSION

It is well established that active cell membrane transport of Gln plays an important role in the Gln-Glu cycle, a pathway that couples Gln production in astrocytes to the synthesis of the neurotransmitters, glutamate and γ-aminobutyric acid (GABA), in neurons. Herein, we corroborate earlier observations of active Gln uptake by cultured astrocytes.[17,27] These previous studies have demonstrated a variable involvement of three sodium-dependent amino acid transport systems in Gln uptake: systems N, ASC, and A. Our preliminary observation that Gln transport in Fischer 344 astrocytes was relatively insignificantly inhibited by ASC or A system competitors (see RESULTS section) turned our focus to system N, which plays a crucial role in native astrocytes.[10] Indeed, we established the uptake to be strongly inhibited by the system N substrate, histidine, and also the expression of SNAT3 mRNA, which within the native CNS is located predominantly—if not exclusively—in astrocytes.[9]

The novel findings of this study are that exposure to acrylamide significantly increases Gln uptake in astrocytes derived from an acrylamide-sensitive rat strain,[20] Fischer 344, and that this increase can, to a significant degree, be attributed to upregulation of system N. The model N system substrate, histidine, fully attenuated the stimulatory effects of acrylamide on astrocytic L-[G-^{3}H]Gln uptake, and this was associated with increased expression of mRNA coding for SNAT3, the predominant astrocytic N system carrier.[9,10] The present study did not consider the role of other systems transporting Gln across cell membranes. Another system worth considering is system ASC, whose ASCT2 variant is strongly expressed in cultured rat astrocytes[14,19] and in a rat astroglioma C6 cell line.[14,15] Our preliminary results indicate that the model ASCT2 substrate, threonine, is a less powerful inhibitor of Gln uptake in Fischer 344 rat astrocytes than histidine.

The acrylamide-induced increase of Gln uptake is consistent with the purported ability of acrylamide to induce astrocytomas in the rat.[20] Nitrogen for a number of important precursors of macromolecule synthesis (including purines, pyrimidines, amino sugars, as well as some amino acids) is provided by Gln.[24] Gln metabolism also furnishes precursors for GSH synthesis, a major store of cellular reducing equivalents.[5] It is also well established that Gln provides fuel for neoplastic cells, with cell-growth rates and the biosynthesis of DNA and protein directly correlating with Gln concentrations in the culture media.[42] Within the context of acrylamide-induced astrocytomas,[20] the present findings are consistent with studies in other neoplasm models in that, as a general rule, malignant cells transport Gln across their plasma membranes at a faster rate than their nonmalignant counterparts (reviewed in ref. 24). Moreover, the increased expression of SNAT3 mRNA observed here as a result of acrylamide treatment is a specific feature of malignant, but not benign human gliomas.[37] We do not imply that astrocytes become malignant upon the treatments carried out in this study; however, the potential of the contribution of acrylamide-produced changes in Gln uptake in a malignant change needs to be considered.

ACKNOWLEDGMENTS

This study was supported by a Scholar Grant of the Foundation for Polish Science (to J. Albrecht). Q. Wu and M. Sidoryk contributed equally to this work.

REFERENCES

1. Albrecht, J., M. Doliska, A. Dybel *et al.* 2001. Glutamine transport in C6 glioma cells: substrate specificity and modulation in a glutamine deprived culture medium. J. Neurosci. Res. **66:** 59–66.
2. Allen, J.W., L.A. Mutkus & M. Aschner. 2000. Isolation of neonatal rat cortical astrocytes for primary cultures. *In* Current Protocols in Toxicology, pp. 12.4.1–12.4.15. Wiley. New York.
3. Aschner, M., C-C. Cao, Q. Wu & M.A. Friedman. 2003. The acute effects of acrylamide on astrocyte functions. Ann. N.Y. Acad. Sci. **993:** 296–304.
4. Aschner, M., Q. Wu & M. Friedman. 2005. Effects of acrylamide on primary neonatal rat astrocyte functions. Ann. N.Y. Acad. Sci. This volume.
5. Bannai, S. & T. Ishii. 1988. A novel function of glutamine in cell culture: utilization of glutamine for the uptake of cystine in human fibroblast. J. Cell. Physiol. **137:** 360–366.
6. Barfknecht, T., D. Mecca & R. Naismith. 1988. The genotoxic activity of acrylamide. Environ. Mol. Mutagen. **11:** 9.
7. Bikales, N.M. 1973. Preparation of acrylamide polymers. *In* Water-Soluble Polymers: Polymer Science and Technology Series Vol. 2, pp. 214–225. Plenum. New York.
8. Broer, S. 2002. Adaptation of plasma membrane amino acid transport mechanisms to physiological demands. Pflüg. Arch. **444:** 457–466.
9. Boulland, J.L., K.K. Osen, L.M. Levy *et al.* 2002. Cell-specific expression of the glutamine transporter SN1 suggests differences in dependence on the glutamine cycle. Eur. J. Neurosci. **15:** 1615–1631.
10. Chaudhry, F.A., R.J. Reimer, D. Krizaj *et al.* 1999. Molecular analysis of system N suggests novel physiological roles in nitrogen metabolism and synaptic transmission. Cell **99:** 769–780.
11. Chauhan, N.B., P.S. Spencer & M.I. Sabri. 1993. Effect of acrylamide on the distribution of microtubule-associated proteins (MAP1 and MAP2) in selected regions of rat brain. Mol. Chem. Neuropathol. **18:** 225–245.
12. Collins, L., M. Wasa, W.W. Souba & S.F. Abcouwer. 1998. Determinants of glutamine dependence and utilization by normal and tumor-derived breast cell lines. J. Cell. Physiol. **176:** 166–178.
13. Crofton, K.M., S. Padila, H.A. Tilson *et al.* 1996. The impact of dose rate on the neurotoxicity of acrylamide: the interaction of administered dose, target tissue concentrations, tissue damage, and functional effects. Toxicol. Appl. Pharmacol. **139:** 163–176.

14. Dolinska, M., B. Zablocka, U. Sonnewald & J. Albrecht. 2004. Glutamine uptake and expression of mRNAs of glutamine transporting proteins in mouse cerebellar and cerebral cortical astrocytes and neurons. Neurochem. Int. **44:** 75–81.
15. Dolinska, M., A. Dybel, B. Zablocka & J. Albrecht. 2003. Glutamine transport in C6 glioma cells shows ASCT2 system characteristics. Neurochem. Int. **43:** 501–507.
16. Endo, H., S. Kittur & M.I. Sabri. 1994. Acrylamide alters neurofilament protein gene expression in rat brain. Neurochem. Res. **19:** 815–829.
17. Friedman, M., L. Dulak & M. Stedham. 1995. A lifetime oncogenicity study in rats with acrylamide. Fundam. Appl. Toxicol. **27:** 95–105.
18. Grant, R. & J.W. Ironside. 1995. Glutathione S-transferases and cytochrome P450 detoxifying enzyme distribution in human cerebral glioma. J. Neurooncol. **25:** 1–7.
19. Heckel, T., A. Broer, H. Wiesinger *et al.* 2003. Asymmetry of glutamine transporters in cultured neural cells. Neurochem. Int. **43:** 289–298.
20. Johnson, K.A., S.J. Gorzinski, K.M. Bodner *et al.* 1986. Chronic toxicity and oncogenicity study on acrylamide incorporated in the drinking water of Fischer 344 rats. Toxicol. Appl. Pharmacol. **85:** 154–168.
21. Knaap, A., P. Kramers, C. Voogd *et al.* 1988. Mutagenic activity of acrylamide in eukaryotic systems, but not in bacteria. Mutagenesis **3:** 263–268.
22. Lafferty, J.S., L.M. Kamendulis, J. Kaster *et al.* 2004. Subchronic acrylamide treatment induces a tissue-specific increase in DNA synthesis in the rat. Toxicol. Lett. **154:** 95–103.
23. Mackenzie, B. & J.D. Erickson. 2004. Sodium-coupled neutral amino acid (system N/A) transporters of the SLC38 gene family. Pflüg. Arch. Eur. J. Physiol. **447:** 784–795.
24. Medina, M.Á. 2001. Glutamine and cancer. J. Nutr. **131:** 2539S–2542S.
25. Miura, M. & T. Sasaki. 1991. Role of glutathione in the intrinsic radioresistance of cell lines from a mouse squamous cell carcinoma. Radiat. Res. **126:** 229–236.
26. Nagane, M., S. Shibui, H. Oyama *et al.* 1995. Investigation of chemoresistance-related genes mRNA expression for selecting anticancer agents in successful adjuvant chemotherapy for a case of recurrent glioblastoma. Surg. Neurol. **44:** 462–468.
27. Nagaraja, T.N. & N. Brookes. 1996. Glutamine transport in mouse cerebral astrocytes. J. Neurochem. **66:** 1665–1674.
28. Pawlik, T.M., W. Souba, T.J. Sweeney & B.P. Bode. 2000. Amino acid uptake and regulation in multicellular hepatoma spheroids. J. Surg. Res. **91:** 15–25.
29. Portais, J., M. Martin, P. Canioni & M. Merle. 1993. Glutathione, but not glutamine, is detected in ^{13}C-NMR spectra of perchloric acid extracts from C6 glioma cells. FEBS Lett. **327:** 301–306.
30. Portais, J., P. Voisin, M. Merle & P. Canioni. 1996. Glucose and glutamine metabolism in C6 glioma cells studied by carbon 13 NMR. Biochimie **78:** 155–164.
31. Rosen, J. & K.E. Hellenas. 2002. Analysis of acrylamide in cooked foods by liquid chromatography tandem mass spectrometry. Analyst **127:** 880–882.
32. Rothstein, J.D. & H. Brem. 2001. Excitotoxic destruction facilitates brain tumor growth. Nat. Med. **7:** 994–995.
33. Rzeski, W., L. Turski & C. Ikonomidou. 2001. Glutamate antagonists limit tumor growth. Proc. Natl. Acad. Sci. USA **98:** 6372–6377.
34. Schafer, F.C., M. Brucke, H.J. Holzhausen *et al.* 2001. Gamma-glutamyl transferase expression in higher-grade astrocytic glioma. Acta Oncol. **40:** 529–535.
35. Schreiber, W. & P. Durre. 1999. The glyceraldehyde-3-phosphate dehydrogenase of *Clostridium acetobutylicum*: isolation and purification of the enzyme, and sequencing and localization of the gap gene within a cluster of other glycolytic genes. Microbiology **145:** 1839–1847.
36. Sega, G., E. Generoso & P. Brimer. 1990. Acrylamide exposure induces a delayed unscheduled DNA synthesis in germ cells of male mice that is correlated with the temporal pattern of adduct formation in testis DNA. Environ. Mol. Mutagen. **16:** 137–142.
37. Sidoryk, M., E. Matyja, A. Dybel *et al.* 2004. Increased expression of a glutamine transporter SNAT3 is a marker of malignant gliomas. Neuroreport **15:** 575–578.
38. Tareke, E., P. Rydberg, P. Karlsson *et al.* 2000. Acrylamide: a cooking carcinogen? Chem. Res. Toxicol. **13:** 517–522.
39. Tilson, H.A. 1981. The neurotoxicity of acrylamide: an overview. Neurobehav. Toxicol. Teratol. **3:** 445–461.

40. TSUDA, H., C. SHIMIZU, M. TAKETOMI *et al.* 1993. Acrylamide; induction of DNA damage, chromosomal aberrations, and cell transformation without gene mutations. Mutagenesis **8:** 23–29.
41. UNITED STATES ENVIRONMENTAL PROTECTION AGENCY. 1994. Chemicals in the Environment: Acrylamide (CAS No. 79-06-01).
42. WASA, M., B.P. BODE, S.F. ABCOUWER *et al.* 1996. Glutamine as a regulator of DNA and protein biosynthesis in human solid tumor cell lines. Ann. Surg. **274:** 189–197.
43. WASA, M., H-S. WANG & A. OKADA. 2002. Characterization of L-glutamine transport by human neuroblastoma cell line. Am. J. Physiol. **282:** C1246–C1253.
44. WEISS, G. 2002. Acrylamide in food: uncharted territory. Science **297:** 27.

Effects of Acrylamide on Primary Neonatal Rat Astrocyte Functions

MICHAEL ASCHNER,[a] QI WU,[b] AND MARVIN A. FRIEDMAN[c]

[a]*Department of Pediatrics and Pharmacology, and the Kennedy Center, Vanderbilt University Medical Center, Nashville, Tennessee, USA*

[b]*Department of Physiology and Pharmacology, Wake Forest University School of Medicine, Winston-Salem, North Carolina, USA*

[c]*Department of Physiology and Pharmacology, University of Medicine and Dentistry of New Jersey, Newark, New Jersey, USA*

ABSTRACT: The present study assessed biochemical endpoints indicative of acrylamide toxicity in astrocyte cultures derived from neonatal rat pups. Given earlier reports on the possible ability of acrylamide to induce astrocytomas in the Fischer 344 rat, we performed studies in neonatal rat astrocyte cultures from the Fischer 344 to assess the ability of acrylamide to induce astrocytic proliferation. Measurements on astrocytic proliferation included [^{3}H]-leucine incorporation, [^{3}H]-thymidine incorporation, and changes in proliferating cell nuclear antigen (PCNA). Although acrylamide (0.1 and 1 mM for 7, 11, 15, or 20 days) did not significantly ($P > 0.05$) affect [^{3}H]-leucine or [^{3}H]-thymidine incorporation, it significantly ($P < 0.05$) increased PCNA protein expression in astrocytes exposed to acrylamide for 15 and 20 days. Additional studies revealed that this effect on PCNA protein expression was not associated with activation of dopamine-2 (D2) receptors, given that quinpirole (10 μM added to cultures for the last hour of 7, 11, 15, or 20 days in culture), a selective D2 receptor agonist, did not produce results analogous to those seen with acrylamide treatment. Cotreatment of astrocytes with acrylamide (7, 11, 15, or 20 days) and the D2 receptor antagonist, sulpiride (1 μM for the last 6 h of exposure), also failed to reverse acrylamide's effect on PCNA protein induction. Taken together, these studies suggest that acrylamide promotes astrocytic cell proliferation in the CNS even though DNA synthesis did not appear stimulated.

KEYWORDS: acrylamide; astrocyte; leucine; neonatal rat; sulpiride; thymidine

INTRODUCTION

There has been much interest in public health fora as to the potential toxicity of acrylamide. In 2002,[7] acrylamide was reported to be present in certain foods cooked at high temperatures. The original Swedish research and subsequent studies in Norway, Switzerland, the United Kingdom, and the United States reported the presence of

Address for correspondence: Michael Aschner, Department of Pediatrics, B-3307 Medical Center North, Vanderbilt University Medical Center, 1162 21st Avenue South, Nashville, TN 37232-2495. Voice: 615-322-8024; fax: 615-322-6541.
michael.aschner@vanderbilt.edu

**Ann. N.Y. Acad. Sci. 1053: 444–454 (2005). © 2005 New York Academy of Sciences.
doi: 10.1196/annals.1344.039**

acrylamide in certain starch-based foods such as potato chips, French fries, cookies, cereals, and bread. Levels of acrylamide in these foodstuffs exceeded the level given in the World Health Organization's Guideline Values for Drinking Water Quality.[7]

Data on the neurotoxicity of acrylamide to the central nervous system (CNS) are too extensive to review here. Acrylamide appears to induce changes in neurofilament distribution and function in the CNS.[3,6] In humans, acrylamide overexposure is associated with fatigue and weight loss. After acute exposure, hallucinations, loss of body temperature control, and coma have been observed.

The major metabolic pathway for acrylamide in rodents is oxidation via hepatic cyp 2e1[18] to glycidamide. This metabolite (glycidamide), unlike the parent compound, reacts with DNA. Acrylamide has been reported to be carcinogenic and genotoxic in rats and mice.[2,8,9] DNA damage in Chinese hamster ovary (CHO) cells was noted at acrylamide concentrations as low as 5 mM, while direct alkylation of 2′-deoxynucleosides was virtually nonexisitent *in vitro* after incubation with acrylamide.[17] DNA breakage in male germ cells[13] and dominant-lethal mutations in male mice[13,14] have been reported following large systemic doses of acrylamide (100 mg/kg/day, ip, for 3 weeks). Johnson *et al.*[9] and Friedman *et al.*[8] described acrylamide induction of benign tumors of the thyroid and mammary glands, and mesotheliomas of the tunica vaginalis testis. The mode of action of induction of these tumors appears to involve partial dopamine agonist activity of acrylamide. However, the ability of acrylamide to induce glial tumors (primarily gliomas and astrocytomas) remains unresolved. By studying a larger number of animals treated at higher doses, Friedman *et al.*[8] failed to demonstrate an increase in acrylamide-induced gliomas and astrocytomas, a finding that contradicted an earlier study.[9]

The present research was undertaken to assess the potential of acrylamide to promote cell proliferation in the CNS. The studies were carried out in astrocytes isolated from the Fischer 344 rat, a strain that has been reported to be susceptible to acrylamide-induced astrocytomas.[9]

GENERAL METHODS

Astrocyte Isolation

Briefly, cerebral cortices were obtained from neonatal (1-day-old) Fischer 344 rats. The meninges were carefully removed, the brain digested with a bacterial neutral protease (dispase, Sigma, St. Louis, MO), and astrocytes were recovered by repeated removal of dissociated cells.[16] The culture medium was changed 24 h after the initial plating to preserve the adherent astrocytes, while at the same time removing less adherent neurons and oligodendrocytes. Astrocytes were maintained for 3–4 weeks in minimum essential medium (MEM) with Earle's salts containing 10% heat-inactivated horse serum, 100 U/mL penicillin, 100 μg/mL streptomycin, and 0.25 μg/mL Fungizone. The medium was changed twice a week. Cells were >95% positive for the astrocytic marker, glial fibrillary acidic protein (GFAP).

Statistical Analysis

Statistical differences in the proposed endpoints between control and treated cells were determined using one-way randomized ANOVA design. When the overall test of significance ($P < 0.05$) led to a rejection of the null hypothesis, post-hoc (Newman-Keuls) comparisons were performed. Statistical analyses were performed with CSS:Statistical software (StatSoft Inc., Tulsa, OK).

EFFECTS OF ACRYLAMIDE ON VARIOUS PARAMETERS OF CELL PROLIFERATION

Protein Synthesis: [^{3}H]-Leucine Incorporation

Initial studies investigated the effects of acrylamide on total protein synthesis in primary neonatal astrocytes. After 7, 11, 15, or 20 days in culture, subconfluent monolayers of astrocytes were treated for 24 h with acrylamide at concentrations of 0.1 and 1.0 mM. Subsequent to treatment, cells were pulsed for 6 h with [^{3}H]-leucine (Amersham Pharmacia, Piscataway, NJ). The experiments were terminated by washing the cells twice with phosphate-buffered saline (PBS) and twice with ice-cold trichloroacetic acid (TCA) (10%). The resulting precipitate was solubilized and counted on a liquid scintillation counter. Each experiment was conducted in triplicate and with separate cultures derived from a minimum of three different litters.

As shown in FIGURE 1, acrylamide (0.1 and 1.0 mM) had no significant effect on [^{3}H]-leucine incorporation into Fischer 344 astrocytes on days 7, 11, 15, or 20 in culture, suggesting that acrylamide does not enhance astrocytic protein synthesis even at concentrations as high as 1 mM.

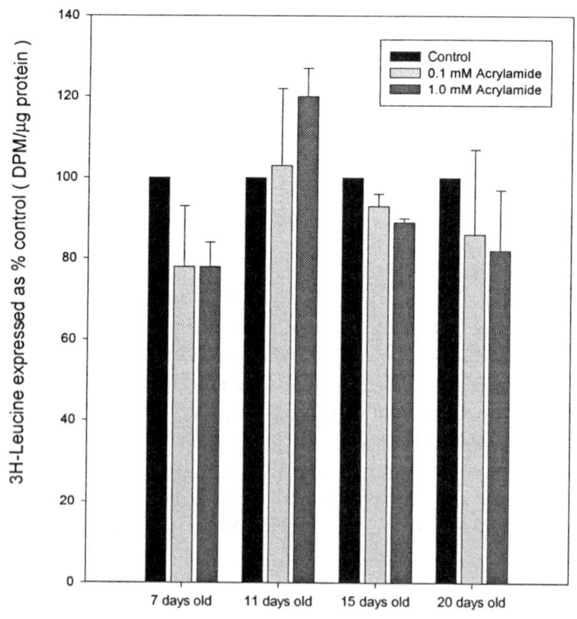

FIGURE 1. [^{3}H]-Leucine incorporation (6 h) in Fischer 344 astrocytes. See text for details.

DNA Synthesis: [^{3}H]-Thymidine Incorporation

Astrocytes were seeded on 12-well plates (22 mm), allowed to grow in standard culture conditions to subconfluency, and subsequently treated with acrylamide (0.1 and 1.0 mM). Twenty-four hours prior to the addition of [^{3}H]-thymidine (Amersham Pharmacia), the medium was removed and fresh medium containing acrylamide, but not serum, was added to the cells. This procedure was carried out to allow for cell cycle synchronization. Subsequently, the medium was removed and fresh medium containing [^{3}H]-thymidine was added for the last 24 h of acrylamide treatment. Cells were washed twice with ice-cold PBS and fixed in methanol for 10 min. Next, cells were washed twice with 10% TCA and once with 0.5% TCA, and dissolved in 0.5 mL of 1 N NaOH for 30 min at room temperature followed by the addition of 0.5 mL of 1 N HCl. Radioactivity was quantitated using a liquid scintillation counter. Each experiment was conducted in triplicate and with separate cultures derived from a minimum of three different litters.

As shown in FIGURE 2, acrylamide had no significant ($P > 0.05$) effect on [^{3}H]-thymidine incorporation into Fischer 344 astrocytes after 7, 11, 15, or 20 days in culture, suggesting that acrylamide did not enhance astrocytic DNA synthesis.

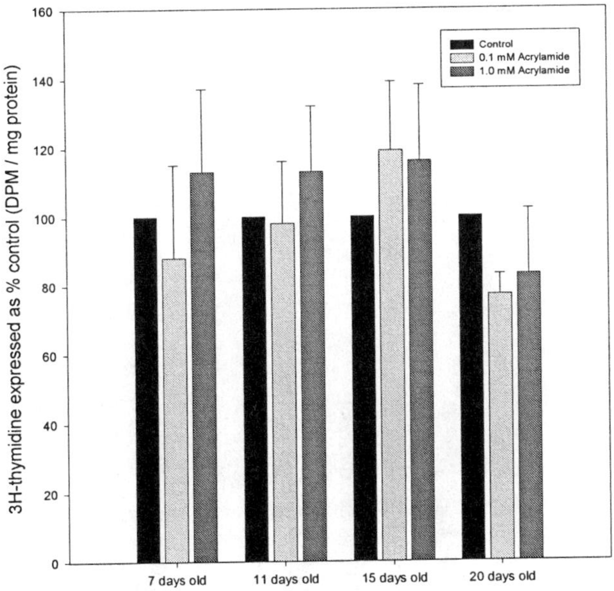

FIGURE 2. [^{3}H]-Thymidine incorporation (6 h) in Fischer 344 astrocytes. See text for details.

Proliferating Cell Nuclear Antigen (PCNA) Assay

PCNA, also known as cyclin, is a 36-kDa nonhistone nuclear protein. It has been demonstrated that PCNA is an auxiliary protein of DNA polymerase-δ and plays a fundamental role in the initiation of cell proliferation.[15] PCNA is a cell cycle–regulated protein that preferentially occurs in dividing cells and is undetectable, or present in small amounts, in resting cells. Its cell cycle distribution has been well described.[15] Elevated expression of PCNA appears in the nucleus during the late G1 phase immediately before the onset of DNA synthesis, becomes maximal during the S phase, and declines again during the G2 and M phases. Thus, its level correlates directly with rates of cellular proliferation and DNA synthesis. PCNA was measured using standard Western blotting techniques in astrocytes isolated from Fischer 344 rats.

Astrocytes in 100-mm dishes were exposed after 7, 11, 15, or 20 days in culture to acrylamide (0.1 or 1 mM) in HEPES buffer for 24 h at 37°C. Subsequently, the cells were washed three times with cold PBS (pH 7.4) and lysed with cold cell lysis buffer (100 mM Tris, pH 7.5, 1% SDS, 1 mM EDTA, 100 mM DTT). Protein content was determined using the bicinchoninic acid assay (BCA) method (Pierce, Rockford, IL). Aliquots of protein were mixed with Laemmli sample buffer and separated by denaturing with SDS-PAGE using 5% stacking and 7.5% resolving polyacrylamide gels. After separation, proteins were electrophoretically transferred (3 h at 60 volts) to a nitrocellulose membrane (Protran BA 83, Schleicher and Schuell, Keene, NH)

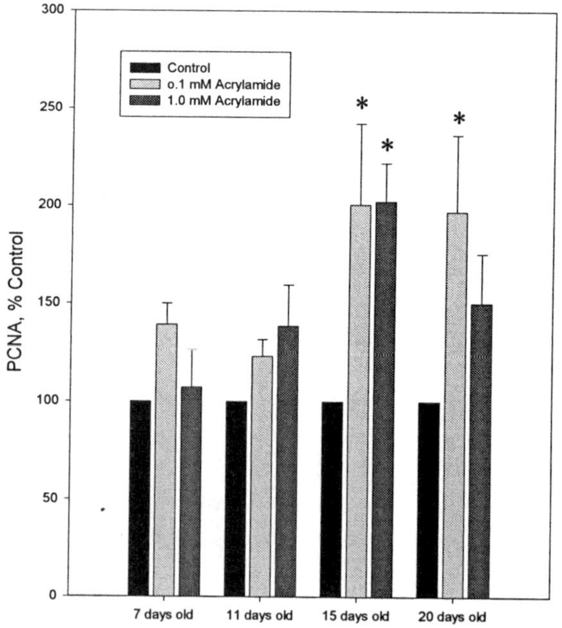

FIGURE 3. PCNA in Fischer 344 astrocytes. See text for details.

in 20% methanol, 0.1% SDS, 25 mM Tris, and 192 mM glycine. Membranes were blocked with 5% (w/v) nonfat powdered milk in Tris-buffered saline with Tween (TBST, 0.1% Tween 20; 150 mM NaCl; 20 mM Tris) for 1 h at room temperature. Next, blots were incubated for 2 h at room temperature with a mouse monoclonal PCNA antibody (1:10 dilution in TBST–5% NFDM; Santa Cruz Biotechnology) followed by incubation for 1 h with a horseradish peroxidase–conjugated anti-mouse secondary antibody (1:1000; Kirkegaard and Perry Laboratories, Gaithersburg, MD). Protein bands were visualized with the Renaissance-enhanced chemiluminescence system (New England Nuclear, Boston, MA) followed by exposure to X-ray film (BioMax MR, Eastman Kodak, Rochester, NY). Films were digitized and band density was determined using the TINA v2.09e (Raytest USA, Inc., Wilmington, NC). Statistical analysis was conducted as previously described.

Each experiment was conducted in triplicate and with separate cultures derived from a minimum of three different litters. The studies were conducted at 7, 11, 15, and 20 days in culture.

As shown in FIGURE 3, treatment of astrocytes with acrylamide (0.1 or 1.0 mM) had no statistically significant ($P > 0.05$) effect on PCNA protein levels after cells were in culture for 7 or 11 days. However, a statistically significant effect ($P < 0.05$) was noted on PCNA protein levels in astrocytes treated with acrylamide (0.1 or 1.0 mM) after cells were in culture for 15 or 20 days (only with 0.1 mM acrylamide). These studies suggest that, in response to acrylamide exposure, "older" astrocytes (15 and 20 days) proliferate at a greater rate than age-matched controls.

Is the Effect of Acrylamide on PCNA Expression Mediated via Dopamine (DA) Receptor Activation?

At least five genes encoding dopamine (DA) receptors have been discovered.[14] These five receptors have distinct pharmacological profiles as well as unique neuro-anatomical distributions. While D1 and D2 receptors are widely expressed in many neural systems, the novel D3 and D4 receptors appear to be concentrated within parts of the limbic system and the D5 receptor has a limited and unusual distribution. The distinct distributions of each of the DA receptors in brain may facilitate understanding the potential neurochemical and neuroanatomical substrates of psychiatric illnesses.

Given that astrocytes have been shown to express mRNA for D2 receptors,[4,5] that acrylamide possesses D2 receptor agonist-like activity,[1] and that D2 receptor activation is known to induce mitogenesis via the extracellular signal–regulated kinases (ERKs) and c-JUN N-terminal kinases (JNKs) activation, it is reasonable to postulate that acrylamide-induced D2 receptor activation might stimulate cell proliferation. D2 receptors have similar regional distributions in rat, monkey, and human brain, with the most intense staining occurring in striatum, olfactory bulb, substantia nigra,[10,12] and prefrontal cortex.[11] The D2 receptor is also expressed in astrocytes.[1] The regional distributions of D2 receptors and astrocytomas[9] allude to the potential involvement of D2 receptor activation and signaling pathways in acrylamide-induced astrocytomas.

To assess the involvement of D2 receptors in PCNA activation, we chose two experimental paradigms. In the first, we assessed whether treatment of astrocytes with quinpirole (in the absence of acrylamide), a selective D2 receptor agonist, would cause changes analogous to those inherent with acrylamide treatment, namely,

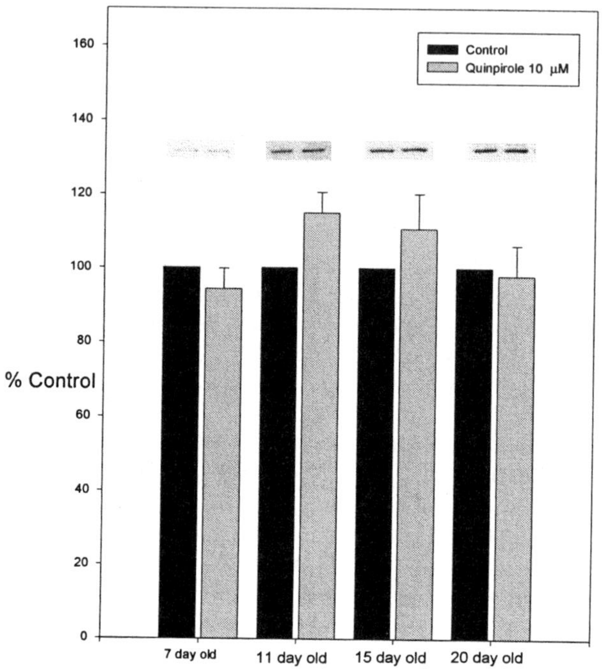

FIGURE 4. PCNA expression levels in Fischer 344 astrocytes treated with 10 μM quinpirole. See text for details.

increased PCNA protein expression as determined by means of routine Western blotting techniques.

As shown in FIGURE 4, it is notable that D2 activation with quinpirole (10 μM added to cultures for the last hour of 7, 11, 15, or 20 days in culture) has no significant ($P > 0.05$) discernible effects on astrocyte proliferation. Thus, it would appear that D2 receptor activation is not a necessary step in acrylamide-induced increased PCNA expression. However, these studies should be extended to cover a broader time course.

If indeed the effect of acrylamide on PCNA expression in astrocytes is mediated via D2 receptor activation, then this effect should be blocked with D2 receptor antagonists. Accordingly, we chose to assess PCNA expression in astrocyte cultures that were treated with acrylamide (0.1 mM; treatment analogous to that described above), in the presence of 1 μmol of the antagonist sulpiride for the last 6 h of exposure.

As shown in FIGURE 5, these studies reinforce the results presented in FIGURE 4 that acrylamide's effect is not likely associated with D2 receptor activation since sulpiride was ineffective in fully reversing the acrylamide-induced increase in PCNA expression. However, it should be noted that the studies were conducted with

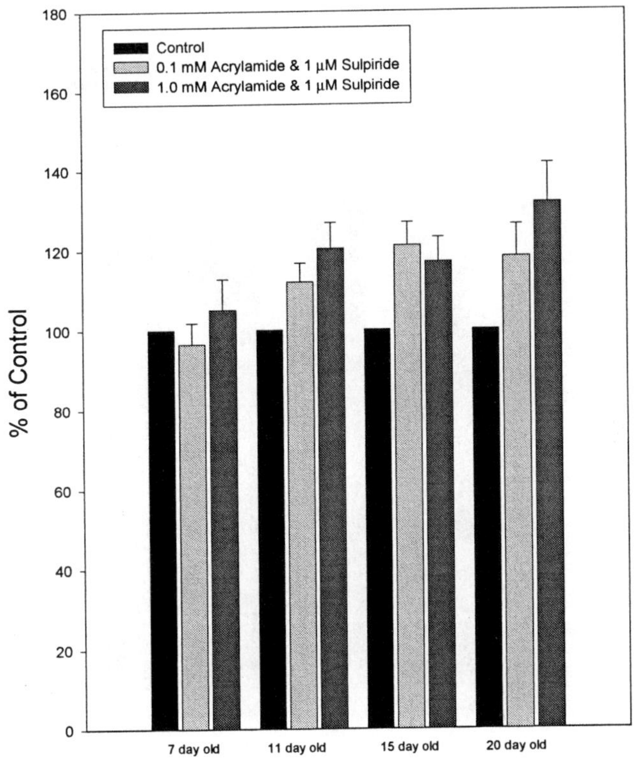

FIGURE 5. PCNA protein expression levels in Fischer 344 astrocytes treated with acrylamide (0.1 and 1 mM) and sulpiride (1 µM for the last 6 h). See text for details.

a single concentration of the antagonist (1 µM) and at a single time point (last 6 h of the treatments), and therefore these studies will have to be expanded in the future. Accordingly, these studies are preliminary in nature and additional studies should be conducted with multiple concentrations of sulpiride, as well as studies at several additional time points.

Is Glycidamide Equally Potent as PCNA Inducer?

Studies were carried out in analogous fashion to those described in FIGURE 1 in order to assess the ability of glycidamide, a postulated active metabolite of acrylamide, to increase the expression of astrocytic PCNA. As shown in FIGURE 6, glycidamide has no significant effect ($P < 0.05$) on PCNA expression at any time points tested, suggesting that the effect of acrylamide on PCNA expression in astrocytes is independent of the generation of glycidamide.

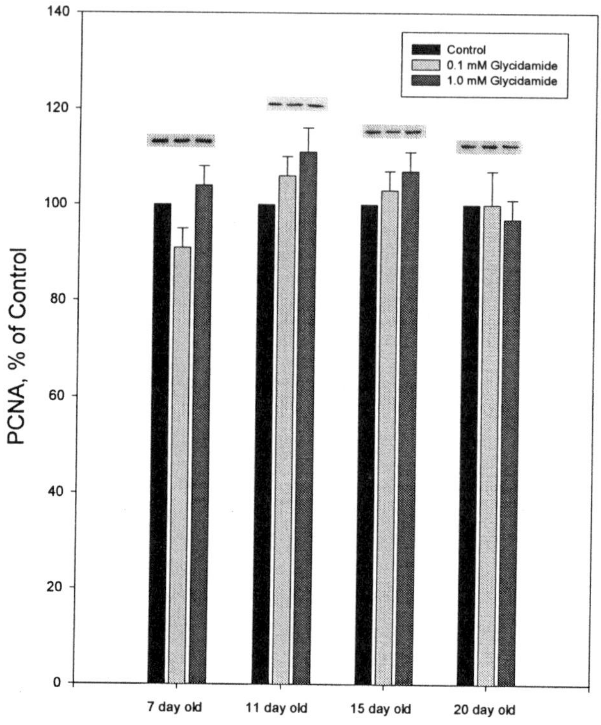

FIGURE 6. PCNA protein expression in Fischer 344 astrocytes treated with glycidamide (0.1 and 1 mM). See text for details.

CONCLUSIONS

The present study indicates that acrylamide increases PCNA expression in astrocytes isolated from Fischer 344 neonatal rats and allowed to grow in optimal conditions for up to 20 days in culture. PCNA was measured using standard Western blotting techniques. Each experiment was conducted with a minimum of triplicate samples derived from separate cultures. The studies were conducted after cells had been in culture for 7, 11, 15, or 20 days. As shown in FIGURE 3, treatment of Fischer 344–derived astrocytes with acrylamide (0.1 and 1.0 mM) led to a significant effect on PCNA protein levels after 15 (at both 0.1 and 1.0 mM concentrations) or 20 days in culture (only with 0.1 mM acrylamide). Comparison between acrylamide's effects on astrocyte PCNA protein expression and its effects on [^{3}H]-leucine (FIG. 1) and [^{3}H]-thymidine incorporation showed more similarities than discrepancies. Nevertheless, discrepancies exist, specifically vis-à-vis acrylamide-treated astrocytes after 15 or 20 days in culture, where increased PCNA protein expression (FIG. 1) indicates enhanced astrocytic proliferation, while no changes in either [^{3}H]-leucine (FIG. 1) or [^{3}H]-thymidine incorporation were noted. A possible explanation for this discrepancy is that acrylamide might affect the rate of uptake of [^{3}H]-thymidine into astrocytes, thus masking a potential difference in [^{3}H]-thymidine incorporation.

Taken together, the high sensitivity of the PCNA assay suggests that acrylamide can stimulate astrocytic proliferation. Notably, and consistent with published data, the studies also suggest that the more mature astrocytes (with a 20-day astrocytic incubation *in vitro* taken as a model of accelerated senescence) are significantly more sensitive to acrylamide compared with immature astrocytes. This effect is most likely not associated with D2 receptor activation, given the inability of quinpirole, a selective D2 receptor agonist, to mimic the effect of acrylamide on PCNA protein expression and the apparent inability of sulpiride (a D2 antagonist) to block the effect of acrylamide. Finally, glycidamide, an active metabolite of acrylamide, does not appear to induce PCNA expression in astrocytes, suggesting that acrylamide's effect is likely independent of this metabolite and not related to DNA binding. Additional studies should be carried out over a wider concentration range and more exposure durations to better define the role of these receptors in acrylamide's effect. Overall, acrylamide was shown to induce PCNA protein expression in astrocytes, and this effect seems selective for "older" astrocytes. The studies support the ability of acrylamide to cause cell proliferation in astrocytes, although the significance is obfuscated by the absence of concomitant increase in DNA synthesis. Future studies could be profitably directed at resolving these issues in *in vivo* models.

ACKNOWLEDGMENTS

This study was supported by funds from SNF S.A., Andrezieux, France. We thank Timothy R. Fennell for the synthesis and provision of glycidamide.

REFERENCES

1. Bal, A., T. Bachelot, M. Savasta *et al.* 1994. Evidence for dopamine D_2 receptor mRNA expression by striatal astrocytes in culture: *in situ* hybridization and polymerase chain reaction studies. Mol. Brain Res. **23:** 204–212.
2. Bull, R.J., M. Robinson, R.D. Laurie *et al.* 1984. Carcinogenic effects of acrylamide in Sencar and A/J mice. Cancer Res. **44:** 107–111.
3. Chauhan, N.B., P.S. Spencer & M.I. Sabri. 1993. Effect of acrylamide on the distribution of microtubule-associated proteins (MAP1 and MAP2) in selected regions of rat brain. Mol. Chem. Neuropathol. **18:** 225–245.
4. Crump, K.S. 1999 (June 11). Consideration of the Potency Classification of Acrylamide Based on the Incidence of Tunica Vaginalis Mesotheliomas (TVMs) in Male Fischer 344 Rats. Prepared for The Acrylamide Monomer Producers Group. The K. S. Crump Group, Inc., Ruston, LA.
5. Crump, K.S. 1999 (December 14). Mechanism of Acrylamide Induction of Benign Mammary Fibroadenomas in the Aging Female Fischer 344 Rat: Relevance to Human Health Risk Assessment. Prepared for The Acrylamide Monomer Producers Group. The K. S. Crump Group, Inc., Ruston, LA.
6. Endo, H., S. Kittur & M.I. Sabri. 1994. Acrylamide alters neurofilament protein gene expression in rat brain. Neurochem. Res. **19:** 815–829.
7. FAO/WHO Consultation on the Health Implications of Acrylamide in Food. 2002 (June 25–27). Summary Report [http://www.who.int/foodsafety/publications/chem/en/acrylamide_summary.pdf]. Geneva.

8. FRIEDMAN, M.A., L.H. DULAK & M.A. STEDHAM. 1995. A lifetime oncogenicity study in rats with acrylamide. Fundam. Appl. Toxicol. **27:** 95–105.
9. JOHNSON, K.A., S.J. GORZINSKI, K.M. BODNER *et al.* 1986. Chronic toxicity and oncogenicity study on acrylamide incorporated in the drinking water of Fischer 344 rats. Toxicol. Appl. Pharmacol. **85:** 154–168.
10. LEVEY, A.I., S.M. HERSCH, D.B. RYE *et al.* 1993. Localization of D1 and D2 dopamine receptors in brain with subtype-specific antibodies. Proc. Natl. Acad. Sci. USA **90:** 8861–8865.
11. LIDOW, M.S., P.S. GOLDMAN-RAKIC, D.W. GALLAGER & P. RAKIC. 1991. Distribution of dopaminergic receptors in the primate cerebral cortex: quantitative autoradiographic analysis using [^{3}H]raclopride, [^{3}H]spiperone, and [^{3}H]SCH23390. Neuroscience **40:** 657–671.
12. MISSALE, C., S.R. NASH, S.W. ROBINSON *et al.* 1998. Dopamine receptors: from structure to function. Physiol. Rev. **78:** 189–225.
13. SEGA, G.A., E.E. GENEROSO & P.A. BRIMER. 1990. Acrylamide exposure induces a delayed unscheduled DNA synthesis in germ cells of male mice that is correlated with the temporal pattern of adduct formation in testis DNA. Environ. Mol. Mutagen. **16:** 137–142.
14. SHELBY, M.D., K.T. CAIN, L.A. HUGHES *et al.* 1986. Dominant lethal effects of acrylamide in male mice. Mutat. Res. **173:** 35–40.
15. SCHUMACHER, B., A. ALPI & A. GARTER. 2003. Cell cycle: check for asynchrony. Curr. Biol. **13:** R560–R562.
16. SHANKER, G., J.L. ASCHNER, T. SYVERSEN & M. ASCHNER. 2004. Free radical formation in cerebral cortical astrocytes in culture induced by methylmercury. Mol. Brain Res. **128:** 48–57.
17. SOLOMON, J.J., J. FEDYK, F. MUKAI & A. SEGAL. 1985. Direct alkylation of 2′-deoxynucleosides and DNA following *in vitro* reaction with acrylamide. Cancer Res. **45:** 3465–3470.
18. SUMNER, S.C., T.R. FENNELL, T.A. MOORE *et al.* 1999. Role of cytochrome P450 2E1 in the metabolism of acrylamide and acrylonitrile in mice. Chem. Res. Toxicol. **12:** 1110–1116.

Neuroprotection by Platelet-Activating Factor Antagonism

XIAOHUA TIAN AND NICOLAS G. BAZAN

LSU Neuroscience Center of Excellence, Louisiana State University Health Sciences Center School of Medicine, New Orleans, Louisiana 70112, USA

KEYWORDS: antagonist; BN 52021; neuroprotection; phospholipase; phospholipid; platelet-activating factor (PAF)

The potent phospholipid messenger platelet-activating factor (PAF) participates in synaptic plasticity as well as pathologic processes. Under physiologic conditions, its synthesis, from arachinoyl (or docosahexaenoyl)–containing membrane phospholipids by phospholipase A2, and degradation by PAF-acetylhydrolases are tightly regulated. This balance is tripped under pathologic conditions, such as ischemia-reperfusion and neurodegenerations: PAF is overproduced and becomes a mediator of inflammation, and becomes neurotoxic when its concentration is enhanced. Physiologically, PAF acts as a retrograde messenger at the synapse, where it enhances long-term potentiation.[1] Administration of PAF pre- or posttraining enhances memory formation, and the PAF membrane-receptor antagonist BN 52021 blocks this effect.[2,3] During ischemia-reperfusion or seizures, phospholipases rapidly release free arachidonic and docosahexaenoic acids from neuronal membrane phospholipids,[4,5] and overproduced PAF contributes to elevated presynaptic glutamate exocytosis. BN 52021 also blocks this effect.[6] Pre- and posthypoxic administration of BN 52021 can decrease the incidence and severity of brain injury in perinatal cerebral hypoxia.[7] A recombinant PAF-acetylhydrolase has been found to protect against NMDA-induced apoptosis in hippocampal neurons in culture.[8]

Likely, the pathologic significance of PAF, in addition to its accumulation, may also be the specific cellular and/or intracellular site where its pool size becomes enlarged. Since PAF is a potent inducer of early gene expression,[9–11] it may, through gene-mediated modulation, elicit both protective or physiologic responses. Insofar as the site(s) of neuroprotection by PAF antagonism is concerned, the cerebrovascular unit is a major target, both in brain ischemia-reperfusion as well as in neurodegenerations. Further studies should define the specificity and potency of PAF antagonists at the level of endothelial cells and astrocytes, as well as in neurons. Accumulated evidence warrants further exploration on the potential clinical usefulness of PAF antagonists in neuroprotection.

Address for correspondence: Nicolas G. Bazan, LSU Neuroscience Center, 2020 Gravier Street, Suite D, New Orleans, LA 70112. Voice: 504-599-0831; fax: 504-568-5801.
nbazan@lsuhsc.edu

Ann. N.Y. Acad. Sci. 1053: 455–456 (2005). © 2005 New York Academy of Sciences.
doi: 10.1196/annals.1344.057

ACKNOWLEDGMENTS

This research was supported by NIH Grant No. NS46741.

REFERENCES

1. KATO, K., G.D. CLARK, N.G. BAZAN & C.F. ZORUMSKI. 1994. Platelet-activating factor as a potential retrograde messenger in CA1 hippocampal long-term potentiation. Nature **367:** 175–179.
2. IZQUIERDO, I., C. FIN, P.K. SCHMITZ *et al.* 1995. Memory enhancement by intrahippocampal, intraamygdala, or intraentorhinal infusion of platelet-activating factor measured in an inhibitory avoidance task. Proc. Natl. Acad. Sci. USA **92:** 5047–5051.
3. BAZAN, N.G., M.G. PACKARD, L. TEATHER & G. ALLAN. 1997. Bioactive lipids in excitatory neurotransmission and neuronal plasticity. Neurochem. Int. **30:** 225–231.
4. HORROCKS, L.A. & A.A. FAROOQUI. 1994. NMDA receptor–stimulated release of arachidonic acid: mechanisms for the Bazan effect. *In* Cell Signal Transduction, Second Messengers, and Protein Phosphorylation in Health and Disease, pp. 113–128. Plenum. New York.
5. SUN, G.Y., J. XU, M.D. JENSEN & A. SIMONYI. 2004. Phospholipase A2 in the central nervous system: implications for neurodegenerative diseases. J. Lipid Res. **45:** 205–213.
6. BAZAN, N.G., E.B. RODRIGUEZ DE TURCO & G. ALLAN. 1995. Mediators of injury in neurotrauma: intracellular signal transduction and gene expression. J. Neurotrauma **12:** 791–814.
7. LIU, X.H., B.L. EUN, F.S. SILVERSTEIN & J.D. BARKS. 1996. The platelet-activating factor antagonist BN 52021 attenuates hypoxic-ischemic brain injury in the immature rat. Pediatr. Res. **40:** 797–803.
8. OGDEN, F., M.A. DECOSTER & N.G. BAZAN. 1998. Recombinant plasma-type platelet-activating factor acetylhydrolase attenuates NMDA-induced hippocampal neuronal apoptosis. J. Neurosci. Res. **53:** 677–684.
9. SQUINTO, S.P., A.L. BLOCK, P. BRAQUET & N.G. BAZAN. 1989. Platelet-activating factor stimulates a fos/jun/AP-1 transcriptional signaling system in human neuroblastoma cells. J. Neurosci. Res. **24:** 558–566.
10. SQUINTO, S.P., P. BRAQUET, A.L. BLOCK & N.G. BAZAN. 1990. Platelet-activating factor activates HIV promoter in transfected SH-SY5Y neuroblastoma cells and MOLT-4 T lymphocytes. J. Mol. Neurosci. **2:** 79–84.
11. BAZAN, N.G., S.P. SQUINTO, P. BRAQUET *et al.* 1991. Platelet-activating factor and polyunsaturated fatty acids in cerebral ischemia or convulsions: intracellular PAF-binding sites and activation of a fos/jun/AP-1 transcriptional signaling system. Lipids **26:** 1236–1242.

Questions and Answers

Session IX: Sensitive Targets for Neurotoxicity and Neuroprotection

QUESTIONS FOR HARI SHARMA

From Naren Banik

You have shown interesting data on the model of spinal cord injury (SCI). Have you looked at evoked potential in the contusion injury model? It was also good to see data on nimodipine, which provides neuroprotection. Have you tried any other Ca^{2+} channel blockers? Last, the indomethacin data were very interesting since it inhibits calpain activity. Have you looked at calpain activity?

ANSWER: Thanks for your comments. We have not seen evoked potentials in the contusion model, but we evaluated spinal cord evoked potentials (SCEPs) in our incision model of SCI. We found that the amplitude of SCEP declines within 2 min after SCI and can recover to some extent after 1 or 2 h. However, the latency of SCEP is increased always. Sometimes, a positive injury potential appears, indicating massive cord injury. Nimodipine is the only drug that prevents the latency increase after SCI. The data on indomethacin also support the idea that the compound, if given before SCI, is neuroprotective. However, we have so far not examined the calpain activity.

From Italo Mocchetti

Did you see any recovery of function following the application of BDNF on ME compounds?

ANSWER: This is a very good question. So far, we have not seen the recovery function after SCI. Due to limitation of our experimental models at the moment, we are unable to conduct such studies. However, we believe that BDNF or melanocortins may influence the functional outcome in our model as well. However, available evidence so far is still unclear regarding the pathological outcome and its correlation with the functional outcome measures. There is evidence that functional outcome improves by some drugs, whereas the spinal cord cell and tissue injury still persists. Thus, it would be interesting to see whether BDNF and melanocortins can influence both motor functions and spinal cord pathology in our model. This is a subject that is currently being examined in my laboratory.

Ann. N.Y. Acad. Sci. 1053: 457–459 (2005).
doi: 10.1196/annals.1344.068

QUESTIONS FOR MICHAEL ASCHNER

From Chia Xi Kuan

You showed that acrylamide induces PCNA and not [^{3}H]thymidine incorporation in astrocytes. Since PCNA can be induced by DNA damage and is not necessarily specific for proliferation, could it be possible that acrylamide induces DNA damage in astrocytes? Have you examined potential single- or double-strand DNA breaks induced by acrylamide?

ANSWER: PCNA, also known as cyclin, is a 36-kDa nonhistone nuclear protein. It has been demonstrated that PCNA is an auxiliary protein of DNA polymerase-δ and plays a fundamental role in the initiation of cell proliferation. PCNA is a cell cycle–regulated protein that preferentially occurs in dividing cells and is undetectable or present in small amounts in resting cells. Its cell cycle distribution has been well described. Elevated expression of PCNA appears in the nucleus during late G1 phase immediately before the onset of DNA synthesis, becomes maximal during S phase, and declines again during G2 and M phases. Therefore, its level correlates directly with the rates of cellular proliferation and DNA synthesis. Having said this, one may not dismiss the possibility that acrylamide induced DNA damage in astrocytes. We have not tested this possibility.

Acrylamide has been reported to be carcinogenic and genotoxic in rats and mice. DNA damage in Chinese hamster ovary (CHO) cells was noted at acrylamide concentrations as low as 5 mM, while direct alkylation of 2′-deoxynucleosides was virtually nonexistent *in vitro* after incubation with acrylamide. DNA breakage in male germ cells and dominant-lethal mutations in male mice have been reported following large systemic doses of acrylamide.

From Naren Banik

The acrylamide-induced astrocytoma is an interesting model. Have you used temozolomide, a cancer treatment drug, to see if this will have some beneficial effects in rats? Have you looked at cysteine sulfinic acid decarboxylase activity? Does retinoic acid promote differentiation of these cells?

ANSWER: Glioblastomas are the most common primary brain tumors in adults. Despite surgical resection and focal radiotherapy, the prognosis is poor, with a median survival of 12 months. Adjuvant chemotherapy with nitrosourea does not have a substantial effect in randomized studies; only a large meta-analysis found a moderate increase in survival. The positive results of a phase III trial of a combination of radiotherapy and temozolomide is thus a major advance in the care of these patients (Carpentier, 2004). As to whether this drug can reduce the incidence of astrocytomas in rats, the answer is that these types of studies have yet to be carried out.

Cysteine sulfinic acid decarboxylase (CSAD), the rate-limiting enzyme in taurine biosynthesis, is known to be present in the brain in multiple isoforms. Given the effects of acrylamide on taurine that I have shown, it would be logical to assess the effect of acrylamide on CSAD and to determine whether it has an effect on taurine synthesis. To date, these studies have not been done.

P19 embryonic carcinoma cells are pluripotent cells that can undergo irreversible differentiation into the derivatives of all three germ layers (i.e., ectoderm, mesoderm, and endoderm) depending on their physical configurations (monolayer culture or cell aggregates) and their environment. The exposure of P19 cell aggregates to retinoic acid (RA) leads to their differentiation into astrocytes and neurons (Rujano *et al.*, 2004), and human malignant glioma cell lines are refractory to RA-mediated differentiation (Schmidt *et al.*, 2000). Hence, with regard to your last question, RA does indeed promote astrocytic differentiation.

From Kenneth Maynard

How does 0.1 nM and 1.0 nM acrylamide compare to blood plasma levels of acrylamide-poisoned patients? Did you measure any changes in cerebral blood flow on the cerebral vasculature since acrylamide poisoning affects peripheral vascular sympathetic contractions as well as SP- and CGRP-induced vasodilatation?

ANSWER: The studies that I have described were conducted *in vitro*; hence, these measurements were not conducted. As you know from studies that you have conducted, acrylamide treatment is not associated with changes in noradrenaline, neuropeptide Y, and calcitonin gene–related peptide tissue content between control and experimental rabbits. However, it causes a slight reduction in catecholamine histofluorescence. In addition, endothelium-dependent relaxant responses to acetylcholine and substance P are attenuated in acrylamide-treated rabbits, whereas relaxant responses mediated by calcitonin gene–related peptide (endothelium-independent) are unaffected. The relationship of these effects to the development of astrocytoma has yet to be defined.

Expression of Prostaglandin E_2 Synthases in Mouse Postnatal Cortical Neurons

VALENTINA ECHEVERRIA,[a] DAVID L. GREENBERG,[a] AND SYLVAIN DORÉ[a,b]

Departments of [a]Anesthesiology/Critical Care Medicine and [b]Neuroscience, Johns Hopkins University School of Medicine, Baltimore, Maryland 21205, USA

ABSTRACT: Eicosanoids and the enzymes associated with their metabolism play an active role in the neuroinflammatory process that is often a hallmark of neurodegenerative disorders. Cerebral cortical neurons constitute a highly affected cell population in neurologic disorders. To obtain a cellular model to analyze prostaglandin action and metabolism in cortical neurons, we developed postnatal neuronal cultures from mouse cortex in a serum-free medium. Cultured cortical cells were highly enriched in neurons containing only 5±2% glial cells. The cultures were assayed for expression of several protein markers of neuronal maturity: synaptic markers (synapsin I and synaptophysin) and glutamate receptor subunits (NMDA receptor 1 and glutamate receptor 1). The protein expression of eicosanoid-metabolizing enzymes, including cyclooxygenase-2 and microsomal and cytosolic PGE_2 synthases, was investigated as well. Postnatal neurons successfully survived for a long term (up to 40 days) *in vitro* in serum-free media, as characterized by the expression of synapsin I, synaptophysin, and microtubule-associated protein 2. Glutamate receptor subunit expression increased over time in cultures, with the highest levels at 15 days. Enzymes involved in the eicosanoid metabolism followed a distinct pattern of expression, suggesting potential regulation of PGE_2 synthesis with time in cultures under basal conditions. Use of postnatal brain cultures offers several advantages, especially regarding degree of neuronal maturation, use of postnatal pups instead of pregnant mice, and potentially increased clinical relevance in models of neuroinflammation processes and prostanoid cellular neurobiology.

KEYWORDS: cell cultures; cyclooxygenase; glutamate receptors; neuroinflammation; prostaglandin E_2; synapsin I; synaptophysin

INTRODUCTION

Over the past decade, it has been determined that eicosanoids, particularly prostaglandins (PGs), participate in several acute or chronic neuropathologic disorders, such as stroke, epilepsy, amyotrophic lateral sclerosis, and Alzheimer's disease.[1–3] PGs are derived from arachidonic acid via the enzymatic action of cyclooxygenases 1 and 2 (COX-1 and COX-2). Published reports are conflicting as to whether COX inhibitors are beneficial or detrimental to patients with these neurologic disorders.[4] Therefore, a better understanding of the role of PGs in these diseases would be

Address for correspondence: Sylvain Doré, Ph.D., Associate Professor, Johns Hopkins University School of Medicine, Dept. ACCM, 720 Rutland Avenue, Ross Research Building 364–365, Baltimore, MD 21205. Voice: 410-614-4859; fax: 410-955-7271.
sdore@jhmi.edu

Ann. N.Y. Acad. Sci. 1053: 460–471 (2005).
doi: 10.1196/annals.1344.040

facilitated by the availability of cellular models. Because several of these neuropathologic conditions affect the cortical neurons, primary cortical cultures provide a useful model with which to study the neurodegeneration and inflammation that accompany them[5–7] and to assay the effects of pharmacologic agents and endogenous molecules on neuronal growth, survival, and synaptic formation.

Although most researchers have used embryonic neurons (because they are easier to culture, more stable, more viable, and longer-lived than cultured adult neurons[5–8]), most neurodegenerative disorders are associated with mature/differentiated neurons and could be more accurately modeled with more mature cells, such as postnatal or adult neurons. Despite the difficulty of culturing adult and postnatal neurons, recently, several protocols have been attempted to maintain postnatal rodent neurons obtained from different brain regions, including the visual cortex,[9] hippocampus,[10,11] and brain stem.[12]

PGE_2 is an eicosanoid that participates in several physiologic responses in the brain, such as synaptic plasticity,[13] neurogenesis,[14] and pyrogenesis,[15] by acting on specific G-protein-coupled receptors.[16] Despite the abundant data reported, both *in vitro* and *in vivo*, concerning the role of COX and PGs, information is incomplete regarding the expression of the numerous enzymes specifically involved in PGE_2 synthesis, such as cytosolic and microsomal PGE synthases (PGESs). Moreover, it is known that neuronal susceptibility to toxic insults changes with time in culture and with degree of cell maturation, and that some of these changes can induce changes in cell signaling[17] and protein expression.[18] We have developed a method by which to culture postnatal mouse cortical cells for use as an *in vitro* neuronal model for analysis of the contribution of eicosanoids in neuroinflammation. We investigated the pattern of expression of several proteins involved in PGE_2 synthesis, such as the PGE_2 synthases not previously characterized in this kind of neuronal culture. Because the culture of mice postnatal neurons in serum-free conditions is not a commonly used technique, we also examined the time course of expression of markers of synapse formation and glutamatergic maturation in these cells using Western blots and immunocytochemistry techniques.

MATERIALS AND METHODS

Animals

All experiments were conducted using C57BL/6 mice that were housed and used in accordance with the National Institutes of Health guidelines for the use of experimental animals. Protocols were approved by the Institutional Animal Care and Use Committee at Johns Hopkins University.

Postnatal Cell Cultures

Cerebral cortical cells were obtained from the brains of 1- to 2-day-old mouse pups. Briefly, brains were removed aseptically and placed into Hibernate™-A medium (Brainbits LLC, Springfield, IL) with B27 at room temperature. Hibernate™-A medium is a Neurobasal-A medium specifically adapted for use with adult neurons because, by virtue of a higher osmolality (280 mOsm/kg H_2O) than traditional media, it enhances the survival of postnatal neurons. The B27 supplement is an optimized serum-free additive (Invitrogen, Carlsbad, CA). After the brains were dissected, the blood vessels and meninges were carefully removed under a dissecting microscope. Brain cortices were isolated and dissociated by digestion with a solution of 0.05% trypsin (Sigma, St. Louis, MO) containing DNase I (0.06%) in Hibernate™-A medium without B27 for 15 min at 37°C. The digestion reaction was stopped with Hibernate™-A/B27 containing 10% fetal bovine serum (Invitrogen) and triturated by repeated passages (<20 times) through a 10-mL pipette. The cell suspension was filtered through a sterile cell strainer (70 μm; BD Biosciences, Bedford, MA) into a 50-mL centrifuge tube. The cells were pelleted by centrifugation at 200*g* for 5 min, and resuspended in Neurobasal-A/B27 medium supplemented with 0.25 mM GlutaMax I (Invitrogen), 0.25 mM glutamine (Invitrogen), and a solution cocktail containing penicillin G (50 U/mL) and streptomycin (50 μg/mL) (Invitrogen). High-density cultures (5×10^5 cells, ~2500 cells/mm^2) were plated onto 20-mm^2 tissue culture wells coated with poly-D-lysine (Sigma). The neurons were kept at 37°C in 95% air/5% CO_2 for various (5–40) days *in vitro* (DIV) and used for cell staining and Western blot analysis. After 4–5 days, half of the conditioned medium was replaced with fresh medium. More frequent changes of culture medium or the use of cytosine arabinoside (Ara-C; Sigma) is not advised because they reduce the cell viability of these postnatal cortical neurons.

Propidium Iodide and Calcein Cell Staining

Cell viability was estimated by calcein and propidium iodide (PI) fluorescent staining of cells cultured for 5, 10, 15, and 30 DIV. After being washed with PBS, the cells were stained by incubation with calcein (1 μM) and PI (5 μM) solutions for 1 h and 15 min, respectively. After the cells were washed, the markers in the cells were analyzed and counted using a fluorescence microscope (Nikon Eclipse TE 2000) and MetaVue imaging software (Universal Imaging Corporation, Downingtown, PA).

Western Blot Analysis

For the analysis of protein expression by immunoblotting, postnatal cortical cells from 5, 10, and 15 DIV were scraped and disrupted by sonication in lysis buffer (Cell Signaling Technology, Beverly, MA) supplemented with 1× complete protease inhibitor cocktail (Roche Molecular Biochemicals, Indianapolis, IN), 1 mM phenylmethyl sulfonyl fluoride (PMSF), and 10 mM NaF (Sigma). After sonication on ice, cell extracts were centrifuged at 20,000*g* for 30 min at 4°C. The resultant supernatants were analyzed for protein concentration, adjusted to 1× Laemmli buffer, and boiled for 10 min. Samples of cell extracts containing equal amounts of protein were separated by SDS-PAGE and transferred to nitrocellulose membranes (BA83 0.2 μm, Bio-Rad, Hercules, CA). The membranes were blocked in Tris-buffered saline with 0.2% Tween 20 (TTBS) containing 10% dry milk. Primary antibody incubations were performed in TTBS with 3% dry milk overnight at 4°C. The following antibodies were assayed: rabbit polyclonal antibodies directed against microsomal prostaglandin E_2 synthase (mPGES-1 and mPGES-2, 1:500, Cayman, Ann Arbor, MI), cytosolic prostaglandin E synthase (cPGES, 1:2000, Cayman), glutamate receptor subunits (anti-NR1, 1:1000, Upstate Cell Signaling Solutions, Charlottesville, VA; anti-GluR1, 1:1000, Upstate), and COX-2 (1:2000, Cayman); and monoclonal antibodies directed against synaptic markers (synapsin I, 1:10,000, BD Biosciences; and synaptophysin, 1:10,000, BD Biosciences). Anti-bIII tubulin (1:10,000, Promega, Madison, WI) monoclonal antibody was used as a loading control. After being washed, the membranes were incubated with the appropriate secondary horseradish peroxidase (HRP)–conjugated antibody for 1 h in TTBS with 3% dry milk. Immunoreactive proteins were visualized as bands with the enhanced chemiluminescence system (ECL; Amersham Biosciences, Piscataway, NJ).

Immunocytochemistry Staining

Fluorescent immunocytochemical staining was used to visualize protein markers of maturity and cell population structure, including microtubule-associated protein 2 (MAP2), glial fibrillary acidic protein (GFAP), synapsin I, and synaptophysin. Briefly, cells were seeded onto 4-well chamber slides coated with poly-D-lysine at a density of 3×10^5/well and cultured for more than a week before analysis. Cells adhering to the slide after being washed twice with PBS were fixed with 4% paraformaldehyde for 15 min, washed with PBS, permeabilized with 0.1% Triton X-100 for 1 min, washed again, blocked in 5% goat serum in PBS for 30 min, and incubated overnight at 4°C in mouse anti-MAP2 (1:250; Sigma), mouse anti-GFAP (1:500; Molecular Probes, Eugene, OR), mouse anti-synapsin I (1:1000; BD Biosciences), or mouse anti-synaptophysin (1:1000; BD Biosciences). After another wash with PBS, the cells were incubated with anti-mouse Alexa Fluor 546 secondary fluorescent antibody (1:2000; Molecular Probes). Some cells were also stained with the fluorescent DNA-binding dye, Hoechst 33258 (1:2000; Molecular Probes), to allow counting of total cell number during MAP2 and GFAP staining. Negative controls were incubated with secondary antibodies, but without primary antibodies. The cellular fluorescence associated with cell nuclei and the specific neuronal and glial markers was visualized under a fluorescence microscope (Nikon Eclipse TE 2000). MAP2- and GFAP-positive cells were counted in 8 separate fields over 3 wells, the percentages of MAP2-positive neurons and GFAP-positive glial cells were determined, and the purity of the neuronal cultures was calculated.

RESULTS

Survival of Cultured Postnatal Mouse Cortical Cells

Immediately after plating, the postnatal mouse cortical cells were spherical and in suspension and began to attach. After a few hours, neurons began to develop growing and branching dendrites and, after 5 DIV, established well-defined dendritic architecture. Over time, extensive development of dendrites and an increase in intercellular connections became evident. FIGURES 1A, 1B, 1C, and 1D show cortical cells stained with calcein and PI after 5, 10, 15, and 30 days in culture, respectively.

Postnatal Mouse Cortical Cells Cultured in Serum-Free Media

Cortical cell cultures in serum-free medium were enriched in neurons, based on analysis of cell morphology and MAP2 and GFAP immunoreactivities. After 15 DIV, the postnatal mouse cortical cell cultures contained 95±2% neurons (FIG. 2) and

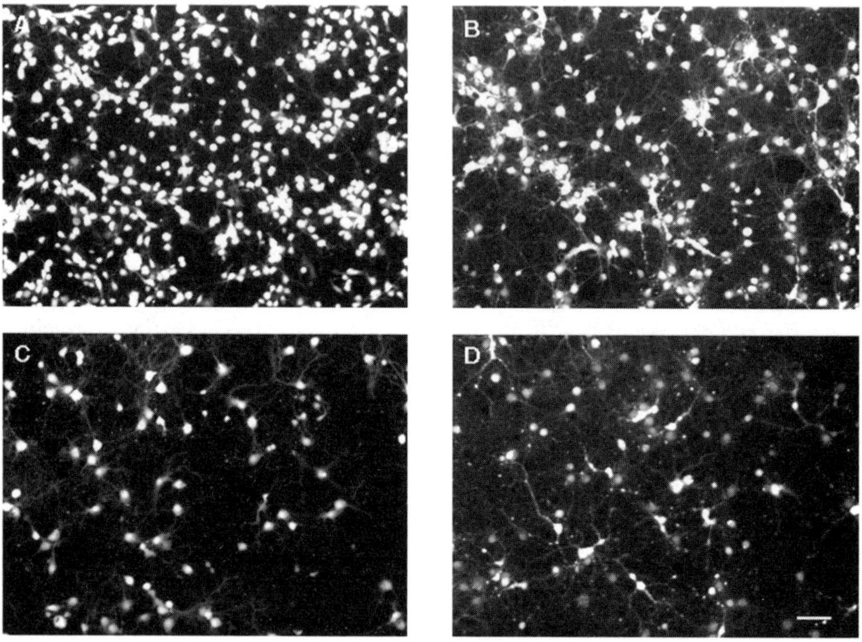

FIGURE 1. **(A–D)** Cell viability and maturation of postnatal mouse cortical cells in serum-free medium. Photomicrographs (×20) of cultured cells at 5 **(A)**, 10 **(B)**, 15 **(C)**, and 30 **(D)** days *in vitro* (DIV) obtained using fluorescent microscopy after staining with calcein and propidium iodide (scale bar: 50 μm). It is possible to observe the development of the dendritic/axonal architecture and the decrease in cell viability of cortical cells in culture from 1 to 15 DIV. [Figure reduced to 52%.]

5±2% glial cells. Highly branched GFAP-positive cells were observed, but they comprised less than 5% of all cells at 15 DIV. Although cell viability decreased with time in culture, living neurons showed a normal architecture, as evaluated with contrast-phase microscopy and fluorescence after staining with MAP2 neuronal markers. Healthy neuronal cultures were maintained as long as 40 DIV with our cell culture methodology.

Expression of Glutamate Receptor Subunits and Synaptic Markers in Postnatal Mouse Cortical Cells

The time course of protein expression of the general glutamate receptor subunits, NR1 (NMDA) and GluR1 (AMPA), and the synaptic markers, synapsin I and synaptophysin, was analyzed from the neuron extracts using Western blot after 5, 10, and 15 DIV. The expected sizes of bands estimated were as follows: NR1, 100 kDa; GluR1, 110 kDa; synapsin I, 80 kDa; and synaptophysin, 33 kDa. The results revealed that NR1, GluR1, synapsin I, and synaptophysin were present from 5 DIV in the cultured cortical cells and increased from 5 DIV to reach a maximum level after 15 DIV (FIG. 3). Immunocytochemical analysis also indicated that postnatal

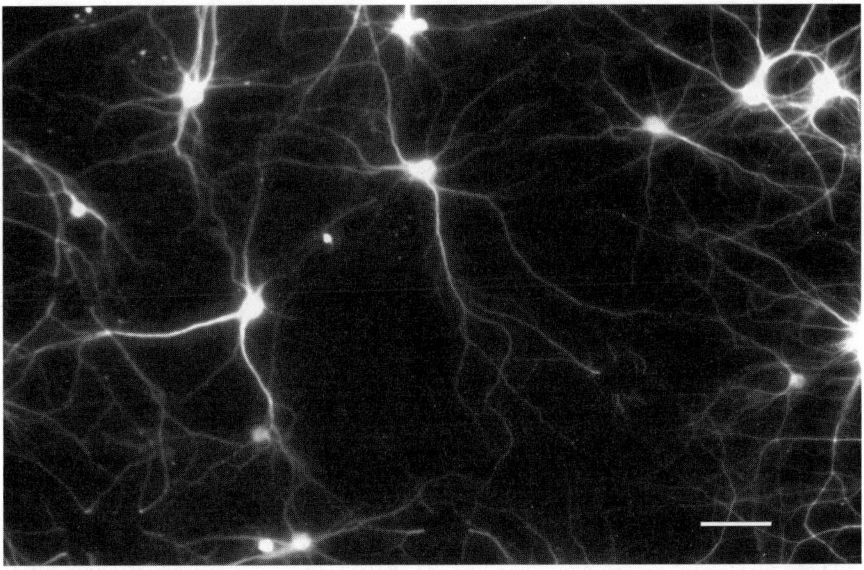

FIGURE 2. Immunostaining of postnatal cortical cells (×20) for microtubule-associated protein 2 (MAP2) after 15 DIV. The cultures of postnatal mouse cortical cells grown in serum-free medium were neuron-enriched and presented an extensively developed neuritic architecture after 15 DIV (scale bar: 50 μm). [Figure reduced to 41%.]

neurons as early as 5 DIV had the typical appearance and distribution of synapsin I (FIG. 4A) and synaptophysin (FIG. 4B) staining and revealed the presynaptic axon terminals (small bright dots) at the axodendritic and axosomatic boutons.

Expression of PGE_2 Synthase and COX-2 in Postnatal Mouse Primary Neurons

The time course of PGES and COX-2 protein expression in postnatal mouse primary neurons at 5, 10, and 15 DIV was analyzed by Western blot. The approximate protein band sizes obtained were as follows: COX-2, 72–74 kDa; microsomal PGES-1, 38 kDa; microsomal PGES-2, 16 kDa; and cytosolic PGES, 23 kDa. We found immunoreactive bands for microsomal and cytosolic PGES in the mouse cortical cells that increased from 5 DIV to 15 DIV (FIG. 3). The antibody directed against COX-2 revealed several immunoreactive bands at around 74 kDa, which could potentially represent posttranslational modifications, as previously reported.[19] The immunoreactive bands were detected at all culture times assayed (FIG. 3).

DISCUSSION

To obtain a cellular model to study neuronal function, the differentiation of embryonic neurons *in vitro* to a more "mature" phenotype has been a constant goal.[5,9] We speculate that substantial functional and molecular differences between

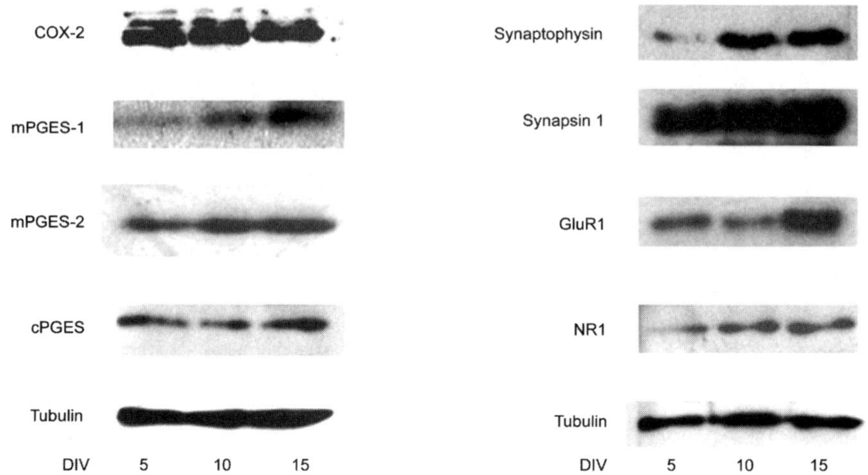

FIGURE 3. Protein maturation and aging of postnatal murine cortical neurons. Molecular changes were evaluated by the protein expression of prostaglandin E_2 synthases (cPGES, mPGES-1, mPGES-2), COX-2, glutamate receptors (GluR1, NR1), and synaptic markers (synapsin I, synaptophysin) over time. Cell extracts (20 μg) obtained from postnatal cortical cells after 5, 10, and 15 DIV were analyzed by Western blot using specific monoclonal and polyclonal antibodies as described in MATERIALS AND METHODS. Results were confirmed by three replicates.

the *in vitro* maturation of embryonic neurons and that of postnatal neurons are likely. During parturition and after birth, neurons are exposed to major hormonal and environmental changes[14] that are difficult to mimic using embryonic neuronal cultures. These differences may have unknown repercussions on the phenotype that exists after one or two weeks in culture, when most studies are performed. Here, we report the successful culture of postnatal mouse cortical cells in serum-free medium and the chronologic characterization of the expression of several proteins, including protein markers involved in the neuronal response to glutamate and synaptic development. We found that the *in vitro* expression of glutamate receptor subunits and synaptic markers in postnatal cortical neurons increased with time during neuron maturation in the culture dish.

Because the investigation of the prostaglandin metabolism in neurons is essential to discover new therapies for diseases that present neuroinflammation, we investigated the time course of expression of enzymes involved in eicosanoid metabolism, especially those related to PGE_2 synthesis,[20] because PGE_2 is one of the most relevant proinflammatory prostaglandins in the brain. A better understanding of arachidonic acid metabolism is of utmost importance because of the undesired side effects, such as an increase in incidence of stroke, associated with the use of COX-2 inhibitors.[21]

It has previously been shown that the expression and function of several proteins, such as trophic factors and neurotransmitter receptors, are differentially regulated during brain development. For example, the expression of brain-derived neurotrophic factor in the cortex and hippocampus is predominantly restricted to the early

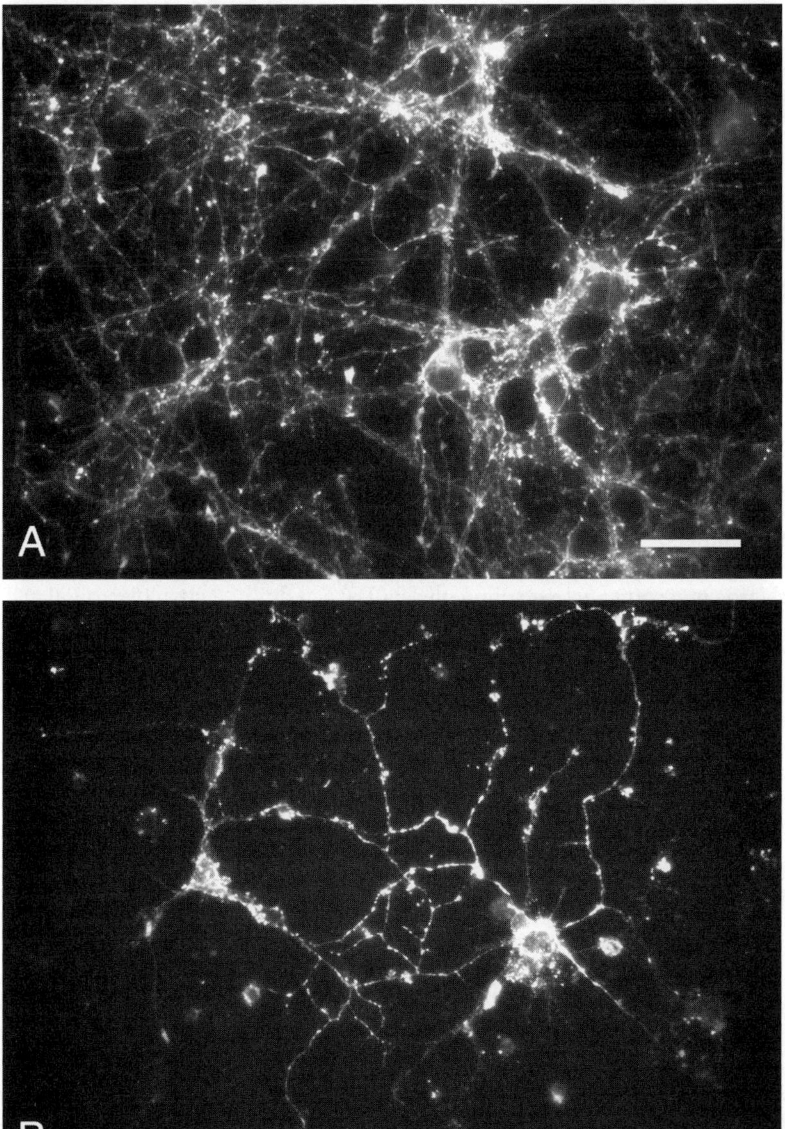

FIGURE 4. Immunocytochemical analysis of the expression of synaptic markers in postnatal cortical cells. Postnatal cortical neurons after 7 DIV were probed with specific antibodies for synapsin I (**A**) and synaptophysin (**B**). Note that the axons and synapses express the characteristic punctate distribution over the dendrites and neuronal cell bodies that seems to correspond with the arriving synaptic boutons. Photo taken at ×30 (scale bar: 50 μm). [Figure reduced to 65%.]

postnatal period.[22] Other developmental hormonal signals, such as estrogen, have been shown to influence maturation and plasticity of embryonic neurons.[23] Changes in the expression of neurotransmitter receptors or ion transporters may change the neuronal response to neurotransmitter and other ligands through brain development. For example, in the adult nervous system, glycine and GABA hyperpolarize the postsynaptic membrane. However, during the embryonic and early postnatal period, GABA and glycine are depolarizing, which increases intracellular calcium concentration and neuronal synaptic activity. This change in their activity results from changes in the expression of a Cl^- transporter named KCC2[24] that provoke a change in GABAergic actions from excitatory to inhibitory,[25] while glutamate gradually becomes the dominant excitatory neurotransmitter at later developmental stages.[26,27]

In general, culturing postnatal neurons offers some advantages over culturing neurons derived from mouse embryos. By sacrificing only pups, we reduce female adult mortality, which is particularly well suited for management of transgenic mouse colonies. Cultures in serum-free media also might increase the reproducibility of the experimental conditions because it is well known that the levels of hormones and glutamate in commercial animal serum vary substantially between batches. The variation in the composition of the media causes differences in cell population and cell viability, and influences the experimental outcome. We also observed that the concentration of glutamate in serum-based cultures is a critical factor for determining postnatal neuronal survival in neuronal cultures (data not shown). Conversely, cultures grown in serum-free medium present less variability and a lower glial cell population, an advantage that allows the performance of functional studies on neurons without the substantial and sometimes confusing influence of nonneuronal cells.

Our results show that postnatal mouse cortical neurons express the glutamate receptor subunits and the synaptic markers as early as 5 DIV. The expression of these synaptic markers at early stages suggests that postnatal cortical cells matured and established synaptic connections at 5 DIV. The regulation of these early-stage synaptic markers is particularly relevant when changes in the synaptic plasticity are being investigated. The temporal changes in NR1 and GluR1 expression levels may be important in neurotoxicity studies that are influenced by glutamate receptor activity. Several reports have described differences in the developmental expression of glutamate receptor subunits during cell culture[28] and in rodent[29,30] and human brains.[31] Previous studies showed that rodent cortical cells are vulnerable to glutamate toxicity after only 11 DIV, a time that correlates with an increase of NMDA receptor subunit expression.[28] Also, differences in glutamate receptor expression may be related to the fact that perinatal and adult brains vary in their vulnerability to excitotoxicity. For example, in rat brains, although it was reported that AMPA receptor subunit GluR1 expression is evident in 20-day-old embryonic brains, it is highly expressed only at postnatal day 15.[32]

Here, we characterized an *in vitro* neuronal system to study PGE_2 metabolism and signaling. PGE_2 synthesis is controlled by the consecutive actions of COX and prostaglandin E synthases (PGESs), which convert arachidonic acid to PGE_2. The two COX enzymes, COX-1 and COX-2, are very similar in structure, but they differ in their kinetic properties, their function in the body, and their intracellular localization. We observed in postnatal neuronal cultures that COX-2-like immunoreactivity revealed several bands that may correspond to previously reported COX-2 glycoforms of calculated molecular masses of 71.2, 72.7, and 73.9 kDa.[19]

COX function in neuroinflammation and brain pathology has received a remarkable amount of attention (for reviews, see refs. 2 and 33). Conversely, only in the last few years has the role of PGES in neuroinflammation been investigated.[34] Three different PGESs have been described: the microsomal PGES-1 (mPGES-1), which would be functionally coupled to COX-2;[35] the PGES-2 (mPGES-2);[36,37] and the cytosolic isoform (cPGES), which was originally reported to be coupled to COX-1.[38] Microsomal PGES-1 is a small oligomeric and membrane-bound protein that can be induced *in vivo* and *in vitro* by several endocrine factors and proinflammatory molecules, such as cytokines and bacterial lipopolysaccharides.[39,40] Microsomal PGES-1 has been postulated to be the major form implicated in COX-2-mediated PGE_2 production and to be involved in several pathologic conditions and neuropathic pain.[41–44] In postnatal neuronal cultures, we detected high levels of expression of cPGES as early as 5 DIV, with no detectable changes with increase in time. On the other hand, the microsomal PGESs, especially mPGES-1, revealed an increase of protein expression over time that was highest at 15 DIV. The easily detectable expression of PGESs in our neuronal cultures by Western blot made them a useful tool with which to investigate the regulation of PGES in physiologic and pathologic models.

In summary, our results suggest that cultures of postnatal mouse cortical neurons are able to acquire a phenotype of high expression levels of synaptic proteins and glutamate receptor subunits as early as 5 DIV. These culture conditions and the expression of several enzymes that participate in prostaglandin metabolism render this type of neuronal culture a feasible and useful tool for the analysis of the role of eicosanoids in neuroinflammation.

ACKNOWLEDGMENTS

This work was supported by research grants from the NIA (AG022971) and the NINDS (NS046400) (to S. Doré). We are grateful to Tzipora Sofare for her assistance in preparing this manuscript.

REFERENCES

1. PASINETTI, G.M. & P.S. AISEN. 1998. Cyclooxygenase-2 expression is increased in frontal cortex of Alzheimer's disease brain. Neuroscience **87:** 319–324.
2. O'BANION, M.K. 1999. COX-2 and Alzheimer's disease: potential roles in inflammation and neurodegeneration. Expert Opin. Invest. Drugs **8:** 1521–1536.
3. XIANG, Z. *et al.* 2002. Cyclooxygenase (COX)–2 and cell cycle activity in a transgenic mouse model of Alzheimer's disease neuropathology. Neurobiol. Aging **23:** 327–334.
4. MUKHERJEE, D., S.E. NISSEN & E.J. TOPOL. 2001. Risk of cardiovascular events associated with selective COX-2 inhibitors. JAMA **286:** 954–959.
5. LESUISSE, C. & L.J. MARTIN. 2002. Long-term culture of mouse cortical neurons as a model for neuronal development, aging, and death. J. Neurobiol. **51:** 9–23.
6. YU, X. & L. AN. 2002. A serum- and antioxidant-free primary culture model of mouse cortical neurons for pharmacological screen and studies of neurotrophic and neuroprotective agents. Cell. Mol. Neurobiol. **22:** 197–206.
7. POTTER, S.M. & T.B. DEMARSE. 2001. A new approach to neural cell culture for long-term studies. J. Neurosci. Methods **110:** 17–24.
8. RAY, J. *et al.* 1993. Proliferation, differentiation, and long-term culture of primary hippocampal neurons. Proc. Natl. Acad. Sci. USA **90:** 3602–3606.

9. HUETTNER, J.E. & R.W. BAUGHMAN. 1986. Primary culture of identified neurons from the visual cortex of postnatal rats. J. Neurosci. **6:** 3044–3060.
10. BREWER, G.J. *et al.* 1993. Optimized survival of hippocampal neurons in B27-supplemented Neurobasal, a new serum-free medium combination. J. Neurosci. Res. **35:** 567–576.
11. EVANS, M.S., M.A. COLLINGS & G.J. BREWER. 1998. Electrophysiology of embryonic, adult, and aged rat hippocampal neurons in serum-free culture. J. Neurosci. Methods **79:** 37–46.
12. KIVELL, B.M., F.J. MCDONALD & J.H. MILLER. 2001. Method for serum-free culture of late fetal and early postnatal rat brainstem neurons. Brain Res. Brain. Res. Protoc. **6:** 91–99.
13. CHEN, C., J.C. MAGEE & N.G. BAZAN. 2002. Cyclooxygenase-2 regulates prostaglandin E_2 signaling in hippocampal long-term synaptic plasticity. J. Neurophysiol. **87:** 2851–2857.
14. AMATEAU, S.K. & M.M. MCCARTHY. 2002. A novel mechanism of dendritic spine plasticity involving estradiol induction of prostaglandin-E_2. J. Neurosci. **22:** 8586–8596.
15. USHIKUBI, F. *et al.* 1998. Impaired febrile response in mice lacking the prostaglandin E receptor subtype EP3. Nature **395:** 281–284.
16. BREYER, M.D. & R.M. BREYER. 2001. G protein–coupled prostanoid receptors and the kidney. Annu. Rev. Physiol. **63:** 579–605.
17. DODGE, M.E., M. RAHIMTULA & K. MEAROW. 2002. Factors contributing to neurotrophin-independent survival of adult sensory neurons. Brain Res. **953:** 144–156.
18. WALSH, G.S. *et al.* 2004. The invulnerability of adult neurons: a critical role for p73. J. Neurosci. **24:** 9638–9647.
19. NEMETH, J.F. *et al.* 2001. Characterization of the glycosylation sites in cyclooxygenase-2 using mass spectrometry. Biochemistry **40:** 3109–3116.
20. ECHEVERRIA, V., D.L. GREENBERG & S. DORÉ. 2004. Characterization of the protein expression profile of eicosanoid metabolism enzymes and prostanoid receptors in postnatal neuronal cultures. Society for Neuroscience, Washington, D.C. Program No. 1021.8. Abstract Viewer/Itinerary Planner, Online.
21. DAVIES, N.M. & F. JAMALI. 2004. COX-2 selective inhibitors cardiac toxicity: getting to the heart of the matter. J. Pharm. Pharm. Sci. **7:** 332–336.
22. IVANOVA, T. & C. BEYER. 2001. Pre- and postnatal expression of brain-derived neurotrophic factor mRNA/protein and tyrosine protein kinase receptor B mRNA in the mouse hippocampus. Neurosci. Lett. **307:** 21–24.
23. TORAN-ALLERAND, C.D. 2004. Estrogen and the brain: beyond ER-alpha and ER-beta. Exp. Gerontol. **39:** 1579–1586.
24. RIVERA, C. *et al.* 1999. The K^+/Cl^- co-transporter KCC2 renders GABA hyperpolarizing during neuronal maturation. Nature **397:** 251–255.
25. KOTAK, V.C. *et al.* 1998. A developmental shift from GABAergic to glycinergic transmission in the central auditory system. J. Neurosci. **18:** 4646–4655.
26. AGUAYO, L.G. *et al.* 2004. Changes on the properties of glycine receptors during neuronal development. Brain Res. Brain. Res. Rev. **47:** 33–45.
27. LIU, B. & J.S. HONG. 2003. Neuroprotective effect of naloxone in inflammation-mediated dopaminergic neurodegeneration: dissociation from the involvement of opioid receptors. Methods Mol. Med. **79:** 43–54.
28. MIZUTA, I. *et al.* 1998. Developmental expression of NMDA receptor subunits and the emergence of glutamate neurotoxicity in primary cultures of murine cerebral cortical neurons. Cell. Mol. Life Sci. **54:** 721–725.
29. AWOBULUYI, M., S.A. LIPTON & N.J. SUCHER. 2003. Translationally distinct populations of NMDA receptor subunit NR1 mRNA in the developing rat brain. J. Neurochem. **87:** 1066–1075.
30. KITAYAMA, T. *et al.* 2004. Regulation of neuronal differentiation by *N*-methyl-D-aspartate receptors expressed in neural progenitor cells isolated from adult mouse hippocampus. J. Neurosci. Res. **76:** 599–612.
31. LAW, A.J. *et al.* 2003. Expression of NMDA receptor NR1, NR2A, and NR2B subunit mRNAs during development of the human hippocampal formation. Eur. J. Neurosci. **18:** 1197–1205.

32. MARTIN, L.J., A. FURUTA & C.D. BLACKSTONE. 1998. AMPA receptor protein in developing rat brain: glutamate receptor-1 expression and localization change at regional, cellular, and subcellular levels with maturation. Neuroscience **83:** 917–928.
33. KAM, P.C. & A.U. SEE. 2000. Cyclo-oxygenase isoenzymes: physiological and pharmacological role. Anaesthesia **55:** 442–449.
34. MURAKAMI, M. *et al.* 2002. Prostaglandin E synthase. Prostaglandins Other Lipid Mediat. **68/69:** 383–399.
35. THOREN, S. *et al.* 2003. Human microsomal prostaglandin E synthase-1: purification, functional characterization, and projection structure determination. J. Biol. Chem. **278:** 22199–22209.
36. TANIKAWA, N. *et al.* 2002. Identification and characterization of a novel type of membrane-associated prostaglandin E synthase. Biochem. Biophys. Res. Commun. **291:** 884–889.
37. BOSETTI, F., R. LANGENBACH & G.R. WEERASINGHE. 2004. Prostaglandin E2 and microsomal prostaglandin E synthase-2 expression are decreased in the cyclooxygenase-2-deficient mouse brain despite compensatory induction of cyclooxygenase-1 and Ca^{2+}-dependent phospholipase A2. J. Neurochem. **91:** 1389–1397.
38. TANIOKA, T. *et al.* 2000. Molecular identification of cytosolic prostaglandin E2 synthase that is functionally coupled with cyclooxygenase-1 in immediate prostaglandin E2 biosynthesis. J. Biol. Chem. **275:** 32775–32782.
39. JAKOBSSON, P.J. *et al.* 1999. Identification of human prostaglandin E synthase: a microsomal, glutathione-dependent, inducible enzyme, constituting a potential novel drug target. Proc. Natl. Acad. Sci. USA **96:** 7220–7225.
40. MURAKAMI, M. *et al.* 2000. Regulation of prostaglandin E2 biosynthesis by inducible membrane-associated prostaglandin E2 synthase that acts in concert with cyclooxygenase-2. J. Biol. Chem. **275:** 32783–32792.
41. YOSHIMATSU, K. *et al.* 2001. Inducible microsomal prostaglandin E synthase is overexpressed in colorectal adenomas and cancer. Clin. Cancer Res. **7:** 3971–3976.
42. KOTNIK, P. *et al.* 2005. Altered expression of COX-1, COX-2, and mPGES in rats with nephrogenic and central diabetes insipidus. Am. J. Physiol. Renal Physiol. Epub ahead of print [http://ajprenal.physiology.org/cgi/reprint/00114.2004v1].
43. TREBINO, C.E. *et al.* 2003. Impaired inflammatory and pain responses in mice lacking an inducible prostaglandin E synthase. Proc. Natl. Acad. Sci. USA **100:** 9044–9049.
44. MABUCHI, T. *et al.* 2004. Membrane-associated prostaglandin E synthase-1 is required for neuropathic pain. Neuroreport **15:** 1395–1398.

Novel Neuroprotective Tripeptides and Dipeptides

ALAN I. FADEN, SUSAN M. KNOBLACH, VILEN A. MOVSESYAN, PAUL M. LEA IV, AND IBOLJA CERNAK

Department of Neuroscience, Georgetown University Medical Center, Washington, District of Columbia, USA

ABSTRACT: It has long been recognized that thyrotropin-releasing hormone (TRH) and certain TRH analogues are neuroprotective in a variety of animal models of CNS trauma. In addition to these neuroprotective actions, TRH and most TRH analogues have other physiological actions that may not be desirable for treatment of acute injury, such as analeptic, autonomic, and endocrine effects. We have developed a series of dual-substituted TRH analogues that have strong neuroprotective actions, but are largely devoid of these other physiological actions. In addition, we have developed a family of cyclized dipeptides (diketopiperazines), structurally somewhat related to a metabolic product of TRH, that appear even more effective as neuroprotective agents *in vitro* and *in vivo*, and may have nootropic properties. Here, we review these novel tripeptide and dipeptide compounds.

KEYWORDS: TRH analogues; dipeptides; tripeptides; CNS injury; neuroprotection

INTRODUCTION

Acute injuries to the central nervous system (CNS) cause not only immediate damage to cells and fiber tracts, but also induce more delayed biochemical changes that lead to secondary cell loss, demyelination, and associated functional deficits.[1] Numerous secondary injury factors have been suggested from experimental studies and occur from minutes to weeks after the insult. These include lipid degradation products, disrupted ionic homeostasis, altered neurotransmitter/receptor function, inflammation, and immune changes, among others.[2] Together, these changes, often occurring in parallel, cause neuronal and oligodendroglial cell death, as well as reactive gliosis and glial scarring.[3]

Address for correspondence: Alan I. Faden, M.D., Department of Neuroscience, Georgetown University Medical Center, 3970 Reservoir Road NW, Research Building, Room EP04, Washington, D.C. 20057. Voice: 202-687-0492; fax: 202-687-4143.
fadena@georgetown.edu

Ann. N.Y. Acad. Sci. 1053: 472–481 (2005).
doi: 10.1196/annals.1344.041

Most neuroprotective strategies have been directed at individual components of this autotoxic reaction, such as inhibiting free radical–induced reactions, excitotoxicity, inflammation, and/or edema.[4] Although such strategies have shown promise in experimental animal models of spinal cord injury, head injury, or stroke, they have shown only modest or no protective effects in humans.[5] In part, this likely reflects the fact that most clinical strategies to date have been aimed at events related to neuronal cell necrosis, which is a relatively early event that largely occurs within 6 h, whereas treatment in patients can only be delivered to a minority of patients within this time frame. Moreover, because most of these therapies have been directed at single components of the complex biochemical cascade, it should not be surprising that minimal effectiveness has been observed.[6] Although most researchers agree that combination treatment strategies, each directed to a different secondary injury component, would likely prove more effective, this has rarely been attempted even experimentally.[7] Yet, such multifactorial treatment strategies have long been successfully implemented in infectious diseases[8] and cancer[9] therapy. In part, this failure reflects the methodological difficulties and costs associated with such strategies in treating neurological disorders.

An alternative approach is to utilize single agents that have multipotential actions on diverse secondary injury pathways.[10] Because the pharmaceutical industry usually develops drugs based upon measurable effects at limited targets such as individual receptors, most multipotential strategies have been developed by academic researchers.[5] In 1981, we demonstrated that a naturally occurring brain hormone, thyrotropin-releasing hormone (TRH), when used at higher than normal physiological concentrations, showed remarkable neuroprotective effects after experimental spinal cord injury.[11] We subsequently found that TRH could limit the actions of multiple identified secondary injury factors, including diminished blood flow, lipid degradation products such as peptidyl leukotrienes[12] and platelet-activating factor,[13] metabolic changes, ionic dyshomeostasis (Na^+, K^+, Ca^{++}, Mg^{++}),[14] and opioids.[15] Moreover, TRH had a therapeutic window for its protective actions of at least 24 h.[16] Subsequently, we found that modifications of either the N-terminal or middle peptide of this tripeptide hormone (pyroglutamyl-histidyl-prolinamide) could yield compounds that were even more effective than native TRH, and had longer biological half-lives and fewer undesirable physiological actions than the natural hormone.[17,18] This work was successfully extended to brain injury models, and the neuroprotective actions of such compounds were confirmed by many laboratories. Indeed, in direct comparison studies, TRH or TRH analogues have been shown to be more effective than many of the other major proposed neuroprotective strategies, including high-dose methylprednisolone,[19–21] opiate antagonists,[21–24] NMDA antagonists,[25] calcium channel blockers,[26] serotonin antagonists,[23] and neurotensin antagonists, among others.[21] In addition, a small clinical trial of TRH suggested protective effects after spinal cord injury in humans.[27]

Over the past 25 years, we have extensively studied the structure-activity relationships of TRH analogues, and more recently have developed a series of novel tripeptides that include single as well as dual substitutions.[28] In addition, we have developed a family of cyclized dipeptides (diketopiperazines), somewhat related to the metabolic product of TRH, cyclo-his-pro (CHP), which itself retains physiological activity.[29] Many of these compounds show remarkable neuroprotective activity *in vitro* and *in vivo*.[18,30,31]

NOVEL TRH ANALOGUES

TRH is metabolized through two pathways: cleavage of the pyroglutamyl moiety by endopeptidases to form cyclo-histidyl-proline diketopiperazine (CHP) or deamidation to form the free acid form of TRH.[32] A number of TRH analogues have been developed that modify one of its amino acids, resulting in compounds that are more resistant to enzymatic degradation,[18,33,34] some of which are also more potent than TRH in terms of CNS activity.[18,35] Importantly, modification of the C-terminus results in compounds devoid of neuroprotective activity, although they retain endocrine, autonomic, and analeptic activity similar to TRH[36] (FIG. 1). In contrast, modification of the amino-terminus yields compounds such as YM-14673, which is longer acting than TRH (8–36 times) and much more potent (10–100 times).[17] However, N-terminal substitutions tend to retain all of the other physiological actions of TRH, that is, endocrine, autonomic, and analeptic (FIG. 1),[37] which may not be

Drug	Structure	Endocrine	Analeptic	Autonomic	Neuroprotection
TRH	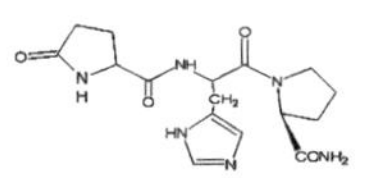	+	+	+	+
CG3509	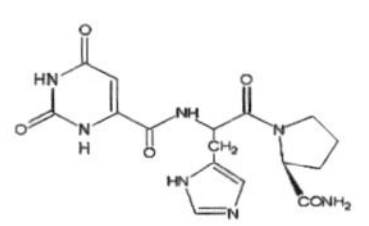	+	+	+	+
CG3703	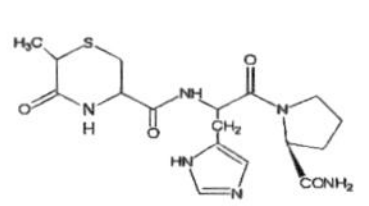	+	+	+	+
RX77368	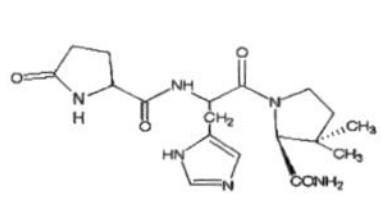	+	+	+	–
MK-771	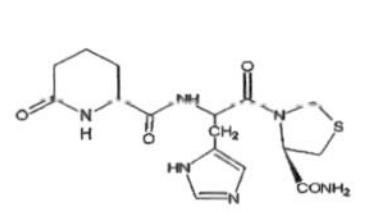	+	+	+	–
YM-14673	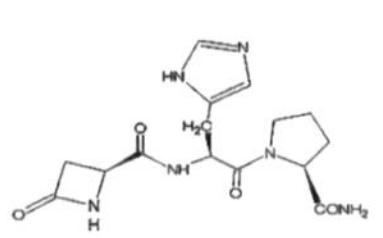	+	+	+	+

FIGURE 1. Comparison of TRH and various substituted TRH analogues that retain the endocrine, autonomic, and analeptic actions of TRH. Modifications of the N-terminus retain neuroprotective activity, whereas modifications of the C-terminus do not. +, positive effect; –, no effect.

Drug	Structure	Endocrine	Analeptic	Autonomic	Neuroprotection
2,4-diiodo (Im)-TRH	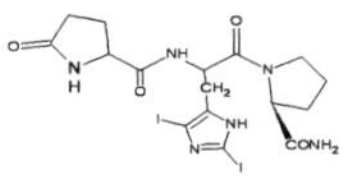	—	NT	—	+
4(5)-NO2 (Im)-TRH	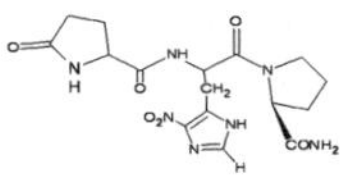	—	NT	+	+
53a	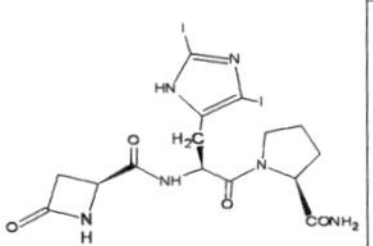	±	—	—	+
57a	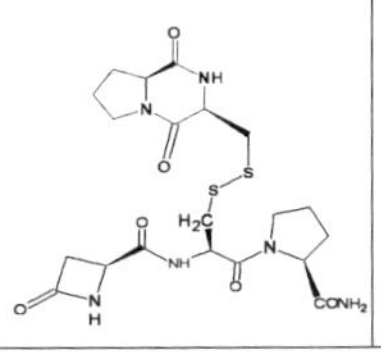	—	—	—	+

FIGURE 2. Comparison of the physiological actions of novel TRH analogues that modify the imidazole structure. These analogues retain neuroprotective activity, but show reduced or absent endocrine, analeptic, and/or autonomic actions. +, positive effect; –, no effect; ±, partial effect; NT, not tested.

optimal for treating CNS injuries. We have also evaluated modifications of the histidyl residue (imidazole substitution) and found that various substitutions reduced the cardiovascular and/or endocrine activity of TRH, while preserving the neuroprotective effects[38] (FIG. 2).

Given these observations, we more recently developed dual-substituted TRH analogues at the N-terminal and histidyl residues. These generated compounds (53a, 57a) that had reduced or even absent endocrine, autonomic, and analeptic effects, while preserving or even enhancing the neuroprotective actions of TRH[18] (FIGS. 2 and 3). Interestingly, based upon a molecular modeling analysis, compound 53a containing an iodo-substitution of the imidazole structure did not significantly alter the conformational profile of the agent. However, 53a proved to be more than two orders of magnitude more hydrophobic than either TRH or YM-14673, based upon their partition coefficients between *n*-octanol and water (log P).[18] This feature should result in increased cellular permeability and improved accessibility to the CNS.

CYCLIZED DIPEPTIDES

As noted above, TRH is metabolized to a cyclized dipeptide (CHP), which retains considerable physiological activity, as do other diketopiperazines. Based upon the remarkable neuroprotective activity of one such prototype compound (35b),[30,39] we

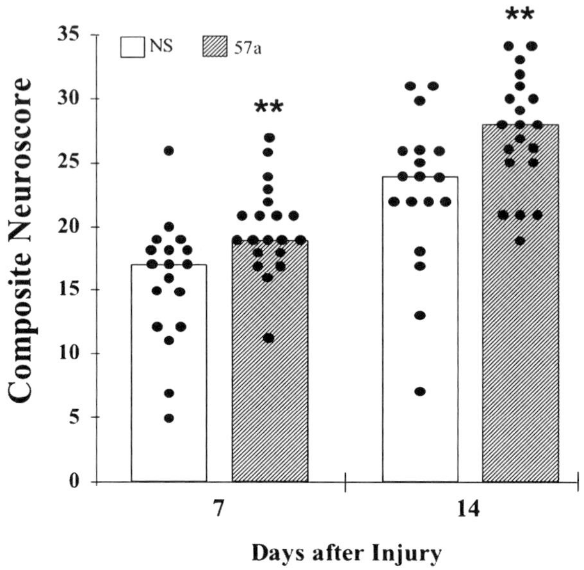

FIGURE 3. Recovery of neurological function measured as a function of treatment after moderate fluid percussion injury (FPI) in the rat. Neurological function was measured using the composite neuroscore. *Histograms* represent median values for each treatment group (NS = *open bars*: FPI + normal saline; 57a = *filled bars*: FPI + 57a), whereas *circles* represent individual animal scores. TRH analogue was administered as a single iv bolus injection at 30 min after trauma. $^{**}P < 0.01$ with respect to FPI + saline.

have developed a series of cyclized dipeptides somewhat related to CHP (FIG. 4). The compound 35b has been extensively studied in a variety of *in vitro* and *in vivo* model systems.[30,39] In neuronal cell culture, 35b shows dose-dependent neuroprotection in both necrotic (maitotoxin, glutamate, punch injury) and apoptotic (staurosporine, β-amyloid) models (FIG. 4). Administered intravenously as a single bolus injection, the compound markedly reduced volumes of brain lesions and improved functional (cognitive, motor) outcomes after either fluid percussion–induced traumatic brain injury (FPI) in rats or controlled cortical impact (CCI) injury in mice.[39] It also significantly reduced apoptotic cell death in ipsilateral hippocampus following FPI. The therapeutic window for 35b was shown to be at least 8 h. It has a relatively flat inverted U-shape dose-response curve between 0.1 and 10 mg/kg. Treatment with 35b in chronic head-injured rats on each of 4 training days before Morris water maze (spatial learning) testing showed that animals recovered to levels of sham-injured controls; this suggests that the compounds may have nootropic activity, as suggested previously for certain diketopiperazines. This drug shows no toxic effects even at more than 100 times the optimal therapeutic dose as demonstrated by preclinical toxicology studies in rats, and is being developed by Research Corporation Technologies for clinical trials in head injury.

The compound 35b has no autonomic analeptic or endocrine effects, and does not bind to either high- or low-affinity TRH receptors. Indeed, based upon screening

Drug	Structure	*In Vitro* Models						
		Glutamate	Maitotoxin	FeSO4	Beta Amyloid	*In Vitro* Trauma	Trophic Factor Removal	Oxygen/Glucose Deprivation
35b	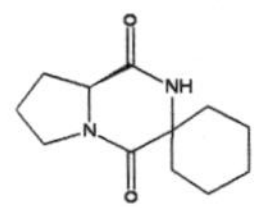	+	+	—	+	+	+	±
144a	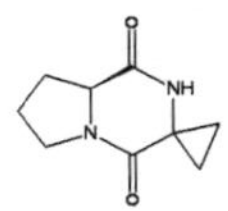	—	NT	NT	—	+	+	NT
606	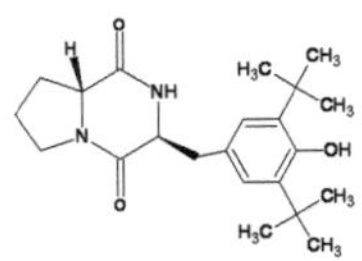	+	+	+	+	+	+	+
807	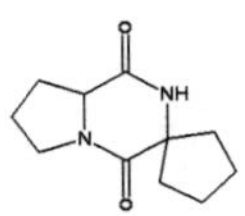	—	NT	NT	—	+	+	NT

FIGURE 4. Comparison of *in vitro* neuroprotection studies on selected tripeptides and dipeptides. +, positive effect; –, no effect; ±, partial effect; NT, not tested.

through the NIMH Psychoactive Drug Screening Program, 35b did not show significant binding affinities for 50 classical receptors, channels, and transporters.[30] With regard to potential mechanism, using Affymetrix microarrays, we found that 35b treatment after FPI upregulated a number of endogenous neuroprotective factors (BDNF, HSP70, HIF1, mGluR7) and downregulated a number of recognized secondary injury factors (cell cycle proteins, calpain, cathepsins) (FIG. 5). These observations were subsequently confirmed by PCR and at the protein level.[31] Perhaps also important are the findings *in vitro* showing that 35b and other diketopiperazines limit the rise in intracellular calcium after glutamate exposure.

At least three other diketopiperazines show neuroprotective effects after CCI in mice that are comparable to those of 35b: 606, 144, and 807, although 35b and 606 show the best neuroprotective profiles *in vitro* (FIG. 3). The compound 606 was

Upregulated	Downregulated
Genes	
4 HRS	
BCl-2-related	Cyclin L
Uncoupling protein 2	Cyclin D1
ApoE	E2F5
Aquaporin 1	c-myc
Aquaporin 5	Rb
24 HRS	
EST (similar to ubiquinine oxidoreductase)	Calpain 6
mGluR7	Cyclin D1
HIF1	Cathepsin C precursor
72 HRS	
HSP 70	Cathepsin H
BDNF	Aquaporin 4

FIGURE 5. Effects of 35b treatment on selected gene expression changes in ipsilateral cortex and/or hippocampus after traumatic brain injury in rats.

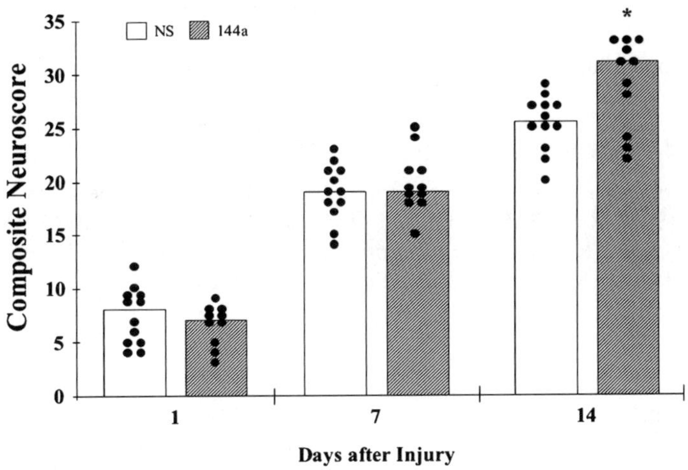

FIGURE 6. Recovery of neurological function measured as a function of treatment after moderate fluid percussion injury (FPI) in the rat. Neurological function was measured using the composite neuroscore. *Histograms* represent median values for each treatment group (NS = *open bars*: FPI + normal saline; 144a = *filled bars*: FPI + 144a), whereas *circles* represent individual animal scores. TRH analogue was administered as a single iv bolus injection at 30 min after trauma. $^*P < 0.05$ with respect to FPI + saline.

derived from CHP, in which the histidine residue was replaced by 3,5-di-*tert*-butyltyrosine (DBT), a phenolic amino acid that serves to trap reactive oxygen species. Indeed, this compound completely blocked free radical–mediated cell death in neuronal cultures induced by $FeSO_4$, whereas 35b did not. The compound 144 also showed substantial neuroprotective actions *in vitro* and *in vivo*, being protective in the FPI as well as CCI models (FIG. 6).

SUMMARY

We have developed and characterized a series of tripeptides and dipeptides related to TRH and its metabolic product, CHP. These compounds show powerful neuroprotective activity *in vitro* and *in vivo*, markedly improve neurological recovery, and reduce lesion volumes/cell loss in rat and/or mouse head injury models. It is noteworthy that these compounds can reduce both necrotic and apoptotic cell death. The fact that 35b can upregulate multiple endogenous neuroprotective factors and reduce induction of multiple classic secondary injury factors indicates a likely multifactorial mechanism of action. Studies are under way to identify potential upstream regulatory targets of these drugs.

Because many similar injury mechanisms appear operative in acute and chronic neurodegeneration, and given the possible nootropic actions of the prototype diketopiperazine, these agents may prove of value for the treatment of such chronic neurodegenerative disorders as Alzheimer's disease or Huntington's disease. It is hoped that the effects of these drugs in animal models of these disorders can be initiated in the near future.

ACKNOWLEDGMENTS

This work was supported by Department of Defense Cooperative Agreement DAMD17-99-2-9007, NIH Grant R01 NS41119, NIH Grant HD40677 (MRDDRC core grant), and a Research Corporation Technologies grant to A. I. Faden. We thank Alan Kozikowski for synthesizing the cyclic dipeptides used.

REFERENCES

1. YAKOVLEV, A.G. & A.I. FADEN. 2004. Mechanisms of neural cell death: implications for development of neuroprotective treatment strategies. NeuroRX **1:** 5–16.
2. ENRIQUEZ, P. & R. BULLOCK. 2004. Molecular and cellular mechanisms in the pathophysiology of severe head injury. Curr. Pharm. Des. **10:** 2131–2143.
3. POVLISHOCK, J.T. & D.I. KATZ. 2005. Update of neuropathology and neurological recovery after traumatic brain injury. J. Head Trauma Rehabil. **20:** 76–94.
4. FADEN, A.I. 2002. Neuroprotection and traumatic brain injury: theoretical option or realistic proposition. Curr. Opin. Neurol. **15:** 707–712.
5. VINK, R. & C. VAN DEN HEUVEL. 2004. Recent advances in the development of multifactorial therapies for the treatment of traumatic brain injury. Expert Opin. Invest. Drugs **13:** 1263–1274.
6. FADEN, A.I. 2001. Neuroprotection and traumatic brain injury: the search continues. Arch. Neurol. **58:** 1553–1555.
7. ROYO, N.C. *et al.* 2003. Pharmacology of traumatic brain injury. Curr. Opin. Pharmacol. **3:** 27–32.
8. CASTAGNOLA, E. *et al.* 2004. Caspofungin associated with liposomal amphotericin B or voriconazole for treatment of refractory fungal pneumonia in children with acute leukaemia or undergoing allogeneic bone marrow transplant. Clin. Microbiol. Infect. **10:** 255–257.
9. CIRONE, P. *et al.* 2004. Combined immunotherapy and antiangiogenic therapy of cancer with microencapsulated cells. Hum. Gene Ther. **15:** 945–959.
10. MAAS, A.I. 2001. Neuroprotective agents in traumatic brain injury. Expert Opin. Invest. Drugs **10:** 753–767.
11. FADEN, A.I., T.P. JACOBS & J.W. HOLADAY. 1981. Thyrotropin-releasing hormone improves neurologic recovery after spinal trauma in cats. N. Engl. J. Med. **305:** 1063–1067.
12. FEUERSTEIN, G. *et al.* 1983. Leukotriene D4–induced hypotension is reversed by thyrotropin-releasing hormone. Prostaglandins **26:** 711–724.
13. FEUERSTEIN, G. *et al.* 1984. Hypotension produced by platelet-activating factor is reversed by thyrotropin-releasing hormone. Circ. Shock **13:** 2552–2560.
14. FADEN, A.I. *et al.* 1990. Effects of TRH-analog treatment on tissue cations, phospholipids, and energy metabolism after spinal cord injury. J. Pharmacol. Exp. Ther. **255:** 608–614.
15. FADEN, A.I. 1988. Role of thyrotropin-releasing hormone and opiate receptor antagonists in limiting central nervous system injury. Adv. Neurol. **47:** 531–546.
16. FADEN, A.I., R. VINK & T.K. MCINTOSH. 1989. Thyrotropin-releasing hormone and central nervous system trauma. Ann. N.Y. Acad. Sci. **553:** 380–384.
17. FADEN, A.I. 1989. TRH analog YM-14673 improves outcome following traumatic brain and spinal cord injury in rats: dose-response studies. Brain Res. **486:** 228–235.
18. FADEN, A.I. *et al.* 1999. Novel TRH analog improves motor and cognitive recovery after traumatic brain injury in rodents. Am. J. Physiol. **277:** R1196–R1204.

19. AKDEMIR, H. *et al.* 1993. Effects of TRH and high-dose corticosteroid therapy on evoked potentials, and tissue Na^+, K^+ and water content in experimental spinal injury. Res. Exp. Med. **193:** 297–304.
20. BEHRMANN, D.L., J.C. BRESNAHAN & M.S. BEATTIE. 1994. Modeling of acute spinal cord injury in the rat: neuroprotection and enhanced recovery with methylprednisolone, U-74006F, and YM-14673. Exp. Neurol. **126:** 61–75.
21. FADEN, A.I. *et al.* 1983. Comparison of thyrotropin-releasing hormone (TRH), naloxone, and dexamethasone treatments in experimental spinal injury. Neurology **33:** 673–678.
22. BEHRMANN, D.L., J.C. BRESNAHAN & M.S. BEATTIE. 1993. A comparison of YM-14673, U-50488H, and nalmefene after spinal cord injury in the rat. Exp. Neurol. **119:** 258–267.
23. PUNIAK, M.A. *et al.* 1991. Comparison of a serotonin antagonist, opioid antagonist, and TRH analog for the acute treatment of experimental spinal trauma. J. Neurotrauma **8:** 193–203.
24. CEYLAN, S. *et al.* 1990. Medical treatment of acute spinal cord injuries. Res. Exp. Med. **190:** 111–119.
25. FADEN, A.I. 1993. Comparison of single and combination drug treatment strategies in experimental brain trauma. J. Neurotrauma **10:** 91–100.
26. CEYLAN, S. *et al.* 1992. Treatment of acute spinal cord injuries: comparison of thyrotropin-releasing hormone and nimodipine. Res. Exp. Med. **192:** 23–33.
27. PITTS, L.H. *et al.* 1995. Treatment with thyrotropin-releasing hormone (TRH) in patients with traumatic spinal cord injuries. J. Neurotrauma **12:** 235–243.
28. PRASAD, C. 1988. Cyclo(His-Pro): its distribution, origin, and function in the human. Neurosci. Biobehav. Rev. **12:** 19–22.
29. PRASAD, C. 1995. Bioactive cyclic dipeptides. Peptides **16:** 151–164.
30. FADEN, A.I. *et al.* 2003. Novel diketopiperazine enhances motor and cognitive recovery after traumatic brain injury in rats and shows neuroprotection *in vitro* and *in vivo*. J. Cereb. Blood Flow Metab. **23:** 3423–3454.
31. FADEN, A.I. *et al.* 2004. Novel small peptides with neuroprotective and nootropic properties. J. Alzheimer's Dis. **6:** S93–S97.
32. REDDING, T.W. & A.V. SCHALLY. 1969. Studies on the inactivation of thyrotropin-releasing hormone (TRH). Proc. Soc. Exp. Biol. Med. **131:** 415–420.
33. PROKAI, L. *et al.* 2004. Centrally acting and metabolically stable thyrotropin-releasing hormone analogues by replacement of histidine with substituted pyridinium. J. Med. Chem. **47:** 6025–6033.
34. BRUNETTI, L. *et al.* 2002. Synthesis and biological evaluation of a novel pyroglutamyl-modified TRH analogue. Farmaco **57:** 479–486.
35. PROKAI-TATRAI, K. *et al.* 2003. Prodrugs to enhance central nervous system effects of the TRH-like peptide pGlu-Glu-Pro-NH_2. Bioorg. Med. Chem. Lett. **13:** 1011–1014.
36. MAPELLI, C., H. VAN HALBEEK & C.H. STAMMER. 1990. Synthesis and conformational studies by ^{1}H- and ^{13}C-NMR spectroscopy of a novel, sterically constrained analogue of thyrotropin-releasing hormone. Biopolymers **29:** 407–422.
37. SZIRTES, T. *et al.* 1986. Synthesis of thyrotropin-releasing hormone analogues. 2. Tripeptides structurally greatly differing from TRH with high central nervous system activity. J. Med. Chem. **29:** 1654–1658.
38. FADEN, A.I., V.M. LABROO & L.A. COHEN. 1993. Imidazole-substituted analogues of TRH limit behavioral deficits after experimental brain trauma. J. Neurotrauma **10:** 101–108.
39. FADEN, A.I. *et al.* 2003. Neuroprotective and nootropic actions of a novel cyclized dipeptide after controlled cortical impact injury in mice. J. Cereb. Blood Flow Metab. **23:** 355–363.

Cocaine Induces a Differential Dose-Dependent Alteration in the Expression Profile of Immediate Early Genes, Transcription Factors, and Caspases in PC12 Cells

A Possible Mechanism of Neurotoxic Damage in Cocaine Addiction

SYED Z. IMAM,[a] HELEN M. DUHART,[b] JOHN T. SKINNER,[b] AND SYED F. ALI[b]

[a]*South Texas Veterans Health Care System and Department of Medicine, University of Texas, Health Science Center, San Antonio, Texas, USA*

[b]*Division of Neurotoxicology, United States Food and Drug Administration/National Center for Toxicological Research, Jefferson, Arkansas, USA*

ABSTRACT: Cocaine is a widely used drug of abuse and psychostimulant that acts on the central nervous system by blocking the dopamine reuptake sites. PC12 cells, a rat pheochromocytoma clonal line, in the presence of nerve growth factor (NGF), multiply and differentiate into competent neurons that can synthesize, store, and secrete the neurotransmitter dopamine (DA). In the present study, we evaluated the effect of increasing doses of cocaine on the expression of immediate early genes (IEGs), *c-fos* and *c-jun*, and closely related transcription factors, SP-1 and NF-kβ, at 24 h after the exposure to cocaine (50, 100, 200, 500, 1000, 2500 μM) in NGF-differentiated PC12 cells. Cocaine (50–500 μM) resulted in significant induction of the expression of *c-fos*, *c-jun*, SP-1, and NF-kβ. However, higher concentrations of cocaine (1000 and 2500 μM) resulted in the downregulation of these expressions after 24 h. To further understand the role of dose-dependent changes in the mechanisms of cell death, we evaluated the protein expression of apoptotic markers. A concentration-dependent increase in the expression of caspase-9 and -3 was observed up to 500 μM cocaine. However, the higher dose did not show any expression. We also evaluated the effect of increasing doses of cocaine on DA concentration and the expression of dopamine transporter (DAT). A significant dose-dependent decrease in the concentration of DA as well as the expression of DAT was observed 24 h after the exposure of PC12 cells to cocaine. Therefore, in the present study, we reported that cocaine has both upstream and downstream regulatory actions on some IEGs and transcription factors that can regulate the mechanism of cell death, and these effects on gene expression are independent of its action on the dopaminergic system.

KEYWORDS: cocaine; psychostimulants; dopamine; immediate early genes; apoptosis; transcription

Address for correspondence: Syed Z. Imam, Ph.D., South Texas Veterans Health Care System and Department of Medicine, University of Texas, Health Science Center, San Antonio, TX 78229; *or* Syed F. Ali, Ph.D., Division of Neurotoxicology, US FDA/NCTR, Jefferson, AR 72079.
simam@satx.rr.com; sali@nctr.fda.gov

**Ann. N.Y. Acad. Sci. 1053: 482–490 (2005). © 2005 New York Academy of Sciences.
doi: 10.1196/annals.1344.042**

INTRODUCTION

The mesolimbic dopaminergic (DAergic) system is an important pathway mediating reinforcement and addiction to psychostimulants.[1] Cocaine potentiates DAergic neurotransmission by binding to the dopamine transporter (DAT) and blocking neurotransmitter uptake, leading to marked elevations in synaptic dopamine (DA).[2] Long-term cocaine abuse leads to neuroadaptive changes in the signaling proteins that regulate DA homeostasis. DAT binding sites are upregulated *in vitro* in the postmortem brain of cocaine addicts[3] and *in vivo* in acutely abstinent cocaine-dependent individuals.[4] Cocaine abuse is also frequently associated with cerebrovascular pathology. Although the cellular and molecular mechanisms of these alterations are not fully understood, they may involve oxidative injury or dysfunction of brain microvascular endothelial cells.[5]

The time course for cocaine addiction in humans and for development of cocaine self-administration in animal models suggests the involvement of alterations in gene expression leading to altered signaling in the brain.[6] Most DA-containing nerve terminals innervate medium spiny neurons in the striatum of the brain.[7] Cocaine enhances DA-mediated neurotransmission by blocking DA reuptake at axon terminals. Chronic exposure to cocaine upregulates several transcription factors that alter gene expression and that could mediate such compensatory neural and behavioral changes.[7] The induction of immediate early genes (IEGs) can also be considered as a tool to study neuronal activation in different brain structures. These genes, which are rapidly and transiently induced in response to diverse extracellular stimulation, coordinate alterations in gene expression underlying neuronal plasticity. Using *in situ* hybridization, we have previously reported that acute ip cocaine (20 mg/kg) injection produced a strong expression of egr-1 and *c-fos* genes in the nucleus accumbens, caudate putamen, and frontal cortex in the rat.[8] Also, cocaine has been reported to activate NF-kβ, AP-1, and TNF-α in human brain microvascular endothelial cells.[5] The present study was designed to understand the gene expression pathway involving interaction of responsiveness of an IEG to the transcription and possible effector apoptotic cascade in the manifestation of cocaine-induced neurotoxic damage.

MATERIALS AND METHODS

Cell Cultures

For the cell culture studies, rat pheochromocytoma (PC12) cells were grown in 75-cm^2 tissue culture flasks at 37°C under an atmosphere of 5% CO_2/95% air in RPMI 1640 medium (Sigma) containing 10% horse serum and 5% fetal bovine serum. The growth medium contained 50 ng/mL of nerve growth factor (NGF). The medium was changed every 3 days and the cells were subcultured once a week. In experiments in which toxicity was assessed, cells were plated in 24-well trays at a cell number of 100,000 cells/well, and the almost confluent cells were used 3 days later for the experiment. Cells were exposed to different doses of cocaine (50–2500 μM) for 24 h.

Determination of Dopamine Concentration

The concentrations of DA were quantified by a modified HPLC method combined with electrochemical detection.[6] The amount of DA was calculated using standard curves that were generated by determining in triplicate the ratio between three different known amounts of the amine or its metabolites and a constant amount of internal standard.

Western Blot Analysis

Analysis of *c-fos*, *c-jun*, SP-1, and NF-kβ protein in the cultures was performed as follows. The cell cultures were homogenized in 10 volumes of extraction buffer containing 20 mM Tris (pH 7.4), 50 mM NaCl, 10% SDS, 1 mM EDTA, 1 mM EGTA, 0.2 mM PMSF, 1 μg/mL pepstatin, 0.5 μg/mL leupeptin, and 5 mM mercaptoethanol. The homogenate was centrifuged at 16,000*g* for 80 min to pellet the insoluble membrane or organelle fraction. Proteins were analyzed for each sample. Samples were diluted 1:1 with sample buffer (125 mM Tris-HCl, 4% SDS, 20% glycerol, 10% 2-mercaptoethanol). Equal amounts of protein (30 μg) were loaded onto a 15% SDS-PAGE gel and separated by the Laemmli method. Proteins were electrophoretically transferred to a nitrocellulose membrane, and the nonspecific sites were blocked in 5% nonfat dry milk in Tris-buffered saline containing 0.3% Tween®-20 for 60 min. Membranes were then incubated in the presence of rabbit anti-*c-fos* (1:1000), rabbit

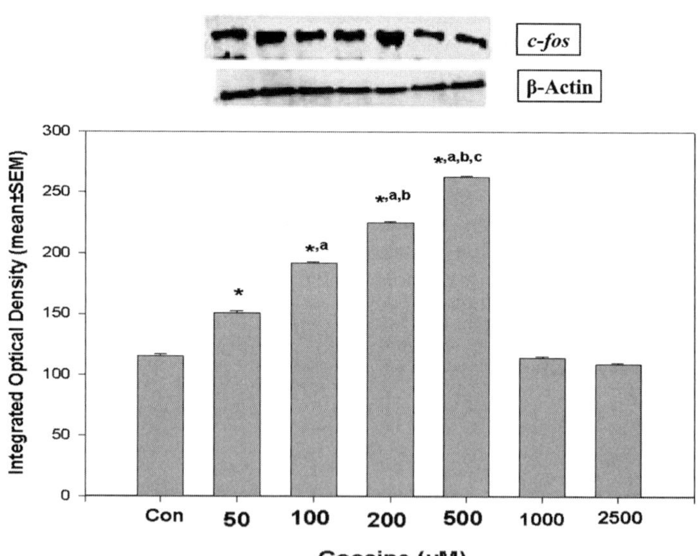

FIGURE 1A. Representative photomicrograph of the immunoblot and integrated optical density units for changes in the expression of *c-fos* in PC12 cells at 24 h after cocaine (0, 50, 100, 200, 500, 1000, 2500 μM); 25 μg protein was loaded in each lane for each group. Each value represents the mean ± SEM derived from three different sets of experiments. $*P < 0.05$, significantly different from control group. $^{a,b,c}P < 0.05$, significantly different from all other groups.

anti-*c-jun* (1:1000), rabbit anti-SP-1 antibody (1:1000), rabbit anti-NF-kβ (1:1000), rabbit anti-caspase-3 and -9 (1:1000), mouse anti-DAT (1:1000), or antibody against β-actin (1:5000). Antibody binding and chemiluminescence enhancement were performed using the Oncogene Western blotting analysis system. Densitometric analysis was performed and calibrated to coblotted dilutional standards of positive control cell lysates using the Scanalytics program (Scanalytics, Billerica, MA).

Statistical Analysis

Analysis of differences between different treatment groups consisted of ANOVA followed by post-hoc comparison (Bonferroni *t* test, all pairwise multiple comparison procedure). Significant differences were defined at $P < 0.05$.

RESULTS

The effect of various doses of cocaine on the expression profile of the IEG, *c-fos*, has been represented in FIGURE 1A. Cocaine (50–500 μM) resulted in a significant induction of *c-fos* expression after 24 h. However, higher doses (1000 and 2500 μM)

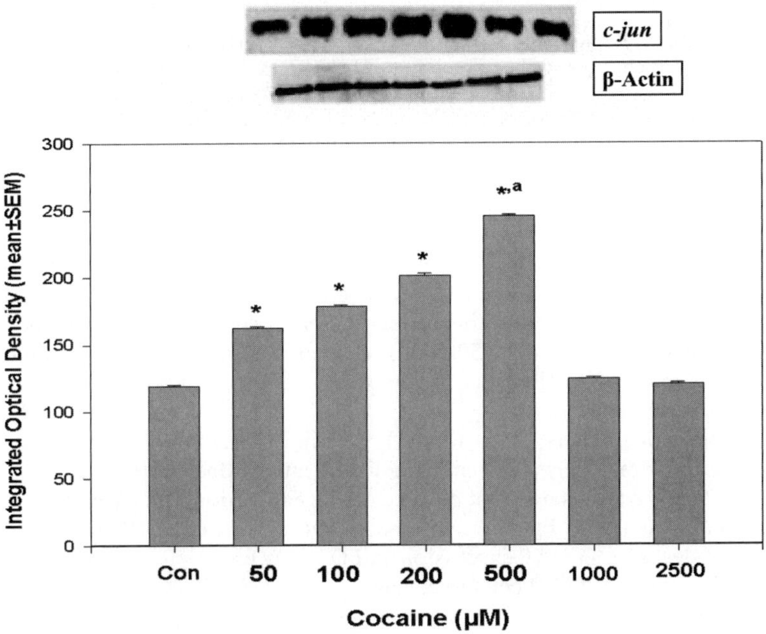

FIGURE 1B. Representative photomicrograph of the immunoblot and integrated optical density units for changes in the expression of *c-jun* in PC12 cells at 24 h after cocaine (0, 50, 100, 200, 500, 1000, 2500 μM); 25 μg protein was loaded in each lane for each group. Each value represents the mean ± SEM derived from three different sets of experiments. *$P < 0.05$, significantly different from control group. $^{a}P < 0.05$, significantly different from all other groups.

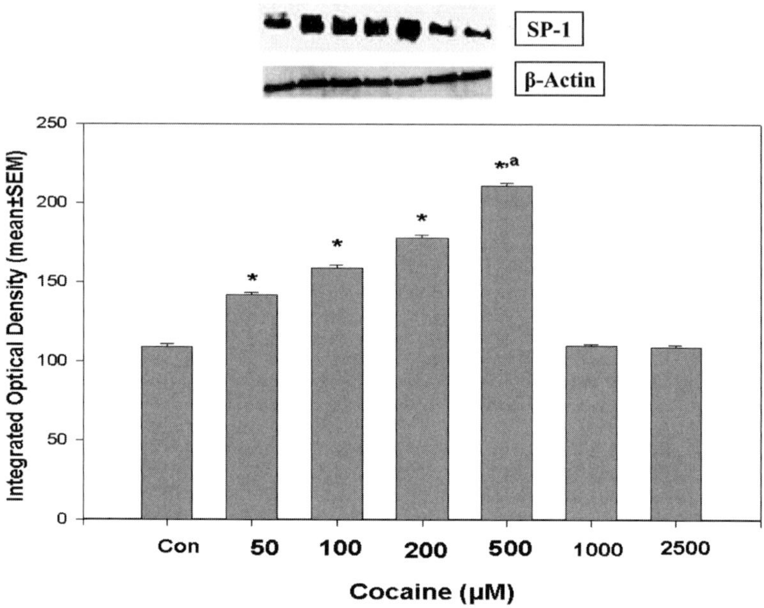

FIGURE 1C. Representative photomicrograph of the immunoblot and integrated optical density units for changes in the expression of SP-1 in PC12 cells at 24 h after cocaine (0, 50, 100, 200, 500, 1000, 2500 μM); 25 μg protein was loaded in each lane for each group. Each value represents the mean ± SEM derived from three different sets of experiments. $^{*}P < 0.05$, significantly different from control group. $^{a}P < 0.05$, significantly different from all other groups.

resulted in a downregulation. A similar pattern of expression was observed in the case of another IEG, *c-jun*, and in the case of SP-1 and NF-kβ, a major part of the transcription family as well as the nuclear factor, as shown in FIGURES 1B, 1C, and 1D, respectively. Cocaine (50–500 μM) resulted in a significant induction of these expressions after 24 h. However, higher doses (1000 and 2500 μM) resulted in a downregulation.

The apoptotic markers, caspase-3 and -9, exhibited a similar pattern of expression as expressed by the IEGs and transcription and nuclear factors (FIG. 2).

The effect of various doses of cocaine on the expression of DAT and DA concentration is represented in FIGURE 2 (*bottom panel*) and FIGURE 3. A significant dose-dependent decrease in DAT expression and DA concentration was observed at 24 h after the exposure of PC12 cells to cocaine.

DISCUSSION

The mechanisms of cocaine-induced DAergic neurotoxicity have yet to be completely understood.[9,10] Motor abnormalities, such as the ones in subclinical parkinsonian-like syndrome that persist over a 3-month period of abstinence, have

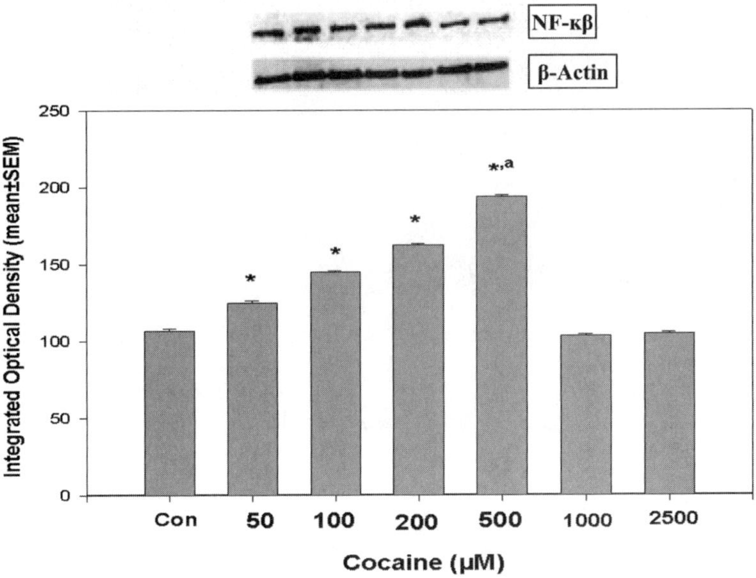

FIGURE 1D. Representative photomicrograph of the immunoblot and integrated optical density units for changes in the expression of NF-kβ protein in PC12 cells at 24 h after cocaine (0, 50, 100, 200, 500, 1000, 2500 μM); 25 μg protein was loaded in each lane for each group. Each value represents the mean ± SEM derived from three different sets of experiments. *$P < 0.05$, significantly different from control group. $^aP < 0.05$, significantly different from all other groups.

been reported in cocaine-dependent subjects.[11] Cocaine administration produces significant DA elevations in the nucleus accumbens and ventral tegmental areas in animal models,[12] and in human chronic users it changes metabolic function and blood flow in terminal regions.[13,14] In animal models, chronic exposure to cocaine induces structural and functional changes in the nucleus accumbens that are presumably mediated by altered gene expression.[15] Cocaine abuse has been associated with a significant decrease in the abundance of Nurr1 and Pitx3 transcription factors in the DA neurons of human midbrain, suggesting that cocaine abuse leads to a partial loss of DAergic phenotype.[16,17] Overexpression of α-synuclein has been reported in the midbrain DA neurons from cocaine abusers, and this overexpression of α-synuclein has been suggested as a neuroadaptive response to cocaine exposure that may put cocaine addicts at risk for degenerative changes in the DA neurons, including the motor abnormalities of Parkinson's disease.[18] In our studies, we observed significant alterations in expression patterns of various IEGs after increasing doses of cocaine to NGF-differentiated PC12 cells. An increase in the expression of IEGs such as *c-fos*, *c-jun*, SP-1, and NF-kβ at lower doses of cocaine, but not at high doses, suggests a possible role of these upregulations in the development of cocaine-dependence. Upregulations in the expression of these IEGs at lower doses of cocaine also suggest a role that these genes might play in the induction of a cell-death cascade that can be a mechanism of cellular damage in long-term cocaine users. Cocaine has been

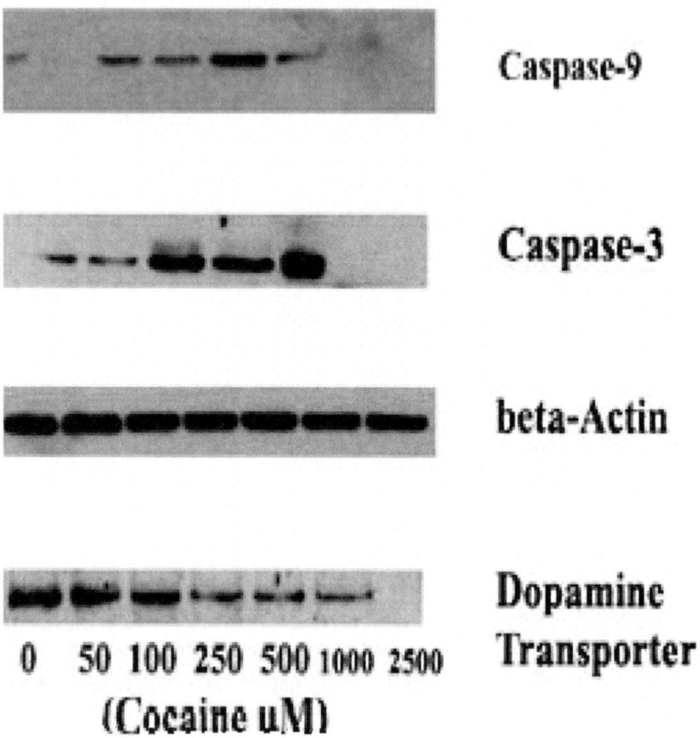

FIGURE 2. Representative photomicrograph of the immunoblot for changes in the expression of caspase-9, caspase-3, and dopamine transporter protein in PC12 cells at 24 h after cocaine (0, 50, 100, 200, 500, 1000, 2500 μM); 25 μg protein was loaded in each lane for each group.

reported to increase *c-fos* expression and cleaved caspase-3 levels in the developing brain in a time- and region-dependent manner,[19] thus relating the expression of *c-fos* to the induction of possible apoptosis in cocaine users. In our studies, we also observed an increased expression of both caspase-3 and caspase-9 at lower doses of cocaine, but not at the higher doses, thus suggesting a dosc-dependent activation of neurotoxic damage induced by cocaine.

The reuptake of DA through a sodium- and chloride-dependent DAT terminates DAergic neurotransmission.[20,21] DAT is a target for cocaine and other psychostimulants.[22,23] Cocaine potentiates DAergic neurotransmission by blocking the reuptake of DA, which leads to marked elevations in the synaptic level of the neurotransmitter.[2] In our studies, we observed a dose-dependent decrease in DAT expression. We also observed a significant decrease in DA content with increasing dose of cocaine, suggesting a decreased uptake of DA by the cells. Our data suggested a significant dose-dependent model of cocaine-induced neurotoxic damage, where we observed an alteration in the DAergic system with increasing dose. However, only lower doses of cocaine were able to upregulate expression of the proapoptotic cascade.

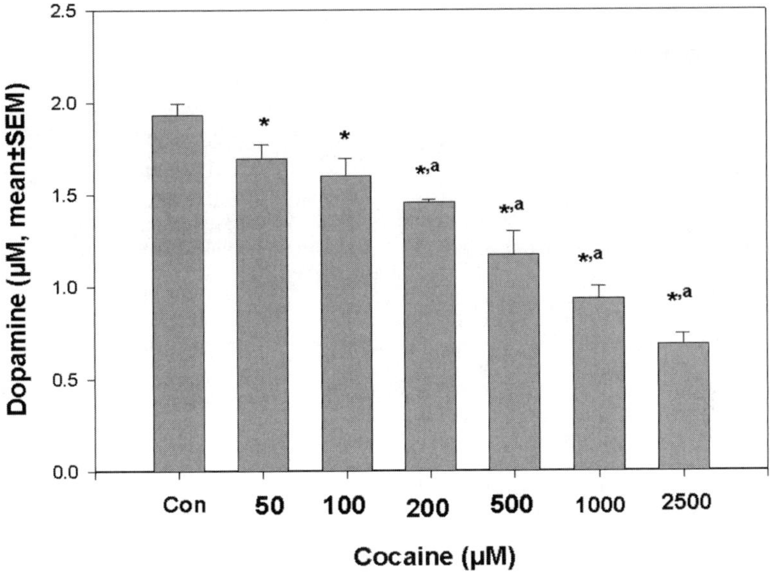

FIGURE 3. Effects of cocaine (0, 50, 100, 200, 500, 1000, 2500 µM) on dopamine depletion in PC12 cell cultures after 24 h. Each value represents the mean ± SEM derived from three different sets of experiments. $^{*}P < 0.05$, significantly different from control group. $^{a}P < 0.05$, significantly different from all other groups.

In summary, although dose-dependent DAergic depletion was observed after the exposure of PC12 cells to cocaine, we also observed a variable spectrum of genetic alterations. The higher doses tend to downregulate the IEGs and transcription and nuclear factors. This might lead to the following hypothesis: although increasing dose of cocaine produces increased DAergic neurotoxicity, the lower dose might result in the activation of various transcriptional gene expression pathways leading to apoptotic cell death as observed in our studies, whereas higher dose can produce necrotic cell death without the activation of any genetic pathways. Further studies are needed for better understanding of these mechanisms, especially the mechanisms for necrotic cell death induced by the higher dose.

REFERENCES

1. Self, D.W. & E.J. Nestler. 1998. Relapse to drug-seeking: neural and molecular mechanisms. Drug Alcohol Depend. **51:** 49–60.
2. Giros, B. & M.G. Caron. 1993. Molecular characterization of the dopamine transporter. Trends Pharmacol. Sci. **14:** 43–49.
3. Mash, D.C., J. Pablo, Q. Ouyang *et al.* 2002. Dopamine transport function is elevated in cocaine users. J. Neurochem. **81:** 292–300.
4. Malison, R.T., S.E. Best, C.H. Van Dyck *et al.* 1998. Elevated striatal dopamine transporters during acute cocaine abstinence as measured by [^{123}I]beta-CIT SPECT. Am. J. Psychiatry **155:** 832–834.

5. LEE, Y.W., B. HENNIG, M. FIALA *et al.* 2001. Cocaine activates redox-regulated transcription factors and induces TNF-alpha expression in human brain endothelial cells. Brain Res. **920:** 125–133.
6. IMAM, S.Z. & S.F. ALI. 2000. Selenium, an antioxidant, attenuates methamphetamine-induced dopaminergic toxicity and peroxynitrite generation. Brain Res. **855:** 186–191.
7. BIBB, J.A., J. CHEN, J.R. TAYLOR *et al.* 2001. Effects of chronic exposure to cocaine are regulated by the neuronal protein Cdk5. Nature **410:** 376–380.
8. THIRIET, N., P. JOUVERT, S. GOBAILLE *et al.* 2001. C-type natriuretic peptide (CNP) regulates cocaine-induced dopamine increase and immediate early gene expression in rat brain. Eur. J. Neurosci. **14:** 1702–1708.
9. BARTZOKIS, G., I.B. GOLDSTEIN, D.B. HANCE *et al.* 1999. The incidence of T2-weighted MR imaging signal abnormalities in the brain of cocaine-dependent patients is age-related and region-specific. Am. J. Neuroradiol. **20:** 1628–1635.
10. BARTZOKIS, G., M. BECKSON, T. NEWTON *et al.* 1999. Selegiline effects on cocaine-induced changes in medial temporal lobe metabolism and subjective ratings of euphoria. Neuropsychopharmacology **20:** 582–590.
11. BAUER, L.O. 1996. Psychomotor and electroencephalographic sequelae of cocaine dependence. NIDA Res. Monogr. **163:** 66–93.
12. CZOTY, P.W., J.B. JUSTICE, JR. & L.L. HOWELL. 2000. Cocaine-induced changes in extracellular dopamine determined by microdialysis in awake squirrel monkeys. Psychopharmacology (Berlin) **148:** 299–306.
13. VOLKOW, N.D., J.S. FOWLER, A.P. WOLF *et al.* 1991. Changes in brain glucose metabolism in cocaine dependence and withdrawal. Am. J. Psychiatry **148:** 621–626.
14. STRICKLAND, T.L., I. MENA, J. VILLANUEVA-MEYER *et al.* 1993. Cerebral perfusion and neuropsychological consequences of chronic cocaine use. J. Neuropsychiatry Clin. Neurosci. **5:** 419–427.
15. NORRHOLM, S.D., J.A. BIBB, E.J. NESTLER *et al.* 2003. Cocaine-induced proliferation of dendritic spines in nucleus accumbens is dependent on the activity of cyclin-dependent kinase-5. Neuroscience **116:** 19–22.
16. BANNON, M.J., B. PRUETZ, A.B. MANNING-BOG *et al.* 2002. Decreased expression of the transcription factor NURR1 in dopamine neurons of cocaine abusers. Proc. Natl. Acad. Sci. USA **99:** 6382–6385.
17. BANNON, M.J., B. PRUETZ, E. BARFIELD & C. SCHMIDT. 2004. Transcription factors specifying dopamine phenotype are decreased in cocaine users. Neuroreport **15:** 401–404.
18. MASH, D.C., Q. OUYANG, J. PABLO *et al.* 2003. Cocaine abusers have an overexpression of alpha-synuclein in dopamine neurons. J. Neurosci. **23:** 2564–2571.
19. MITCHELL, E.S. & A. SNYDER-KELLER. 2003. c-fos and cleaved caspase-3 expression after perinatal exposure to ethanol, cocaine, or the combination of both drugs. Brain Res. Dev. Brain Res. **147:** 107–117.
20. MCELVAIN, J.S. & J.O. SCHENK. 1992. Studies of the mechanism of inhibition of the dopamine uptake carrier by cocaine *in vitro* using rotating disk electrode voltammetry. Ann. N.Y. Acad. Sci. **654:** 480–482.
21. MCELVAIN, J.S. & J.O. SCHENK. 1992. A multisubstrate mechanism of striatal dopamine uptake and its inhibition by cocaine. Biochem. Pharmacol. **43:** 2189–2199.
22. AMARA, S.G. & M.J. KUHAR. 1993. Neurotransmitter transporters: recent progress. Annu. Rev. Neurosci. **16:** 73–93.
23. RITZ, M.C. & M.J. KUHAR. 1993. Psychostimulant drugs and a dopamine hypothesis regarding addiction: update on recent research. Biochem. Soc. Symp. **59:** 51–64.

Neuroprotection in the PNS: Erythropoietin and Immunophilin Ligands

AHMET HÖKE AND SANJAY C. KESWANI

Department of Neurology, Johns Hopkins University School of Medicine, Baltimore, Maryland, USA

ABSTRACT: Many illnesses that affect the peripheral nervous system (PNS) lead to distal axonal degeneration rather than loss of neuronal cell bodies. Strategies aimed at promoting survival of injured neurons (i.e., preventing cell death) may not be applicable to many PNS illnesses. We have developed *in vitro* and *in vivo* animal models to study mechanisms of acquired peripheral neuropathies and used these models to evaluate the therapeutic potential of novel compounds. In recent years, erythropoietin (EPO) has been recognized as a novel neuroprotectant in the central nervous system. In the PNS, we recently showed that Schwann cell–derived EPO acts as an endogenous neuroprotectant and that it is most effective in preventing distal axonal degeneration seen in models of peripheral neuropathy. Similarly, we showed that immunophilin ligands are also neuroprotective in the PNS and prevent axonal degeneration seen in models of peripheral neuropathies. Both EPO and non-immunosuppressive immunophilin ligands are in early clinical development for the treatment of acquired peripheral neuropathies.

KEYWORDS: axonal degeneration; immunophilin ligands; GPI-1046; EPO; erythropoietin

INTRODUCTION

Peripheral neuropathies are common and cause significant morbidity. The vast majority of peripheral neuropathies, including diabetic and human immunodeficiency virus (HIV)–associated neuropathy, are "dying back" axonopathies, characterized by degeneration of the most distal portions of axons, with centripetal progression.[1,2] Although most published *in vitro* studies of neurotoxicity and neuroprotection in the peripheral nervous system (PNS) have focused on neuronal apoptosis as the sole outcome measure, neuronal death, in contrast to distal axonal loss, is not a prominent pathological feature of most human peripheral neuropathies. Furthermore, the signaling pathways mediating axonal degeneration are distinguishable from those mediating neuronal apoptosis.[3–6] Thus, in considering whether a particular "neuroprotective" agent may have therapeutic relevance to human peripheral neuropathies

Address for correspondence: Ahmet Höke, M.D., Ph.D., Department of Neurology, Johns Hopkins University, 600 North Wolfe Street, Path 509, Baltimore, MD 21287. Voice: 410-614-1196; fax: 410-614-1008.
ahoke@jhmi.edu

Ann. N.Y. Acad. Sci. 1053: 491–501 (2005). © 2005 New York Academy of Sciences.
doi: 10.1196/annals.1344.043

(and to other neurological diseases where axonopathy is prominent), it is important to discover if it robustly prevents axonal degeneration, independent of neuronal death.[7]

In order to study mechanisms underlying axonal and neuronal injury in peripheral neuropathies, we developed *in vitro* models of HIV-associated neuropathies.[8,9] Using these models, we demonstrate that immunophilin ligands and erythropoietin (EPO) are potent neuroprotectants that prevent axonal degeneration in sensory neurons.[8,10,11] We also show that neuronal nitric oxide acts an "injury" signal and stimulates production of Schwann cell–derived EPO, which in turn acts as an endogenous neuroprotectant against axonal injury.

IN VITRO MODELS OF HIV-ASSOCIATED NEUROPATHIES AND IMMUNOPHILIN LIGANDS

HIV-associated neuropathies are the most common neurological complications of HIV infection in the current era of highly active antiretroviral therapy. Main types of neuropathies associated with HIV are sensory neuropathies that are either due to the HIV infection itself (distal symmetric polyneuropathy) or to the neurotoxicity of a class of antiretroviral drugs (antiretroviral toxic neuropathy) (reviewed in refs. 12 and 13). The exact mechanisms of these neuropathies are being elucidated. Recently, we demonstrated that nucleoside analogue reverse-transcriptase inhibitors (NRTIs) that cause neuropathy in HIV patients also lead to dysfunction and axonal degeneration in sensory neurons *in vitro* (FIG. 1).[8] This neurotoxicity was due to a rapid loss of mitochondrial membrane potential as measured by JC-1, a bifluorescent mitochondrial dye that reports on the mitochondrial membrane potential differential in live cells.[14,15] Loss of mitochondrial membrane potential led to a reduction in ATP production and energy failure, resulting in necrotic cell death.[8] This neurotoxicity of NRTIs was preventable by coadministration of an immunophilin ligand, FK-506, but not by cyclophilin ligand, cyclosporine (CSA) (FIG. 2). Since CSA and FK-506 share a calcineurin-binding domain that is thought to mediate their immunosuppressive activities, this finding raised the possibility that in this sensory neuronal injury paradigm the neuroprotective activity of FK-506 may be independent of its immunosuppressive properties. Nonimmunosuppressive analogues of FK-506 have been developed and shown to be neuroprotective in various injury paradigms.[16–21] In our NRTI-induced neurotoxicity paradigm, GPI-1046, one of the FK-506 analogues, prevented axonal degeneration in primary sensory neurons (data not shown).

In addition to the toxic neuropathy associated with antiretroviral therapy, HIV patients suffer from a predominantly sensory polyneuropathy that is due to the HIV infection per se. The pathogenic mechanism of this neuropathy is not well understood and is likely to be complex. In the nervous system, there is minimal, if any, direct infection of the neurons or the glial cells. Most of the neurological dysfunction in HIV infection is likely to be due to indirect mechanisms. A potential candidate for this is the infiltration of the nervous system with HIV-infected macrophages. Over the years, there have been many models of neurotoxicity developed using secreted viral envelope proteins and central nervous system (CNS) neurons (reviewed in refs. 22 and 23). In a recent study, we expanded on the potential role of gp120, one of the main secreted envelope proteins of HIV, in HIV neuropathogenesis and demonstrated that gp120 can cause axonal degeneration in sensory neurons in an indirect manner

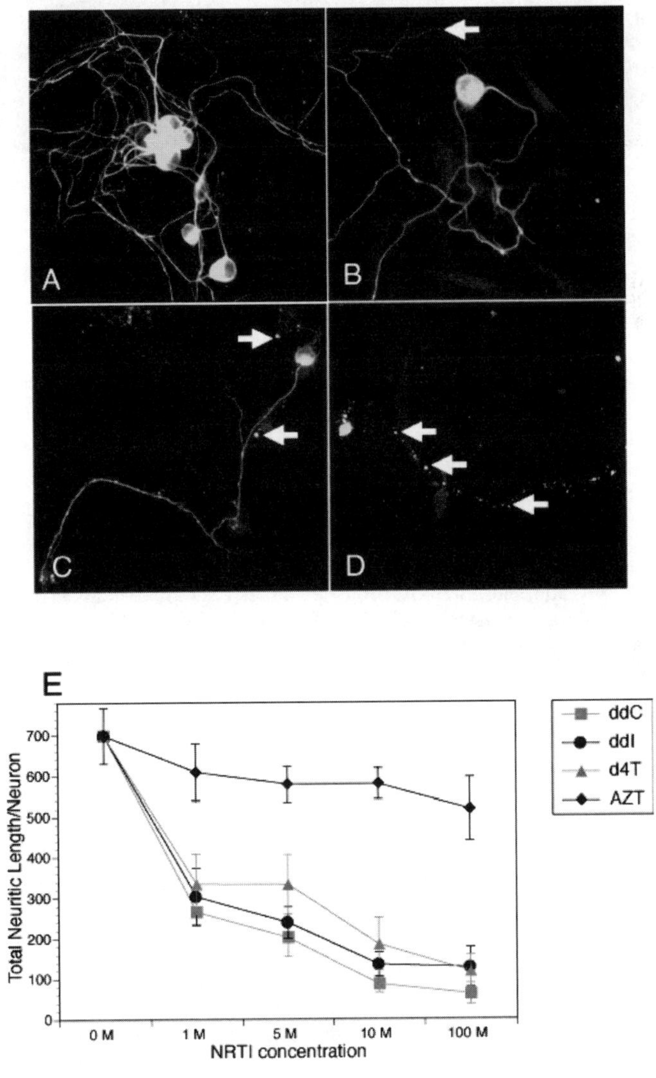

FIGURE 1. NRTI-induced neurotoxicity in primary DRG sensory neurons. NRTIs that cause neuropathy in HIV patients (ddC, ddI, and d4T), but not AZT, cause degeneration of axons in primary sensory cultures in a dose-dependent manner **(E)**. **(A)** Control. **(B)** ddC at 1 μM. **(C)** ddC at 10 μM. **(D)** ddC at 100 μM. *Arrows* point to axonal degeneration. (Adapted from ref. 8.)

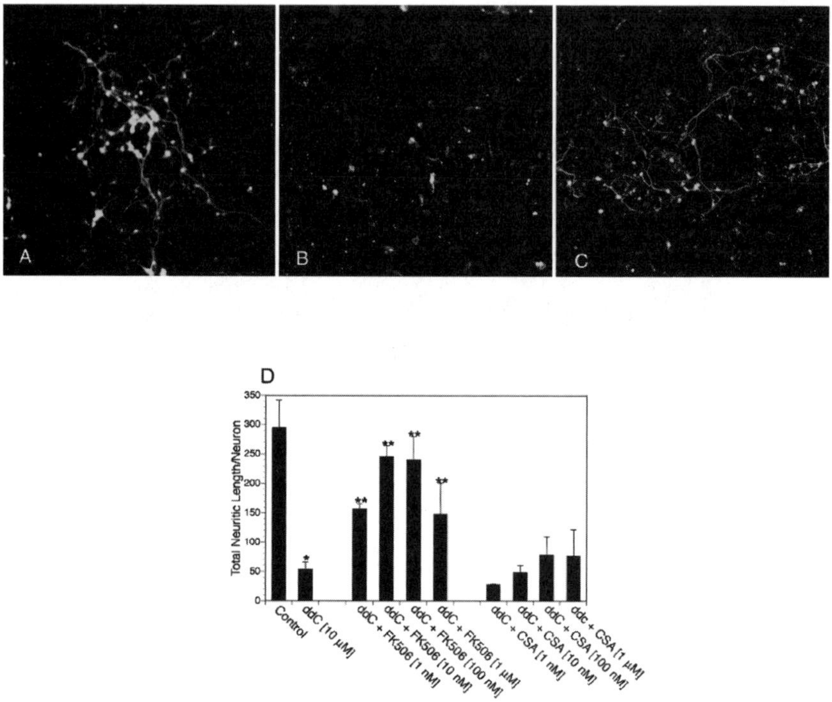

FIGURE 2. FK-506, but not CSA, protected against ddC-induced neurotoxicity. DRG sensory neurons had long neurites in vehicle (**A**) and ddC + FK-506 (**C**) treated cultures, but not in ddC alone (**B**). FK-506, but not CSA, protected against ddC-induced reduction in total neuritic length (**D**) per neuron (*$P < 0.05$, ddC vs. control; **$P < 0.05$, ddC vs. ddC + FK-506). (Adapted from ref. 8.)

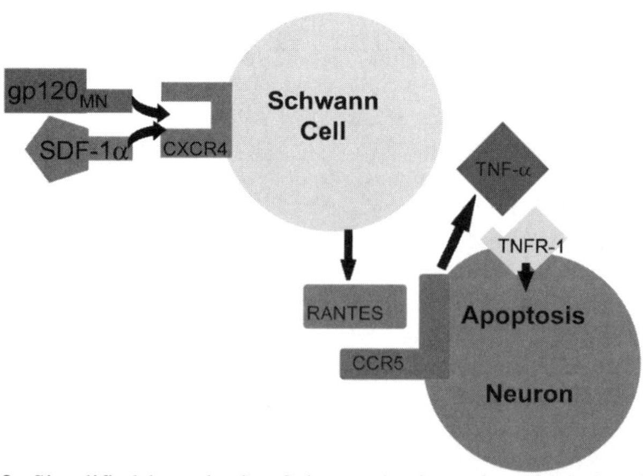

FIGURE 3. Simplified hypothesis of the mechanism of gp120-induced DRG neurotoxicity. CXCR4 binding on Schwann cells by SDF-1α or gp120 results in the release of RANTES, which induces TNF-α production by DRG neurons, and subsequent TNFR1-mediated neurotoxicity in an autocrine/paracrine fashion. (Adapted from ref. 9.)

through activation of chemokine receptors on Schwann cells, the main supporting glial cells in the PNS (FIG. 3).[9] In this model, gp120 binds to chemokine receptor CXCR4 on Schwann cells and induces secretion of chemokine RANTES, which in turn binds to its receptor, CCR5, on sensory neurons and causes TNF-α-mediated apoptotic neuronal death. Using this model, we were able to show neuroprotection by the nonimmunosuppressive immunophilin ligands, GPI-1046 and GPI-1485 (unpublished observations), and EPO (see below).[11] Based on the data in both the NRTI-induced axonal degeneration and gp120-induced neurotoxicity paradigms, a phase I clinical trial is being planned with GPI-1485.

SCHWANN CELL–DERIVED EPO-MEDIATED ENDOGENOUS NEUROPROTECTIVE PATHWAY IN THE PNS

The glycoprotein, EPO, is a very promising neuroprotective agent, whose anti-apoptotic properties have been thoroughly evaluated by several investigators. The administration of EPO prevents CNS neurons from death caused by a variety of insults, including hypoxia, hypoglycemia, glutamate toxicity, growth factor deprivation, and free radical injury.[24–28] Recently, Campana and coworkers also demonstrated that EPO administration prevented apoptosis of dorsal root ganglion (DRG) sensory neurons.[29] As shown by Campana's group and us,[10] in the DRG, Schwann cells are the predominant cell type that expresses EPO, and the sensory neurons express EPO receptor (EPO-R). In response to axonal transection or axonal toxic injury, perineuronal Schwann cells increase their expression of EPO and the neurons increase their expression of EPO-R both *in vitro* and *in vivo*.[10] This increase in Schwann cell EPO expression was only seen in Schwann cells in close proximity to injured axons, suggesting the presence of a "sick neuron" signal from the injured neuron.

What is the identity of the neuronal/axonal "injury factor" that stimulates EPO production by neighboring Schwann cells? We screened a number of promising candidates, including β-neuregulin-1 and insulin growth factor-1 (IGF-1), without success. Finally, we discovered that nitric oxide (NO) might be the relevant signaling molecule, on the basis of the following observations. All the agents that we noted had caused dying back axonal degeneration in our cultures, including gp120, ddC, and acrylamide, and increased neuronal intracellular NO production (FIG. 4A). This observation correlates with previous studies showing that neuronal nitric oxide synthase (nNOS) gene expression is significantly increased at 4 h in ipsilateral DRG samples following sciatic nerve injury in a rat tourniquet model.[30] We also noted that NO donors, such as SNAP and NOR-3, increased EPO mRNA levels in pure Schwann cell cultures as early as 30 min after administration, with a 3- to 4-fold increase being noted at 1 h (FIG. 4B). This was mirrored by an increase in intracellular EPO production by Western blotting (FIG. 4C) and a large increase in EPO content in the supernatants of these cultures, as measured by ELISA (FIG. 4D). Coadministration of L-NAME, a nonspecific NOS inhibitor, almost completely obliterated the ability of gp120 to induce EPO release into the supernatants of DRG cultures (FIG. 4E). Moreover, TRIM, a specific nNOS inhibitor,[31] completely prevented the 18-fold induction of EPO mRNA by gp120 in these cultures, suggesting that NO generated by nNOS was responsible for triggering EPO production by surrounding glial cells. In

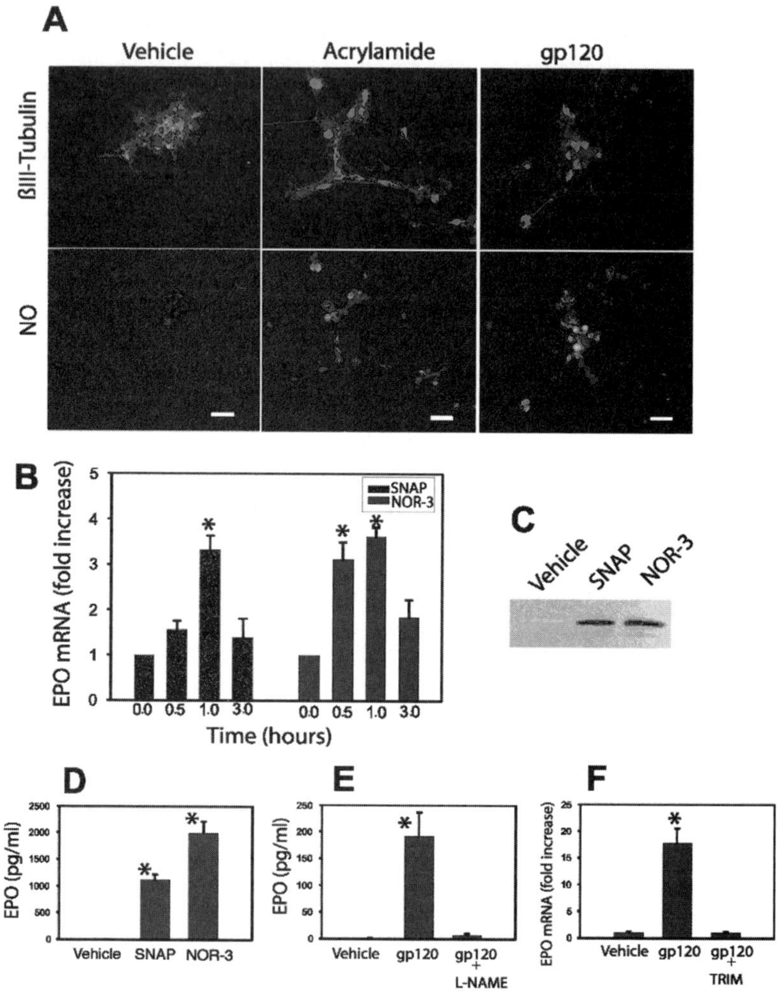

FIGURE 4. Axonal injury stimulates Schwann cell production of EPO via nitric oxide (NO): **(A)** Exposure of DRG cocultures to agents causing axonal degeneration, including gp120 (1 pg/mL) and acrylamide (1 mM), induces NO production (green) at 6 h in beta III tubulin–labeled neurons (red), as assayed by DAF-2T fluorescence. Scale bar: 100 mm. **(B)** NO donors, SNAP (10 mM) and NOR-3 (100 nM), induce increased EPO mRNA levels (3- to 4-fold at 1 h, $*P < 0.05$) in pure Schwann cell cultures. **(C)** Cell lysates of pure Schwann cell cultures treated for 6 h with SNAP (10 mM) or NOR-3 (100 nM) have increased EPO protein by Western blotting, compared to those treated with vehicle control. **(D)** Supernatants of pure Schwann cell cultures treated for 24 h with SNAP (10 mM) or NOR-3 (100 nM) have markedly increased EPO content by ELISA, compared to vehicle control treatment ($*P < 0.05$). **(E)** L-NAME (100 mM) coadministration prevents gp120-induced EPO release from DRG neuron/Schwann cell cocultures as measured by EPO ELISA ($*P < 0.05$). **(F)** TRIM (100 mM) coadministration abrogates gp120-induced (18-fold) increase in Schwann cell EPO mRNA in DRG neuron/Schwann cell cocultures ($*P < 0.05$). (Adapted from ref. 10.)

our dissociated DRG cultures, immunostaining for nNOS only occurred in neurons, in contrast to iNOS staining, which was present in both neurons and Schwann cells.

What is the relevance of this Schwann cell–derived EPO? When we prevented Schwann cell–derived EPO production by transfecting Schwann cells with siRNA constructs prior to coculturing, sensory axons were far more vulnerable to degeneration by ddC and gp120.[10] The "axonoprotective" efficacy of endogenous EPO was further suggested by similarly increased axonal degeneration by ddC and gp120 when antagonist antibodies to EPO or to EPO-R were coadministered. No associated increase in neuronal death was observed by ethidium homodimer staining (which would detect both apoptotic and necrotic death), suggesting that the increased axonal degeneration by EPO/EPO-R antagonism was not due to neuronal death.

Similar to the effect of endogenous EPO antagonism in the DRG cocultures, the application of TRIM, a specific nNOS inhibitor, resulted in markedly increased axonal degeneration induced by gp120 (1 pg/mL). As in previous experiments, TRIM coadministration with gp120 did not result in increased neuronal death. These findings, in combination with our previous observations (FIG. 4), suggest the importance of nNOS in the endogenous EPO "axonoprotective" response to axonal injury. The dual role of NO with respect to neurotoxicity and neuroprotection has been commented on in the literature.[32,33] While NO-mediated neurotoxicity has been explored by several groups over the years, NO-mediated neuroprotection is poorly understood. In our study, nNOS inhibition exacerbates the axonal degeneration induced by gp120. This correlates with prevention by TRIM of Schwann cell–derived EPO production in response to axonal injury. Of some relevance to this discussion is a study by Keilhoff *et al.*, which showed that nNOS knockout mice had worsened axonal degeneration following sciatic nerve transection compared to wild-type mice.[34] FIGURE 5 summarizes our model of endogenous "axonoprotection" by Schwann cell–derived EPO.

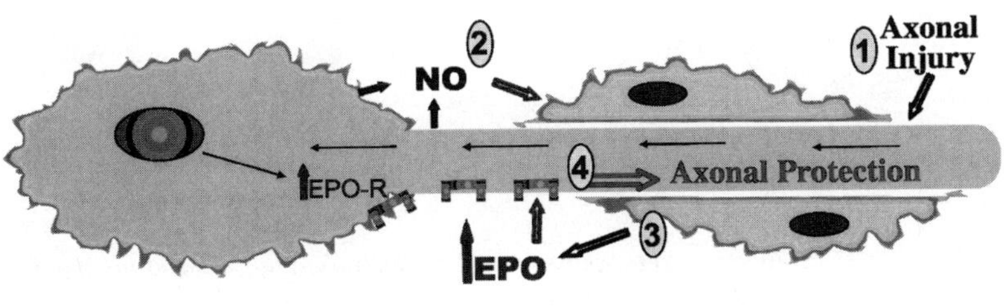

FIGURE 5. Schematic diagram of the EPO-mediated intrinsic axonoprotective pathway. Based on our data, we hypothesize the following: Axonal injury (1) induces nitric oxide (NO) production (2) within neurons. This neuron-derived NO stimulates EPO production (3) by neighboring Schwann cells. This Schwann cell–derived EPO results in activation of an "axonoprotective" pathway (4) via EPO-R ligation on neurons. (Adapted from ref. 10.)

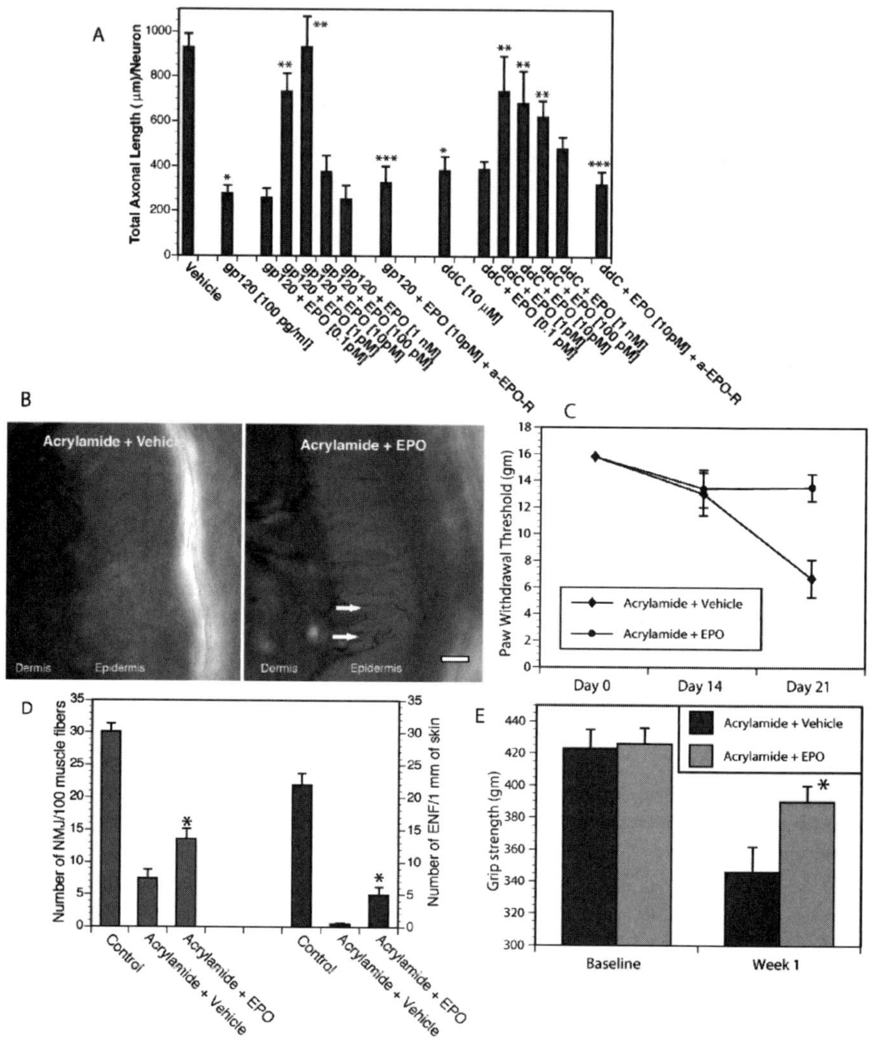

FIGURE 6. Exogenous EPO prevents axonal degeneration *in vitro* and *in vivo*. **(A)** Administration of EPO prevents gp120- and ddC-induced DRG axonal degeneration in a dose-dependent fashion. Coapplication of anti-EPO-R antibodies blocks this neuroprotection (**P* < 0.05, vehicle control vs. gp120 or ddC; ***P* < 0.05, EPO + gp120/ddC vs. gp120/ddC alone; ****P* < 0.05, EPO + gp120/ddC vs. EPO + gp120/ddC + anti-EPO-R antibody). Systemic coadministration of EPO in acrylamide-treated rats prevents degeneration of distal sensory innervation in the skin **(B, D)** and in motor terminals **(D)**, and reduces hyperalgesia and loss of grip strength **(E)** (**P* < 0.05). **(C)** Decreased mechanical hyperalgesia on von Frey filament testing. Scale bar (B): 100 mm. (Adapted from refs. 10 and 11.)

EXOGENOUS EPO PREVENTS AXONAL DEGENERATION IN MODELS OF HIV-ASSOCIATED NEUROPATHIES AND IN ACRYLAMIDE-INDUCED NEUROPATHY

Can this endogenous "axonoprotective" pathway be therapeutically exploited by systemic administration of EPO? First, we used our *in vitro* models of HIV-associated neuropathies and examined neuroprotection afforded by coadministration of recombinant human EPO in ddC- and gp120-induced axonal degeneration.[11] As seen in FIGURE 6A, at low picomolar concentrations, EPO prevented axonal degeneration induced by ddC and gp120. Since there were no reliable animal models of HIV-associated peripheral neuropathies,[1,13] we used a well-established model of peripheral neuropathy characterized by distal axonal degeneration, namely, the rat acrylamide toxicity model.[35–38] In this model, oral acrylamide administration to Sprague-Dawley rats results in severe "dying back" degeneration of both sensory and motor fibers, in the absence of significant neuronal death.[38,39] Affected rats characteristically have distal limb weakness and an ataxic gait.[37,40] Furthermore, we noted that acrylamide-treated rats developed mechanical hyperalgesia, a correlate of neuropathic pain behavior. As shown in FIGURE 6B and quantified in FIGURE 6D, acrylamide-treated rats given EPO had significantly less sensory axonal degeneration as indicated by greater cutaneous innervation (increased epidermal nerve fiber density) on PGP 9.5 immunohistochemistry, compared to those given placebo. This correlated with decreased mechanical hyperalgesia on von Frey filament testing (FIG. 6C). Furthermore, EPO-treated rats had significantly less motor axonal degeneration as demonstrated by a higher innervated neuromuscular junction density in the intrinsic foot muscles using α-bungarotoxin binding (FIG. 6D). This correlated with greater grip strength (FIG. 6E).

CONCLUSIONS

Progressive "dying back" degeneration of the distal regions of long axons, rather than neuronal loss, is the predominant pathological change in the most common peripheral neuropathies afflicting humans, such as diabetic sensorimotor polyneuropathy, HIV-associated sensory neuropathy, and toxic neuropathies.[1,2,13,36] Furthermore, progressive axonal loss is observed in multiple sclerosis and is now thought to highly correlate with disability.[41,42] Consequently, agents with "axonoprotective" properties may be very helpful therapeutically. However, often only the antiapoptotic properties of putative neuroprotective agents are evaluated, with little or no attention paid to whether axonal degeneration can be prevented. It does not necessarily follow that an agent that prevents neuronal apoptosis will prevent axonal degeneration as it is now well recognized that the two processes may employ different signaling pathways.[3–6,43]

In this review, we described experiments designed to provide insights into mechanisms of HIV-associated peripheral neuropathies and an endogenous EPO-mediated pathway that prevents axonal degeneration. We also showed that immunophilin ligands and recombinant human EPO can prevent axonal degeneration associated with various toxic injuries in sensory neurons. These findings suggest that both immunophilin ligands and EPO may be therapeutically useful in a wide variety of human neurological diseases characterized by axonopathy.

ACKNOWLEDGMENTS

This work was supported by grants from the National Institutes of Health (NS43991, NS46262, NS47972); by the Center for AIDS Research, Johns Hopkins University; and by a contract from the R. W. Johnson Pharmaceutical Research Institute.

REFERENCES

1. Pardo, C.A., J.C. McArthur & J.W. Griffin. 2001. HIV neuropathy: insights in the pathology of HIV peripheral nerve disease. J. Periph. Nerv. Syst. **6:** 21–27.
2. Sidenius, P. 1982. The axonopathy of diabetic neuropathy. Diabetes **31:** 356–363.
3. Ehlers, M.D. 2004. Deconstructing the axon: Wallerian degeneration and the ubiquitin-proteasome system. Trends Neurosci. **27:** 3–6.
4. Glass, J.D. *et al.* 2002. Very early activation of m-calpain in peripheral nerve during Wallerian degeneration. J. Neurol. Sci. **196:** 9–20.
5. Raff, M.C., A.V. Whitmore & J.T. Finn. 2002. Axonal self-destruction and neurodegeneration. Science **296:** 868–871.
6. Zhai, Q. *et al.* 2003. Involvement of the ubiquitin-proteasome system in the early stages of Wallerian degeneration. Neuron **39:** 217–225.
7. Coleman, M.P. & V.H. Perry. 2002. Axon pathology in neurological disease: a neglected therapeutic target. Trends Neurosci. **25:** 532–537.
8. Keswani, S.C. *et al.* 2003. FK506 is neuroprotective in a model of antiretroviral toxic neuropathy. Ann. Neurol. **53:** 57–64.
9. Keswani, S.C. *et al.* 2003. Schwann cell chemokine receptors mediate HIV-1 gp120 toxicity to sensory neurons. Ann. Neurol. **54:** 287–296.
10. Keswani, S.C. *et al.* 2004. A novel endogenous erythropoietin mediated pathway prevents axonal degeneration. Ann. Neurol. **56:** 815–826.
11. Keswani, S.C., G.J. Leitz & A. Höke. 2004. Erythropoietin is neuroprotective in models of HIV sensory neuropathy. Neurosci. Lett. **371:** 102–105.
12. Höke, A. & D.R. Cornblath. 2005. Peripheral neuropathies in human immunodeficiency virus infection. *In* Peripheral Neuropathy, Vol. 2. Saunders. Philadelphia. In press.
13. Keswani, S.C. *et al.* 2002. HIV-associated sensory neuropathies. AIDS **16:** 2105–2117.
14. Mathur, A. *et al.* 2000. Evaluation of fluorescent dyes for the detection of mitochondrial membrane potential changes in cultured cardiomyocytes. Cardiovasc. Res. **46:** 126–138.
15. Reers, M., T.W. Smith & L.B. Chen. 1991. J-aggregate formation of a carbocyanine as a quantitative fluorescent indicator of membrane potential. Biochemistry **30:** 4480–4486.
16. Emborg, M.E. *et al.* 2001. Systemic administration of the immunophilin ligand GPI 1046 in MPTP-treated monkeys. Exp. Neurol. **168:** 171–182.
17. Harper, S. *et al.* 1999. Analysis of the neurotrophic effects of GPI-1046 on neuron survival and regeneration in culture and *in vivo*. Neuroscience **88:** 257–267.
18. Khan, Z. *et al.* 2002. The non-immunosuppressive immunophilin ligand GPI-1046 potently stimulates regenerating axon growth from adult mouse dorsal root ganglia cultured in Matrigel. Neuroscience **114:** 601–609.
19. Sauer, H. *et al.* 1999. Systemic treatment with GPI 1046 improves spatial memory and reverses cholinergic neuron atrophy in the medial septal nucleus of aged mice. Brain Res. **842:** 109–118.
20. Steiner, J.P. *et al.* 1997. Neurotrophic immunophilin ligands stimulate structural and functional recovery in neurodegenerative animal models. Proc. Natl. Acad. Sci. USA **94:** 2019–2024.

21. TANAKA, K. *et al.* 2002. GPI1046 prevents dopaminergic dysfunction by activating glutathione system in the mouse striatum. Neurosci. Lett. **321:** 45–48.
22. DEWHURST, S., H.A. GELBARD & S.M. FINE. 1996. Neuropathogenesis of AIDS. Mol. Med. Today **2:** 16–23.
23. YOSHIOKA, M. *et al.* 1995. Role of immune activation and cytokine expression in HIV-1-associated neurologic diseases. Adv. Neuroimmunol. **5:** 335–358.
24. CHONG, Z.Z., J.Q. KANG & K. MAIESE. 2002. Erythropoietin is a novel vascular protectant through activation of Akt1 and mitochondrial modulation of cysteine proteases. Circulation **106:** 2973–2979.
25. DIGICAYLIOGLU, M. & S. LIPTON. 2001. Erythropoietin-mediated neuroprotection involves cross-talk between Jak2 and NF-kappaB signalling cascades. Nature **412:** 641–647.
26. GORIO, A. *et al.* 2002. Recombinant human erythropoietin counteracts secondary injury and markedly enhances neurological recovery from experimental spinal cord trauma. Proc. Natl. Acad. Sci. USA **99:** 9450–9455.
27. RUSCHER, K. *et al.* 2002. Erythropoietin is a paracrine mediator of ischemic tolerance in the brain: evidence from an *in vitro* model. J. Neurosci. **22:** 10291–10301.
28. SIREN, A.L. *et al.* 2001. Erythropoietin prevents neuronal apoptosis after cerebral ischemia and metabolic stress. Proc. Natl. Acad. Sci. USA **98:** 4044–4049.
29. CAMPANA, W.M. & R.R. MYERS. 2003. Exogenous erythropoietin protects against dorsal root ganglion apoptosis and pain following peripheral nerve injury. Eur. J. Neurosci. **18:** 1497–1506.
30. MIZUSAWA, I. *et al.* 2003. Expression of cytokines, neurotrophins, neurotrophin receptors, and NOS mRNA in dorsal root ganglion of a rat tourniquet model. Leg. Med. (Tokyo) **5**(suppl. 1): S271–S274.
31. HAGA, K.K. *et al.* 2003. The neuronal nitric oxide synthase inhibitor, TRIM, as a neuroprotective agent: effects in models of cerebral ischaemia using histological and magnetic resonance imaging techniques. Brain Res. **993:** 42–53.
32. BOLANOS, J.P., P. GARCIA-NOGALES & A. ALMEIDA. 2004. Provoking neuroprotection by peroxynitrite. Curr. Pharm. Des. **10:** 867–877.
33. WIGGINS, A.K., P.J. SHEN & A.L. GUNDLACH. 2003. Neuronal-NOS adaptor protein expression after spreading depression: implications for NO production and ischemic tolerance. J. Neurochem. **87:** 1368–1380.
34. KEILHOFF, G., H. FANSA & G. WOLF. 2002. Differences in peripheral nerve degeneration/regeneration between wild-type and neuronal nitric oxide synthase knockout mice. J. Neurosci. Res. **68:** 432–441.
35. CROFTON, K.M. *et al.* 1996. The impact of dose rate on the neurotoxicity of acrylamide: the interaction of administered dose, target tissue concentrations, tissue damage, and functional effects. Toxicol. Appl. Pharmacol. **139:** 163–176.
36. GOLD, B.G., J.W. GRIFFIN & D.L. PRICE. 1985. Slow axonal transport in acrylamide neuropathy: different abnormalities produced by single-dose and continuous administration. J. Neurosci. **5:** 1755–1768.
37. KO, M.H. *et al.* 1999. Age-dependent acrylamide neurotoxicity in mice: morphology, physiology, and function. Exp. Neurol. **158:** 37–46.
38. LOPACHIN, R.M., JR. & E.J. LEHNING. 1994. Acrylamide-induced distal axon degeneration: a proposed mechanism of action. Neurotoxicology **15:** 247–259.
39. FULLERTON, P.M. & J.M. BARNES. 1966. Peripheral neuropathy in rats produced by acrylamide. Br. J. Ind. Med. **23:** 210–221.
40. DEGRANDCHAMP, R.L. & H.E. LOWNDES. 1990. Early degeneration and sprouting at the rat neuromuscular junction following acrylamide administration. Neuropathol. Appl. Neurobiol. **16:** 239–254.
41. BJARTMAR, C. & B.D. TRAPP. 2001. Axonal and neuronal degeneration in multiple sclerosis: mechanisms and functional consequences. Curr. Opin. Neurol. **14:** 271–278.
42. BJARTMAR, C., J.R. WUJEK & B.D. TRAPP. 2003. Axonal loss in the pathology of MS: consequences for understanding the progressive phase of the disease. J. Neurol. Sci. **206:** 165–171.
43. KORHONEN, L. & D. LINDHOLM. 2004. The ubiquitin proteasome system in synaptic and axonal degeneration: a new twist to an old cycle. J. Cell Biol. **165:** 27–30.

Questions and Answers

Session X: Novel Approaches to Neuroprotection

QUESTIONS FOR AHMET HOKE

From Philip Lazarovici

To keep alive *in vitro* the DRG Schwann cell model, you need NGF/DNF in the medium. Thus, can you claim that the neurotoxic/neuroprotective effects measured are observed under a "maintenance influence of the neurotrophins"?

ANSWER: Yes, and that would be the normal condition *in vivo*. In our culture system, we try to model the *in vivo* conditions as closely as possible.

From Moussa Youdim

I was not aware of the mechanisms of neuroprotective action of immunophilin GPI 1046 and whether its actions on the cell surface membrane receptor are on the mitochondrial permeability transition (MPT) pore. Does it act on a different site than cyclosporin A?

ANSWER: Yes, the nonimmunosuppressive immunophilin compounds do not have the calcineurin-binding domain and do not act on the MPT pore.

From Naren Banik

Do you think that similar dysfunction occurs in GBS as you have shown in HIV neuropathy?

ANSWER: It is possible that secondary axonal damage that occurs in GBS is also due to indirect toxicity from Schwann cells, but there are no data on it yet.

QUESTIONS FOR ALAN FADEN

From Sylvain Doré

You mentioned that neurons that are entering into cell cycle will progressively die by apoptosis. Is it possible that BrdU-positive cells (colabeled with neuronal markers), which several researchers are using, will gradually die through an apoptotic-like pathway?

ANSWER: Yes, BrdU-positive neurons may reflect aberrant cell cycle reentry, which leads to apoptosis in postmitotic cells like neurons. Thus, BrdU-positive cells do not necessarily reflect neurogenesis, raising an important caveat for studies examining neurogenesis after CNS injury.

Ann. N.Y. Acad. Sci. 1053: 502–504 (2005). © 2005 New York Academy of Sciences.
doi: 10.1196/annals.1344.069

From Naren Banik

Your studies with cyclic dipeptides and flavonoid compounds on brain injury are very promising and exciting. Have you looked at the effects of these compounds in spinal cord injury (SCI)?

ANSWER: Yes. In preliminary studies, both classes of compounds also show neuroprotection or neuroprotective trends after experimental SCI.

QUESTIONS FOR VICTOR MARCHESELLI

From Sylvain Doré

How does 10,17(*S*)-docosatriene act? Does it bind to membrane or intracellular receptors? Does it have affinity on known receptors in the similar extended family members?

ANSWER: Neuroprotection by NPD1 is stereospecific (only the *S*-isomers are active), which is a good indicator that specific receptors are involved. However, at present, no receptors have been identified.

From Philip Lazarovici

The NPD1 neuroprotection approach *in vivo* is supplementing a neuroprotective DHA lipid mediator. How will this therapeutic approach affect lipid metabolism?

ANSWER: Because DHA is an essential fatty acid, which is under extremely tight control in terms of distribution and metabolism, therapeutic administration will create a rapid alteration of free DHA pools, and increased incorporation of DHA into membrane phospholipids could modify membrane fluidity. As we have shown in response to cell injury, this will facilitate the synthesis of NPD1. Those effects also could change the balance of other lipid metabolic pathways and favor the formation of neuroprostanes (DHA oxidation products), but no adverse effects have been found in animals after low-dose DHA treatment.

From Gregory Oxenkrug

Schizotypal personality disorder patients suffer an abnormal adaptation of retinal cells to light signal. This is recorded by the ERG. Four weeks of treatment by DHA reversed this abnormality. Could you comment on this?

ANSWER: DHA administration to humans has been studied for some time. For example, in early child development, DHA prevents visual-acuity defects. More recently, epidemiologic studies imply that diets enriched in DHA are associated with reduced risk of cognitive deficits and Alzheimer's disease. In age-related macular degeneration (AMD), there is an inverse relationship between diets high in DHA and the risk for AMD.

QUESTION FOR SILVIA MANDEL

From Ashraf Virmani

Are polyphenols found only in green tea and how much do you need to drink for neuroprotective action?

ANSWER: Polyphenols are natural substances present in beverages obtained from plants, fruits, and vegetables, such as olive oil, red wine, and tea. Fresh tea (*Camellia sinensis*) leaves contain a high amount of catechins, a group of flavonoids (the largest group of polyphenols), known to constitute 30–45% of the solid green tea extract. Tea consumption varies between individuals, but there is a consensus of 3–6 cups per day. High tea concentrations have been shown to be detrimental to cell viability and function.

Improving Predictive Modeling in Pediatric Drug Development: Pharmacokinetics, Pharmacodynamics, and Mechanistic Modeling

WILLIAM SLIKKER, JR.,[a] JOHN F. YOUNG,[b] RICHARD A. CORLEY,[c] DAVID C. DORMAN,[d] RORY B. CONOLLY,[d] THOMAS B. KNUDSEN,[e] BRIAN L. ERSTAD,[f] RICHARD H. LUECKE,[g] ELAINE M. FAUSTMAN,[h] CHARLES TIMCHALK,[c] AND DONALD R. MATTISON[i]

[a]*Office of Research and* [b]*Division of Biometry and Risk Assessment, National Center for Toxicological Research/FDA, Jefferson, Arkansas, USA*

[c]*Center for Biological Monitoring and Modeling, Pacific Northwest National Laboratory, Richman, Washington, USA*

[d]*CIIT, Centers for Health Research, Research Triangle Park, North Carolina, USA*

[e]*Birth Defects Center, Systems Analysis Laboratory, University of Louisville, Louisville, Kentucky, USA*

[f]*Department of Pharmacy Practice and Science, College of Pharmacy, University of Arizona, Tucson, Arizona, USA*

[g]*Department of Chemical Engineering, University of Missouri–Columbia, Columbia, Missouri, USA*

[h]*Institute for Risk Analysis and Risk Communication, University of Washington, Seattle, Washington, USA*

[i]*National Institute of Child Health and Human Development, National Institutes of Health, Bethesda, Maryland, USA*

ABSTRACT: A workshop was conducted on November 18–19, 2004, to address the issue of improving predictive models for drug delivery to developing humans. Although considerable progress has been made for adult humans, large gaps remain for predicting pharmacokinetic/pharmacodynamic (PK/PD) outcome in children because most adult models have not been tested during development. The goals of the meeting included a description of when, during development, infants/children become adultlike in handling drugs. The issue of incorporating the most recent advances into the predictive models was also addressed: both the use of imaging approaches and genomic information were considered. Disease state, as exemplified by obesity, was addressed as a modifier of drug pharmacokinetics and pharmacodynamics during development. Issues addressed in this workshop should be considered in the development of new predictive and mechanistic models of drug kinetics and dynamics in the developing human.

Address for correspondence: William Slikker, Jr., Office of Research, National Center for Toxicological Research, 3900 NCTR Road, Jefferson, AR 72079-9502. Voice: 870-543-7950; fax: 870-543-7576.

wslikker@nctr.fda.gov

Ann. N.Y. Acad. Sci. 1053: 505–518 (2005). © 2005 New York Academy of Sciences. doi: 10.1196/annals.1344.044

KEYWORDS: **PBPK; pharmacokinetics; pharmacodynamics; pediatrics; children; modeling**

INTRODUCTION

Over the past decade, regulatory agencies in developed countries have recognized that infants, children, and adolescents handle drugs and chemicals differently than adults. Some of these differences are innate (e.g., inborn differences in xenobiotics metabolism), while others arise from inherent life-stage-dependent differences in physiology and development. Recognition of these differences has focused attention on the design of preclinical and clinical studies; however, restrictions on the testing of chemicals in pediatric populations create persistent data gaps. The concepts of efficacy and safety must be reformulated in the context of development, and new approaches for preclinical and clinical testing (including clinical trial designs) must be developed and validated in immature animals and immature humans. These testing methods must be grounded on an understanding of normal developmental trajectories, as well as the impact of disease and treatment on development of healthy individuals. Clearly, constraints on pediatric human testing will require development of alternative approaches to preclinical and clinical testing specifically for pediatric pharmacology and toxicology.

The use of physiologically based (PB) pharmacokinetic/pharmacodynamic (PK/PD) models improves thinking about mechanism, efficacy, and toxicity in pediatric pharmacology. The complexity of development including changing body composition, changing expression of targets, metabolic systems, protein binding, and so forth demands the design and use of sophisticated models to improve development of efficacious drugs and the prediction of risk to children. Particular issues or concerns include the potential for impaired drug efficacy or increased toxicity. Since dosing regimens for children may be quite different from those for adults, model development will thus aid in the selection of age-appropriate dosing regimens.

In addition to developmental effects, environmental concerns including disease state are known to influence the PK or PD of a drug. Childhood obesity, currently reaching epidemic proportions, has a major influence on appropriate drug administration to children. As we understand more about gene and environment interactions and move in the direction of personalized medicine, PBPK/PD models incorporating pharmacogenomic information will be necessary. The workshop participants addressed these issues, and models were proposed that begin to incorporate these features in an attempt to improve drug administration to children.

In order to achieve the goal of predictive PK/PD models for children and adolescents, a number of research needs were identified and summarized.

WORKSHOP OUTLINE

PBPK/PD Models for Developing Humans: Risk Assessment Strategies and Research Recommendations

Session 1: Extrapolation between stages of development

(*a*) Prenatal vs. postnatal models.
(*b*) Children aren't small adults for drug therapy!
(*c*) When do infants/children start becoming small adults for PBPK considerations?

Session 2: Use of imaging in model development

(*a*) What types of data can be gathered by an imaging approach?
(*b*) What types of imaging are appropriate?
(*c*) What is the level of quantitation?

Session 3: Inclusion of "omics" data in model development

(*a*) Is this more than understanding mechanisms?
(*b*) How to incorporate "omics" into PBPK/PD models.

Session 4: Incorporation of disease state in model development

(*a*) Modeling on a lean body mass basis.
(*b*) Obesity as a disease state?
(*c*) Practical issues related to dosimetry with regard to childhood obesity.

Session 5: The next generation of models: vision of the future and research recommendations

WHEN DO INFANTS/CHILDREN START BECOMING SMALL ADULTS FOR PBPK CONSIDERATIONS?

Therapeutic dogma is that children are not small adults![1] However, from a physiologically based pharmacokinetic (PBPK) modeling basis, how early can adult models be applied to children? Can adult models be scaled based on weight and applied to children? Is a 70-kg 15-year-old equivalent to a 70-kg adult? What about a 30-kg 10-year-old? Or a 10-kg 1-year-old?

Ginsberg and colleagues[2] have compiled a database of 45 drugs across development from the neonate to the adult and concluded that clearance and/or elimination half-life were equivalent to the adult value by 6 months of age. Scheuplein *et al.*[3] investigated sensitivity to chemical toxicity between children and adults and concluded that, by 6 months of age, children were usually no more sensitive to chemical toxicity than adults. Several authors have noted that most metabolic systems were reasonably mature in people by 6 to 12 months of age.[3–7]

There are sufficient data in the literature on human growth in both males and females to mathematically (e.g., polynomials) relate individual organ/tissue/fluid developmental weight to the overall age or weight of a person, in a normally developing individual. Specific organ weight data are available at birth and then at 1- to 2-month intervals through the first year of life and at half-year intervals through puberty in healthy children.[8] Price *et al.* have described both time-dependence and interindividual variation in human physiological and biochemical parameter values relevant to PBPK modeling.[9] Such growth equations have already been successfully incorporated into PBPK models.[10]

Present PBPK models, however, do not address the time-sensitive emergence of metabolic or elimination capabilities, or impact of disease processes. As noted earlier, these capabilities generally approach adult levels by 1 year of age. However, some P-450 isozymes involved in oxidative metabolism do not mature until somewhat later in development. Even though the developmental timelines for all metabolic enzymes are not fully defined, they are sufficiently described to assign simple mathematical relationships for functionality.

Theoretically, adult PBPK models could be scaled to infants of 6 months to 1 year of age or older based on weight alone. Infants younger than 6 months of age will require additional consideration of altered absorption, metabolism, and elimination capabilities.

However, there is the additional caution of idiosyncratic metabolic and/or adverse reactions that do not follow normal scaling that must always be considered [e.g., theophylline to caffeine conversion that occurs only in the neonate].[6,11] Prandota[12] noted that the neonate may handle drugs differently and cautioned about generalizing about drug excretion in the young infant.

Although some data sets do exist, obviously lacking are sufficient PBPK data sets derived in the neonatal/infant time frame to fully test these assertions.

INCORPORATION OF MEDICAL IMAGING AND SUPERCOMPUTING IN THE DEVELOPMENT AND VALIDATION OF BIOLOGICALLY BASED EXPOSURE-DOSE-RESPONSE MODELS: AN EXAMPLE FROM THE RESPIRATORY SYSTEM

Medical imaging technologies such as magnetic resonance imaging (MRI), X-ray computed tomography (CT), and positron emission tomography (PET) have resulted in numerous breakthroughs in recent years in the detection, diagnosis, and treatment of disease. As with the "omics", advances in computing hardware and software have facilitated our ability to manage and manipulate the enormous quantities of digital information that imaging produces. A significant by-product of these advances is that health scientists now have extraordinarily useful new tools for obtaining quantitative anatomical and functional information on humans and animal models at various stages of development or under conditions of toxicity or disease. Such information will enable the development and validation of more robust predictive models of responses to environmental challenges or therapeutic interventions.

An example of the convergence between imaging and computational technologies in health research has been the development of "4-dimensional" (3-D geometry plus time) computational models of the respiratory system. The respiratory tract is a highly complex organ that must protect the body from atmospheric chemical or biological agents while fulfilling its role in gas exchange. Biologically based models are currently being developed at several institutions to study gas, vapor, and particulate dosimetry from the organ to the cellular level, the potential impacts of toxicity and disease on respiratory function and subsequent exposures to environmental agents, and the growth and development of the respiratory system. As the imaging techniques are refined and computational methods are developed that span the scales of information from the cellular to the whole organ level for the respiratory system, one can expect that similar multidimensional models for other organ systems may someday be linked as proposed by The Physiome Project (www.physiome.org) to develop a more quantitative understanding of animal and human physiology and pathophysiology.

Imaging methods can also be applied to dosimetry studies as well. For example, MRI has emerged as a noninvasive approach to evaluate brain manganese levels in people and animals. A consistent hallmark of these neuroimaging studies is the observation of symmetrical high intensity T1 MRI signals in the globus pallidus. Since manganese is paramagnetic, its distribution within the brain can be appreciated by MRI. Newland and coworkers were among the first to use MRI to assess brain manganese delivery.[13] Subsequent MRI studies in people have shown that increased manganese exposure or reduced hepatobiliary excretion of manganese can result in appreciable hyperintensities in the pallidum and other brain regions that accumulate manganese.[14–18] One measure of the signal hyperintensity is the so-called pallidal index (PI), which reflects the relative signal intensity in the T1 MRI of the globus pallidus versus the adjacent subcortical frontal white matter.[19] Despite growing interest in the use of the PI as a biomarker of manganese exposure,[14,15] there are few data available demonstrating that changes in the PI reflect brain manganese concentrations. Data presented at the workshop related to a recently completed study showed that changes in the PI and pallidal manganese concentration were correlated. The results of these studies are being used to develop a predictive, PBPK model for inhaled manganese that relates lung, brain, and other tissue manganese concentrations to exposure concentrations of manganese during inhalation.

"OMICS" DATA AND COMPUTATIONAL MODELING OF DOSE RESPONSES AT THE MOLECULAR, CELLULAR, TISSUE, AND WHOLE ORGANISM LEVELS

Knowledge of the dose-response curve must extend to levels at which humans are typically exposed to accurately assess the risk of adverse health effects of environmental chemicals. Experimental data are usually sparse at environmental levels of exposure, and computational models have been relied on to estimate both chemical disposition (i.e., pharmacokinetics) and tissue responses (i.e., pharmacodynamics). PK modeling has become increasingly sophisticated, with current models incorporating physiological and anatomical information to provide accurate estimates of target tissue doses.[20] In contrast, the PD relationship between a chemical at its target site and the ultimate biological effect is usually described empirically or semi-empirically (e.g., Sheiner and Steimer;[21] Moolgavkar *et al.*[22]). Molecular-level descriptions of PD mechanisms would provide a better understanding of dose-response curves and would reduce uncertainty in safety and risk assessments. Systems biology, which combines the high-throughput "omics" technologies with computational modeling, provides the toolbox needed to develop the molecular-level descriptions. This approach is currently being used to examine how intracellular signal transduction pathways influence dose- and time-response behaviors in response to xenobiotic exposure.

To identify components of specific signaling pathways, a number of research groups have begun to utilize large-scale reverse genetic screens.[23–26] In these screens, cell-based assays are constructed with various cellular endpoints or reporter genes that indicate activation of a specific pathway. Robotic systems individually screen thousands of full-length genes to identify which genes, when overexpressed, alter the signaling of the pathway of interest. Similarly, the pathway of interest can be stimulated using a ligand or constitutively active mutant, and individual inhibitory RNAs are screened to identify which genes, when knocked out inside the cell, also alter the signaling of the pathway of interest. The results from these screens are integrated with additional molecular and biochemical information to develop a directed graph that places the genes contextually within the signaling network.

Given a directed graph representation of the signaling network, the next logical step is to convert the graphical information into a computational model that is capable of describing the dynamical behavior of the network. Computational models of biological systems are by their nature integrative—the models specify how components interact at lower levels of organization to produce behavior at a higher level. The end result is a unique insight into the behavior of the system that may not be intuitively obvious. For example, Albert and Othmer[27] found that the gene regulatory network controlling segment polarity development in *Drosophila* is robust with respect to changes in parameter values and that its behavior is largely determined by its topology. The robust nature of the pathway evolved to correct for small errors in timing during development, thereby providing the species with an evolutionary advantage. In contrast, computational models of the MAPK signaling pathway demonstrate a highly nonlinear, switchlike dose-response behavior that is capable of bistability. The behavior of the MAPK signaling pathway is dependent on both parameter values and overall network structure.[28] From a toxicological perspective, environmental chemicals that target pathways similar to these examples would have significantly different dose-response behaviors. Signaling networks with robust structures may be relatively resilient to chemical perturbation, while highly nonlinear systems that rely on a delicate balance to maintain normal signaling behavior may be more sensitive.

Computational models for signaling pathways such as MAPK[28] and NF-κB[29] generate a suite of interesting dynamic behaviors at the level of individual cells. These include oscillations, bistability, history-dependence, and switchlike dose response. While the available data describing the scale-up of these behaviors to all the cells in a tissue are limited, some reports suggest that signaling-mediated behaviors across large numbers of cells are coordinated. For example, Tritscher *et al.*[30] used histochemical staining to show that the induction of hepatic CYP1A1 and CYP1A2 in rats exposed to TCDD spread from the central vein outwards as the dose of TCDD was increased. The interface between induced and uninduced cells was distinct, indicating that the responses of individual cells were coordinated. This behavior is consistent with bistable behavior of the network that controls CYP1A1 and CYP1A2 levels in rat liver, with TCDD providing the extracellular signal that coordinates the responses of individual cells.[31]

Scale-up of the dose- and time-response behaviors of molecular networks will determine dose and time responses at the level of tissues and of even higher-level physiological systems and will ultimately link changes at the molecular level with clinical disease. Ingolia and Murray[32] and Ting and Endy[33] have considered some of the challenges involved in the computational modeling of these biochemical networks and in the scale-up of these descriptions to higher levels of organization.

Integrating functional genomic tools and computational models can define a path towards eventual molecular-level descriptions of PD mechanisms. This capability as it develops will do much to explain how environmental stressors exert adverse health effects. It will eventually become possible to link sophisticated dosimetry and PD models together to replace less rigorous assumptions about the safety of drugs and the toxicity of environmental stressors.

COMPUTATIONAL SYSTEMS ANALYSIS OF A DISEASE NETWORK

Integration of PK/PD modeling, transcript profiling, and phenotype analysis can be a powerful force in the search for key changes that invoke irrevocable disease. This concept was illustrated in the pathogenesis of eye malformations with early mouse embryos exposed to 2CdA, a stable 2-chloro analogue of 2′-deoxyadenosine, which is a metabolic toxin in the early postimplantation uterus. 2CdA is an ocular teratogen through hyperactivation of the p53 pathway.[34] The 2CdA benchmark dose modeled for 5% increased risk in microphthalmia (BMD_5) is 2.5 mg/kg on day 8 of gestation.[35] PK analysis with HPLC revealed rapid accumulation (0.25 h) of 2CdA in the maternal plasma and complete clearance within 3.0 h. This rapid PK profile, coupled to the specificity of target organ response to the optic pit of the day-8 embryo, provides a useful model system to pursue the intervening steps in the exposure-disease continuum. The BMD_5 for 2CdA exposure resulted in 1.8 μM C_{max} for 2CdA in the embryo at 0.25 h postexposure, a concentration consistent with the limited bioactivation of 2CdA by mitochondrial deoxyguanosine kinase (dGK-3) in the mitochondrion. Transitory accumulation of 2CdATP in 2CdA-exposed embryos correlated with NADH depletion between 0.5 and 2.0 h postexposure and with upregulation of mitochondrial DNA (mtDNA) genomic expression by 3.0 h postexposure. This implies interference of 2CdA with mitochondrial function(s) as a possible consequence of 2CdA exposure. Pax6, a master regulator gene of eye development, declined in expression significantly at 3.0 h postexposure, and the p53 tumor suppressor protein accumulated in the embryo between 3.0 and 4.5 h postexposure.[34] The mitochondrial benzodiazepine receptor (PBR) antagonist PK11195 blocked p53 protein induction and microphthalmia, and was effective before the time of p53 protein induction, but not after.[36] The PBR agonist (Ro5-4864) did not block p53 protein induction nor rescue eye development. We can therefore define a series of steps from 2CdA exposure involving bioactivation by mitochondrial dGK-3, interference with NADH-dependent processes, compensatory upregulation of mtDNA biogenesis, dysregulation of Pax6 expression, and p53 protein induction. By 4.5 h postexposure, the embryo is "committed" to the disease phenotype (microphthalmia).

To connect this PK/PD model with changes in gene expression, we performed three kinds of microarray-based experiments in which patterns of gene expression were correlated with (1) dose-response profiles at the BMD_5 dose, just above this dose, and just below this dose; (2) trajectory profiles at 1. 5 h, 3.0 h, and 4.5 h post-exposure, corresponding to time points before, during, and after irrevocable disease; and (3) trajectories during pharmacological intervention with PBR ligands that rescue (PK11195) or do not rescue (Ro5-4864) normal eye development. Preliminary analysis of differentially regulated genes implies compensatory regulation of the embryonic transcriptome that is optimal as the applied dosage approaches the threshold for disease. Furthermore, the temporal trajectory is dramatically altered at a critical time during exposure preceding p53 protein induction. Signaling pathways upstream to p53 protein induction appear to be highly relevant to the adaptive response of embryos to 2CdA exposure. Using these genes as a framework, efforts are under way to build a computational biological regulatory network for modeling the critical event leading to irrevocable disease. Efforts to combine these networks with other chemical classes and target embryonic systems are now under way.[37]

CHALLENGES IN DESIGNING MEDICATION REGIMENS FOR OBESE CHILDREN

The frequency of adverse drug events associated with inappropriate dosing regimens in children is almost certainly underestimated in the United States since the common techniques (e.g., voluntary incident reporting and episodic chart reviews) used for detecting such problems are susceptible to underreporting. There are a variety of reasons for this underreporting, and there have been recent calls for improvements in postmarketing surveillance of new medications. However, until such changes are made, it is much more important that adequate research is performed at the front end of the development process in order to establish optimal dosing regimens for a range of clinical conditions. There are substantial challenges in developing whole body or PBPK/PD models for pediatric drug development that take into account potential differences in the pathophysiology of disease processes between adults and children, and the effects of changing body composition and function issues during growth. These challenges, though, are not insurmountable and have great potential for designing medication regimens in children that are likely to maximize the benefits and minimize the risks of therapy.

One of the major factors involved in designing a dosing regimen for a child is the choice of an appropriate size descriptor. While body weight is most commonly used in the clinical setting, an ideal descriptor in children would account for age, gender, height/weight (relative to growth charts), and some measure of body composition. Some indicator of body composition is needed to account for factors not indicated by height and weight determinations. For example, assume a 10-year-old female patient is 53 inches tall and weighs 50 kg (>95th percentile based on growth charts) and needs a medication that has a large volume of distribution. Assuming factors such as clearance and protein binding were known to be similar between children and adults for this medication, the dosing regimen could still vary substantially depending on at least four common clinical scenarios: a low percentage of fat relative to lean tissue, a high percentage of fat relative to lean tissue, a large amount of third-spaced (edematous) fluid, and a combination of high fat stores and third-spaced fluid retention. Unfortunately, medical literature is often not available to help the clinician in such a situation even if the excess weight is attributed to obesity.

There are relatively few studies, particularly in subjects with more extreme forms of obesity, and most involved adults given a single dose of a medication with subsequent recommendations based on an ideal, adjusted, or total body weight.

In addition to frequent alterations in fluid status, there are other factors that can complicate the PBPK/PD modeling process in critically ill patients. In many cases, it is desirable to have medications with rapid onset and rapid offset in the intensive care unit (ICU) setting since patients' conditions change quickly. Such medications may have effects that are only indirectly linked to plasma concentrations. Additionally, therapeutic drug concentration monitoring is not possible for most medications used in the ICU, and the optimal PD and patient assessment tools are not always established. Thus, the clinician must base medication dosing on general principles involving available PK parameters such as clearance and Vd, along with broad indicators of medication response. Hopefully, improved dosing regimens will result from state-of-the-art modeling techniques and advances in pharmacogenomics.

PBPK/PD MODELS FOR EFFECTS OF OBESITY

Therapeutic dose sizes for obese patients, both adults and children, may be different from the norm. PBPK models have the potential to assist in the determination of proper doses of medicines for patients, either children or adults, of nonnormal weight. Body weights are central variables in PBPK models; other parameters such as organ weights and blood flow rates can be calculated as functions of body weight. Partition coefficients, which govern the storage capacity of chemicals in various organs and tissues (including adipose tissue), are commonly calculated using empirical methods based on the structure of the drug.

Using this approach, a PBPK simulation was made for chlorpyrifos, an organophosphate pesticide. Chlorpyrifos is of interest because it is very lipophilic. A simulation with normal body weights was compared to a second one with the same set of parameters except the amount of fat was increased by a factor of about eight. The simulations showed significant effects of obesity, particularly at lower doses where larger fractions of the chemical were absorbed and stored in adipose tissue. PBPK models show also the effects of complicated internal interactions.

However, is this the whole story? A PBPK simulation was made for lean and obese rats and compared to laboratory data from Todd and Abernethy.[38] These authors indicated that the amount of adipose tissue was only one of several important differences between lean and obese rats. The weight of some organs changed as did some partition coefficients. Other organ weights and partition coefficients changed very little. However, using all these reported changes for obesity, it was not possible to fit the blood concentration data in obese rats for verapamil from a model based on lean rats. To fit the concentration data for the obese rats, a fourfold reduction in the liver elimination rate constant for obese rats was also required. At present, there is no a priori way to predict this rate constant change.

Prediction of dosages for obese patients from dosage for normal weight patients remains an uncertain and unsatisfactory process. What can be done? There is extensive literature comparing the response of obese patients to subjects of normal weight for a wide variety of drugs and chemicals. Seldom are these data cast in terms that allow simple or easy extraction of parameters needed for PBPK simulation. However, a great deal of quantitative information is embedded in these reports. These reports should be intensively examined and analyzed using PBPK models to delimit parameters where possible and combinations of parameters in other cases. Combined with empirical methods such as partition coefficient prediction techniques, some generalized guides for obesity dosimetry are likely to emerge. PBPK models represent a way to quantitatively mine these data as well as to effectively organize them in terms of parameters.

MODELING DEVELOPMENTAL PROCESSES IN ANIMALS: APPLICATIONS IN UNDERSTANDING MECHANISMS OF NEURODEVELOPMENTAL TOXICOLOGY

Biologically based dose-response models can provide a framework for incorporating mechanistic information into assessments of neurotoxicity.[39–42] In order to highlight work on toxicokinetic and dynamic models for developmental neurotoxicity, models have been constructed for normal midbrain and neocortex development. These models of neurodevelopment have been extended to evaluate the effects of various toxicants on these developmental processes. Using such modeling approaches, hypothesized modes of action for ethanol on sensitive target tissues such as the neocortex have been tested. Specifically, ethanol's effects on neocortical neurogenesis have been compared to the exacerbation of apoptosis during the synaptogenesis period.[43,44] These studies highlight the particular significance of assessing early impacts of ethanol on neurogenesis at biologically relevant exposures. The need for evaluating both qualitative and quantitative kinetic and dynamic factors was illustrated in order to understand the impacts of neurodevelopmental toxicants such as ethanol. Cross-species considerations in normal and ethanol-impacted neurodevelopment was illustrated with rodent and primate models. Development of such biologically based models allows testing of hypothesized modes of action and identifying critical mechanistic pathways in neurodevelopmental toxicity.[42]

DEVELOPMENT AND USE OF PREDICTIVE PBPK/PD MODELS FOR CHILDREN AND ADOLESCENTS

Biological modeling across the continuum from molecular to whole organisms has and will continue to play an increasingly important role in helping to understand how complex biological systems (like humans) interact with their environment. A major element of many future research programs will be the development of a new generation of advanced biological models that closely couple high performance computing with imaging technologies (molecular, cellular, organ), and experimental research. To accomplish this, an infrastructure must be developed that supports interactive, collaborative investigations that engage a broad base of scientific disciplines, including those that have not historically been engaged in biological research. These future biological models will effectively integrate both structural and functional data, over a broad continuum of complexity (cells to whole organism). The computational framework will serve to integrate functional, genomic, proteomic, and metabonomic data and could be viewed as a computational repository of the collective knowledge for a given cellular or organ system (i.e., virtual cell or virtual organ). To accomplish this goal, a number of challenges exist, including the need to develop and consolidate databases for model parameterization, the need to develop a user-friendly software platform architecture to facilitate model integration and cross-model communication, and the need to be able to link models hierarchically so that it is feasible to integrate across scales from molecules to cells to organs and systems, as well as across species. Although there are substantial challenges, it is clear that the next generation of biologically based models will provide researchers, clinicians, and risk assessors with a unique set of tools to better understand the intricacies of how the human body functions and, most importantly, how to prevent and mitigate human disease.

Studies on the pharmacokinetics of a xenobiotic provide critically useful insights into the toxicological response associated with a given agent. An important application of pharmacokinetics within toxicology has been to estimate risk by predicting the amount of absorbed dose under realistic exposure conditions.[45]

Toxicology studies are designed to provide a quantitative assessment of toxicity based on what the chemical agent does to the test animals, whereas pharmacokinetics focuses on what the animal (or human) does to the chemical. Clearly, toxicity and pharmacokinetics are integrally related since the extent of absorption, retention, metabolic activation, or detoxification will be ultimately responsible for delivering a dose to a target tissue, resulting in observed effects. PK models are critically important tools that, if used correctly, can quantitatively establish a unifying model that describes dosimetry and can be related to biological response across exposure routes, species, and chemical agents. The further linkage of pharmacokinetics with pharmacodynamics (i.e., measure of response) is particularly useful.

Unlike compartment modeling approaches, PBPK/PD models utilize biologically meaningful compartments that represent individual organs such as liver and kidney or groups of organ systems (i.e., well perfused/poorly perfused). The general model structure is based on an understanding of comparative physiology and xenobiotic metabolism, a chemical's physical properties that define tissue partitioning, the rates of biochemical reactions determined from both *in vivo* and *in vitro* experimentation, the physiological characteristics of the species of interest, any maternal factors, and some understanding of the mode of action that results in an observed dynamical response.[46] PBPK models have been developed to describe target tissue dosimetry for a broad range of environmental contaminants such as solvents, heavy metals, and pesticides.[47–52] A number of reviews have been published on the development, validation, application, and limitations of these models in human health risk assessment.[45,53–58]

RESEARCH NEEDS

(1) Development of computational dose-response models across multiple levels of biological organization. These multiscale models are needed to understand the implications of the behavior of biochemical networks in individual cells and their relationship to dose-response behaviors at the levels of tissues and organisms.

(2) Increase emphasis on computational dose-response modeling of signal transduction and biological regulatory networks. A key need is to under-

stand the level of biological detail required to obtain qualitatively accurate and, eventually, quantitatively accurate predictions.

(3) Continue the development of PBPK and anatomically based airway dosimetry models to provide the necessary base for PD models. Together, the dosimetry and PD models provide a complete exposure response (or dose-response) description.

(4) Development and testing of PBPK/PD models for infants/children and geriatrics based on adult PBPK/PD models. Development and testing of congruent models in laboratory animals that include immature animals and postnatal growth to help evaluate dosimetry windows in terms of concentrations at internal sites of action.

(5) Development of PBPK/PD models for specific disease states such as obesity for both infants/children and adults. Again, congruent models for laboratory animals that include postnatal growth may allow more effective transfer of animal obesity data to human problems. Growth parameters for the obese individual need to be compiled and parameterized.

REFERENCES

1. National Research Council. 1993. Pesticides in the Diets of Infants and Children. Chapter 2, pp. 23–47. National Academy Press. Washington, D.C.
2. Ginsberg, G., D. Hattis, B. Sonawane *et al.* 2002. Evaluation of child/adult pharmacokinetic differences from a database derived from the therapeutic drug literature. Toxicol. Sci. **66:** 185–200.
3. Scheuplein, R., G. Charnley & M. Dourson. 2002. Differential sensitivity of children and adults to chemical toxicity. I. Biological basis. Reg. Pharmacol. **35:** 429–447.
4. Cresteil, T. 1998. Onset of xenobiotic metabolism in children: toxicological implications. Food Addit. Contam. **15**(s)**:** 45–51.
5. Hines, R.N. & D.G. McCarver. 2002. The ontogeny of human drug-metabolizing enzymes: phase I oxidative enzymes. J. Pharmacol. Exp. Ther. **300**(2)**:** 355–360.
6. McCarver, D.G. & R.N. Hines. 2002. The ontogeny of human drug-metabolizing enzymes: phase II conjugation enzymes and regulatory mechanisms. J. Pharmacol. Exp. Ther. **300**(2)**:** 361–366.
7. Gentry, P.R., T.R. Covington & H.J. Clewell III. 2003. Evaluation of the potential impact of pharmacokinetic differences on tissue dosimetry in offspring during pregnancy and lactation. Reg. Toxicol. Pharmacol. **38:** 1–16.
8. Report of the Task Group on Reference Man. 1974. International Commission on Radiological Protection, W. S. Snyder, Chairman. Pergamon. New York.
9. Price, P.S., R. Conolly, C. Chaisson *et al.* 2003. Modeling inter-individual variation in physiological factors used in PBPK models of humans. Crit. Rev. Toxicol. **33:** 469–503.
10. Luecke, R.H., W.D. Wosilait, B.A. Pearce *et al.* 1994. A physiologically based pharmacokinetic computer model for human pregnancy. Teratology **49:** 90–103.
11. Kauffman, R.E. 2004. Drug action and therapy in the infant and child. *In* Neonatal and Pediatric Pharmacology: Therapeutic Principles in Practice. Third edition, chapter 3, pp. 20–31. Lippincott/Williams & Wilkins. Philadelphia.
12. Prandota, J. 1985. Clinical pharmacokinetics of changes in drug elimination in children. Dev. Pharmacol. Ther. **8:** 311–328.
13. Newland, M.C., T.L. Ceckler, J.H. Kordower *et al.* 1989. Visualizing manganese in the primate basal ganglia with magnetic resonance imaging. Exp. Neurol. **106:** 251–258.
14. Rose, C., R.F. Butterworth, J. Zayed *et al.* 1999. Manganese deposition in basal ganglia structures results from both portal-systemic shunting and liver dysfunction. Gastroenterology **117:** 640–644.
15. Sato, K., H. Ueyama, R. Arakawa *et al.* 2000. A case of welder presenting with parkinsonism after chronic manganese exposure. Rinsho Shinkeigaku **40**(11)**:** 1110–1115.

16. NAGATOMO, S., F. UMEHARA, K. HANADA *et al.* 1999. Manganese intoxication during total parenteral nutrition: report of two cases and review of the literature. J. Neurol. Sci. **162:** 102–105.
17. IKEDA, S., Y. YAMAGUCHI, Y. SERA *et al.* 2000. Manganese deposition in the globus pallidus in patients with biliary atresia. Transplantation **69:** 2339–2343.
18. SADEK, A.H., R. RAUCH & P.E. SCHULZ. 2003. Parkinsonism due to manganism in a welder. Int. J. Toxicol. **22:** 393–401.
19. KRIEGER, D., S. KRIEGER, O. JANSEN *et al.* 1995. Manganese and chronic hepatic encephalopathy. Lancet **346:** 270–274.
20. KIMBELL, J.S., R.P. SUBRAMANIAM, E.A. GROSS *et al.* 2001. Dosimetry modeling of inhaled formaldehyde: comparisons of local flux predictions in the rat, monkey, and human nasal passages. Toxicol. Sci. **64:** 100–110.
21. SHEINER, L.B. & J.L. STEIMER. 2000. Pharmacokinetic/pharmacodynamic modeling in drug development. Annu. Rev. Pharmacol. Toxicol. **40:** 67–95.
22. MOOLGAVKAR, S.H., E.G. LUEBECK, J. TURIM *et al.* 1999. Quantitative assessment of the risk of lung cancer associated with occupational exposure to refractory ceramic fibers. Risk Anal. **19:** 599–611.
23. BERNS, K., E.M. HIJMANS, J. MULLENDERS *et al.* 2004. A large-scale RNAi screen in human cells identifies new components of the p53 pathway. Nature **428:** 431–437.
24. CHANDA, S.K., S. WHITE, A.P. ORTH *et al.* 2003. Genome-scale functional profiling of the mammalian AP-1 signaling pathway. Proc. Natl. Acad. Sci. USA **100:** 12153–12158.
25. LUM, L., S. YAO, B. MOZER *et al.* 2003. Identification of hedgehog pathway components by RNAi in *Drosophila* cultured cells. Science **299:** 2039–2045.
26. MICHIELS, F., H. VAN ES, L. VAN ROMPAEY *et al.* 2002. Arrayed adenoviral expression libraries for functional screening. Nat. Biotechnol. **20:** 1154–1157.
27. ALBERT, R. & H.G. OTHMER. 2003. The topology of the regulatory interactions predicts the expression pattern of the segment polarity genes in *Drosophila melanogaster*. J. Theor. Biol. **223:** 1–18.
28. BHALLA, U.S., P.T. RAM & R. IYENGAR. 2002. MAP kinase phosphatase as a locus of flexibility in a mitogen-activated protein kinase signaling network. Science **297:** 1018–1023.
29. HOFFMANN, A., A. LEVCHENKO, M. SCOTT *et al.* 2002. The I-kappaB-NF-kappaB signaling module: temporal control and selective gene activation. Science **298**(5596)**:** 1241–1245.
30. TRITSCHER, A.M., J.A. GOLDSTEIN, C.J. PORTIER *et al.* 1992. Dose-response relationships for chronic exposure to 2,3,7,8-tetrachlorodibenzo-*p*-dioxin in a rat tumor promotion model: quantification and immunolocalization of CYP1A1 and CYP1A2 in the liver. Cancer Res. **52:** 3436–3442.
31. ANDERSEN, M.E., L.S. BIRNBAUM, H.A. BARTON *et al.* 1997. Regional hepatic CYP1A1 and CYP1A2 induction with 2,3,7,8-tetrachlorodibenzo-*p*-dioxin evaluated with a multicompartment geometric model of hepatic zonation. Toxicol. Appl. Pharmacol. **144:** 145–155.
32. INGOLIA, N.T. & A.W. MURRAY. 2002. Signal transduction: history matters. Science **297:** 948–949.
33. TING, A.Y. & D. ENDY. 2002. Signal transduction: decoding NF-kappaB signaling. Science **298**(5596)**:** 1189–1190.
34. WUBAH, J.A., M.M. IBRAHIM, X. GAO *et al.* 1996. Teratogen-induced eye defects mediated by p53-dependent apoptosis. Curr. Biol. **6:** 60–69.
35. WUBAH, J.A., R.W. SETZER, C. LAU *et al.* 2001. Exposure-disease continuum for 2-chloro-2′-deoxyadenosine, a prototype ocular teratogen. I. Dose-response analysis. Teratology **64:** 154–169.
36. CHARLAP, J.C., R.J. DONAHUE & T.B. KNUDSEN. 2003. Exposure-disease continuum for 2-chloro-2′-deoxyadenosine, a prototype ocular teratogen. 3. Intervention with PK11195. Birth Defects Res. (Part A) **67:** 108–115.
37. SINGH, A.V., K.B. KNUDSEN & T.B. KNUDSEN. 2005. Computational systems analysis of developmental toxicity: design, development, and implementation of a birth defects systems manager (BDSM). Reprod. Toxicol. **19:** 421–439.
38. TODD, E.L. & D.R. ABERNETHY. 1986. Pharmacokinetics and dynamics of (±)-verapamil in lean and obese Zucker rats. J. Pharmacol. Exp. Ther. **238**(2)**:** 642–647.

39. Lewandowski, T.A., R.A. Ponce, J.S. Charleston *et al.* 2003. Changes in cell cycle parameters and cell number in the rat midbrain during organogenesis. Dev. Brain Res. **141:** 117–128.
40. Gohlke, J.M., W.C. Griffith, S.M. Bartell *et al.* 2002. A computational model for neocortical neuronogenesis predicts ethanol-induced neocortical neuron number deficits. Dev. Neurosci. **24**(6)**:** 467–477.
41. Lewandowski, T.A., R.A. Ponce, J.S. Charleston *et al.* 2003. Effect of methylmercury on midbrain cell proliferation during organogenesis: potential cross-species differences and implications for risk assessment. Toxicol. Sci. **75:** 124–133.
42. Faustman, E., M. Gohlke, N. Judd *et al.* 2005. Modeling developmental processes in animals: applications in neurodevelopmental toxicology. Environ. Toxicol. Pharmacol. **19**(3)**:** 615–624.
43. Gohlke, J.M., W.C. Griffith & E.M. Faustman. 2004. The role of cell death during neocortical neurogenesis and synaptogenesis: implications from a computational model for the rat and mouse. Dev. Brain Res. **151**(1–2)**:** 43–54.
44. Gohlke, J.M., W.C. Griffith & E.M. Faustman. 2005. A systems-based computational model for dose-response comparisons of two mechanistic hypotheses for ethanol-induced neurodevelopmental toxicity. Toxicol. Sci. In press.
45. Clewell, H.J., III. 1995. The application of physiologically based pharmacokinetic modeling in human health risk assessment of hazardous substances. Toxicol. Lett. **79**(1–3)**:** 207–217.
46. Krishnan, K. & M.E. Andersen. 2001. Physiologically based pharmacokinetic modeling in toxicology. *In* Principles and Methods of Toxicology. Third edition, pp. 193–241. Raven Press/Taylor & Francis. New York/London.
47. Poet, T.S., A.A. Kousba, S. Dennison *et al.* 2004. Physiologically based pharmacokinetic/pharmacodynamic model for the organophosphate pesticide diazinon. Neurotoxicology **25**(6)**:** 1013–1030.
48. Timchalk, C., R.J. Nolan, A.L. Mendrala *et al.* 2002. A physiologically based pharmacokinetic and pharmacodynamic (PBPK/PD) model for the organophosphate insecticide chlorpyrifos in rats and humans. Toxicol. Sci. **66:** 34–53.
49. O'Flaherty, E.J. 1995. PBPK modeling for metals: examples with lead, uranium, and chromium. Toxicol. Lett. **82/83:** 367–372.
50. Sultatos, L.G. 1991. Metabolic activation of the organophosphorus insecticides chlorpyrifos and fenitrothion by perfused rat liver. Toxicology **68**(1)**:** 1–9.
51. Corley, R.A., A.L. Mendrala, F.A. Smith *et al.* 1990. Development of a physiologically based pharmacokinetic model for chloroform. Toxicol. Appl. Pharmacol. **103:** 512–527.
52. Andersen, M.E., H.J. Clewell III, M.L. Gargas *et al.* 1987. Physiologically based pharmacokinetics and the risk assessment process for methylene chloride. Toxicol. Appl. Pharmacol. **87:** 185–205.
53. Andersen, M.E. 1995. Physiologically based pharmacokinetic (PB-PK) models in the study of the disposition and biological effects of xenobiotics and drugs. Toxicol. Lett. **82/83:** 341–348.
54. Andersen, M.E. 2003. Toxicokinetic modeling and its applications in chemical risk assessment. Toxicol. Lett. **138:** 9–27.
55. Frederick, C.B. 1995. Summary of panel discussion on the "advantages/limitations/ uncertainties in the use of physiologically based pharmacokinetic and pharmacodynamic models in hazard identification and risk assessment of toxic substances". Toxicol. Lett. **79**(1–3)**:** 201–206.
56. Leung, H.W. & D.J. Paustenbach. 1995. Physiologically based pharmacokinetic and pharmacodynamic modeling in health risk assessment and characterization of hazardous substances. Toxicol. Lett. **79**(1–3)**:** 55–65.
57. Clewell, H.J., III & M.E. Andersen. 1996. Use of physiologically based pharmacokinetic modeling to investigate individual versus population risk. Toxicology **111**(1–3)**:** 315–329.
58. Mason, H. & K. Wilson. 1999. Biological monitoring: the role of toxicokinetics and physiologically based pharmacokinetic modeling. Am. Ind. Hyg. Assoc. J. **60**(2)**:** 237–242.

Index of Contributors